HANDBOOK FAMILY MEDICINE

VOLUME 2

INTEGRATED CARE ACROSS THE LIFESPAN

Prof. (Dr.) Sujata K. Das

ALLIED HEALTH PRESS

Handbook Family Medicine
Volume 2: Integrated Care Across the Lifespan

Author: **Prof. (Dr.) Sujata K. Das**

Allied Health Press
4164 Lakeshore Road
Burlington ON L7L 1A4
Canada
www.alliedhealthpress.com
Email: orders@arclereducation.com

ISBN: 978-1-77956-853-3

ABOUT THE AUTHOR

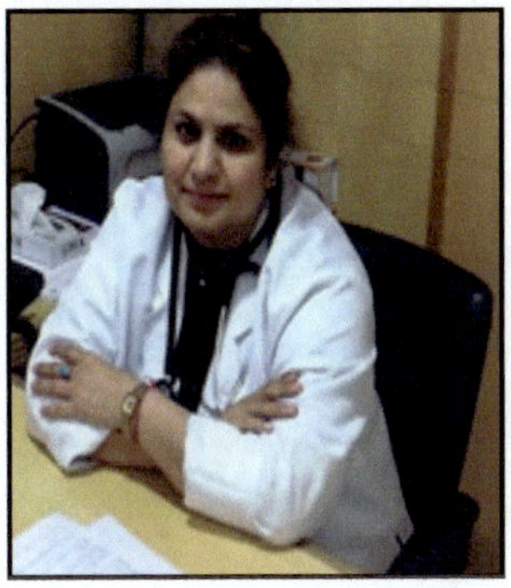

Prof (Dr) Sujata K. Dass, M.B.B.S, D.N.B, Ph.D. (Medicine) is a distinguished neuro-physician and academician, currently serving as an Attending Consultant in the Department of Neurology, B.L. Kapur Hospital, a renowned super-specialty medical institution in the New Delhi. Her illustrious career in medicine and research spans over three decades, characterized by her profound contributions to neurology and her unwavering commitment to medical education. Dr. Dass began her educational journey at Flushing High School in New York, USA, and completed her High School Diploma thereafter she joined Queens College of the City University of New York as an undergrad student. With a passion for medicine, she pursued her MBBS degree at King George Medical College, Lucknow, U.P., India. Her academic prowess and dedication to medicine were evident early on, setting the stage for a remarkable career. Dr Dass worked under the supervision of Dr M.S. Bains, M.D. as a Visiting Fellow in cardio-thoracic surgery at Memorial Sloan Kettering Cancer Research Center, New York, USA. Dr. Dass furthered her medical training by obtaining a D.N.B. (Family Medicine) and conducted significant research on hematological changes in malaria. Her quest for knowledge and excellence led her back to New York, where she completed her Ph.D. (Medicine) at the Department of Obstetrics & Gynecology, The New York Hospital-Cornell University Medical Center under the mentorship of Prof. Brij B. Saxena. Her groundbreaking work on Sn-Proto and Sn-Mesoporphyrin and the chemoprevention of neonatal jaundice culminated in the award of her D.Sc. (Medicine). Dr. Sujata Dass joined as the BR Ambedkar Chair Professor in July 2002 in the Institute of Biomedical Sciences, Faculty of Medicine, Bundelkhand University, Jhansi. Her tenure was marked by her dedication to advancing medical research and education. She also served as UGC National Research Award (Professor) at V.P. Chest Institute, University of Delhi. Throughout her career, Dr. Dass has received numerous awards and accolades on a global level. Notable among these are the UGC Research Award, the Fast Track Young Scientist Award from the Department of Science and Technology (DST), and the Women's Award of Highest Honour from Soka University, Japan. She has also received numerous research grants from DST, DBT and ICMR, UGC etc. These awards and grants underscore her exceptional contributions to medical science and research. Dr. Dass is a respected member of various scientific and administrative bodies like Planning Board (IGNOU), Executive Council - Bhagat Phool Singh Mahila Vishwavidhlaya, Haryana (2008-2011) where she continues to influence the medical community with her insights and expertise. Her commitment to guiding and mentoring students in their master's and doctoral thesis highlights her dedication to nurturing the next generation of medical professionals. Dr. Dass remains a beacon of excellence and a role model for aspiring medical professionals worldwide.

Brief Table of Contents

Getting Started with This Book

Chapter Openers

A list of Chapter Outline is presented providing a brief Introduction to what will be covered in the chapter.

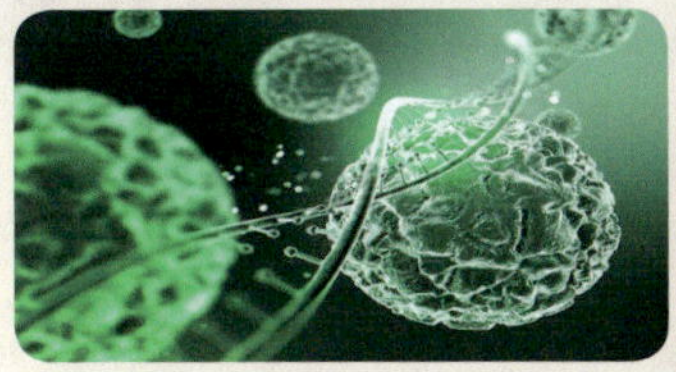

Introduction

Often referred to as the science of life, biology is a broad field of study aimed at comprehending the several kinds of life on Earth, from tiny creatures to sophisticated multicellular entities. Comprising several subfields, including molecular biology, ecology, and evolutionary biology, each of which advances our knowledge of living systems, this field clarifies the mechanisms controlling life events, including development, reproduction, and interaction with the surroundings, which is the central goal of biology. Moreover, biology fills in the void between the natural sciences and medicine by offering a necessary understanding of health, illness, and the interactions between organisms and their environments. Dealing with urgent global issues such as climate change, biodiversity loss, and new diseases depends on an awareness of these complex biological interactions, therefore highlighting the critical part biology plays in modern civilization. Fundamentally, biology explores and tests ideas about the living world using the scientific method. Through methodical observation and experimentation,

LEARNING OBJECTIVES

After studying this chapter, you will be able to:

1. Discuss the scientific method in biology;
2. Explain the cell theory;
3. Discuss the genetics and heredity;
4. Evolution and natural selection;
5. Focus on ecology and ecosystems;
6. Learn about human biology;
7. Evaluate the plant biology;
8. Explain the microbiology;
9. Focus on current trends in biology.

1.1. The Scientific Method in Biology

Learning Outcome

1. Describe the steps of the scientific method;
2. Focus on hypothesis formation;
3. Learn about experimental design.

Learning Outcomes

The beginning of each section of every chapter contains a set of Learning Outcomes that inform students of concepts they should understand. These outcomes help students understand what they should be able to do if they have mastered the material in that section.

Test Your Knowledge

Throughout each chapter, Test Your Knowledge cues you to note which topics have been covered and to self-test your understanding of the material presented.

Test Your Knowledge

1. Explain why correlation does not imply causation in scientific experiments.
2. How does the scientific method help reduce the influence of personal opinions in research?

Chapter Summary

The Summary Section appear at the end of each chapter and summarize main concepts covered throughout the chapter. These points provide key concepts in an engaging and meaningful way.

Summary

The investigation of biological principles highlights the importance of a comprehensive view of life by reflecting the intricate interactions that occur within living systems. The complexity of biology goes beyond individual species or systems, as this essay highlights; it also includes the interactions that mold ecosystems and affect biodiversity. Researchers can conduct in-depth analyses of metabolomic data using sophisticated technologies like MetaboAnalyst, which offer insights into the molecular mechanisms underlying these interactions. As demonstrated by the developments in MetaboAnalyst, for example, the integration of diverse omics data promotes a thorough understanding of metabolic pathways and helps identify important biological markers necessary for research on development and disease (Chong et al., 2018). Additionally, the phenomenon of ecological invasions is a key component of biological research and a vital field of study. The introduction of non-native species into unfamiliar habitats has significant ramifications and calls for multidisciplinary management strategies. Examining the origins and effects of these biological incursions, invasion science has become a crucial field that highlights the need to comprehend ecological dynamics and community interactions. As interest in biological invasions increases, new findings are emerging that put conventional ecological theories and practices to the test. The importance of incorporating various scientific viewpoints is shown by this developing discipline, which also highlights how invasive species shape ecosystems and advances our knowledge of ecological resilience (David et al., 2013). When taken as a whole, these discoveries from invasion science and metabolomics highlight the value of multidisciplinary biology research. Fostering cross-disciplinary collaboration and utilizing technological breakthroughs to improve our comprehension of intricate biological interactions are crucial as we look to the future of biological research. In addition to deepening our understanding of the complexities of life, this method lays the groundwork for tackling urgent environmental issues. Future studies can ensure the continued relevance of biology in a world that is constantly changing by acknowledging the interconnection of biological systems and opening the door to creative solutions that support sustainability and biodiversity conservation. We might imagine a thorough comprehension of life that serves both academia and society at large through ongoing investigation and integration of scientific knowledge.

Knowledge Assessment

The chapter includes material designed to review and reinforce each content. It includes Critical Thinking Questions to help test of your understanding of information presented in the chapter and Short answer Questions to review your understanding of the key concepts presented in the chapter.

Critical Thinking Questions

1. **Who is known as the "Father of Modern Biology"?**
   a. Aristotle
   b. Charles Darwin
   c. Gregor Mendel
   d. Louis Pasteur
2. **What is the basic unit of life?**
   a. Atom
   b. Molecule
   c. Cell
   d. Organism
3. **Which branch of biology studies the interaction of organisms with their environment?**
   a. Genetics
   b. Ecology
   c. Physiology
   d. Botany
4. **Which macromolecule is the main source of energy for living organisms?**
   a. Proteins
   b. Lipids
   c. Carbohydrates
   d. Nucleic acids
5. **DNA is primarily responsible for which function in living organisms?**
   a. Energy production
   b. Protein synthesis
   c. Storing genetic information
   d. Regulating body temperature

Short Answer Questions

1. What is biology, and why is it important to study biology?
2. What are the three main domains of life, and how are they different from one another?
3. Define homeostasis and give an example of how it works in living organisms.
4. What is the cell theory, and why is it fundamental to biology?
5. How do autotrophs and heterotrophs differ in the way they obtain energy?
6. What is the scientific method, and how is it applied in biological research?
7. Discuss how biology helps address global challenges such as climate change, disease, and food security.
8. Explain the levels of biological organization from the smallest unit to the largest. Provide examples at each level.
9. Describe the relationship between structure and function in biology, giving specific examples from cells or organs.
10. How has the discovery of genetics shaped our understanding of inheritance and variation among organisms?

Supplementary Materials

Key Terms: A list of key terms is given for quick reference

KEY TERMS FROM THIS CHAPTER

Annotation enrichment analysis	Biological structure	Cell
Cell theory	Cellular structure	Ecology
Ecosystems	Genetics	Human biology
Microbiology	Natural selection	Organism
Plant biology		

Further Resources: Recommendations for additional readings, websites, and multimedia resources.

References

1. Argelaguet, R., Velten, B., Arnol, D., Dietrich, S., Zenz, T., Marioni, J. C., Buettner, F., et al. (2018). Multi-omics factor analysis—A framework for unsupervised integration of multi-omics data sets. *Molecular Systems Biology, 14.* https://doi.org/10.15252/msb.20178124.
2. Bacher, S., Blackburn, T. M., Essl, F., & Genovesi, P. (2017). *Socio-Economic Impact Classification of Alien Taxa (SEICAT).* https://core.ac.uk/download/286567949.pdf (accessed on 8th March 2025).
3. Barnett, R., Brace, S., Cucchi, T., & Dobney, K. (2013). *Divergent Evolutionary Processes Associated with Colonization of Offshore Islands.* https://core.ac.uk/download/20664364.pdf (accessed on 8th March 2025).

Detailed Table of Contents

CHAPTER 6

Palliative and End-of-Life Care 173

CHAPTER 7

Acute Care in Family Practice 203

LIST OF FIGURES

PREFACE

People's and populations' health and happiness are largely determined by the care they receive throughout their lifetimes. Primary care settings are the first line of treatment for both short- and long-term health issues, integrating preventive care with ongoing management. Family medicine holds an important place in this continuum, specifically. It provides holistic, continuous, and patient-focused care that is available to every age group, sex, organ system, and disease. The scope of the knowledge required in practice is broad, and practitioners must be able to recognize complex patterns of health, coordinate care across multiple specialties, and facilitate patients in negotiating myriad physical, emotional, and social challenges.

As populations grow older and more diverse, family physicians carry heavier loads of responsibility for chronic disease, mental health, rehabilitation, and palliative care. These are combined with newer challenges from the environment, substance misuse, and the increasing burden of non-communicable disease. Modern family physicians also need to remain plastic, putting into practice new clinical evidence, patient-led innovation, and evolving public health agendas. With the increasing adoption of holistic and community-based healthcare models, the family doctor's role is further augmented by the need for a solid foundation and ongoing replenishment of knowledge.

The *Handbook of Family Medicine – Volume 2* is an exhaustive guide that encompasses this broad spectrum of practice. Based on the core pillars of family-centered care, this volume extends its reach to encompass such fundamental issues that confront contemporary practitioners, such as psychosocial dynamics and environmental medicine. This handbook provides evidence-based guidance in managing patients through the various phases of life and illness. Each chapter combines clinical experience with practical advice, highlighting areas often encountered in daily practice but sometimes missing from standard medical texts. The book complements Volume 1, and the two volumes together offer healthcare professionals an educated, thorough approach to primary care.

Chapter 1 gives a clinical overview of disorders of mental illness, with an emphasis on presenting symptoms such as depression, anxiety, and personality disorders, with a focus on screening tools and primary care management.

Chapter 2 addresses substance abuse and addiction, presenting identification, brief intervention, and referral, as well as continuing relapse and withdrawal management strategies.

Chapter 3 shifts to the area of geriatric mental health, addressing dementias, late-life depression, and delirium, and addressing how to manage confounding cognitive and physical impairments in the aging population.

Chapter 4 covers chronic disease management, including diabetes, hypertension, cardiovascular disease, and asthma, with attention to long-term monitoring, patient education, and decision-making.

Chapter 5 covers the care of older adults, with attention to functional assessment, medication management, and comprehensive care planning.

Chapter 6 covers palliative and end-of-life care, including strategies for symptom management, ethical decision-making, and family support in advanced disease or terminal illness.

Chapter 7 discusses acute care in family practice, including the treatment of acute-onset illness and urgent conditions requiring immediate diagnosis and treatment within a primary care setting.

Chapter 8 discusses trauma and injury care, such as management of minor injuries, fracture assessment, wound dressing, and identification of injuries requiring referral to secondary services.

Chapter 9 introduces allergy and immunology, including assessment of allergic reactions, an overview of immunotherapy, and autoimmune related primary care problems.

Chapter 10 covers infectious diseases, including common and emerging infections, vaccination strategies, and antibiotic stewardship principles.

Chapter 11 covers occupational and environmental medicine, addressing work-related illnesses, exposure assessments, and the physician's role in advising on workplace modifications.

Chapter 12 covers rehabilitation medicine, addressing recovery from injury, stroke, or surgery and promoting physical function and independence in people with chronic disability.

Chapter 13 speaks about trends in the future of family medicine, reflecting on breakthroughs such as telehealth, individualized medicine, artificial intelligence-based diagnosis, and altered models of care delivery. It offers reflections on how family physicians can be prepared for shifting roles, introduce new tools responsibly, and enhance overall health system functioning.

This book is for a wide audience engaged in healthcare. Medical learners and trainees will find foundational knowledge and practical schemes that link academic theory to practice. Family practice physicians and general practitioners can use it as a working manual to refresh or broaden their clinical knowledge within specific areas. Nurse practitioners, physician assistants, and allied health professionals will also find value in its interdisciplinary scope and practical focus. Furthermore, policymakers and instructors can learn from the book's overall outlook on the position of family medicine in contemporary healthcare systems.

MENTAL HEALTH DISORDERS

1

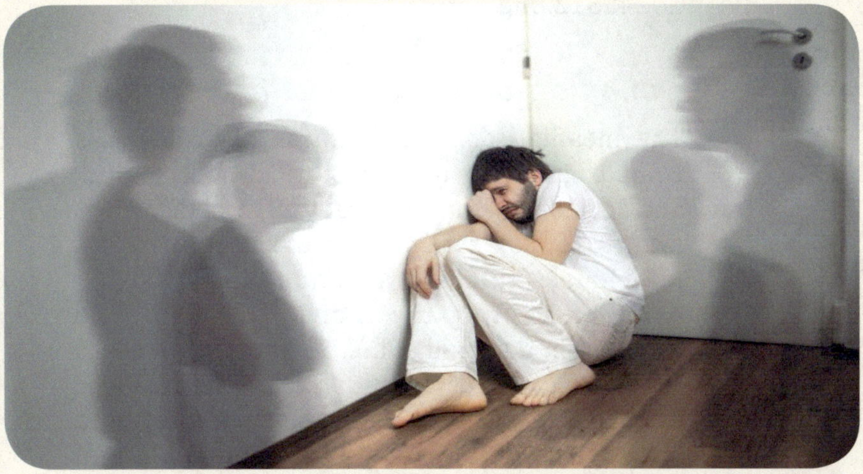

LEARNING OBJECTIVES

After studying this chapter, you will be able to:

1. Describe the types of mental health disorders
2. Understand the causes of mental health disorders
3. Understand the symptoms and accurate diagnosis of mental health disorders
4. Know the treatment options for mental health disorders
5. Know the impact of mental health disorders on daily life
6. Understand the importance of prevention and awareness in addressing mental health disorders

Introduction

The field exposure of mental health disorders is essential in understanding the complexity of these diseases. Mental health disorders are a wide range of diseases that affect the emotional, psychological, and social well-being of an individual. Mental health disorders are now widely recognized to be significant causes of global disease burden that affect millions of people across different populations. The stigmatization of mental illness then results in underdiagnosis and inadequate treatment, contributing to the sophistication of mental health care provision. Complex public health strategies and awareness campaigns are needed to overcome these issues, create understanding, and request help. Through wide-ranging research and analysis, the content of this chapter attempts to illuminate the intricate interplay among various mental illness disorders, treatment adherence, and the social issues of these diseases overall, finally casting light on the causes of mental illness problems in contemporary society. Among the most significant domains that are omitted from research into mental illness is the interplay between other psychiatric illnesses and social issues. For instance, studies like those conducted in mental health centers describe the impact socioeconomic status has on treatment compliance by those suffering from schizophrenia diagnoses. Treatment compliance in this case is a significant prognostic factor, as evidenced by strong correlations among social support, self-awareness, and compliance. Specifically, those patients who possessed more information about their illness and were raised in supportive homes reported greater treatment compliance. This highlights the need for intensive intervention that addresses clinical treatment as well as social elements of health. Understanding such connections is crucial for developing integrative treatment plans that consider not only the individual's psychological needs but also the social environment, paving the way for more favorable outcomes. Mental illness conditions cross individual experience, being symbolic of more pervasive concerns of society as a whole, including stigma, access to treatment, and policy reform.

Conditions like intellectual disability often increase vulnerability to a series of health states, including malnutrition, which makes overall wellness more complicated. The problems are pervasive among specific populations, particularly children and youth with intellectual disabilities across the globe. Analysis of health trends among such groups yields disconcerting statistics suggesting that malnourishment can increase exposure to other health conditions, thereby creating a cycle of disadvantage and poor health. Turning these disparities around will require specific efforts to develop effective interventions relevant to the needs of vulnerable groups. By examining the intricate interplay among physical health, socio-economic factors, and mental health, this chapter aims to contribute to an understanding of the systemic problems that must be addressed to improve mental health outcomes for all (Figure 1.1).

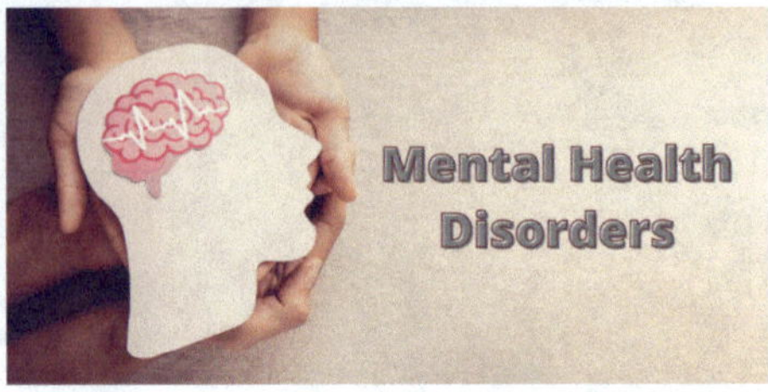

Figure 1.1. Mental health disorders.

Source: https://www.psypathy.com/wp-content/uploads/2022/08/Mental-Health-Disorders-1-1024x512.png.

Definition of Mental Health Disorders

The meaning of mental illness disorders is a complex interplay of psychological, neurological, and social elements. Typically, mental disorders manifest as severe disturbances in an individual's thinking, emotion, and behavior, hence disrupting the individual's ability to function in day-to-day life. Such definitions are required in order to understand the nuances of illnesses such as depression, anxiety, and schizophrenia. The Diagnostic and Statistical Manual of Mental Disorders (DSM-5) gives standardized criteria, but the assignment is to describe the typicality effects inherent in mental health disorders. Each disorder has variations that defy fixed categorizations and, therefore, demand a dynamic process of thinking of mental health as a spectrum rather than a binary division. With the advancement of science, definitions of mental disorders are more precise, trying to explain in the midst of the intricacies of human life. Even further, understanding mental illness may be achieved by recognizing the biological underpinnings shared by certain maladies. Drug dependence is an excellent case in illustrating how a mental illness can be caused by psychological vulnerability and neurobiological mechanisms. The compelling desire to consume substances is most often the result of an intricate interplay between pharmacological effects and individual neurological histories. Thus, drug dependence relies not only on behavioral assessment but also on comprehension of those neurobiological mechanisms of addiction. The research within the branch underscores the need to combine pharmacotherapy with psychological treatment, resulting in more effective treatment regimens. This dual reaction highlights that mental disorders require solution alternatives that accept the multifaceted quality that addresses both the mind as well as the underlying physiological attributes (Baconi et al., 2015). Furthermore, the representation of mental disorders avoids the traditional medical typologies that rely on individual variables of diversity and complexity in human psychology. As cognitive scholarship has noted, the majority of medical concepts—especially mental disorders—resist categorical definition in terms of necessary and sufficient conditions. This raises an essential issue in artificial intelligence and computer science, where knowing representation needs to be as close to the real-world complexity of such diseases as possible. The combination of geometric knowledge representations with classical ontological systems enables researchers to preserve more of the nuances of psychiatric concepts. This blended approach allows for a more expansive grasp of mental health disorders, one that enables representation that accounts for typical features and the interpersonal variation that defines each disorder (Lieto et al., 2019). Lastly, this evolving understanding is consistent with the broader goal of enhancing diagnosis, treatment, and prevention strategies in mental health disorders.

Importance of Mental Health Awareness

The value of mental health awareness cannot be overstated, for it is the foundation for education in mental health disorders and promotes overall wellness. Awareness is the impetus to reduce stigma, a barrier that has kept individuals from seeking help for years. Mental illness has a tendency to thrive under the guise of misinterpretation and critique, preventing affected individuals from acknowledging their problems and seeking proper treatment. By creating awareness, communities can ensure settings in which discussing mental health is alright, enabling people to come forward and access aid without the risk of facing discrimination. Such open discourse can lead to improved mental health, as people are more likely to use beneficial resources when they are embraced and understood. This transformation in society may have a direct effect on the consumption of mental health care, as seen through evidence linking increased awareness to increased access among groups, namely postpartum women (Rawal, 2025). In addition, the synergy between early intervention and awareness of mental health is pivotal to effective management of mental health diseases. As more people become aware, individuals are likely to recognize early symptoms in themselves or others and seek intervention and support early enough. Early intervention is most often associated with better prognosis and recovery rates, significantly reducing the long-term impacts of mental health diseases. In the medical field, mental health experts and AI experts are increasingly noting the potential benefits of integrating innovative technologies for the prediction and treatment of mental health conditions. But that has to be done with a commitment towards ethical concerns and sensitivity towards the constraints posed by such technologies (Lashari et al., 2025). With an awareness of the fine balance between intervention and awareness, stakeholders can design appropriately focused programs that not only promote information sharing but also build trust towards innovative mental health interventions. Lastly, facing the impediments to mental health treatment—rooted in an ignorance—is essential to expanding access to treatment. Most remain ignorant of what assistance is accessible, thereby perpetuating cycles of distress and solitude. Mental illness awareness involves not just a broader understanding of mental illness disorders but also an active combat against stigma, misconceptions, and fiscal limitations that limit access. Evidence suggests that targeted, evidence-based interventions such as community-based education and outreach programs can significantly increase awareness among marginalized groups, ultimately enhancing service utilization (Rawal, 2025). The growth of awareness and understanding can empower the community to fight for their mental health needs and insist on improved services, which, in turn, can bring about a change in society's perceptions of mental health. In total, the importance of mental health awareness goes beyond individual profit; it is essential to support a compassionate, informed society that cares about mental health for all (Figure 1.2).

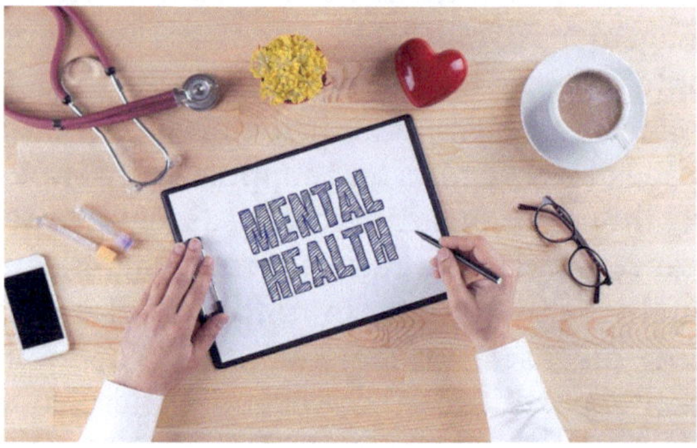

Figure 1.2. Importance of mental health awareness.

Source: https://sa1s3optim.patientpop.com/assets/images/provider/photos/2617086.jpg.

1.1. Types of Mental Health Disorders

Learning Outcome

1. Understand the anxiety disorders
2. Describe the mood disorders
3. Describe the classification of psychotic disorders

The landscape of mental illness disorders is both complex and diverse, as these disorders take various forms and are grouped according to symptoms as well as causes. The most prevalent forms include anxiety disorders that consist of generalized anxiety disorder, panic disorder, and social anxiety disorder. The disorders are characterized by unusually high levels of fear and worry that greatly impair an individual's everyday activities. They have been stated to be triggered by environmental stressors in reports given in research and may lead to health-bad consequences if left untreated. The need to treat anxiety disorders cannot be overstated since they are not only common but also greatly influence total health and productivity, portraying the need for appropriate therapeutic interventions within the community (Ajeh et al., 2024). The other critical category of mental illness disorders is mood disorders, primarily encompassing depression and bipolar disorder. Mood disorders may have a very important impact on the emotional life of a person and are typically attributed to biological, psychological, and social reasons. Major depressive disorder is a predominant subtype wherein there is continuous sadness, loss of interest, and various physical symptoms. Similarly, bipolar disorder illustrates periodic depression with episodes of mania, bringing to the limelight the two-faced nature of the illness. Interestingly, further studies are indicating that mood disorders are increasingly becoming prevalent, and particularly so among working populations, where lifestyle and stress may act as precipitating factors (Ajeh et al., 2024). It is vital to learn about these disorders as they can functionally debilitate interpersonal and working relationships, highlighting the importance of intensive mental health services. In addition to mood and anxiety disorders, personality disorders represent an essential category of mental health. These conditions, such as borderline personality disorder, narcissistic personality disorder, and antisocial personality disorder, are characterized by persistent patterns of behavior and internal experience that are significantly different from societal expectations.

They will be expressed through maladaptive coping mechanisms, and social dysfunction and impaired interpersonal relationships will result. The subtlety and ubiquitous nature of the personality disorders make it difficult to diagnose and treat them, and they will not view their behavior as pathological. According to more recent studies, some personality disorders have a gender-specific incidence and vary significantly in men and women, which makes appropriate means in diagnostic and therapeutic processes necessary (Izydorczyk et al., 2017). Such complex disorders need to be managed to develop psychological resilience and improve quality of life in patients (Figure 1.3).

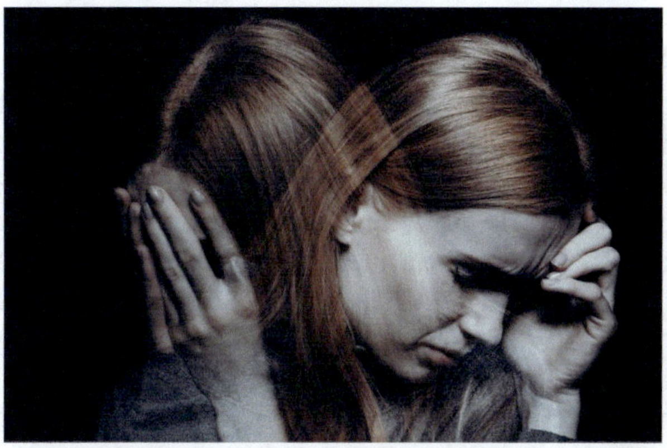

Figure 1.3. Types of mental health disorders.

Source: https://alterbehavioralhealth.com/wp-content/uploads/2021/04/What-Are-the-7-types-of-Mental-Disorders.jpg.

1.1.1. Anxiety Disorders

Anxiety disorders are a category of mental diseases characterized by heightened worry or fear, which could significantly hamper functioning. Prevalence in these disorders is on the rise, particularly among young people, reflecting a critical public health problem that demands immediate attention. Anxiety disorders have been shown to emerge either during childhood or adolescence and, therefore, making it essential to establish early intervention systems. The successful treatment modalities, such as cognitive-behavioral therapy (CBT), are in demand at the present time, which may provide individuals with coping strategies to manage anxiety effectively. Furthermore, the understanding of the biopsychosocial variables implicated in anxiety disorders would assist in formulating a particular therapeutic approach meeting the unique needs of every patient, ultimately resulting in better mental health status among individuals. The interaction between physical health states and anxiety disorders can complicate management, requiring more intense models of combined care. For instance, a review demonstrates that comorbid illnesses such as hypertension are more likely to occur together with depression and anxiety, leading to adverse health outcomes. Patients suffering from anxiety disorders may struggle to adhere to treatment for both their mental and physical conditions, further deteriorating their overall condition. It is worthwhile to treat these comorbidities; simultaneous care that attacks anxiety and associated health issues can lead to immense increases in treatment adherence and patient satisfaction. This multidisciplinary care not only treats the psychological aspects of anxiety disorders, but it also respects the interconnected nature of physical and mental health, thereby permitting more totalistic approaches to care. Drop-in mental health services have become trendy as a new approach to addressing the growing demand for timely treatment of anxiety disorders, particularly among children and adolescents. Evaluations of these services have been marked by high clinical utility, as reflected in reductions in anxiety symptoms and improvements in quality of life. For instance, a study reported significant decreases in emotional and behavioral problems among youth with access to drop-in services, along with higher overall satisfaction with the care they received. Such care models are not merely cost-efficient but also achieve high levels of patient participation, indicating their potential to expand access to evidence-based treatments for mental illnesses. While health systems keep seeking ways to address issues of mental health, integrating such readily available services in children's hospitals can also significantly enhance the availability of coverage for teenagers with anxiety disorders, enabling early intervention and better long-term outcomes(Roach et al., 2025; Urmi et al., 2025) (Figure 1.4).

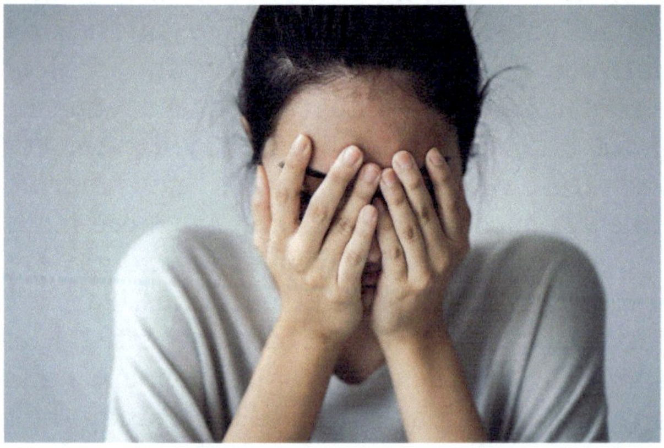

Figure 1.4. Anxiety disorders.

Source: https://www.homage.com.my/wp-content/uploads/sites/2/2021/08/Article-Images-8-scaled.jpg.

1.1.2. Mood Disorders

Mood disorders represent a significant category of mental illnesses that consist of many conditions, such as depression and bipolar disorder. Mood disorders are characterized by a chronic disturbance in mood that can significantly impair an individual's functioning and quality of life. Depression, for example, may manifest as sadness, hopelessness, and loss of interest in normal activities, and bipolar disorder by phases of cyclical mania and depression. The staggering impact of mood disorders extends beyond the individual to affect social relationships, work output, and overall societal production. Further, it should be noted that mood disorders do not stand alone; they have a tendency to worsen when accompanied by other diseases, for example, chronic pain disorders, thereby emphasizing the correlation between the state of the body and mind. The prevalence of mood disorders in the general population emphasizes the necessity of effective treatment strategies. Current research has demonstrated that almost one in five adults suffers from some form of mood disorder during their lifespan, placing an overwhelming burden on society. When it comes to chronic pain syndromes, such as temporomandibular disorder (TMD), the occurrence of mood disorders is exceedingly high, with patients being at heightened risk for depression and anxiety. Chronic pain not only adversely affects physical health but also causes emotional distress as well as neuroanatomical structural modification, leading to a mutual relationship between them. To control mood disorders effectively, particularly in chronic pain patients, involves the integration of psychological and physical health interventions to facilitate patients' overall outcomes and well-being among affected populations (Afaque et al., 2025). Additionally, the world continues to advance in ways that make mood disorders increasingly prevalent, particularly among susceptible groups such as refugees. The psychological well-being of victims who have experienced displacement due to war, such as the ongoing war in Ukraine, points towards this deteriorating problem. Studies show that refugees are subjected to nearly twice the rate of mood and anxiety disorders compared to non-refugee immigrants, pointing to the extensive psychological trauma caused by forced migration. Stress from war and resettlement, subsequently, can result in deteriorating mental health, complicating prior mood disorders or bringing on new ones. With such challenges confronting health systems, there is a need to adopt an integrated approach that accounts for the intricate relationship between individual circumstances and the social determinants of health, and to make therapy patient-specific to the experience of those undergoing conflict and displacement (Ramos et al., 2024) (Figure 1.5).

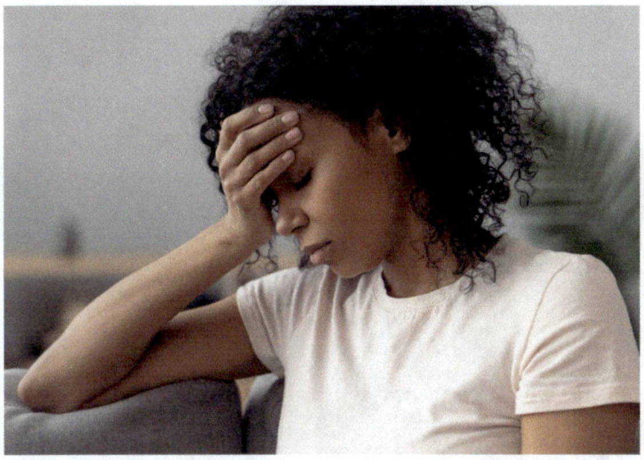

Figure 1.5. Mood disorders.

Source: https://wexnermedical.osu.edu/-/media/images/wexnermedical/pages/patient-care/healthcare-services/mental-behavioral/mood-disorders/depressed-woman.jpg.

1.1.3. Psychotic Disorders

Diagnosis of psychotic disorders is vital in the field of mental health and encompasses all disorders that play a significant role in a person's thoughts, perceptions, and overall reality. Among the eminent psychotic disorders, the most prevalent one is schizophrenia, which is commonly accompanied by a combination of hallucinations, delusions, and disorganized thinking. These symptoms can seriously affect a person's daily performance, impacting their social relationships and occupational activities. An important aspect of the management of psychotic disorders is early intervention and good management, which can significantly reduce the severity of the symptoms. The complex interplay among genetic, environmental, and neurobiological factors underscores the need for long-term studies in these disorders to inform the development of effective therapeutic approaches that improve patient care. Moreover, the physiological impact of psychotic disorders does not merely extend to mental health, having a tendency to unveil severe comorbidities that make the issue worse for the patient. Studies have indicated a dramatic association of psychotic disorders with a higher rate of metabolic syndrome incidence, including obesity, hypertension, dyslipidemia, and hyperglycemia. Evidence establishes that individuals with psychotic disorders not only have a risk for these metabolic disturbances but are also shorter-lived than the general population. Most terrifyingly, however, most of these patients remain untreated for these metabolic disorders, and guidelines in existence today emphasize the importance of regular monitoring and intervention.

This treatment failure underscores the urgent need for the mental health care system to be more compliant with the established guidelines, so that patients are treated for all the psychological and physiological impacts on their well-being (Bartels-Velthuis et al., 1977). The co-occurrence of mental illness is also prevalent among individuals diagnosed with psychotic illnesses, which renders it harder to treat and recover overall. The high levels of comorbidity, especially in substance use treatment settings, highlight the need for integrated interventions that treat both psychotic symptoms and any accompanying mental health problems. For instance, evidence recently emerged that over 19% of individuals in community alcohol and other drug treatment have a psychotic disorder, presenting starkly against lower rates of prevalence among the broader population (Mortlock et al., 2016).

That prevalence indicates an urgent requirement for mental health clinicians to enhance screening processes for co-occurring disorders to facilitate support within an integrated treatment environment. Effective management requires collaboration between alcohol and drug services and mental health services, with the potential of improved therapeutic outcomes, plus increased awareness of the complexity of psychotic disorders (Figure 1.6).

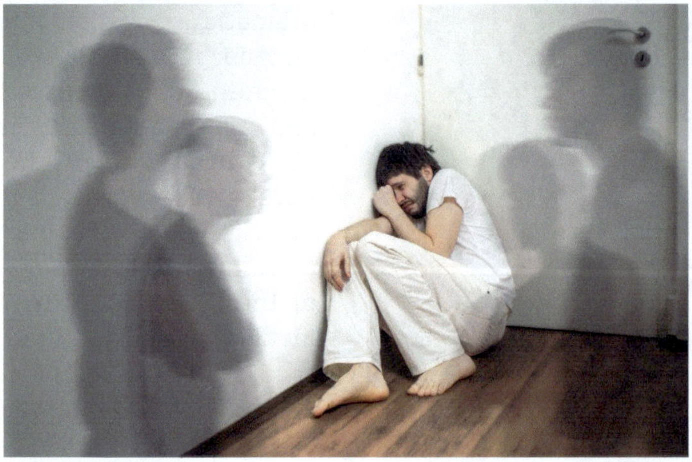

Figure 1.6. Psychotic disorders.

Source: https://advancedpsychiatrydfw.com/wp-content/uploads/2019/06/schizophrenia.jpeg.

Test Your Knowledge

1. What are the anxiety disorders?
2. What are the mood disorders?

1.2. Causes of Mental Health Disorders

Learning Outcome

1. Understand the genetic factors
2. Know the environmental influences on mental health disorders;
3. Describe the psychological factors of mental health disorders

Understanding the etiologies of mental illness is crucial in planning prevention and effective treatment strategies. Several factors can contribute to the onset of these diseases, often interacting in a complex pattern. Biological predispositions, such as genetic influences, can provide the basis for susceptibility to mental illness. For example, individuals with a history of depression, anxiety, or other mental disorders in their relatives will be more likely to develop similar conditions. In addition, neurochemical imbalance and structural brain changes may play an important role in a person's mental state. While biological determinants are more intrinsic, they do not operate independently of external pressures; environmental stress has a great impact upon the mental health landscape, augmenting or diminishing risk to a greater extent than genetic vulnerability, and thus emphasizing the importance of an overarching understanding of causal determinants in the context of individual experience. Psychosocial factors serve as pivotal causal determinants in the causation of mental health disorders. One's history, including trauma at an early stage in life, bullying, and significant life changes, may have a strong influence on their psychological well-being. Studies on the lives of adolescents have indicated that several factors, like life dissatisfaction, low teacher support, and family support, are good predictors of psychoneurological disorders among students, which indicates the role played by external influences in mental health (Kuchma et al., 2025). Also, the pressures of modern life do have the effect of loading on these issues, and over-reliance on screens and sedentary life has been associated with higher rates of mental illness. These psychosocial stressors are significant to consider because they have the tendency to aggravate an existing vulnerability and perpetuate a cycle of mental illness, one that needs interventions and prevention directed at these issues. Parent mental health also has a wide impact on children's mental development and has a big role to play in the causation of mental health disorders. Research has shown that anxious parents affect children's early schooling and socialization, which can hinder speech development and emotional well-being (Saleem et al., 2024). For instance, when parents are low in responsiveness, most notably towards sons, it may result in attention disorders and other disabilities. Family dynamics, such as varying degrees of emotional support, socio-economic challenges, and parenting styles, give the next generation determining conditions for mental health outcomes. These familial factors should be understood because they underscore the importance of addressing not only parental mental health but also family functioning in interventions to promote psychological resilience in children (Figure 1.7).

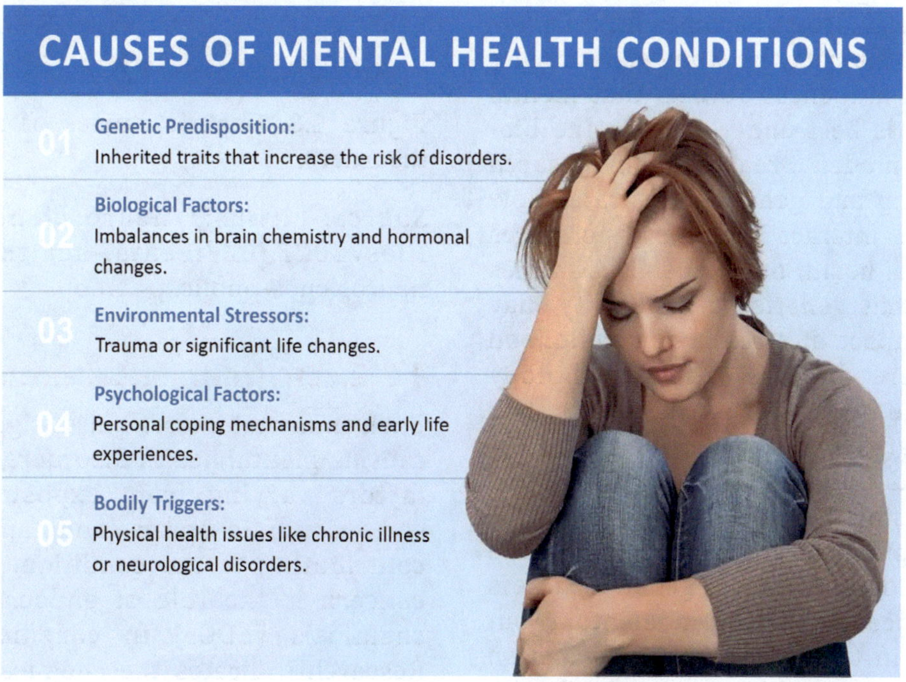

Figure 1.7. Causes of mental health conditions.

Source: https://whitelightbh.com/wp-content/uploads/Causes-Mental-Health-Conditions-1536x1056.webp.

1.2.1. Genetic Factors

Understanding genetic factors is crucial in the exploration of mental health disorders, as these biological components can significantly influence an individual's susceptibility to various psychiatric conditions. Research has increasingly highlighted the intricate relationship between genetics and mental health, revealing that certain disorders, such as schizophrenia and bipolar disorder, exhibit heritability patterns that suggest a strong genetic component. These findings emphasize the fact that while environmental factors are indispensable, there is a substantial contribution of genetic predisposition to the causation and etiology of mental disorders. Secondly, the identification of genes associated with psychiatric disorders is paving the way for personalized treatment approaches, enhancing the possibility of tailoring interventions to an individual's genetic makeup, which can revolutionize the treatment of mental health disorders (Nair et al., 2014). As the biological underpinnings of mental health are further explored, the integration of genetic information with psychosocial factors becomes increasingly important. The interplay between genetics and environmental influences reveals that mental health disease is best understood by the bio-psycho-social model. Breakthrough research in neuroimaging and genetics illustrates how inherited traits interact with life experiences to shape mental health outcomes. DNA studies have shown that genetic susceptibility may amplify the impact of stressors or childhood trauma. Where biology and psychology converge in the domain of mental health, this transdisciplinary approach can better direct prevention initiatives and treatment protocols aimed at reversing risk and fostering resilience in high-risk populations (Smith et al., 2008). The search for the identification of genetic markers for mental illness is gaining momentum, but issues persist in translating such information into effective clinical interventions. Though there has been some progress toward understanding specific genetic contributions to conditions like depression and autism, polygenic inheritance complicates identifying straightforward causal pathways. Additionally, public health education on the importance of genetics remains inadequate, affecting research and funding. Merging new science with clinical practice is essential, encompassing not only robust research but also public engagement in de-stigmatizing speech about mental illness and genetics. It is essential to collaborate with neuroscientists, clinicians, and policymakers to ensure that genetic research ultimately leads to evidence-based approaches, thereby enhancing the quality of care for patients with mental health disorders (Nair et al., 2014) (Figure 1.8).

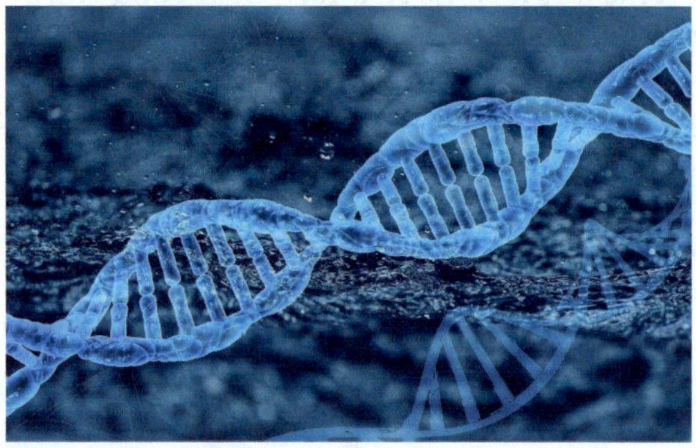

Figure 1.8. Genetic causes of mental health disorders.

Source: https://neurosciencenews.com/files/2022/02/mental-health-genetics-ai-neurosicnes-public.jpg.webp.

1.2.2. Environmental Influences

Environmental factors play a significant role in causing mental health disorders, with external factors varying from exposure to toxins, socioeconomic status, and family dynamics contributing to the condition. Of significant concern is the role of endocrine-disrupting chemicals (EDCs) in consumer products. Research indicates the chemicals play a role in compromising the central nervous system's function and are increasingly being implicated in major depressive disorder (MDD) in affected individuals. The biological actions of the interactions of EDCs with hormone receptors are capable of disrupting critical neurological processes and thus possibly being responsible for the growing incidence of MDD on a global level. Secondly, sensitivity to these effects varies widely across groups, underscoring environmental contaminants as central factors in mental health. This growing body of evidence underscores the importance of addressing environmental toxins as a component of a comprehensive approach to mental health treatment and prevention (Ehsanifar et al., 2025). The home environment is also a crucial environmental influence on mental health. Evidence illustrates that children's development is directly impacted by parents' mental health, which usually results in an intergenerational pattern of mental health illness. Kids growing up in families with parents who suffer from mental disorders are at risk of developing the same. This is compounded by the accumulation of environmental stressors such as poverty and lack of social support, which further erode family functioning. A survey of clinical samples of children and parents reported significant interactions among various risk factors, suggesting that these environmental and interpersonal stresses tend to accumulate, creating complex issues for families. Hence, in response to these risks, one must utilize a holistic treatment approach that includes not just individual therapy but also family-based interventions (Stolper et al., 2024). Finally, the overall social milieu also plays a role in mental health disorder severity and prevalence, particularly through structural disparities and system determinants. Social determinants of health, such as socioeconomic status, access to healthcare, and community resources, are essential for shaping the outcomes of mental health. The inhabitants of marginalized communities are likely to be exposed to additional stressors such as discrimination and poverty, which may amplify the severity of prior mental health disorders. Environmental factors such as noise pollution, poor housing conditions, and safety in the residential areas also exert direct impacts on mental well-being. Keeping such factors in view, it is evident that treatment for mental illness requires an interdisciplinary approach that encompasses public health measures, policy reform, and community activities. By improving the environments in which individuals live and transcending system-based obstacles, mental health disparities can be significantly reduced, ultimately resulting in a healthier society overall (Stolper et al., 2024; Ehsanifar et al., 2025) (Figure 1.9).

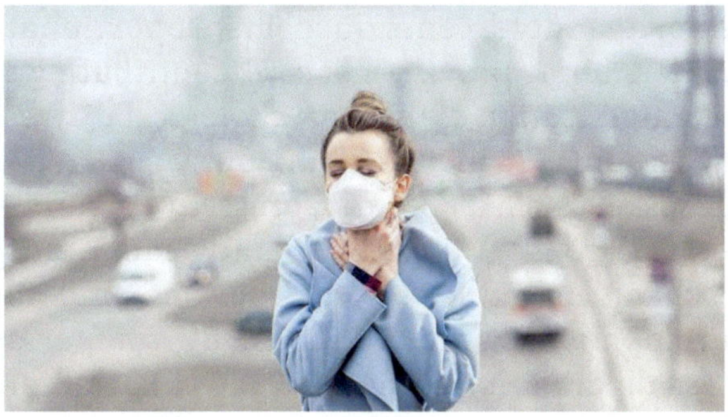

Figure 1.9. The impact of the environment on mental health.

Source: https://ghost-cms.s3.ap-south-1.amazonaws.com/2023/04/How-Does-Your-Environment-Affect-Your-Mental-Health-1.jpg.

1.2.3. Psychological Factors

The relationship between psychological problems and mental disorders is complicated, influencing not just the development of such conditions but the efficacy of intervention as well. Research indicates that children with various psychological ailments, including anxiety and depression disorders, are likely to develop strange behaviors and emotional displays. These are critical indicators of internal mental health problems and can be a prime focus for intervention. For instance, the prevalence of somatic complaints usually comes along with anxiety, and the latter requires psychological interventions that address underlying issues and not merely symptom suppression. As quoted in the literature, those treatment interventions that prove effective must place such psychological foundations first and foremost, especially in populations such as primary school-age children, because the emergence of adverse mental health consequences can have severe implications on their overall health and social functioning (Smith et al., 2008). Mental health disparities also complicate the scenario of those psychological factors influencing mental health disorders. Both ethnicity and race have deep effects on mental health as well as mental health treatment access. Science explains that minority adolescents face disproportionate barriers to the provision of care, contributing to the amplification of their psychological distress and the adverse mental health outcomes. When addressing such disparities, protective factors—healthy family dynamics and community mechanisms—must be incorporated into the development of interventions. By comparing these differences, researchers and clinicians are able to identify specific psychological factors that not only lead to mental illness disorders but also play key roles in developing an effective prevention and treatment strategy (Green et al., 2015). Furthermore, understanding psychological resilience can further the development of individualized interventions in individuals with mental health disorders. Psychological resilience involves the adaptation to stressors and adversity, partially shaped by internal factors and external support networks. Enhancing resilience in individuals, particularly those at risk for mental disorders, can be a protective factor against the development or exacerbation of disorders. Interventions with a psychological focus, such as developing coping skills, enhancing social networks, and providing cognitive-behavioral interventions, could be particularly effective. Taking into account the dynamic interplay among these elements can improve individual outcomes and promote mental well-being in diverse populations globally (Smith et al., 2008) (Figure 1.10).

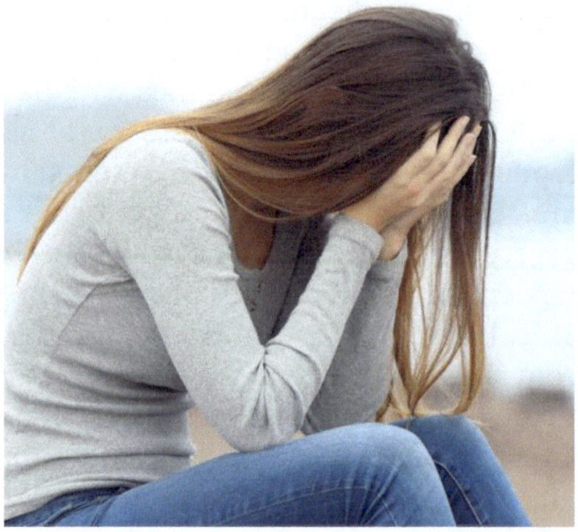

Figure 1.10. Psychological factors and mental health disorders.

Source: https://sp-ao.shortpixel.ai/client/to_webp,q_glossy,ret_img,w_768,h_512/https://care24.co.in/wp-content/uploads/2016/07/48.jpg.

Test Your Knowledge

1. What are genetic factors?
2. What are the psychological factors of mental health disorders?

1.3. Symptoms and Diagnosis

Learning Outcome

1. Learn about common symptoms of mental health disorders
2. Understand diagnostic criteria and tools for mental health disorders
3. Understand the importance of early diagnosis in the management of mental health disorders

Understanding the signs and accurate diagnosis of mental illness disorders is key to providing effective treatment approaches. In the case of managing mental illness disorders like anorexia nervosa and atypical anorexia nervosa, mental health providers would predominantly apply patient presentations, which would significantly vary based on physical considerations like body weight. Specifically, research revealed that clinicians are more reactive to diagnosing and detecting eating disorders when the patient is thin, being biased towards not noticing people with greater body weights who present the same symptoms. These findings suggest an imperative of immediacy for practitioners in the mental health field to adopt a more nuanced understanding of the diverse ways in which eating disorders manifest themselves among patients of all weight conditions so that each one is properly treated regardless of appearance or state (Silbiger, 2024). In addition to the nuances of eating disorder diagnosis, mental health in caregivers for individuals with disorders like bipolar disorder is also a significant concern. Review of literature has actually demonstrated that caregivers themselves develop higher levels of psychiatric symptoms and psychiatric disorders compared to the general population. With respect to these revelations, though, there remains a critical paucity of research concerning the application of the right diagnostic tools in assessing these caregivers' mental health status. The review emphasizes the need for systemic examination and the use of the right diagnostic tools to screen for psychiatric disorders among caregivers because neglecting to work on their mental health has the unfortunate consequence of affecting both their own health and patient outcomes that they support (Prates et al., 2024). Consequently, symptom and diagnosis convergence of mental health disorders is intricate with profound implications to both patients and care systems. Development of comprehensive knowledge of symptoms is crucial, not only for the correct identification of mental health disorders but also for the development of effective interventions that are appropriate for the needs of different patients and caregivers. Ensuring that diagnostic protocols can account for the complexity of these conditions will require ongoing education and training of mental health professionals to decrease bias and enhance caregivers' awareness of their own requirements, ultimately creating a more robust approach to mental health treatment that can engage all stakeholders (Prates et al., 2024; Silbiger, 2024).

1.3.1. Common Symptoms of Mental Health Disorders

Mental illness is exhibited in the form of a variety of symptoms that can potentially have serious effects on one's daily life and overall well-being. Some of the usual symptoms will often include long-standing feelings of hopelessness or anxiety, mood swings, and fluctuations of energy. The person feels hopeless or is burdened with an overwhelming feeling of fear that affects the capacity to interact with others or perform daily tasks. For instance, a person suffering from depression may struggle to get out of bed in the morning, while a person with an anxiety disorder may excessively worry about trivial matters. These symptoms not only affect individuals' health but also put pressure on relationships as a cause and an effect of poor mental health. Identification of these symptoms is crucial for early identification and effective intervention strategies in the case of mental health illnesses. Prolonged intrusive recall, or involuntary autobiographical memories (IAMs), are also significant symptoms of mental health illnesses. Research has indicated that although such memories might be an integral aspect of living, they become pathological when they are associated with mental health impairments. For example, individuals with post-traumatic stress disorder (PTSD) will have memories of their trauma, and these can lead to debilitating problems such as flashbacks or emotional dysregulation. In consideration of this, the specific content of the memories—traumatic experiences or negative relationship histories, for example—has been linked to worse mental health outcomes, including depression and anxiety disorders. By examining the frequency and content of these recurrent IAMs, mental health clinicians can develop tailored therapeutic interventions that consider the particular aspects of a patient's experience (Yeung et al., 2023). In addition to long-standing effects and symptoms of memory, patients with mental illness may present with changes in physical and behavioral states. For instance, worried individuals will exhibit avoidance behaviors in the sense that they will shun those situations that distress them.

There are physical symptoms such as sleep disturbances, appetite alterations, and fatigue without an organic cause that are common, often exacerbating the psychological challenge that presents with individuals. Physical symptoms have been shown by research to impact an individual's quality of life, further complicating the maintenance of mental health. Digital mental health interventions have been shown to be a possible solution to address these complex symptoms, particularly in low-resource settings, through improved access and treatment efficiency (Karyotaki et al., 2023). Overall, recognition and diagnosis of the wide range of symptoms of mental health conditions are imperative to the delivery of effective care and intervention for individuals affected (Figure 1.11).

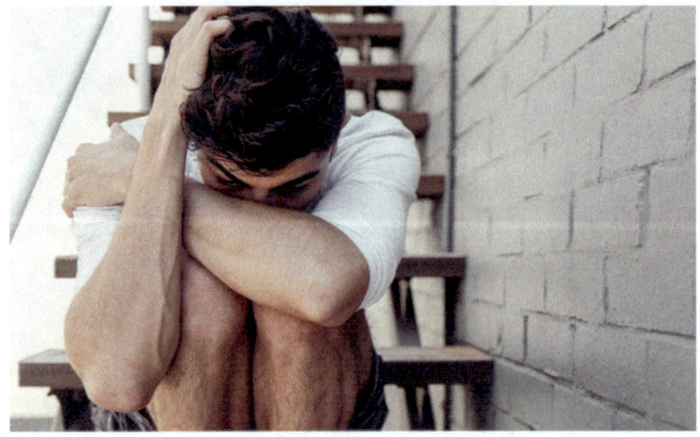

Figure 1.11. Symptoms of mental illness.

Source: https://parashospitals-web.s3.ap-south-1.amazonaws.com/blogs/July2024/1721126178mental%20ilness.jpg.

1.3.2. Diagnostic Criteria and Tools

Diagnostic criteria and tools for mental illness are a must to know in order to detect and treat with accuracy. These criteria normally stem from widely used guidelines such as the Diagnostic and Statistical Manual of Mental Disorders (DSM) and the International Classification of Diseases (ICD). These manuals provide systematic guidelines for diagnosing various mental illnesses in the same manner across populations. For instance, standardized measures like structured interviews or self-report scales are effective in translating difficult behavioral symptoms into numerical data, which in itself may be essential in determining the presence of conditions such as attention deficit hyperactivity disorder (ADHD) or autism spectrum disorder (ASD). With the introduction of standardized screening tools, the diagnosis has become highly accurate, revealing previously undiscovered disorders, especially in institutions like prisons where mental illness goes undetected, as established by research applying diverse assessment methods (Asherson et al., 2015). The role of screening and diagnostic tools cannot be overstated in the understanding of neurodevelopmental disorders

(NDD). Recent research focuses on the effective use of such instruments in diagnosing disorders like ADHD and ASD among those who are likely to receive suboptimal mental health care. An example is a study on a group of male prisoners, which used the ADHD self-report scale among other tests and found that several prisoners had undiagnosed NDD. Such findings underscore the value of access to and knowledge of systematic screening, which can influence appropriate treatment regimens and interventions. Moreover, the overwhelming statistics obtained through these measurements show the prevalence and extent of mental health disorders among certain groups of people, emphasizing the necessity for more precise diagnostic methods to address the requirements of those who are likely to fall through the cracks in mainstream mental health systems (Asherson et al., 2015).

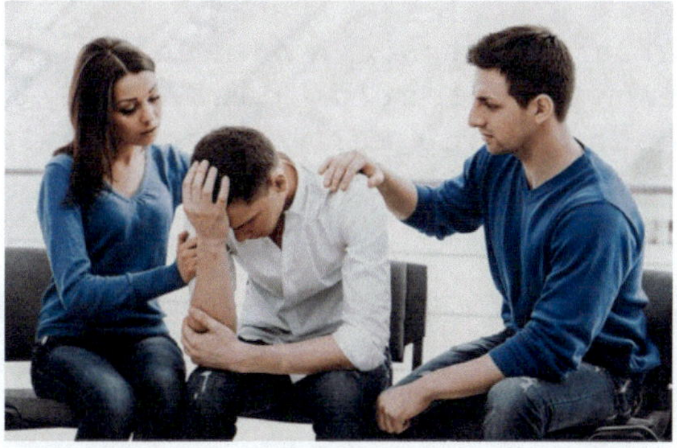

Figure 1.12. Mental illness diagnosis.

Source: https://www.aspirefrisco.com/wp-content/uploads/2024/12/Getting-treatment-for-mental-illness-updated.png.

In global mental health research, diagnostic instrument and criterion differences can lead to fluctuation in prevalence rates across regions. A meta-analysis of the autism spectrum disorder (ASD) rate in mainland China revealed substantial evidence by way of the application of strict screening instruments. The study revealed a pooled ASD rate, indicating a discrepancy relative to rates in other countries. This disparity raises significant questions about the consistency and cross-cultural applicability of diagnostic tests, revealing the probable bias entrenched in their construction and use. Such disparities highlight the need for additional research to create diagnostic criteria that take cultural factors into consideration, thus remaining meaningful and useful in multicultural populations. Knowledge of these differences is fundamental to the development of sound mental health policy on an international basis, upholding the need for standardization while allowing room for flexibility to accommodate cultural variations (Figure 1.12).

1.3.3. Importance of Early Diagnosis

Early detection plays a crucial role in the treatment of mental illnesses, significantly impacting treatment and the patient's quality of life. Early detection of depression, anxiety, and bipolar illness at their initial stage allows early intervention, which prevents symptom exacerbation. This reduces the likelihood of co-occurring illness, hence improving the effectiveness of therapeutic interventions. By emphasizing early detection, healthcare practitioners can also implement interventions to better fit individualized patient needs—crucial for illnesses that encompass a wide extent of severity and expression. Directed treatment not only maximizes results but also could minimize the stigma traditionally associated with treatment and pursuit of care for mental illness, encouraging more individuals to seek care and intervention when early signs of distress are detected. Besides, emerging technologies, particularly those artificial intelligence-based, are promising to facilitate early diagnosis of mental illness. Natural language processing and machine learning can analyze patient information more effectively than human methods, perhaps even detecting warning signs before they become full-blown illnesses. For instance, predictive analytics can detect patterns in behavioral data, alerting physicians to changes that indicate deteriorating mental health. Through the use of such technological innovations, professionals are not only able to detect problems in advance but also to keep track of patients in real-time, allowing management plans to adapt to the patient's condition. Through the incorporation of such digital solutions into everyday practice, the healthcare environment becomes more adaptive and responsive, eventually changing how mental health disorders are treated and viewed in society (Bhalsing et al., 2025). Additionally, the importance of early diagnosis applies to the manner in which mental health illnesses impact aspects of daily living, including work performance and social functioning. Conditions like dental fear, along with other mental illnesses, have an extensive ability to impair patients' health-seeking behavior, thereby creating secondary medical complications (Bejarano, 2024). In essence, if not treated, mental illness has a tendency to escalate issues in terms of personal relationships, employment continuity, and well-being. By diagnosing and treating these disorders early, individuals are more likely to engage with the treatments they require, reducing the likelihood of chronic disease development. Early engagement inspires not only healthier results but a sense of empowerment as well in individuals as they navigate their mental illness journeys. As a result, the emphasis on early diagnosis is vital to both personal and public health initiatives (Figure 1.13).

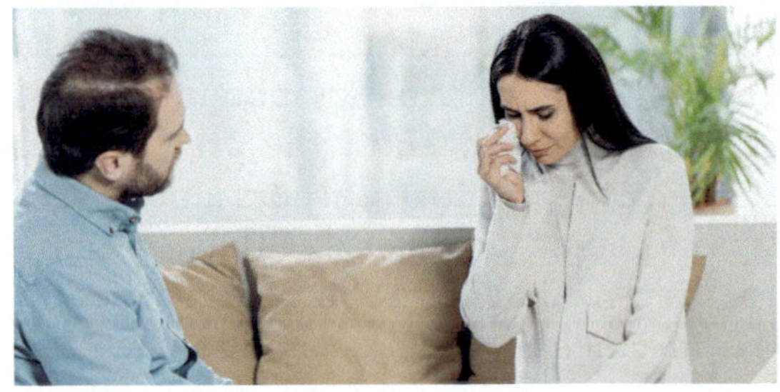

Figure 1.13. Importance of early mental health treatment.

Source: https://www.aspirefrisco.com/wp-content/uploads/2024/09/woman_getting_early_mental_health_treatment-e1727388354699.jpg.

Test Your Knowledge

1. What are the common symptoms of mental health disorders?
2. What are the diagnostic tools for mental health disorders?

1.4. Treatment Options

Learning Outcome

1. Describe the psychotherapy
2. Understand the role of medication in the management of mental health disorders
3. Describe the alternative therapies

In the landscape of mental illness, treatment available can be diverse, reflecting the complexity of these illnesses. The type of treatment plan will often change with the disorder, severity, and requirements of the individual patient. Psychotherapy, pharmacotherapy, and complementary treatments are usual procedures. Psychotherapy, or talking therapy, takes the form of various techniques, such as cognitive behavioral therapy (CBT) and dialectical behavioral therapy (DBT), designed to alter unwanted thoughts and behavior. Pharmacotherapy, on the other hand, entails the use of medication such as antidepressants, antipsychotics, and mood stabilizers, which achieve their effect in symptom diminution and regulation of the biological basis of mental illnesses. A personalized approach—integrating psychological and pharmacological treatments—can lead to more effective outcomes for individuals who suffer from complex mental illness disorders. The network model of psychopathology has emerged as a new paradigm for the conceptualization and treatment of mental illness disorders. This method assesses intercorrelations among individual symptoms and approximates the effects of various treatments through network analyses. Literature presents an extensive application of this framework in intervention research, demonstrating that common methodological practices preclude the assessment of treatment effectiveness (Schumacher et al., 2024).

Conducting symptom network analyses prior to, during, and after treatment provides researchers with valuable information about the influence of interventions on not only overall mental health but also on specific symptoms. For instance, therapeutic interventions that alter connectivity in symptom networks could reduce disorder severity and, by extension, inform treatment tailoring to improve patient outcomes. In particular, treatment of ED is one such critical space where multidisciplinary approaches really pay off. Pregnant and postpartum women of childbearing age, especially those with a history of EDs, also present with their own issues, necessitating multimodal management of their conditions. An effective treatment modality is reported to be a collaborative effort between clinicians, psychologists, nutritionists, and hospitalists, emphasizing attention to the psychological and physiological aspects of these conditions (Fontaine et al., 2024). Early intervention and detection can reduce the risks of EDs in this population to a significant degree, leading to better fetal and maternal health. Further research on treatment modalities focused on the postpartum period is significant, as this field is underexplored and, if studied more, might improve the overall health of affected women at a vulnerable time of life (Figure 1.14).

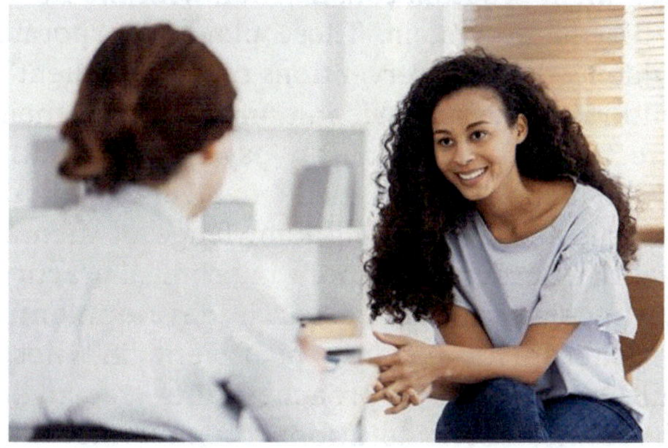

Figure 1.14. Understanding mental health disorders and various treatment options.

Source: https://sa1s3optim.patientpop.com/assets/images/provider/photos/2713254.jpg.

1.4.1. Psychotherapy

Psychotherapy is a mainstay in the management of mental health disorders, providing a structured and therapeutic environment for individuals seeking help. By engaging in therapeutic dialogue with clients, psychotherapists work to establish the causative factors behind distressing mental states, facilitating the exploration of thought, emotion, and action. Beyond facilitating insight and self-awareness, this also empowers clients to develop coping strategies tailored to their specific circumstances. It relies heavily on the therapeutic relationship between therapist and client, which is key to creating a healing, supportive, and developmentally supportive atmosphere. As mental health issues continue to rise, it is essential to see the value of this therapeutic relationship in the treatment of disorders ranging from depression and anxiety to more severe issues such as post-traumatic stress disorder. Perhaps the most significant aspect of psychotherapy is that it can be adaptable when applied in diverse cultures and with variable client needs, so that treatment programs are not only client-centered but also culturally relevant. Educational systems for mental health counselors promote this adaptability by stressing treatment program construction with the DSM-5 diagnostic system. These plans incorporate evidence-based interventions tuned to a client's cultural values and orientation to enhance their effectiveness. Importantly, psychotherapeutic practice must continually evolve to reflect the constantly changing knowledge of mental health disorders, incorporating clinical practice advancements and research developments. As therapists become proficient in these culture-sensitive approaches, they reconcile the ethical considerations of implementing manualized therapeutic techniques, ensuring that standardized treatment is matched with individualized care (Hittner et al., 2015).

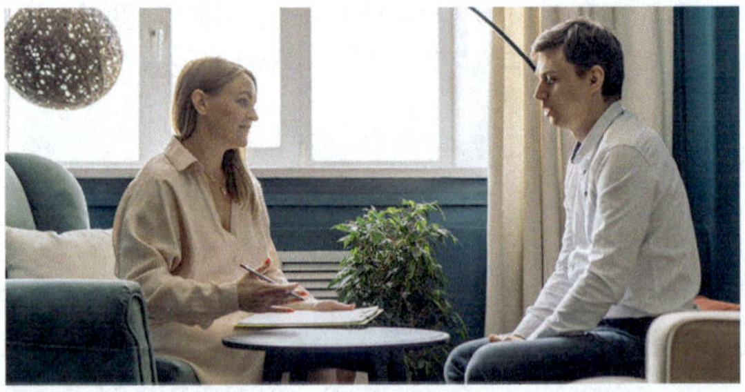

Figure 1.15. Psychotherapy.

Source: https://www.apa.org/images/psychotherapy-topic-landing-page-tile_tcm7-311728.jpg.

Lastly, evidence-based practice in psychotherapy is essential in providing effective treatment outcomes in clients who have a multitude of mental illnesses. Mental health counselor education programs emphasize the application of evidence-based interventions, not just for the quality of care, but also for treatment planning and accountability. Evidence-based interventions have been shown to significantly reduce symptoms and improve overall functioning. The evaluation process is also important for therapists in that it allows them to measure client progress and adjust treatment methods accordingly. This psychotherapy cycle promotes an ongoing dialogue between client and therapist, fostering a collaborative environment in which healing can emerge. With the mental health industry constantly evolving, the role of psychotherapy remains vital to creating meaningful effects on people's lives (Baltrinic et al., 2016) (Figure 1.15).

1.4.2. Medication

The role of medication in mental illness has grown in recent decades, and it has proven to be essential in treatment protocols for various psychiatric disorders. Psychotropic medications like antidepressants, antipsychotics, and mood stabilizers are at the forefront of controlling symptoms, enhancing quality of life, and enhancing functionality for patients. These medications target the neurotransmitter systems directly that are most frequently dysregulated in psychiatric illness and thereby restore balance to the brain's chemistry. But the caveat is ensuring that medication regimens are optimized and tailored to individual patients, particularly regarding differential drug responses. As underscored by the Neurological and mental health Global Epidemiology Network (NeuroGEN), there is a significant need to investigate medication use and medical outcomes to better evaluate the efficacy of treatment across different populations (Bazelier et al., 2020). Despite the advantage, medication compliance is still a complex issue in mental health treatment. Several barriers, including side effects, stigma, and a lack of knowledge about the disease, are common causes of patient non-adherence. New methods to increase adherence rates are being explored, including monetary incentives. Early findings suggest that offering incentives to improve adherence can yield significant gains for patients with psychotic disorders, for example, in recent trials involving hard-to-reach community patients (Priebe et al., 2009). Not only do these interventions operate to enhance adherence, but they also operate to reduce the broader health burden for untreated mental disorders. Therefore, a setting that has the potential to enhance medication compliance is crucial to achieving optimal treatment outcomes and quality of life for the patients. The impact of medication on psychiatric disease extends beyond symptom management; it has occupational and social functioning as well. For individuals suffering from serious and chronic mental illness, consistent and effective medication can facilitate their rehabilitation into society, make it possible to participate in schooling and work, and reduce the incidence of crises that require more severe interventions, such as hospitalization. From the studies conducted by NeuroGEN, understanding the long-term medical and social consequences of medication adherence is important for developing combined treatment schedules for psychiatric disorders (Bazelier et al., 2020). Additionally, addressing these consequences creates avenues for policy formulation and practice approaches that not only advocate for medication adherence but also overall recovery for persons who are caught up in the web of mental illness (Figure 1.16).

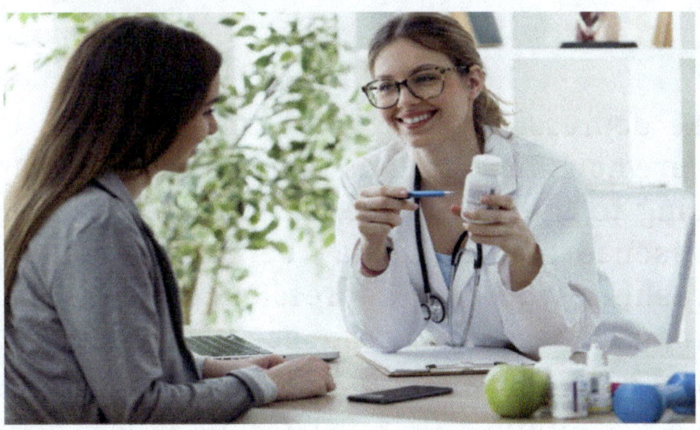

Figure 1.16. Medication management for mental health.

Source: https://connectionswellnessgroup.com/wp-content/uploads/2024/03/Screen-Shot-2024-03-19-at-11.06.37-AM-1024x682.png.

1.4.3. Alternative Therapies

The landscape of mental health treatment has undergone significant shifts, with complementary therapies becoming increasingly accepted as viable adjuncts to conventional pharmacological treatment. Among these therapies, gut microbiota modulation is a promising area of research for the management of mental health disorders. The evidence shows that gut health can influence mental health through bidirectional signaling between the brain and gut. Interventions with gut microbiota modulators (GMMs), such as probiotics and prebiotics, have shown promise in the treatment of many mental diseases, suggesting that dietary interventions and microbiome manipulation could be beneficial adjunct therapies to conventional therapies. But their clinical application needs further research to establish safety and efficacy across different patient populations, based on the emerging literature on GMMs and their implications for mental health outcomes (Wadan et al., 2025). Thus, the combination of these complementary therapies could offer more choices for patients looking for integrative care. In addition to gut microbiota modulation, neuropeptides like oxytocin have been in the limelight for their therapeutic application in mental disorders. Oxytocin has been found to promote social bonding and reduce anxiety, and hence has been looked up to as a candidate for treating disorders like autism spectrum disorder and post-traumatic stress disorder. Research has indicated that intranasal administration of oxytocin can enhance emotional regulation, foster social interaction, and build trust among people. These findings suggest the possibility of the use of endogenous neuropeptides in the clinical treatment of mental disorders for their management. However, as the translation of oxytocin therapy into clinical practice advances, personalized treatment protocols must take center stage to maximize effectiveness. The proper definition of the specific mechanisms of action of oxytocins and the identification of target populations of patients likely to benefit most are critical steps toward its further refinement in therapeutic usage (Chaulagain et al., 2025). The potential of oxytocin opens the door to new ways of managing mental illness. The complementary and alternative treatments of meditation and mindfulness have also become integral parts of comprehensive mental health treatment protocols. These methods aim at emotional strength and self-awareness, effectively remediating symptoms of depression and anxiety. Mindfulness-based treatments encourage participants to cultivate awareness in the here and now and construct acceptance that is capable of buffering negative thinking patterns so characteristic of mental illness. There has been demonstrated capability in these methods to promote psychological functioning and enhance quality of life. While non-conventional treatments cannot replace conventional medical interventions, they can be effective adjuncts, promoting a comprehensive approach that encompasses both physiological and psychological well-being. By adding these integrative modalities to mental health treatment plans, clinicians can enhance their therapeutic arsenal and tailor interventions to meet the complex needs of their patients, thereby maximizing outcomes and enabling recovery (Figure 1.17).

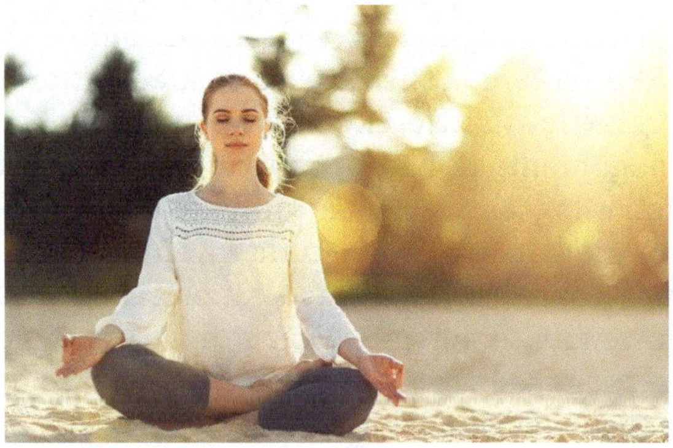

Figure 1.17. Alternative mental health therapies.

Source: https://www.bridgestorecovery.com/wp-content/uploads/2018/10/do-alternative-therapies-really-work-855x570.jpg.

Test Your Knowledge

1. What is psychotherapy?
2. What are the medications used to treat mental health problems?

1.5. Impact on Daily Life

Learning Outcome

1. Understand the effects of mental health disorders on personal relationships
2. Know the influence of mental health disorders on academic and work performance
3. Know the social stigma and its consequences

The impact of mental illness on daily living is extensive and serious, permeating most areas of one's life. For a person suffering from conditions like depression or anxiety, daily tasks can be overwhelming. Tasks as simple as waking up, going to the workplace, or even being in the presence of others may be discouraged by crushing waves of depression or fear. Also, mental illness has a tendency to disrupt one's ability to maintain relationships extensively, since symptoms may drive individuals away from family and friends. The loneliness will also lead to further replenishment of feelings of hopelessness and loneliness, creating a cycle that adversely affects both physical and mental health. As studies have highlighted, the cyclical nature of this pattern demands holistic intervention, including psychological treatment, to improve not only mental health but also daily life (Pilarczyk et al., 2025). Furthermore, the consequences of mental illness are not limited to the patient. Caregivers and family members experience secondary stress and issues with coping with their loved ones' problems. In cases like pediatric epilepsy, for example, there are indeed reported high emotional burden and social stigma from the child's mental illness issues, which can frequently co-exist with the physical manifestation of the disorder (Pilarczyk et al., 2025). Intra-family dynamics can change sharply as family members become caregivers and assume added responsibility, and potentially experience burnout. Additionally, its effect on family life may include financial strain, given that treatment and healthcare for mental illness are expensive, making the stability of the family even more difficult. The acknowledgment of these shared issues means that there is an imperative for mental health services that not only treat the needs of the suffering individual but also take into account the welfare of the entire family involved. In addition, psychiatric conditions like benign prostatic hyperplasia (BPH) in men also clarify the interdependent relationship between mental and physical health. While predominantly characterized by urinary symptoms, BPH can also create emotional distress in terms of anxiety and depression due to fear of embarrassment and compromised quality of life. Such psychological distress can lead to avoidance of necessary medical treatment in men, fueling the vicious cycle of unawareness and aggravated symptoms. Stigma attached to urinary conditions can ensure that individuals cannot openly share their condition with others, thus forcing them to suffer and be lonely for a long time. As the link between chronic disease and mental health becomes apparent, there is a requirement to adopt an integrative model in treatment regimens. The integrative model should include mental health assessment and supportive counseling in addition to standard medical care to improve patients' quality of life when dealing with chronic health problems (Figure 1.18).

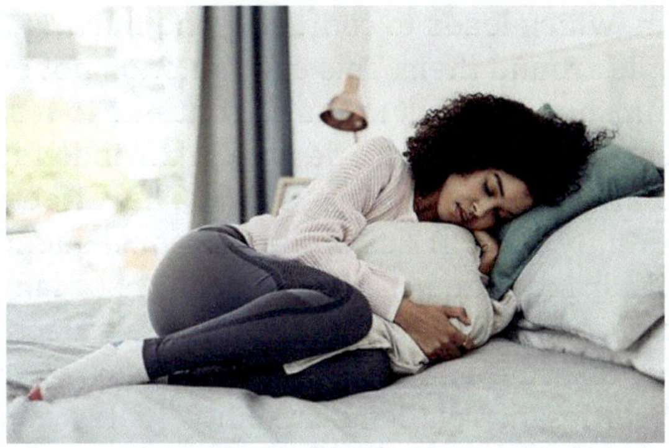

Figure 1.18. Impact of mental health problems on daily life.

Source: https://sa1s3optim.patientpop.com/assets/images/provider/photos/2634363.jpg.

1.5.1. Effects on Personal Relationships

The impact of mental illness on inter-personal relationships is substantial and multifaceted, and has a propensity to impose serious disruption in inter-personal dynamics. The suffering patient with conditions such as depression, anxiety, or borderline personality disorder typically becomes impaired in developing and sustaining relationships. The reasons for impairment stem from the symptoms that can alter emotional availability, communication style, and levels of trust. For instance, anxious individuals may become avoidant or hyper-vigilant for social cues, isolating themselves from loved ones who cannot recognize these reactions. Therefore, the interplay of the mental health issues has the potential to lead to a cycle of confusion and emotional estrangement, ultimately undermining relationships that were once healthy. In particular, in borderline personality disorder (BPD), the inconsistency of interpersonal relationships is normal and troubling. BPD is marked by intense emotional reactions and acting on impulse that can lead to unstable relationships with family members and friends. According to research, BPD patients move in between idealizing individuals and devaluing them, which leads to confusing and hurting the people around them. This contradiction not only diminishes trust but may also continue to foster a sense of isolation and despair in the individual and in their support system. The affective instability in BPD has spill-over consequences in other individuals, as the responses of family and friends outside can determine the trajectory of the disorder and access to care, with resultant difficulties in relational stability (Salas et al., 2024). Further, the lives of people who have gone through psychedelic therapies exhibit complex interactions with mental health and relationships, and both positive and negative possibilities. Many of the subjects in studies evaluating psychedelic experiences reported personal growth and better relationships following their experience.

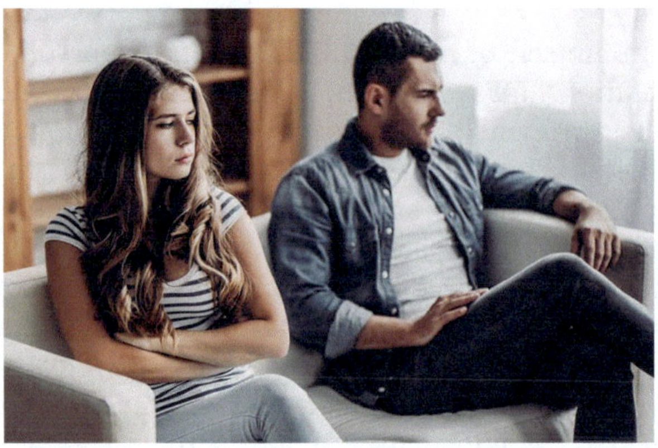

Figure 1.19. Impact of mental health disorders on personal relationships.

Source: https://herway.net/wp-content/uploads/2019/01/unhappy-couple-sitting-on-the-couch-1.jpg.

Nevertheless, a considerable percentage mentioned adverse effects like the exacerbation of symptoms and relationship difficulties due to the unanticipated emotional responses. These findings underscore the complicated role that mental illness serves in shaping relational processes; although healing and reunification are realized by some, others suffer adverse effects from having been exposed and now with current mental illness problems. Interestingly, the research points out that personal growth usually takes place alongside possible adverse experiences and thus warrants consideration of therapeutic tactics and their personal relationship aspects (Torre et al., 2024) (Figure 1.19).

1.5.2. Influence on Academic and Work Performance

The intersection of mental illness disorders and academic and occupational performance is a valuable study area, particularly due to the fact that more and more people are suffering from these disorders. The disorders such as anxiety, depression, and attention-deficit/hyperactivity disorder (ADHD) will badly affect one's concentration, memory, and control over tasks. Students with mental illness cannot go to classes, meet deadlines, and engage fully in class. This can lead to a cascade of adverse consequences, including lower grades and higher dropout rates, ultimately jeopardizing their future academic aspirations and career prospects. As the International Labor Organization (ILO) has pointed out, the recognition of mental health as an illness that severely reduces individuals' chances of advancing to a suitable occupation underscores the necessity for specially tailored interventions in schools among vulnerable learners (Gabriel et al., 2000). Additionally, the impacts of mental illness extend to workplaces, where they exert considerable influence on work performance and company interactions. These patients are often plagued by interpersonal relationship issues and difficulties in group work, which leads to low job performance and satisfaction. The resulting absenteeism and presenteeism, in which an employee is present but less effective due to mental distress, lead to low overall productivity. The ILO's encouragement of work practices that incorporate individuals with mental disorders underscores the essential necessity for the creation of supportive workplaces that not only assist individuals with mental disorders but also make a recognition of mental well-being central to organizational effectiveness (Gabriel et al., 2000). Organizational training and workplace interventions in mental health can increase resilience and adaptability in the workforce. Besides, closing mental health gaps among different groups is crucial to promote equitable performance in academia and the workplace. Research indicates huge disparities in mental health status and access to care based on race and ethnicity, citing structural issues that minority youth experience in schools and workplaces. Disparities can drive isolation and ineffectiveness, further threatening performance. By looking at individualized support systems that address these imbalances, employers and educators can create an environment in which individuals of all backgrounds have a fair opportunity to succeed. Research in this field must continue to advance to develop effective interventions that narrow mental health disparities and, ultimately, lead to greater academic success and workplace productivity for all (Figure 1.20).

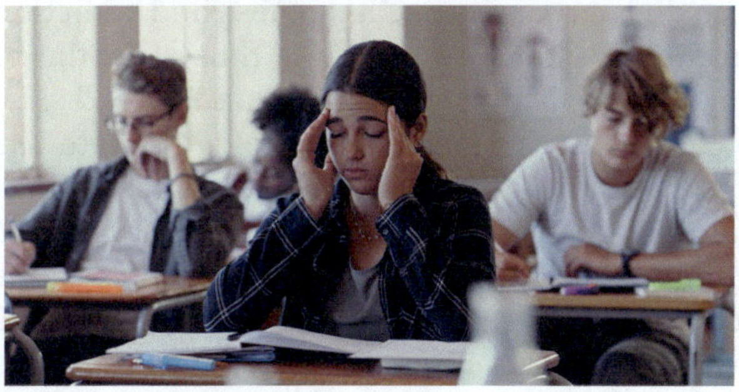

Figure 1.20. Understanding the impact of mental health on academic performance.

Source: https://isminc-public-assets.s3.amazonaws.com/public/2023-02/article-page-sharing-1200x630-understand-i.png.

1.5.3. Social Stigma and Its Consequences

Social stigma for mental health conditions stems from deeply ingrained societal misconceptions and attitudes, which have extensive effects on those who are in pursuit of care. It is usually articulated through labeling, social isolation, and discrimination, particularly against those with more complex conditions such as schizophrenia and bipolar disorder. According to mental health workers in Malaysia, stigma is most frequently encountered across various populations and articulated at the family and social levels. Such discriminatory acts not only bar individuals from access to required treatment but also make them feel isolated and less worthy. Lastly, social stigma is an extremely powerful barrier, digging in ill-grace stereotypes that sustain misunderstanding and fear around mental illness, which gives rise to the need to address these assumptions in order to provide a healing and support-nurturing environment, as per stigma in mental health results (Hanafiah et al., 2015). The impact of stigma on mental health extends well beyond the individual; it overflows into families and communities with pervasive psychological, economic, and social consequences. Individuals with mental health disorders find themselves trapped in a cycle of discrimination where their challenges are met with confusion rather than sympathy. Consequently, these stigmatizing attitudes will dissuade individuals from reporting their conditions or accepting help, exaggerating their symptoms, and getting in the way of healing. The effects of stigma also spill over into working relationships, where individuals with mental conditions are destined to be rejected or dismissed due to their conditions, and thus affect their financial stability. Thus, it is apparent that breaking down the stigma surrounding mental health conditions is not a personal issue but a social one that requires effort to raise awareness and knowledge among the general population (Hanafiah et al., 2015). In addition, the impact of social stigma depends on the types of mental illnesses, more importantly, in cases of co-occurring conditions like mental illness and drug use. Research has indicated that individuals with substance abuse conditions suffer from more stigma than those with mental illness alone. Stigma results in discrimination, which symbolizes the intricacy of stigma in mental health, as alcohol and drug addiction and mental illness can make it difficult to understand an individual's experience in treatment and the world. Stigmatization is diverse in its levels and types, requiring focused intervention to address these twin deficits. With the integration of anti-stigma strategies, mental health clinicians can design a more welcoming and embracing climate, empowering individuals to reclaim their stories and pursue recovery without the stigma of community disapproval. Such attempts are crucial in shattering barriers established by stigma, eventually enhancing the quality of care for mentally ill patients (Figure 1.21).

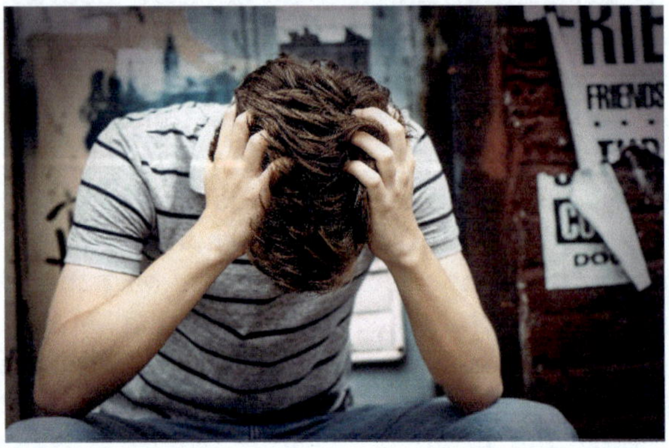

Figure 1.21. Social stigma surrounding mental health disorders.

Source: https://newsnetwork.mayoclinic.org/n7-mcnn/7bcc9724adf7b803/uploads/2015/10/shutterstock_320788322.jpg.

Test Your Knowledge

1. How does mental health affect personal relationships?
2. What is social stigma?

1.6. Prevention and Awareness

Learning Outcome

1. Understand the importance of mental health education
2. Describe the community support programs
3. Understand the role of media in promoting mental health awareness

Prevention and awareness play a vital role in addressing mental health disorders in the age of ubiquitous digital technology. Increased online activity has bred a society in which mental illness, such as anxiety and depression, is on the rise due to reasons like loneliness and addiction to the internet. Prevention is thus essential to reverse these impacts. Families and schools play a central role in making technology safe to use and laying the ground for the individual to make rational choices regarding their mental health. Prioritizing skill development and programs for awareness-raising can empower individuals with the abilities required to manage challenges in digital settings and reduce the rates of cases of mental health disorders caused by technology misuse (Abudalu, 2025). In addition to education programs, effective dissemination of information regarding Digital Mental Health Interventions (DMHIs) is also critical. Research indicates that low familiarity among the target audience, such as medical students, deters the use of these advanced preventive measures. Thus, targeted information strategies directed toward the respective groups can ensure awareness and understanding of DMHIs. For example, medical students like to receive information through peer networks and newer sources such as social media. We can ensure that future health care professionals are properly equipped to recognize and treat mental health diseases through user-centric approaches, thus fostering a culture of vigilance and active management among medical practitioners (Bau et al., 2024). Long-term policy will also be required to ensure sustained awareness and foster mental health resilience. Education systems, policymakers, and healthcare practitioners owe it to themselves and their publics to implement comprehensive mental health education programs that address the evolving issues posed by technology. These programs must focus on prevention through early intervention, destigmatization, and advocacy for available resources.

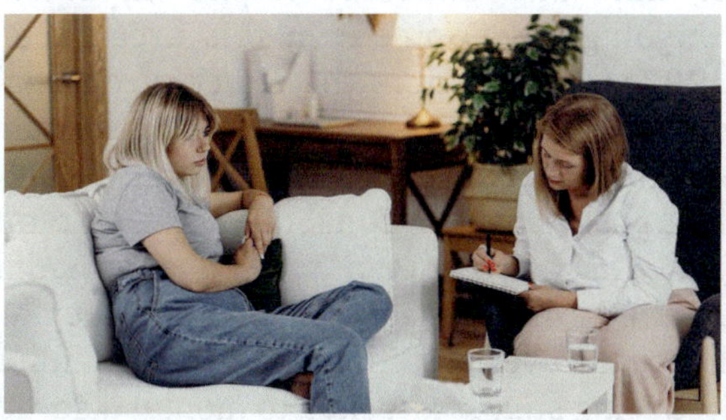

Figure 1.22. Mental health awareness therapy session.

Source: https://www.betterup.com/hs-fs/hubfs/Blog%20Images/mental-health-awareness-therapy-session.jpg?width=800&name=mental-health-awareness-therapy-session.jpg.

Encouraging awareness among communities on mental health issues can empower individuals to take action on the need for assistance instantly and reduce the burden of unresolved disorders. Furthermore, lobbying for government policies that support mental health awareness campaigns can further increase preventive measures, leading to a healthier society that is better equipped to recognize and treat the symptoms of mental distress (Abudalu, 2025) (Figure 1.22).

1.6.1. Importance of Mental Health Education

Education for mental health is crucial in minimizing and managing mental health disorders in communities. Greater awareness and understanding of mental illness prompt educational courses to wipe out the stigma that tends to be generated by mental illness. It then becomes easier for individuals to seek help on their own or from someone else, thereby promoting improved mental health outcomes. For example, increased awareness in Ethiopia demonstrates a shift where the family now easily facilitates members who are mentally ill to seek medical attention without significant reluctance. Thus, mental health education promotes not just an open setting but also helps individuals better comprehend the complexities of mental health illnesses, enhancing the health of the overall community (Appunni et al., 2011). Besides, education in mental health is a preventive measure to prevent the development of mental illness. Initiatives that equip individuals, especially youths, with coping skills and emotional regulation competency significantly reduce the likelihood of catching serious mental illness later in life. Education programs that emphasize resilience and emotional intelligence are thus important for fostering healthier communities. In Brazil, the economic burden of mental illness is significant, since patients with disorders contribute to extra health expenditure and lost productivity at individual and societal levels (Filho et al., 2025). Maintaining mental health education as a priority will allow societies to promote a prevention culture, lowering the economic and psychological burden of untreated mental illnesses. Finally, integrating mental health education into broader health curricula is required to create an educated citizenry. Not only does such a policy prepare people to deal with their own potential mental health problems, but it also prepares them to look after peers appropriately. Curriculum inclusion in schools ensures that mental health becomes part of mainstream politics, leading to earlier detection and treatment of disorders. The need for such integration is also underscored by studies on health expenditure due to mental disorders, which indicate huge societal expense in terms of untreated conditions (Filho et al., 2025). By incorporating mental health education in schools, we can lay the foundation for a future where mental health would rank high on everybody's agenda, eventually resulting in a healthier, more resilient society that is better capable of confronting mental illness with courage and determination.

1.6.2. Community Support Programs

Community support programs are a vital component of the mental disorder landscape in that they provide assets and social supports to those who have mental disorders. Community support programs are set up to offer a variety of services, such as peer support, counseling, and activity-based skill building in order to enhance coping abilities. By incorporating those who have had similar experiences, these types of programs provide a sense of belonging as well as empathy among members. Significantly, such actions help to reverse feelings of loneliness that are normally associated with mental health conditions, thereby enhancing social interaction and community engagement. Evidence indicates that supportive environments like these can have measurable effects on an individual's well-being, resilience, and overall mental health outcomes, making it critical to include support structures within communities in holistic mental health plans. As mental health continues to be a significant public health concern, ongoing investment in and evaluation of such programs becomes critical. Additionally, evidence of the effectiveness of community support programs comes from systematic reviews that have identified their positive outcomes. Specifically, peer support programs, a major component of community support systems, have proved to be beneficial to personal empowerment and quality of life for individuals with severe mental illnesses. In keeping with the results, although overall global impact on depressive and psychiatric symptomatology was modest, specifically on self-efficacy, it was significant, suggesting that these programs produce a sense of mastery in participants. The evidence from the research, as evidenced in randomized controlled trials, favors the effectiveness of these programs in providing a supportive environment where individuals can share experiences and coping strategies for maintaining their mental well-being. Beyond all doubt, self-efficacy development through community interventions can be a catalyst for significant transformations in individuals' mental health over time and underscores the importance of ongoing development in this area (Lee et al., 2024). In addition, the effect of optimally designed community support programs extends from immediate benefits to the individual to encompass societal consequences. Not only do they have a tendency to fill the immediate mental health care requirements, but they also enhance the overall well-being of the community by reducing stigma attached to mental disorders and facilitating frank conversation about mental illness. Interventions with communities and family members are successful at expanding their reach and influence, working to deal with the underlying causes of mental health problems. Research emphasizes the value of tailoring interventions to cultural environments, making them more relevant and useful to diverse groups. The merging of early intervention services and community support services through strategic planning can lead to a comprehensive mental health care strategy aimed at prevention, in addition to the long-term management of disorders (Katas et al., 2023). With continuing development in mental health programs, the position of community support programs has to be the priority when shaping policies and practices for healthy and thriving communities (Figure 1.23).

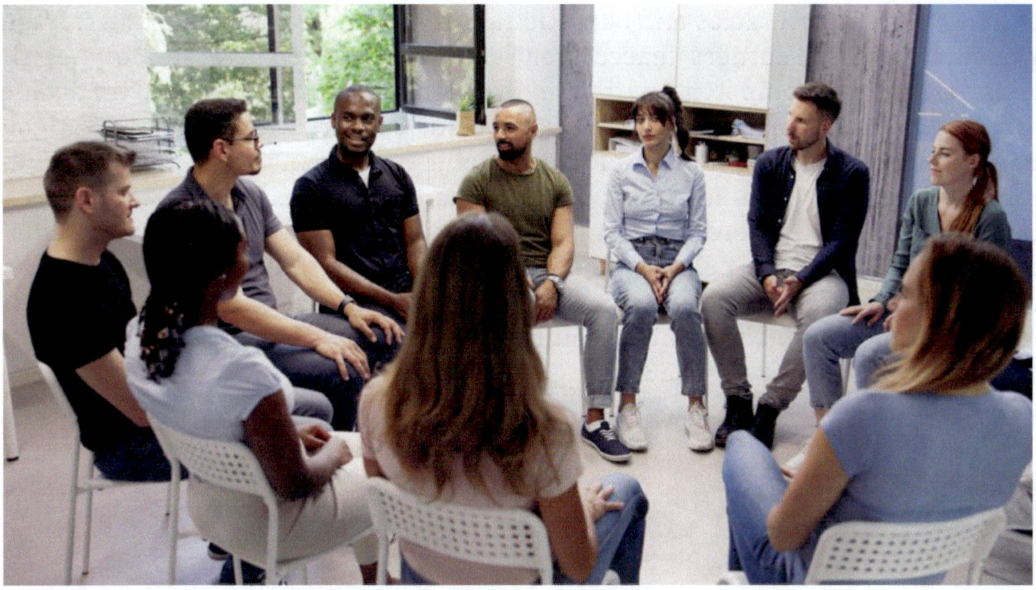

Figure 1.23. The vital role of community in improving mental health.

Source: https://i0.wp.com/mdforlives.com/blog/wp-content/uploads/2023/10/community-mental-health-group-1024x581.jpg?resize=1024%2C581.

1.6.3. Role of Media in Promoting Mental Health Awareness

The media is at the forefront of molding public perception of mental health conditions, hence instilling consciousness and eradicating stigmatization. The narrative on mental health has been redefined from being taboo to becoming part of the popular discourse on various platforms, including social media, television shows, and documentaries. The portrayal of mental illness and recovery in common environments can be a strong source of reassurance for those suffering from such illnesses, since it reminds them that such illnesses are common and manageable. Celebrity endorsement and everyday experience can also facilitate the contact of large numbers of people and encourage individuals to become forthcoming in talking about their mental illness, which can be the stimulus for initiating early intervention and treatment. Accordingly, as negative stereotypes decrease, a more educated and empathetic public emerges, which eventually results in a more responsive society to mental health needs (Wasserman et al., 2023). In recent years, the surge of digital media has redefined the reception and dissemination of mental health information. Instagram and TikTok, although widely bashed for being superficial, have emerged as useful platforms for mental health education and advocacy. Members share personal experiences, coping mechanisms, and work facts, making it simpler to discuss mental health and more credible. Furthermore, organizations working in mental health use these platforms to share evidence-based information efficiently. Visual stories, along with user-generated content, give a sense of community and enable people to search for support and help. Additionally, during crises such as the COVID-19 pandemic, media have been instrumental in broadcasting mental health help and coping strategies, putting into the spotlight the importance of mental wellness as much as physical health. Passing on information is particularly important because it helps address the rising need for mental health services among pandemic-hit communities (Rousseau et al., 2020). However, the media's portrayal of mental illness is not without its flaws, since inaccuracies and sensationalism may increase stigma and misconceptions. Portraying mental illness disorders inaccurately can generate negative stereotypes that depict individuals as violent or incompetent, detracting from the actuality of living with such disorders. Additionally, media sensationalization of mental health concerns might further stigmatize and marginalize concerns, potentially overshadowing genuine experience and meaningful discussion. Mental health professionals and advocates should thus critically examine media representations and advocate for responsible, ethical reporting. Through such collaborations with media agencies, mental health professionals can help shape a more realistic narrative that fosters understanding and empathy. These partnerships could enable campaigns that not only raise awareness but also challenge the population to place mental health as a core aspect of well-being at the forefront of their priorities (Wasserman et al., 2023).

Test Your Knowledge

1. What is the importance of mental health education?
2. What is the role of media in promoting mental health awareness?

SUMMARY

The culmination of the mental health disorder research reveals the intricate play between psychological health and factors in the environment. Above all, traffic noise research has revealed strong correlations with various outcomes for mental health, most significantly depression. A meta-analysis of aircraft noise exposure revealed a striking 12% increased risk of depression for every 10 dB of sound, suggesting that environmental noise not only disrupts daily life but also etiologically contributes to mental illness. Conversely, though, evidence surrounding road and railway noise failed to show statistically significant effects on depression and anxiety, indicating the complexity of these interactions. Thus, public policy interventions to address environmental conditions such as noise pollution can take center stage in enhancing mental health outcomes and preventing disorders arising from exposure to unhealthy auditory environments (Hegewald et al., 2020). Aside from environmental considerations, stress on frontline healthcare workers during emergencies like the COVID-19 pandemic underscores the necessity of treating mental health in high-stress jobs. An integrative review showed that such workers experience a range of mental health challenges because of a lack of appropriate personal protective equipment, stigma, and overwhelming feelings of fear. The condition has caused more emotional distress and can lead to long-term mental illnesses if not managed accordingly. Interventions to minimize emotional burnout are critical, especially given that cultural and geographical settings can alter responses to such emergencies. By understanding these dynamics, interventions can be crafted specifically to meet the needs of healthcare staff, in the long term creating an improved work environment and preventing adverse effects on mental health (Paiano et al., 2020). Overall, mental health disorders are typically aggravated by a combination of occupational and environmental stressors and need multidimensional prevention and treatment. The findings on traffic noise effects illustrate the broader applicability of environmental health to mental well-being, while healthcare workers' experiences during the pandemic confirm the importance of addressing occupational sources of stress. Future work should continue examining these connections and justifying policies aimed at mitigating the effects of noise pollution and expanding professional mental health care. By promoting conditions favorable for mental well-being, society can easily reverse the rising levels of mental health disorders, thereby achieving healthier communities. Full comprehension of the determinants of mental health disorders is hence fundamental in designing effective intervention strategies and enabling individuals to manage their mental health disorders.

In research into the intricate nature of mental health disorders, it is evident that these disorders impose a significant influence not only on individual well-being but also on societal trends. A lot of research leads towards the interconnection of mental health disorders and organizational phenomena such as Absenteeism and Presenteeism. Particularly, research shows that a past history of mental illness elevates both Absenteeism—when workers are absent from work—and Presenteeism—when workers show up to work but function at reduced levels. This similarity underscores the compelling need for organizational policies that support mental health programs and provide assistance to affected employees. The implications of these findings extend beyond the individual, underscoring the need for comprehensive workplace mental health interventions to mitigate the adverse effects of these disorders on employee productivity and retention (Monroy et al., 2025). In addition, public attitudes regarding mental health also play a significant role in how people view and manage their conditions. Stigma for mental illness is a key motivator that encourages greater Absenteeism because individuals may avoid work out of fear of discrimination or judgment. This underscores the importance of fostering a warm, welcoming workplace where mental health can be discussed openly, without fear of judgment. Studies also indicate that participation in therapy effectively reduces Presenteeism by at least 36 percentage points, further underpinning the effectiveness of expert intervention in promoting workplace engagement. This accords with the hypothesis that active mental health interventions not only bring relief to individuals but also maximize organizational health and productivity, and consequently generate a virtuous cycle of support and performance (Monroy et al., 2025). Also, the shifting landscape of mental health treatment has been shaped to a great extent by policy reform concerns for access to other forms of therapy, including cannabis. In recent studies, it has been established that those states where medical or recreational cannabis is legalized have seen notable shifts in the prescribing of conventional medication in the management of mental illness. For instance, dispensing of benzodiazepines has gone down significantly, which would suggest that cannabis is serving as a substitute therapy in certain instances. That being said, this trend is accompanied by a rise in the consumption of other psychotropic drugs, which would suggest an all-around relationship between access to cannabis and treatment for mental illness. It is important that policymakers and health care professionals grasp these dynamics as they strive to reconcile the twin imperatives of optimizing mental health outcomes with the control of drugs in increasingly complicated moral and legal landscapes.

KEY TERMS FROM THIS CHAPTER

- Anxiety disorders
- Cognitive research
- Discrimination
- Malnutrition
- Mood disorders
- Personality disorder
- Physical health
- Bipolar disorder
- Depression
- Intellectual disability
- Mental health
- Panic disorder
- Pharmacotherapy
- Public health

CRITICAL THINKING QUESTIONS

1. **Which of the following is a core symptom of major depressive disorder (MDD)?**
   a. Racing thoughts
   b. Hyperactivity
   c. Loss of interest or pleasure (anhedonia)
   d. Delusions
2. **Which neurotransmitter is primarily implicated in anxiety disorders?**
   a. Dopamine
   b. Serotonin
   c. Acetylcholine
   d. Glutamate
3. **What is the first-line pharmacological treatment for generalized anxiety disorder (GAD)?**
   a. Benzodiazepines
   b. Tricyclic antidepressants
   c. Selective serotonin reuptake inhibitors (SSRIs)
   d. Antipsychotics
4. **Which of the following is a positive symptom of schizophrenia?**
   a. Apathy
   b. Hallucinations
   c. Social withdrawal
   d. Cognitive deficits
5. **Which condition is characterized by alternating periods of mania and depression?**
   a. Major depressive disorder
   b. Schizoaffective disorder
   c. Bipolar disorder
   d. Cyclothymia

Short Answer Questions

1. What are the mental health disorders?
2. Why is mental health awareness important?
3. List the types of mental health disorders.
4. What are the causes of mental health disorders?
5. What are the treatment options for mental health disorders?

Answer to Critical Thinking Questions

1. (c); 2. (b); 3. (c); 4. (b); 5. (c).

REFERENCES

1. Abudalu, A. (2025). The psychological diversity in the treatment of mental disorders associated with technology. *International Journal for Scientific Research*. https://www.semanticscholar.org/paper/4bfdf3c52f169c47c6ad3100ded2259781513e2f (accessed on 14th July 2025).
2. Afaque, S., Saxena, V. S., Agarwal, N., Shukla, S., Chaudhary, K., & Fatima, S. (2025). Temporomandibular Joint Disorders and Mental Health: Unleashing the veiled bond. *DENTAL JOURNAL OF INDIRA GANDHI INSTITUTE OF MEDICAL SCIENCES, 4*, 63–66. https://doi.org/10.25259/djigims_1_2025Ajeh, Rogers, Anastos, K., Barrington, C., et al. (2024). Factors influencing integration of mental health screening and treatment at HIV clinic settings in Cameroon: A qualitative study of health providers' perspectives. https://core.ac.uk/download/624146965.pdf (accessed on 14th July 2025).
3. Appunni, S. S. (2011). Mental health services in Ethiopia: Emerging public health. https://core.ac.uk/download/62634424.pdf (accessed on 14th July 2025).
4. Asherson, P., Chaplin, E., Forrester, A., et al. (2015). Screening and diagnostic assessment of neurodevelopmental disorders in a male prison. https://core.ac.uk/download/77011521.pdf (accessed on 14th July 2025).
5. Baconi, D. L., Bălălău, C., Ciobanu, A. M., et al. (2015). Current concepts on drug abuse and dependence. https://core.ac.uk/download/144552331.pdf (accessed on 14th July 2025).
6. Baltrinic, E. R. (2016). *CE 652 Syllabus: Treatment Planning*. https://core.ac.uk/download/483393831.pdf (accessed on 14th July 2025).
7. Bartels-Velthuis, A. A., Bruggeman, R., Bruins, J., et al. (1977). *Progress in Drug Metabolism, Volume 1*. Edited by J. W. Bridges and L. F. Chasseaud. John Wiley and Sons. https://core.ac.uk/download/pdf/82174066.pdf (accessed on 14th July 2025).
8. Bau, J., Vomhof, M., Braun, P., Calo, S., Stehl, S., Haastert, B., Schuster, L., et al. (2024). P-078 How to inform medical students about digital mental health interventions? A discrete choice experiment. *Occupational Medicine*. https://www.semanticscholar.org/paper/d210ff656c72e2b8598f968b69016d358b2bf31d (accessed on 14th July 2025).
9. Bazelier, M., Bell, J. S., Brauer, R., et al. (2020). Application of healthcare 'big data' in CNS drug research: The example of the Neurological and Mental Health Global Epidemiology Network (NeuroGEN). https://core.ac.uk/download/326711929.pdf (accessed on 14th July 2025).
10. Bermúdez Bejarano, E. (2024). Importance of early diagnosis of mental disorders, anxiety and dental fear, to improve management in the dental office. *Austin Journal of Public Health and Epidemiology*. https://www.semanticscholar.org/paper/88435c35ebc1b117703a9005d7a2ccb5b13926d9 (accessed on 14th July 2025).
11. Bhalsing, A. R., & Kul, S. R. (2025). AI-driven behavioral insights for personalized mental health. *International Journal on Science and Technology*. https://www.semanticscholar.org/paper/18158806bb7b1b4d138fb35a63d94859b10af893 (accessed on 14th July 2025).
12. Bradford, A. C., Lozano-Rojas, F., Shone, H., Bradford, W. D., & Abraham, A. J. (2024). Cannabis laws and utilization of medications for the treatment of mental health disorders. *JAMA Network Open, 7*. https://www.semanticscholar.org/paper/729fe1255398d1e9b8a6b52a0fd8d4afd23b15b6 (accessed on 14th July 2025).

13. Byrne, T. H., Corrigan, P., Harnish, A., et al. (2016). A comparison of substance uses stigma and health stigma in a population of veterans with co-occurring mental health and substance use disorders. https://open.bu.edu/bitstream/2144/22787/1/FINAL%20DRAFT%20AH%20edits%208%201%202016_TB.pdf (accessed on 14th July 2025).
14. Cao, X. L., Hou, C. L., Jia, F. J., et al. (2018). The prevalence of autism spectrum disorders in China: A comprehensive meta-analysis. https://core.ac.uk/download/213607690.pdf (accessed on 14th July 2025).
15. Chaulagain, R. P., Shrestha, Y., Shrestha, H., Bhandari, R., & Gurung, P. (2025). The neurobiological impact of oxytocin in mental health disorders: A comprehensive review. *Annals of Medicine and Surgery, 87*, 1479–1486. https://www.semanticscholar.org/paper/9553732a72b68052cf9fc080df8d570ec3ca3d1f (accessed on 14th July 2025).
16. Chiavegatto Filho, A. D. P., Malik, A. M., Campino, A. C. C., Andrade, L. H., Viana, M. C., & Wang, Y. P. (2025). Incremental health expenditure and lost days of normal activity for individuals with mental disorders: Results from the São Paulo Megacity Study. https://core.ac.uk/download/pdf/81891128.pdf (accessed on 14th July 2025).
17. Ehsanifar, M., Gholami, A., & Esmaeili, A. (2025). Mental health disorders following exposure to endocrine disruptor chemicals. *OBM Neurobiology*. https://www.semanticscholar.org/paper/46c586dd95b837a500f395178fcc5a9887d811f3 (accessed on 14th July 2025).
18. Farah, N., Essafi, A., Eschater, S., Benhaddouch, Y., & El Ammouri, A. (2024). Therapeutic adherence in a population of patients treated for schizophrenia at the Hospital for Mental Health and Psychiatric Disorders in Tangier. *International Journal of Advanced Research*. https://www.semanticscholar.org/paper/af7abb1e62693577dd5fe552902c98e186f04654 (accessed on 14th July 2025).
19. Fontaine, A., & Meale, E. (2024). A review of risk factors, adverse outcomes, and counseling strategies among pregnant individuals with eating disorders. *Research Posters*. https://www.semanticscholar.org/paper/7129ecb7747f3a5a70df06aefbd705e7fccf3a7c (accessed on 14th July 2025).
20. Gabriel, P., & International Labor Office. (2000). Mental health in the workplace: Situation analyses, United States. https://core.ac.uk/download/5129345.pdf (accessed on 14th July 2025).
21. Green, J. G., McLaughlin, K. A., Alegria, M., & Loder, S. (2015). Disparities in child and adolescent mental health and mental health services in the U.S. https://core.ac.uk/download/75780891.pdf (accessed on 14th July 2025).
22. Hanafiah, A. N., & Van Bortel, T. (2015). A qualitative exploration of the perspectives of mental health professionals on stigma and discrimination of mental illness in Malaysia. https://core.ac.uk/download/77406952.pdf (accessed on 14th July 2025).
23. Hegewald, J., Schubert, M., Freiberg, A., Romero Starke, K., Augustin, F., Riedel-Heller, S., Zeeb, H., et al. (2020). Traffic noise and mental health: A systematic review and meta-analysis. *International Journal of Environmental Research and Public Health, 17*. https://www.semanticscholar.org/paper/67731044745b074640c1d47a26f1f2a3eb03b50b (accessed on 14th July 2025).
24. Hittner, J. (2015). *CE 652 Syllabus: Treatment Planning*. https://core.ac.uk/download/490623141.pdf (accessed on 14th July 2025).

25. Izydorczyk, B. (2017). Mental condition and specificity of mental disorders in a group of workers from southern Poland: A research report. https://core.ac.uk/download/149239765.pdf (accessed on 14th July 2025).

26. Karyotaki, E., Miguel, C., Panagiotopoulou, O., Harrer, M., Seward, N., Sijbrandij, M., Araya, R., et al. (2023). Digital interventions for common mental disorders in low- and middle-income countries: A systematic review and meta-analysis. *Cambridge Prisms: Global Mental Health, 10*. https://www.semanticscholar.org/paper/54b1e1a7699162277ef866b6a8b44834b89f440b (accessed on 14th July 2025).

27. Kato, J. K. (2024). The psychological impact of chronic prostate disorders: Addressing mental health in BPH patients. *IDOSR Journal of Scientific Research*. https://www.semanticscholar.org/paper/4dd7c92f3d8e91e8abcad60c0005cfa9fa8b1408 (accessed on 14th July 2025).

28. Kuchma, V., Sokolova, S., Sedova, A. S., Rapoport, I. K., Chubarovsky, V. V., Tikashkina, O., & Boldyreva, M. G. (2025). Identification of prognostic risk factors associating with lifestyle contributing to the development of health disorders in 9–11 grades students. *Hygiene and Sanitation*. https://www.semanticscholar.org/paper/ebb72fe29c326ef1aa143fd995d7cb3956025dee (accessed on 14th July 2025).

29. La Torre, J. T., Gallo, J., Mahammadli, M., Zalewa, D., & Williams, M. T. (2024). Experiences of psychedelic drug use among people with psychotic symptoms and disorders: Personal growth and mystical experiences. *Journal of Psychedelic Studies*. https://www.semanticscholar.org/paper/9a56fc72c019ac8a99c3e881705ed451d12dfd32 (accessed on 14th July 2025).

30. Lashari, U. G., Shabbir, S., Shahbaz, T., & Kayani, H. W. (2025). The role of AI in predicting mental health disorders: A clinical psychology perspective. *Journal of Medical & Health Sciences Review*. https://www.semanticscholar.org/paper/2b3bbbec96147c7ce25875e8c535a395575d4fbd (accessed on 14th July 2025).

31. Lee, S. N., & Yu, H. (2024). Effectiveness of peer support programs for severe mental illness: A systematic review and meta-analysis. *Healthcare, 12*. https://www.semanticscholar.org/paper/33b03ef664f8daf73e2337e86416337199ad43dc (accessed on 14th July 2025).

32. Lieto, A., American Psychiatric Association, American Psychiatric Association, Lieto, A., Boorse, C., Machery, E., Rosch, E., et al. (2019). Ontologies, mental disorders and prototypes. https://core.ac.uk/download/186331620.pdf (accessed on 14th July 2025).

33. Mohamed, S., Soo, K., & Vanoh, D. (2021). Malnutrition and its risk factors among children and adolescents with intellectual disability (ID) in Asian countries: A scoping review. *Malaysian Journal of Nutrition, 27*, 027–040. https://www.semanticscholar.org/paper/840ac222aef4a101a2c53f10eb2a1d5b1a9c3474 (accessed on 14th July 2025).

34. Monroy, V., & Michel, E. (2025). Mental health disorders and productivity: Which is the risk and mitigating factors of absenteeism and presenteeism? Evidence from the U.S. tech sector. *Investigacion & Desarrollo*. https://www.semanticscholar.org/paper/1889b5030c8d265075e635dfe5748ff07b73a834 (accessed on 14th July 2025).

35. Mortlock, K. S. (2016). Screening for mental disorder comorbidity in Australian alcohol and other drug residential treatment settings. https://core.ac.uk/download/81225313.pdf (accessed on 14th July 2025).

36. Nair, A., & Pariante, C. (2014). Neuroscience and mental illness. https://core.ac.uk/download/79498993.pdf (accessed on 14th July 2025).

37. Paiano, M., Jaques, A., Nacamura, P. A. B., Salci, M. A., Radovanovic, C. A. T., & Carreira, L. (2020). Mental health of healthcare professionals in China during the new coronavirus pandemic: An integrative review. *Revita Brasileira de Enfermagem, 73*(Suppl 2), e20200338. https://www.semanticscholar.org/paper/bf43ccde1b32f092bc8dbcd78eb9166e9c824c95 (accessed on 14th July 2025).

38. Pilarczyk, K., Grzesik, K., Rabęda, A., Klepacz, N., Adamska, H., Sawczuk, H., Nowak, W. E., et al. (2025). Epilepsy in children: Coexistence of mental disorders and the impact of social factors. *Medical Science Pulse.* https://www.semanticscholar.org/paper/b8b11c70bc30ced6d388ecac0b024e0c5fc93337 (accessed on 14th July 2025).

39. Prates, S., Troesch, M., Magalhães-Britto, R., Dallalana, C., Studart-Bottó, P., Léda-Rêgo, G., Socorro-Casqueiro, J., et al. (2024). Diagnosis of mental disorders in caregivers of patients with bipolar disorder: A gap in the scientific literature. *Trends in Psychiatry and Psychotherapy.* https://www.semanticscholar.org/paper/ad19f8e1eadf89cb05a8e8e8f69a30fc2b7b6162 (accessed on 14th July 2025).

40. Priebe, S., Burton, A., Ashby, D., Ashcroft, R., Burns, T., David, A., Eldridge, S., et al. (2009). Financial incentives to improve adherence to anti-psychotic maintenance medication in non-adherent patients: A cluster randomized controlled trial (FIAT). https://core.ac.uk/download/212831.pdf (accessed on 14th July 2025).

41. Ramos, A. L., & Salgado, H. (2024). War and migration–When mental health is left behind. *European Psychiatry, 67*, S614–S614. https://www.semanticscholar.org/paper/487d8da148c03d568897e9b3e5eb09aa3acb9360 (accessed on 14th July 2025).

42. Rawal, S. (2025). Mental health awareness and access to services in postpartum women. *Journal of Pharmacy & Bioallied Sciences, 17*, S417–S419. https://www.semanticscholar.org/paper/544fba1a82ae1a024ac62ef3823392bef19aab5c (accessed on 14th July 2025).

43. Roach, A., Bennett, S. D., Heyman, I., Coughtrey, A., Batura, N., Gonzalez, L., Astle, N., et al. (2025). Clinical effectiveness of drop-in mental health services in pediatric healthcare settings: A non-randomized multi-site study for children, young people and their families. *BMC Health Services Research, 25.* https://www.semanticscholar.org/paper/bee4030c845d4b44946c4250a2a211cc0db454be (accessed on 14th July 2025).

44. Rousseau, C., & Miconi, D. (2020). Protecting youth mental health during the COVID-19 pandemic: A challenging engagement and learning process. *Journal of the American Academy of Child & Adolescent Psychiatry, 59*, 1203–1207. https://doi.org/10.1016/j.jaac.2020.08.007 (accessed on 14th July 2025).

45. Salas, F., Nvo-Fernández, M., Leiva-Bianchi, M., Avello Sáez, D., Sepúlveda Páeza, G., Via García, M., & Villacura-Herrera, C. (2024). Components of event-related potentials and borderline personality disorder: A meta-analysis. *European Journal of Psych Traumatology, 15.* https://www.semanticscholar.org/paper/780600a4ea921cd4e9e8a44be008b9d02a2eeb2c (accessed on 14th July 2025).

46. Saleem, S., & Hussain, M. S. (2024). A psychoanalytic probe into pre-birth vs. post-birth learning and discourse disorders in young children: Reasons and remedies. *Human Nature Journal of Social Sciences.* https://www.semanticscholar.org/paper/bbba9acfffb41ae726aab937504627a1f1f1f3b5 (accessed on 14th July 2025).

47. Schumacher, L., Burger, J., Echterhoff, J., & Kriston, L. (2024). Methodological and statistical practices of using symptom networks to evaluate mental health interventions: A review and reflections. *Multivariate Behavioral Research, 59*, 663–676. https://www.semanticscholar.org/paper/e968129831afca13ce92d4382a70197a963d0a40 (accessed on 14th July 2025).

48. Silbiger, K. (2024). Mental health providers' perceptions of restrictive eating disorders: Relationship with client body weight. *The International Journal of Eating Disorders*. https://www.semanticscholar.org/paper/fbc9b78f45c739f78a6b158c3158e0da98f7b586 (accessed on 14th July 2025).

49. Smith, M., & Storey, P. (2008). Methods and approaches to improving the emotional health and well-being of children: A briefing paper concerning interventions to prevent internalizing disorders. https://core.ac.uk/download/pdf/82102.pdf (accessed on 14th July 2025).

50. Stolper, H., van der Vegt, M., van Doesum, K. V., & Steketee, M. (2024). The integrated family approach in mental health care services: A study of risk factors. *International Journal of Environmental Research and Public Health, 21*. https://www.semanticscholar.org/paper/48159169f38eb05d5ec0a8668afba17fbd35dcfa (accessed on 14th July 2025).

51. Udemezue, K., Nwankwo, E. I., Igwama, G. T., Olaboye, J. A., & Anyanwu, E. C. (2023). Evaluating the impact of early intervention programs on substance abuse prevention in adolescents: A comprehensive review. *International Journal of Applied Research in Social Sciences*. https://www.semanticscholar.org/paper/ae59566c2299ee07c404c2c63106855bb8378500 (accessed on 14th July 2025).

52. Urmi, B. R., Islam, S., Karim, A., Hasan, M., Rashed, M. J. R., Hasan, M. M., Das, A., et al. (2025). Recognizing and addressing mental health comorbidities in hypertension care strategies: A narrative review. *International Journal of Innovative Science and Research Technology*. https://www.semanticscholar.org/paper/06803ce714c9bc876319334bfaf661e660504f09 (accessed on 14th July 2025).

53. Wadan, A. H. S., Abd El-Aziz, M. K., & Ellakwa, D. (2025). The microbiota-gut-brain-axis theory: Role of gut microbiota modulators (GMMs) in gastrointestinal, neurological, and mental health disorders. *Naunyn-Schmiedeberg's Archives of Pharmacology*. https://www.semanticscholar.org/paper/a0ebed85e51635c8fd5fe205536604011fba30d0 (accessed on 14th July 2025).

54. Wasserman, D., Arango, C., Fiorillo, A., Levin, S., Peters, A. C., Rao, P. G., Sanchez-Villanueva, T., et al. (2023). Improving mental health through fostering healthy lifestyles in young people: One of the targets in the *WPA* Action Plan 2023-2026. *World Psychiatry, 22*, 488–489. https://doi.org/10.1002/wps.21146 (accessed on 14th July 2025).

55. Yeung, R. C., & Fernandes, M. A. (2023). Specific topics, specific symptoms: Linking the content of recurrent involuntary memories to mental health using computational text analysis. *NPJ Mental Health Research, 2*. https://www.semanticscholar.org/paper/f22e5485431628a53d35157db27b6b93b8f6c0bd (accessed on 14th July 2025).

SUBSTANCE ABUSE AND ADDICTION

2

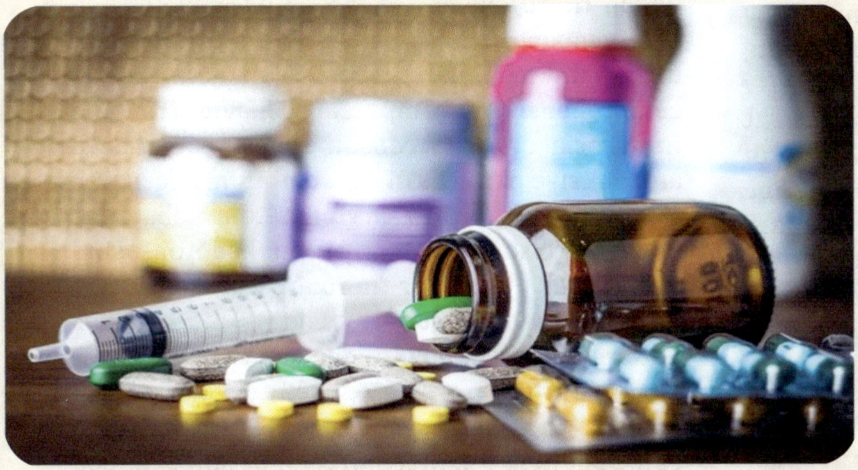

LEARNING OBJECTIVES

After studying this chapter, you will be able to:

1. Describe the types of substances abused
2. Understand the causes of substance abuse
3. Recognize the signs and symptoms of addiction
4. Know the impact of substance abuse on individuals
5. Describe the societal implications of substance abuse and addiction
6. Describe the treatment and recovery options for substance abuse and addiction

Introduction

Substance abuse and addiction are both real public health issues that require urgent attention and intervention based on knowledge. As societies deal with the complexities of these issues, it is essential to understand the various substances and their impacts on communities and individuals. The evolution of trends in substance use has witnessed the rise of new psychoactive substances (NPS) as a rising concern that has not been explored until now in recent years. NPS, not subject to existing international drug control treaties, have grown in popularity at a fast rate and pose severe health consequences. According to the United Nations Office of Drugs and Crime (UNODC), the evaluation of health risks among NPS users has been shockingly low, reflecting public unawareness and medical preparedness for addressing such rapidly spreading drugs (Crnić et al., 2020). The demographic landscape of substance abuse continues to evolve, particularly with regard to youth engagement in both legal and illegal substance use. Over the past two decades, while there has been a general decline in illicit drug use, a perplexing trend has emerged: youth perceptions regarding the safety of certain substances, such as marijuana and e-cigarettes, are shifting towards normalization. This change is especially concerning, as it conceals the potential for addiction and long-term health effects of these drugs. Youth Substance Abuse: A Reference Handbook places a unique focus on the history of drug use and addiction and how drug use and addiction become more important as their role in social, psychological, and economic problems in contemporary societies grows (Newton, 2016). Recognizing this multifaceted environment is a priority in creating viable prevention and treatment strategies. Due to the pervasive nature of addiction, addressing substance abuse must be addressed in a holistic and multi-disciplinary manner. Successful strategies include education, early intervention, and customized treatment programs that take into account individual needs and circumstances.

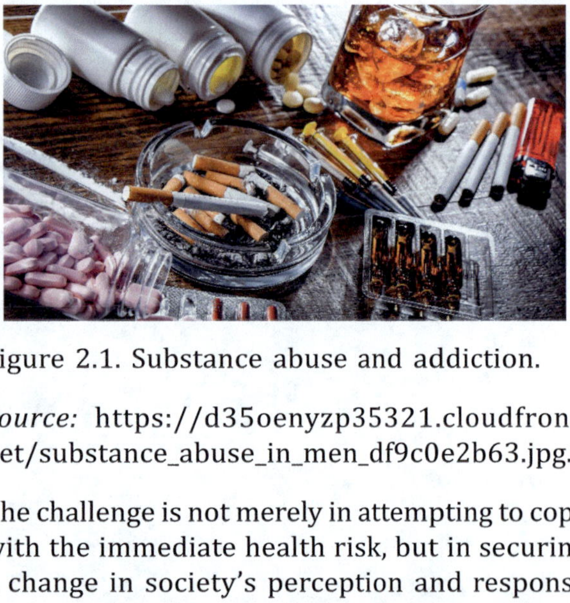

Figure 2.1. Substance abuse and addiction.

Source: https://d35oenyzp35321.cloudfront.net/substance_abuse_in_men_df9c0e2b63.jpg.

The challenge is not merely in attempting to cope with the immediate health risk, but in securing a change in society's perception and response to drug-related issues. Because the prevalence and character of drug abuse are in a state of flux, it becomes obvious that an interactive response among healthcare providers, educators, policymakers, and society is necessary. More surveillance and collaboration with agencies engaged in monitoring and regulating NPS are required to minimize the threats of substance abuse and provide public health protection. Preventive action can generate greater benefits for people and society as a whole, thereby reducing the effects of addiction on groups (Figure 2.1).

Definition of Substance Abuse

Substance abuse is a multifaceted condition in which there exists dangerous or harmful use of psychoactive drugs, including alcohol, illicit drugs, and legal medications. This definition is comprehensive, encompassing behaviors ranging from social or casual consumption to compulsive and abusive patterns of consumption. According to the World Health Organization, substance abuse is observed when people keep on using substances even after there are adverse social, legal, or medical consequences. This broader understanding highlights the fact that addiction is not only a physical dependence problem but also includes psychological and emotional components. Furthermore, substance abuse is commonly found in conjunction with other mental health issues, further complicating diagnosis and treatment and thus necessitating an integrated strategy for both prevention and intervention methods throughout society, given the huge individual and community cost it imposes. A critical aspect of understanding the nature of substance abuse is identifying the patterns of behavior that typify this disease. Patients will typically be fixated on drug-seeking activity, and therefore, occupational or academic performance can decline, and interpersonal relationships can become strained. The Diagnostic and Statistical Manual of Mental Disorders (DSM) categorizes these behaviors by severity, ranging from mild to severe, based on the number of criteria met. These parameters can include tolerance, withdrawal syndrome, and unsuccessful efforts to cut back on use. These dichotomizations not only provide more accurate diagnostic procedures but also aid in the modification of some of the treatment modalities corresponding to the severity of the patients' substance use disorder. With treatment still evolving, such a multidimensional understanding of these behavioral signs is still crucial in facilitating effective intervention and long-term recovery. Also, socialization plays a very big role in the prevalence and attitude towards substance abuse, suggesting that it is not only a failure of the individual but a reflection of cultural and economic forces. For instance, regions with limited mental health services will tend to have increased rates of substance abuse because individuals use substances as a means of coping rather than turning to professionals. Additionally, stigmatization of addiction keeps individuals away from treatment, thereby leading to the cycle of abuse. To effectively design public health interventions, substance abuse should be understood as it is influenced by many factors. These interventions can address not only the addiction symptoms but also social determinants that contribute to the dissemination of addiction, ultimately influencing a well-informed and humane public response towards alcohol addiction and drug abuse (Sohn et al., 2019; Dwivedi et al., 2022) (Figure 2.2).

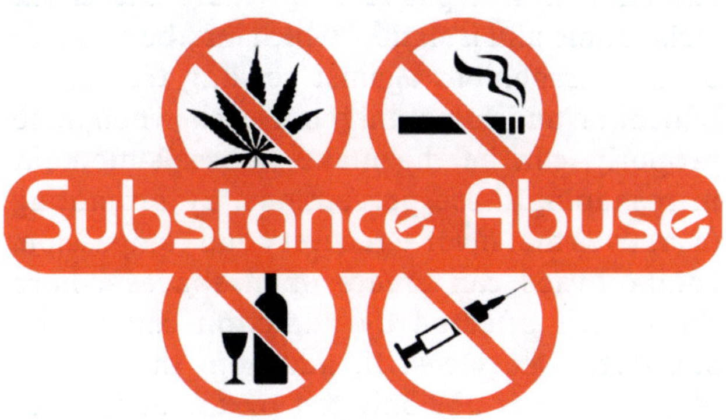

Figure 2.2. Substance abuse.

Source: https://publichealthnotes.com/wp-content/uploads/2020/10/drugs_alcohol_problems.png.

Overview of Addiction

Addiction is a multifaceted process that entails a heightened engagement in activities or the use of chemicals despite detrimental outcomes. Essentially, it is a series of alterations in the structure and function of the brain, particularly in the areas concerned with reward, motivation, and impulse regulation. The etiology of addiction is typically established through the interaction of genetic, environmental, and psychosocial factors. These influences might predispose individuals to start using substances and become addicted. Moreover, the addiction cycles tend to be complicated by the co-existence of mental health disorders, which points towards the need for integrated treatment plans addressing both the substance use and the psychological disorders. One of the key features of addiction is the role of psychological processes such as psychological inflexibility (PI) and psychological flexibility (PF). PI, characterized by rigorous commitment to feelings and thoughts, has been related to SUDs, which inhibit one's capacity to successfully manage stressors. In contrast, PF, involving the adaptation of an individual's thoughts and behaviors in accordance with changing circumstances, has been related to lower rates of substance abuse. A meta-analysis discovered that experiential avoidance—a component of PI—had a positive and moderate correlation with substance abuse ($r = 0.34$), while mindfulness—tied to PF—showed low and negative correlation with substance abuse ($r = -0.25$) (Barrado-Moreno et al., 2025). They point out the necessity for cultivating psychological flexibility in prevention and addiction treatment. In addition, addiction's impact transcends the self, affecting various aspects of life, from social relationships to physiological well-being. SUDs have proven to trigger severe sexual dysfunction, raising significant barriers to intimacy and quality of life for victims. Loss of libido and erectile dysfunction are common among SUD patients, attributed to underlying physiological changes and hormone dysregulation induced by the abuse of substances. These consequences not only heighten psychological suffering from addiction but also isolate individuals further, potentially perpetuating the vicious cycle of addiction (Soltaninejad et al., 2024). The reversal of such multifaceted consequences calls for an interrelated solution that involves healthcare practices and therapeutic procedures, thus achieving recovery and overall well-being (Figure 2.3).

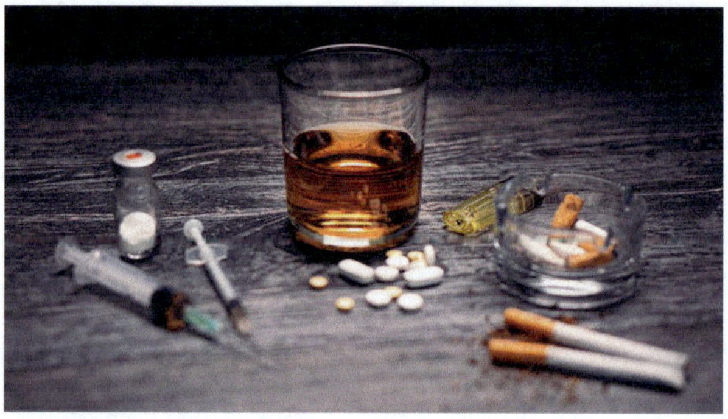

Figure 2.3. Addiction.

Source: https://www.brainfacts.org/-/media/Brainfacts2/Diseases-and-Disorders/Addiction/Article-Images/introduction-to-addiction.jpg.

Importance of Addressing the Issue

It is important to realize the necessity for treating substance abuse and addiction, particularly with these issues on the rise in the older demographic. Having a possible increase in the 60-and-older population, communities are faced with an urgent need to realize the impact of addiction on this subgroup. The National Institute on Drug Abuse stresses that elderly individuals can often present certain hazards relating to drug and alcohol abuse, including physiological frailties and co-occurring disease states. This age group's growing propensity toward addiction only serves to underscore the necessity of special interventions and training for health care workers, family members, and caregivers. By promoting awareness and knowledge regarding the complexities of addiction in older populations, society can more effectively tailor care systems to decrease health risks and enhance the quality of life in addiction sufferers and make society healthier overall. Moreover, substance abuse and addiction have far-reaching economic impacts that need to be urgently addressed. Societal addiction costs in the US have been estimated at more than $700 billion annually, including criminal justice, healthcare, and lost productivity expenses (Baysinger et al., 2015). These staggering figures place policymakers and public health professionals under intense pressure to fund prevention interventions and rehabilitative approaches. Addressing addiction not only improves individual health outcomes but also moves toward economic stability as a whole. Identification and implementation of evidence-based treatment strategies can significantly reduce the burden of addiction and, consequently, free resources for other significant societal needs. This comprehensive strategy for addressing addiction is fundamental for the development of a healthier and more robust public. Lastly, drug abuse and addiction treatment are necessary to produce an enabling social environment that fosters recovery and discourages stigma. Socially, the perception of addiction is a negative one, where the client feels shame and isolation, which may be a source of discouragement against seeking treatment. Education and community outreach, when done properly, can be the make-or-break moment in reshaping these perceptions. By promoting narratives that involve recovery and compassion, communities can create open spaces where the clients affected by addiction can access supportive services. In addition, the impact of addiction is not only felt by the addict but typically extends to the family and society at large, highlighting the need for comprehensive support systems that attenuate emotional and psychological burdens. Addressing this issue comprehensively can ultimately lead to a more compassionate and cohesive society, creating a setting conducive to healing and resilience.

2.1. Types of Substances Abused

Learning Outcome

1. Describe the alcohol
2. Describe the prescription medications
3. Understand the illicit drugs

The arena of substance abuse contains a vast array of substances that individuals resort to for all sorts of reasons, from escapism and social integration to underlying psychological problems. Arguably, the most prevalent varieties are depressants, stimulants, and hallucinogens. Depressants such as alcohol and benzodiazepines are used inappropriately frequently enough for their tranquilizing effects. While the majority of individuals take these drugs to cut back on anxiety or insomnia, dependency and severe health risk, including overdose, is created after long-term use. Stimulants such as cocaine and amphetamine create increased energy and excitement and can lead to death via physical and psychological effects. Hallucinogens such as LSD and mushrooms of psilocybin alter reality and perception, producing uncontrollable and potentially dangerous experiences. Familiarity with these categories is crucial to comprehending the sophistication of substance use and addiction, as well as in formulating effective interventions. Opiates are a very problematic category of substances that have been abused in modern society, with prescription drugs such as oxycodone and hydrocodone often at the forefront of abuse. Initially prescribed for legitimate medical purposes, the potential for abuse of these drugs has led to rampant abuse and addiction. The United States, among others, has been experiencing an opioid epidemic characterized by rampant overdose and death rates related to prescription opioids and illicit opioids like heroin and fentanyl. The rapidly evolving dynamics of drug misuse patterns demand integrated research and intervention strategies commensurate with the particularities of opioid addiction. An excellent Indian study by Ghuman et al. brought into focus the high prevalence of opioid and cannabis derivatives among their consumers, further emphasizing their family life, community health, and well-being concerns (Karki, 2024). Such drugs require targeted policy interventions to counteract their growing threat among different populations. Substance abuse extends beyond illegal drugs and prescription drugs to include legally available and common drugs, such as alcohol and tobacco, that can be abused. While alcohol is socially accepted and in most societies widely utilized, its potential for addiction is high and usually underestimated. Long-term abuse of alcohol leads to a variety of physical health issues, such as liver disease and neurologic damage, in addition to aggravating mental health conditions.

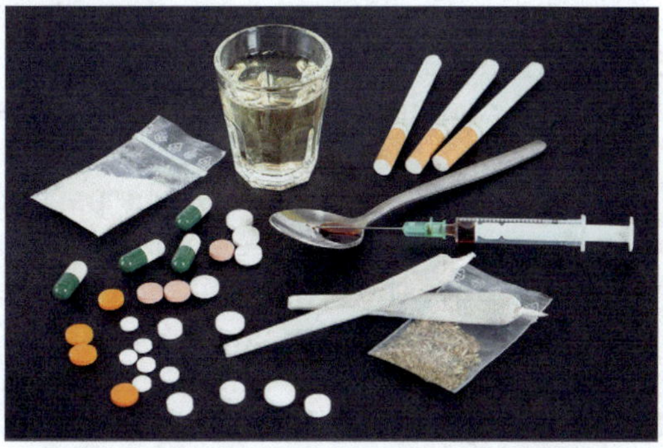

Figure 2.4. Types of substances abused.

Source: https://www.libertybayrecovery.com/wp-content/uploads/2015/03/Types-Of-Drug-Abuse-in-Portland-ME.jpeg.

Tobacco use, mainly via cigarette smoking, continues to be a major preventable cause of death worldwide. The fact that nicotine is addictive presents significant obstacles to quitting. In addition, the growing popularity of vaping devices has added new threats and unforeseen public health effects. As has been observed in recent research, observing the dynamics of psychological flexibility can uncover the processes involved in such substance use and provide new directions for more effective treatment models (Barrado-Moreno et al., 2025). As substances continue to evolve patterns of use, public health must respond with targeted strategies to confront these issues (Figure 2.4).

2.1.1. Alcohol

The complex interaction between alcohol use and adolescent development plays an important role in contributing to the overall problem of substance misuse and addiction. Adolescence is characterized by big biological, psychological, and social changes that tend to result in hazardous behaviors, including the misuse of substances. Research indicates that unhealthy behaviors, including alcohol use, tend to develop during adolescence, which presents huge public health problems. The combined effects of drug use disorders have the ability to severely undermine mental and physical health, not only for individuals but for their families and communities as well. Besides, it has been shown through research that there exists a subtle interaction between parenting and drug use; e.g., an indulgent maternal style is shown to reduce the likelihood of adolescents altering their drinking behavior, while more authoritative parenting is shown to promote healthier lifestyles, which is indicative of the role of family in substance outcomes (El-Shiekh et al., 2024). Social media is also one of the contributing factors towards how alcohol is viewed and used, particularly among youths. The glorification of alcohol on platforms like Instagram and TikTok has the potential to normalize and glamorize alcohol use behaviors, causing increased use among vulnerable users. Research illustrates how content creators, including social media influencers, are most likely to frame alcohol use in ways that emphasize social contact and enjoyment, hence shaping general perceptions towards alcohol use. This emphasizes the applicability of Social Cognitive Theory, which argues that television portrayals in the media provoke imitation in viewers. In contrast to traditional advertising, social media photos allow ordinary users to leave comments and record drinking experiences with alcohol, institutionalizing these accounts further as cultural ideals about drinking (Döring et al., 2022). While glorification of alcohol consumption is the norm, there is also more prominent anti-alcohol content on social media seeking to counteract the numerous health hazards of alcohol consumption and addiction. Such negative portrayals of drinking provide a counter-narrative that acknowledges the importance of harm reduction, better behaviors, and the worth of abstinence. Nevertheless, the scale and potency of such anti-alcohol messages need to be investigated.

Studies indicate that, while there are negative portrayals, comprehensive assessments of their spread and effectiveness remain to be conducted. Through understanding both the glorification and negative portrayals of alcohol on social media, health agencies can develop enhanced substance abuse and addiction plans for addressing such problems, particularly among vulnerable groups like young people (Döring et al., 2022) (Figure 2.5).

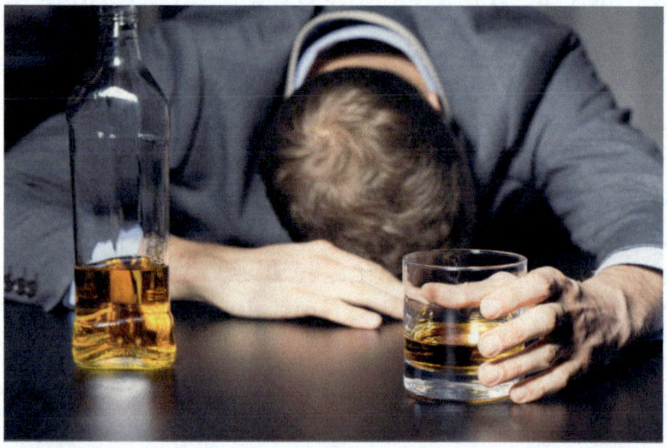

Figure 2.5. Alcohol.

Source: https://w3ins.com/wp-content/uploads/2021/01/iStock-507250010-1024x683.jpg.

2.1.2. Prescription Medications

The misuse of prescription medications is a major contributor to the growing epidemic of abuse and addiction. Opioids, benzodiazepines, and stimulants, prescribed for legitimate sickness, have addiction potential when misused outside their intended purposes. The convenience of use of these medications encourages individuals to perceive them as safe alternatives to illegal drugs, thus being more appealing. This is a dangerous mindset that can perpetuate an unhealthy cycle of abuse where the users would raise their doses or combine these drugs with other drugs to gain more intense experiences. These harmful habits can cost them their health, for instance, in the event of an overdose, which calls for stringent regulation and education about the risks of prescription drugs when abused and used in addiction. Also, the overlap of psychiatric disorders and abuse of prescription drugs is a key area of concern. Most patients suffering from chronic illnesses end up being prescribed medication to alleviate their symptoms; however, overlap of mental disorders such as depression and anxiety can complicate the situation. Research has shown that such patients with comorbidities are at high risk for abuse of drugs, particularly when their self-efficacy for treatment is low or diminished. Further, the relationship between prescribed medications and chronic liver disease depicts the dangers inherent in this crossover because mental distress amplifies the severity of the physical impact of substance use. Handling these complexities with convergent treatment approaches is imperative since it has the potential to improve patient outcomes and reduce prescription drug abuse rates among vulnerable populations (Holmes et al., 2022). Lastly, the opioid epidemic has put into perspective the growing issue with prescription drugs and their role in addiction. Opioids, on the other hand, have been associated with an estimated half a million overdose fatalities, with prescription-related deaths accelerating at spectacular rates. The COVID-19 pandemic has also worsened this scenario with decreased access to addiction treatment and support services, while simultaneously increasing stress levels among those who were already struggling with substance use disorders. Because health systems are challenged with the legacy of pandemics, it is important to prioritize new ways of addressing addiction that consider the complexity of abuse of prescription medicine. Reform policies intended to expand access to medication-assisted treatment and ongoing research into the impact of prescription medication on addiction will be key in preventing this disaster and further discovering recovery from substance abuse (Wen et al., 2020) (Figure 2.6).

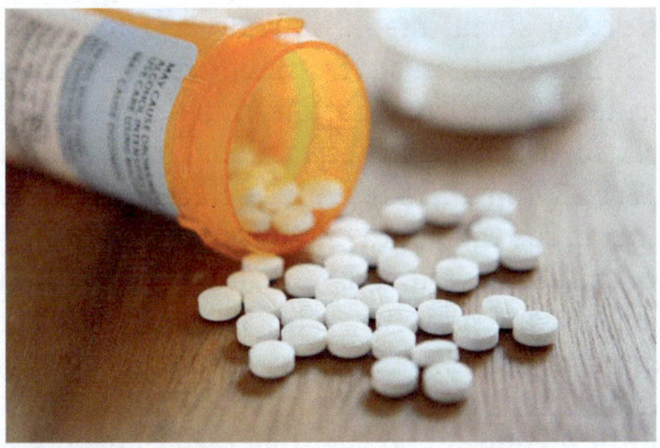

Figure 2.6. Prescription drug use and abuse.

Source: https://ranchatdovetree.com/wp-content/uploads/2017/12/prescription-drug-use-and-abuse.jpg.

2.1.3. Illicit drugs

The complex interplay between illegal drugs and social structures is a major factor in the abuse of substances and addiction. Illicit drug use begins during adolescence, a period characterized by high levels of risk-taking behavior and peer influence. A study shows that during this developmental stage, one tends to experiment with drugs without a comprehensive appreciation of the long-term impact on their physical and psychological health. This experimentation can lead to substance addiction, and emotional regulation deficits, and low perceived risk are among the most significant factors fueling the drug use (Bozzola et al., 2022). Furthermore, the fact that these drugs are easily available, combined with a culture that frequently glamorizes drug use, renders the situation all the more critical, calling for prevention and intervention interventions aimed at addressing it from various perspectives. This rise in the use of the internet and social media has also been attributed to increasing vulnerabilities among the youth regarding substance abuse. Research indicates that the spread of screen time fueled by the pandemic also coincided with rising mental health issues, anxiety, and depression, primarily among young people driven by social media narratives (Bozzola et al., 2022). Such an environment can be used as a ground for normalization of drug use and as a platform for destructive behaviors, such as cyberbullying and substance-related discussion that coerces the youth. Such issues require vigil and collective effort by health professionals, teachers, and parents, who would have to be trained to identify the signs of drug abuse and discuss the harms of drug abuse in an era of open information. Preventive interventions for illegal drug use must incorporate a network of great support involving family, community, and individual factors. A systemic risk and protective factor analysis of adolescent drug use underscores the role of family influence, school involvement, and neighborhood resources (Nawi et al., 2021). For example, increased parental involvement and monitoring can counteract the vulnerability of drug use through the creation of a healthy environment. Education about the risks of drug use and life skills can similarly enable adolescents to make sounder choices. As the environment surrounding drug abuse continues to shift, specialized prevention programs capable of targeting these trends are essential in reducing the incidence and impact of illicit drugs on public health (Figure 2.7).

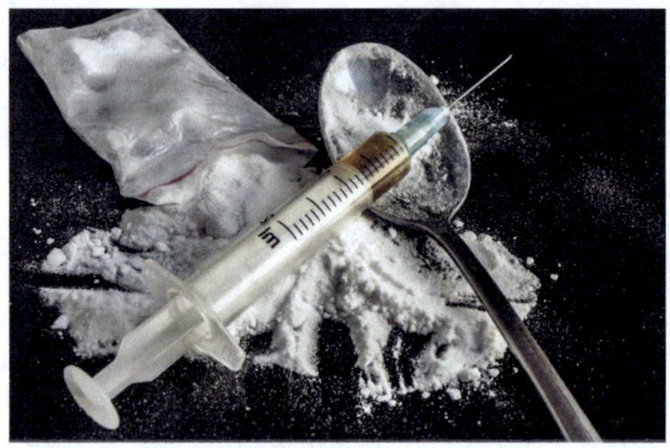

Figure 2.7. Illicit drugs.

Source: https://www.drugfreekidscanada.org/wp-content/uploads/2016/08/heroin.jpg.

Test Your Knowledge

1. What is a prescription medicine?
2. What is the most common drug used by adolescents?

2.2. Causes of Substance Abuse

Learning Outcome

1. Understand the genetic predisposition
2. Understand the role of environmental factors in the dynamics of substance abuse and addiction
3. Describe the psychological influences on substance abuse

Understanding the etiology of substance abuse requires the unraveling of intricate factors through which biology, psychology, and environment are entangled. Inherited predispositions highly increase one's likelihood for addiction, insofar as those who have a tendency for substance abuse in their lineage are likely to do the same. Moreover, neurobiological changes in the brain's reward system can enhance sensitivity to pleasurable stimuli, so that the individual seeks the drug to evade pain or to become high. This interface between genetics and neurobiology is a fundamental foundation for comprehending why some people will become ill in their alcohol and drug use patterns, setting the stage for addiction and associated health problems like liver and cardiovascular disease (Charuni, 2024). Social environments play an equally crucial role in the prevalence of drug and substance abuse within particular communities. Peer pressure, financial status, and exposure to substance use can increase the susceptibility to developing addictive behavior. For example, research confirms that adolescents are more susceptible to risk factors such as disrupted interpersonal relationships and low self-esteem, which drive them toward pursuing the instant fulfillment associated with drug use (Tarantino et al., 2022). This creates a vicious cycle, wherein drug use initially for enjoyment can turn into addiction through environmental stress and the desire to discontinue dependence on mental distress. The social influence landscape is therefore imperative in assessing the larger setting of drug abuse and demanding the required intervention strategies. Mental illness is frequently linked to drug and alcohol consumption, which can then serve as a cause and effect of addiction. Individuals who struggle with conditions such as depression, anxiety, or bipolar disorder can utilize drugs or alcohol as a form of self-medication in an attempt to temporarily eliminate their distress. This maladaptive coping mechanism typically exacerbates the underlying mental health issues, leading to worsening of the overall level of well-being as well as further increasing the addiction dependency (Charuni, 2024). The relationship between substance use and mental health is intricate; while the administration of addictive drugs alters the brain's chemistry, it can exacerbate the mental health disorder, and the process goes on in a cycle of feedback that is difficult to break. Therefore, treating mental health issues comprehensively together with substance abuse treatment is key to successful recovery and long-term health stability (Figure 2.8).

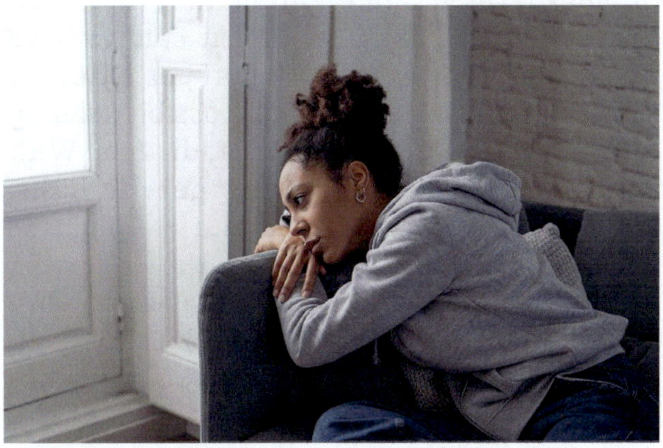

Figure 2.8. Causes of substance abuse.

Source: https://mlfhdmqocr7f.i.optimole.com/cb:lWqs.35cfa/w:1200/h:800/q:mauto/ig:avif/https://thewillowsatredoak.com/wp-content/uploads/2020/09/5-Causes-of-Substance-Abuse-in-Women.jpg.

2.2.1. Genetic Predisposition

A discussion of substance abuse and addiction cannot overlook the influence of genetic predisposition. Increasingly, evidence is presented that illustrates how genes are involved in a person's vulnerability to developing substance use disorders. Certain variations in genes have the ability to influence the body's processing of substances, for instance, alcohol, to produce varying levels of vulnerability to addiction. The interaction of genes and the environment generates a complex landscape in which an individual's risk is determined not only by his or her genetics but also by sociocultural determinants. This complexity prohibits the traditional description of addiction as simply a behavior issue and confirms the definition of addiction as a disease having biological determinants interwoven with social determinants. By embracing this wider knowledge, we can better address the holistic challenge of prevention and treating addiction. Furthermore, the genetic underpinnings of alcohol addiction underscore the importance of multifaceted intervention in prevention and treatment programs. Recent studies have illustrated that certain genotypes affect a person's response to alcohol, possibly leading to greater consumption and addiction. With such evidence supporting this genetic basis, public health interventions must implement genetic screening to identify those at risk more effectively. For instance, individuals with variants that are implicated in sensitivity to the reward aspect of alcohol would require targeted preventive interventions. In addition, understanding these genetic factors paves the way for personalized medicine approaches to treating addiction, in which pharmacogenetics can enhance the effectiveness of treatment plans. Such developments highlight the need for incorporating genetic studies into general addiction research and practice. Ultimately, continued research into the genetic factors of substance abuse represents a paradigm shift in societal attitudes and treatment of addiction. As Morse points out, the disease model of addiction argues that numerous behaviors frequently stigmatized are actually expressions of underlying biological processes shaped by genetic disposition (Morse et al., 2006). This is especially crucial when considering the moral and legal considerations of addiction, where the person can be considered less blameworthy based on their genetic inclinations. Additionally, taking this study a step further into the genetic aspects of alcohol dependence reveals complex interactions within reward systems, which indicate that individuals will be more vulnerable to alcohol consumption and the dangers that come with it at birth (Ferraguti et al., 2015). If we couple genetic insight with compassionate public policy, we can foster a more informed conversation about addiction that resists stigma and invites compassion, enabling effective interventions tailored to individuals' unique genetic profiles (Figure 2.9).

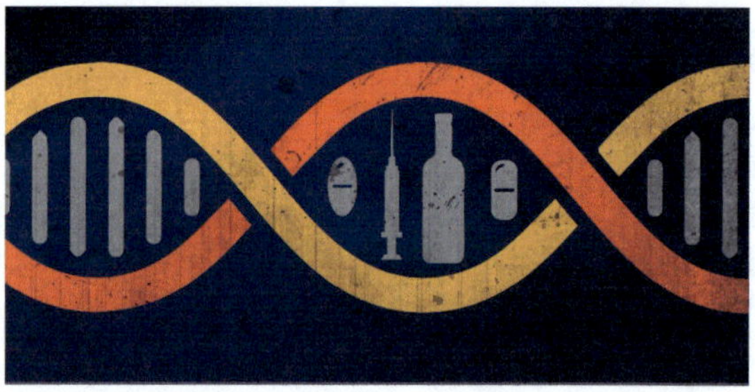

Figure 2.9. Genes and addiction.

Source: https://dhyy726gu6a89.cloudfront.net/wp-content/uploads/2017/12/08122946/Genes-feature-image-2.jpg.

2.2.2. Environmental Factors

Environmental factors play a prevailing role in the cycle of substance abuse and addiction, serving as catalysts that can facilitate or inhibit patterns of substance use. Situational environments such as peer influence, family, and social norms tend to dictate an individual's level of exposure to alcohol and drugs. For instance, individuals who are raised in environments where substance use is accepted may be more likely to establish the same type of behavior in their lives. This phenomenon highlights the importance of understanding the social contexts that contribute to the onset and course of drug use, considering that awareness of these factors can enable the formulation of targeted prevention strategies. As has been noted in studies among university students, family background and social interaction with friends both have important effects on the prevalence of drug use, illustrating the broader nature of one's environmental context on addiction outcomes (Agrawal et al., 2018). In addition, environmental aspects include both the availability of substances and the characteristics of an individual community that can make a population more susceptible to addiction. An illustrative case in point is the commonality of alcohol and drug availability in urban environments, which can promote higher rates of use among residents, particularly youth. The overlap between opportunity and frequency of use is brought out by findings that genetic influences on the abuse/dependence on cannabis overlap to a large extent with those on opportunity and frequency of use (Agrawal et al., 2018). Therefore, a good understanding of addiction demands that these environmental factors be investigated in order to understand how they establish the contexts under which individuals take drugs. Furthermore, the social environment is responsible for shaping attitudes toward substance use and triggering behavior patterns leading to addiction. Educational level, socioeconomic status, and peer culture are determinants of an individual's probability of engaging in substance use. For example, university students who co-reside with peers who drink heavily are likely to drink heavily as well, indicating the powerful impact of social networks on the use of substances. In addition, the mediating effect of alcohol abuse on the relationship between tobacco use and drug use illustrates how multifaceted and interconnected these environmental factors are (Cño et al., 2020). By targeting these elements in prevention and intervention strategies, stakeholders can better prepare individuals to abstain from substance use and design healthier communities (Figure 2.10).

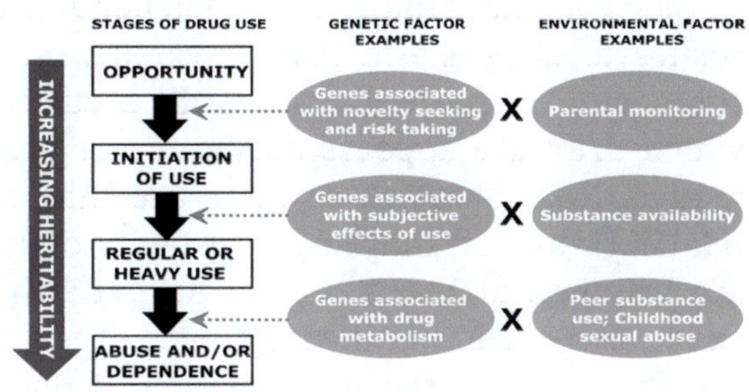

Figure 2.10. Diagram of stage-sequential drug use, depicting plausible stage-specific genetic and environmental influences, and the increasing magnitude of genetic influences on later stages.

Source: https://media.springernature.com/full/springer-static/image/art%3A10.1007%2Fs40429-015-0049-8/MediaObjects/40429_2015_49_Fig1_HTML.gif?as=webp.

2.2.3. Psychological Influences

The intricate web of psychological considerations and substance abuse identifies the importance of mental health being at the core of risk factors for addiction. Psychological forces such as trauma, stress, and emotional turmoil are able to prompt the onset of substance use when individuals try to escape emotional distress. For instance, people who experience depression or anxiety may turn to the use of drugs or alcohol as self-medication. This coping mechanism, nevertheless, also tends towards dependence instead of addressing the underlying psychological problems. It is crucial to comprehend these effects so as to develop effective prevention and intervention measures geared at alleviating substance-related issues in society in general, but mostly in vulnerable groups. Research finds that treating the psychological causes of addiction can potentially result in more successful treatment, eventually lowering the risk of relapse and promoting better coping mechanisms (Taha et al., 2024). Moreover, the social environment in which one develops can most likely have substantial control over psychological vulnerability to drug dependence. Exposure to drug use in family systems, peer cultures, and broader society instills a culture in which drug use appears normative or even attractive. Normalization of drug use may be a manifestation of adapting to psychological or environmental stress, hence perpetuating the addiction cycle. Significantly, peer pressure also plays a role in the perpetuation of drug-seeking behavior, particularly among young people during the adolescent years, where the psychological and emotional basis is formed for subsequent drug use. By examining such socio-environmental determinants, treatments can be developed not only to cure the abuse itself but also to address the psychological environment that supports such behavior (Aız et al., 2024). Treating the psychological aspects of drug use is a multidisciplinary process. Cognitive-behavioral therapy (CBT) and trauma-informed treatment are effective methods of treating the psychological conditions that cause addiction. These two interventions allow patients to learn healthier ways of coping, hence being able to cope with their emotions without drugs. Secondly, as was the case in S.A., the treatment of trauma—whether individually or in a group—has a crucial component in the recovery process. This entire model of addiction recognizes that, while drugs provide temporary relief, only when patients confront their emotional hurts and learn to adopt healthy coping mechanisms can they recover. By acting on these variables, society can work together not only to cure existing issues of drug abuse but also to build a healthier psychological environment for future generations (Aız et al., 2024).

Test Your Knowledge

1. What is the role of environmental factors in addiction?
2. What are the psychological influences on substance abuse?

2.3. Signs and Symptoms of Addiction

Learning Outcome

1. Understands the behavioral changes associated with substance abuse and addiction
2. Know the physical health issues
3. Describe the emotional and mental health effects of substance abuse

Recognition of the signs and symptoms of addiction is crucial for early intervention and effective treatment. These include some of the most frequent indicators, which are behavioral alterations that manifest in various ways. Individuals with addiction become more secretive, back away from social relationships, and are more preoccupied with obtaining and using substances. These tendencies usually go hand in hand with a change of priorities, whereby formerly satisfying or enjoyable activities are skipped for drug use. In addition, physical manifestations—e.g., alterations in hunger, insomnia, and variations in weight—are also indicative of underlying addiction. Combined, these signs can create a general picture of the plight of the individuals, showing the need for a thorough understanding of addiction and its effects on both personal and societal levels, as depicted in the conversation of Neonatal

Abstinence Syndrome (Chandler et al., 2018). Psychological symptoms of addiction usually develop alongside physical and behavioral symptoms, depicting a complicated picture of the condition's intensity. They can also suffer from mood swings, depression, and anxiety that, on the one hand, make things worse and, on the other hand, provide an incentive to take drugs. The link between addiction and mental health is widely established, contrary to the prevailing myth that it is purely a matter of willpower. As the historical perceptions have shifted from moral denunciation to viewing addiction as a disease, it has become starkly apparent that such mental symptoms are not merely personal failures but signs of a syndrome. This shift is attributed to the efforts of early doctors who adopted a disease perspective, emphasizing care over denunciation, thereby laying the groundwork for current strategies toward addiction (Reeves et al., 2019). The implications of failure to diagnose and treat signs and symptoms of addiction not only have direct effects on the patient but also on families and communities. A case in point is that of Neonatal Abstinence Syndrome, which illustrates the way that addiction can have intergenerational effects, as children born to substance-dependent mothers will immediately have health complications and long-term development complications (Chandler et al., 2018). This interlinking highlights the need for awareness and intervention at both the individual and population levels. Moreover, since the stigma of addiction exists, numerous individuals may avoid approaching help, again feeding a cycle of pain that not only harms them but also impacts the people around them. It is therefore essential to develop an environment that is supportive, where free discussion of addiction and its manifestations is encouraged to help build recovery and healing in every area of affected lives, making the community resilient against the far-reaching consequences of addiction and drug abuse (Figure 2.11).

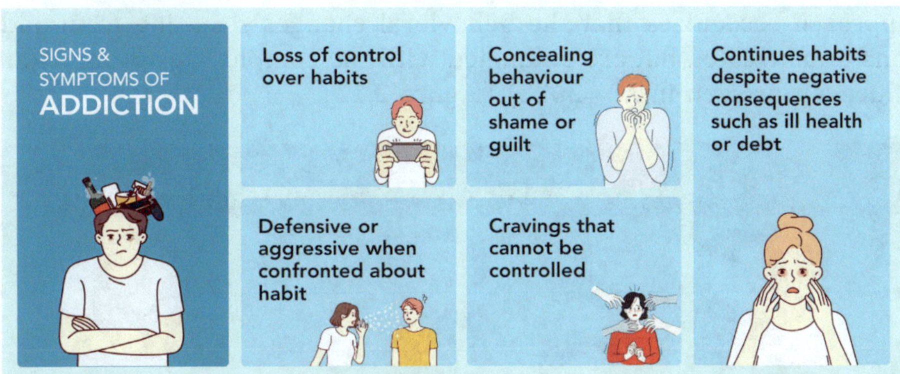
SIGNS & SYMPTOMS OF
ADDICTION
Loss of control over habits
Concealing behaviour out of shame or guilt
Continues habits despite negative consequences such as ill health or debt
Defensive or aggressive when confronted about habit
Cravings that cannot be controlled

Figure 2.11. Signs and symptoms of addiction

Source: https://www.imh.com.sg/Mental-Health-Resources/Conditions-and-Challenges/PublishingImages/Addictions_signs_and_symptoms.jpg.

2.3.1. Behavioral Changes

Behavioral change from addiction and drug abuse is considered a major lifestyle change, as well as a change in social relationships and mental health. As individuals become more involved in addictions, they start to value substances over mandatory obligations, and therefore, duties at work, in school, and in social relationships are avoided. This shift can create a cycle of manipulation and deception, wherein the subject will resort to dishonest activities in order to obtain drugs or to conceal their drug dependence. Further, the quest for intoxicants can frequently dominate productive coping mechanisms, which further enhances the erosion of a person's social relations and mental well-being. As explained by Taha et al. (2024), this brain function alteration results in drug-seeking compulsivity, underlining the complexity of addiction as a chronic disorder. This chronicity not only alters individual behaviors but also compels families and communities into chronic impairment, hence reinforcing the need for integrated intervention strategies. In addition, the drug addiction influence is not only limited to the addict but also to the effects of society that amplify increasing problems in communities. Community values and norms are changed by the presence of drug addiction. As substance use becomes more common, the more peer pressure increases, and it encourages an unhealthy phenomenon. Such normalization can lead to more tolerance for such abnormal behavior, and thus more frequency of violence, crime, and health emergencies in such societies. As emphasized by Taha et al. (2024), the consequences of such behavioral modification are dire, with the entire society, including economic stability and security, affected. Accordingly, it is crucial to reverse such patterns through education and community intervention to develop resistance to substance dependence and safeguard future generations from such a fate. Lastly, the knowledge of the origins of behavioral change related to drugs is also critically vital while developing effective treatment plans. Facilitators like genetic predisposition, environmental influences, and early drug exposures significantly raise the risk of addiction and related behavior modification. Evidence-based intervention practices are important in relation to such factors overall. Education schemes that inform potential users of the dangers of drug abuse can reverse early exposure, while treatment approaches tailored to individuals guarantee that the concerned get care tailored to their situation. Through methods utilizing preventative measures as well as effective treatments, society is able to reverse the adverse effects of drug abuse. This multi-faceted approach recognizes that the behavioral changes resulting from addiction are not merely conditions to be treated but are entangled with the complexities of individual experiences and societal influences, as seen in Ali (2023) (Figure 2.12).

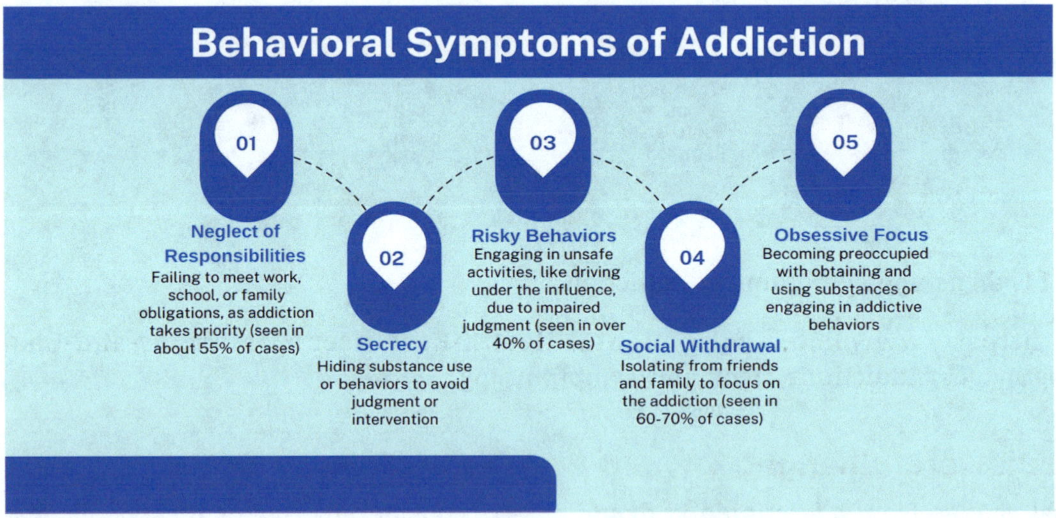

Figure 2.12. Behavioral symptoms of addiction.

Source: https://www.innovodetox.com/wp-content/uploads/2025/02/Behavioral-Symptoms-1200x600.jpg.

2.3.2. Physical Health Issues

Substance abuse and addiction are responsible for a vast array of physical health issues that significantly impact individuals and society as a whole. The physiological price of drug use is best illustrated via the example of opioid addiction, which has been a significant public health issue in the United States. The patients mostly develop various ailments, such as impaired cardiovascular status, liver injury, and respiratory disease, primarily due to the drugs taken and mode of consumption. Apart from that, addiction leads to unsafe behavior, such as unsafe sex, which makes them more prone to acquiring sexually transmitted diseases.

The complex interplay of these health issues in physical health highlights the need for a rounded solution in meeting the war against substance abuse because most of the health consequences will also perpetuate the addictive cycle and make the recovery prospects complicated while people struggle to get care under tragic conditions (Wooton et al., 2021). To respond to the physical health issues of drug abuse appropriately, it is important to understand the two-way relationship between addiction and worsening health. Many victims of already existing physical or psychological illness may develop a dependency on drugs as self-medication, making their health more complex and difficult to recover from. For instance, people suffering from chronic pain may misuse opioids to alleviate their suffering, leading to a dependence that further aggravates the underlying health issues. Integrated care methods that address these underlying health issues have been demonstrated by research to decrease the consequences of addiction and improve overall health. Moreover, the treatment of underlying disorders simultaneously with substance abuse provides assistance in eliminating addiction stigma and promoting less stigmatized healthcare settings, which is crucial for successful interventions (Cannon et al., 2019). The social impacts of substance abuse-induced physical illnesses extend beyond the individual to affect public health systems and economic stability. The current opioid crisis has strained healthcare resources to the breaking point, leading to increased emergency room visits and hospitalizations, and ultimately placing a greater burden on healthcare providers and taxpayers. As addiction continues to erode physical health, the subsequent spike in healthcare costs places the broader economy squarely in the financial strain column, as documented by job loss directly attributed to addiction-related causes. Utilizing prevention programs and prioritizing early interventions has the capability to minimize long-term physical outcomes of alcohol and other drug abuse. Implementing preventive interventions through existing health systems, such as children's Medicaid, provides an opportunity to promote protective practices that lower addiction risk and ultimately lay the groundwork for improved public health outcomes (Cannon et al., 2019) (Figure 2.13).

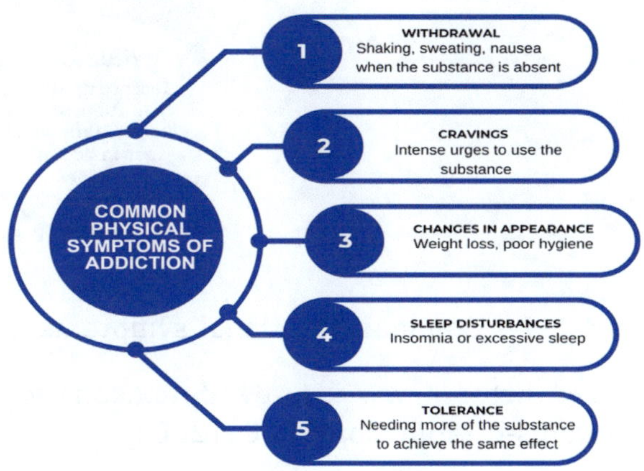

Figure 2.13. Common physical symptoms of addiction.

Source: https://www.innovodetox.com/wp-content/uploads/2025/02/Common-physical-symptoms-of-addiction--1200x1200.jpg.

2.3.3. Emotional and Mental Health Effects

The psychological and emotional impact of drug abuse is quite adverse, not only on the abuser but also on his/her interpersonal relationships. Substance use disorders can create a vicious cycle of emotional distress in terms of feelings of guilt, shame, and hopelessness. Drugs serve as an escape mechanism for emotional pain for the majority, but this only exacerbates the problems and generates additional psychological distress. When individuals keep substances around, they might ignore valuable relationships that make them feel isolated and lonely. Isolation has a feedback loop of feelings where a lack of social support can amplify their addiction since they will feel like they cannot seek help or trust others. Therefore, it is critical to understand the emotional implications in order to develop effective intervention and treatment strategies since addressing the psychological roots of addiction can result in recovery and improved relationships. Aside from this, maternal drug use transfers into parenting, influencing children's attachment styles and emotional development to a significant extent.

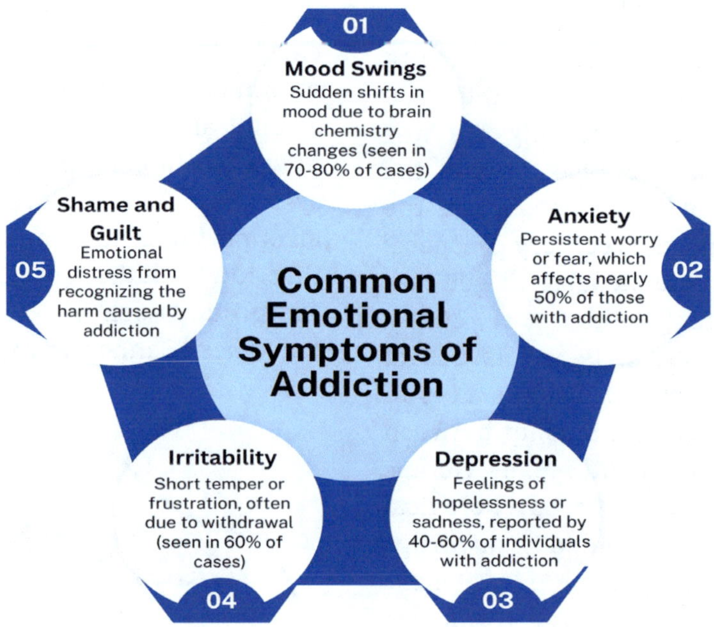
Common Emotional Symptoms of Addiction
01
Mood Swings
Sudden shifts in mood due to brain chemistry changes (seen in 70-80% of cases)
02
Anxiety
Persistent worry or fear, which affects nearly 50% of those with addiction
03
Depression
Feelings of hopelessness or sadness, reported by 40-60% of individuals with addiction
04
Irritability
Short temper or frustration, often due to withdrawal (seen in 60% of cases)
05
Shame and Guilt
Emotional distress from recognizing the harm caused by addiction

Figure 2.14. Common emotional symptoms of addiction.

Source: https://www.innovodetox.com/wp-content/uploads/2025/02/Common-Emotional-Symptoms-of-Addiction-1200x1200.jpg.

Research has indicated that mothers with substance use disorder are more likely to show insecure styles of attachment, which interfere with their capacity to connect and take care of their children. Such impairment creates a cycle of emotional neglect, leading to developmental problems in the child, including higher anxiety and behavioral problems. In addictions-debilitated care environments, the Attachment Theory dictates that the dissolution of relational development may ensue, ultimately affecting the emotional health of mothers and offspring. Through interventions fortifying the mother-child relationship, treatment programs can reverse such negative tendencies and promote healthier emotional connections, thereby guaranteeing positive consequences for future generations of substance-addicted individuals (Parolin et al., 2016). The intergenerational transfer of trauma highlights a critical dynamic in the situation of drug abuse and its emotional impact. Mothers exposed to childhood trauma are more likely to develop alcohol and other drug use disorders, transferring the cycle of dysfunction they experienced deeply into their parenting. Through qualitative interviews, research has indicated that such mothers internalize their own traumatic experiences and bring them to bear on self-concept and parent strategies, ultimately leading to dysfunctional family relationships. Trauma coupled with drug abuse presents a cycle wherein earlier emotional pain gets construed as aversive relationship patterns towards their children, further complicating recovery. Thus, addressing both the trauma and substance abuse in treatment programs is crucial, with the priority being the need for integrated, trauma-informed treatments that can break this intergenerational cycle of trauma and facilitate healing and healthier emotional outcomes for affected families (Pauw et al., 2019) (Figure 2.14).

Test Your Knowledge

1. What are the behavioral changes of substance abuse?
2. What are the emotional and mental health effects of substance abuse?

2.4. Impact on Individuals

Learning Outcome

1. Know the impact of substance abuse on personal relationships
2. Know the impact of substance abuse on employment and education
3. Describe the financial consequences of substance abuse and addiction

The consequences of substance addiction for individuals extend far beyond their physical well-being, primarily eroding mental well-being and day-to-day functioning. Untreated addiction will likely leave the individual with a complex interaction among psychological disorders, leading to functional disabilities interfering with effective functioning in work, social, and personal settings. The majority of individuals with substance use disorders present with comorbid conditions such as depression and anxiety, which form a cycle of impairment in their social and occupational responsibilities. This complex is the rationale for the necessity of whole interventions that will address not just the addiction but also the psychological and social impacts it has, as pointed out by recent studies that examine these forces in greater depth (Sivaprakash et al., 2025). Moreover, substance addiction has also been linked with sleep disorders, which have complicated underlying conditions and further complicate recovery processes. It is reported, through research, that a significant percentage of individuals suffering from addiction have suffered from sleep disorders that have entrenched people in a cycle of dependence and incapacitation. Insomnia and circadian rhythm disorders are most readily found among substance abusers, effectively reducing their quality of life. The negative consequences of such sleeping disorders can lead to heightened irritability, reduced cognitive functioning, and more difficulty managing relationships, highlighting the ruinous impact of substance consumption on an individual's everyday functioning and emotional regulation (Siddiqui et al., 2025). Lastly, the stigma associated with substance consumption can deeply influence individuals, intruding on their sense of self-identity and leading to social isolation. The majority of those with an addiction suffer judgment from others and society, which translates into a sense of shame that prevents them from seeking help. Stigma can perpetuate an addiction cycle, as individuals disconnect from support circles and can slip back into use of substances. Elimination of substance abuse stigma is critical in establishing a conducive recovery and rehabilitation environment. By comprehending the diverse impact of addiction on the individual, society can begin making a case to debunk negative stereotypes and promote a more compassionate and supportive disposition toward treatment and recovery (Figure 2.15).

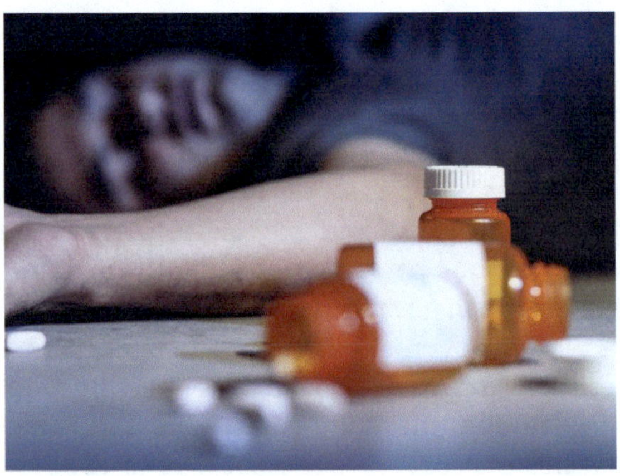

Figure 2.15. Effects of drug abuse.

Source: https://media.post.rvohealth.io/wp-content/uploads/sites/3/2020/02/323461_2200-732x549.jpg.

2.4.1. Personal Relationships

The relationship between personal relationships and drug abuse is a sophisticated phenomenon that must be viewed carefully. In most cases, the addicted person's personal relationships are strained or ruptured due to his/her behavior and the consequent outcomes of drug consumption. The family and friends are frustrated, enraged, or helplessness-motivated, and thus they establish a pattern of suffering for all the persons involved. As these relationships disintegrate, the addict becomes increasingly isolated from support, fueling their urge to escape reality through drug or alcohol consumption. This process not only illustrates the personal effects of addiction, but also highlights the need for support systems in the rehabilitation of the addicted. Interaction with trusted others can greatly influence the path of recovery by instilling a sense of responsibility and belonging. Furthermore, personal relationships are both risk and protective factors in terms of substance abuse. Such positive relationships are likely to be important for recovery-seekers since they can motivate and encourage them not to use alcohol or drugs. In contrast, neglectful or enabling relationships can perpetuate addiction. For instance, where friends are promoting dangerous behaviors or not directly tackling the abuse of drugs and alcohol, it can reinforce the user's addiction. The comprehension of the I-PACE model brings into focus the importance of personal interactions in drug addiction. This model recognizes that individual susceptibility interacts with environmental and social contingencies, which may imply that poor relationship patterns might trigger or condition drug use patterns, thereby making recovery difficult (Brand et al., 2016). Thus, helping relationships are critical in recovery and treatment processes. Education and increased awareness regarding substance abuse can also transform the relationships in one's own life. Health care providers' attitude towards substance use patients significantly determines their therapeutic relationships, as established by recent studies. Those who work in supportive roles—friends, relatives, and doctors—can make the environments more conducive by comprehending the complexity of addiction. Improved attitudes that recognize substance abuse as a health issue rather than personal failure can lead to more compassionate interactions, which would potentially enhance the impact on outcomes (Clarke et al., 2015). Education interventions involving family and friends can also empower them with the skills necessary to assist the person they care about who has an addiction. This transformation of awareness can eventually give rise to healthier interpersonal relationships, processes of resilience and recovery less obstructed by misunderstanding and stigma (Figure 2.16).

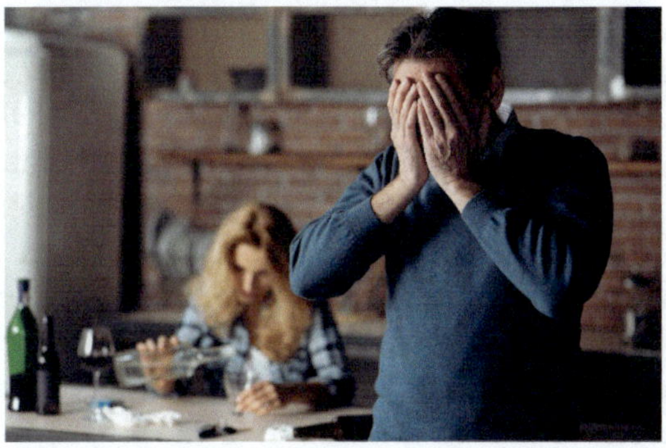

Figure 2.16. Substance use affects relationships.

Source: https://diamondhousedetox.com/wp-content/uploads/2021/05/realtionships.jpeg.

2.4.2. Employment and Education

The connection between education and working is thus pivotal to the development of one's immunity against drug use and addiction. Academic success is typically coupled with the provision of employment and financial independence, both of which underlie the avoidance of drug abuse. Learners exposed to academic pressure can be victims of negative coping behaviors, such as drug use, that further compromise their studies and lead to chronic unemployment. The impact extends to broader battles; when school failure in education increases the likelihood of school dropout, this results in a less capable workforce with the required skills. The economic burden is therefore amplified, with governments facing billions in lost employment capacity and extra healthcare expenditure, particularly on the treatment of drug and alcohol abuse and associated societal effects (Pascoe et al., 2019). Additionally, the recognition of stigma about drug use has far-reaching implications for education and labor outcomes. Stigma acts as a deterrent, frequently discouraging individuals from accessing help and, in turn, lessening their capacity to pursue education or stable employment to any degree. This stigma is interlocking with other social factors such as race, gender, and socioeconomic status, further complicating the recovery process for those trying to overcome drug addiction. An in-depth understanding of this stigma's extensive scope emphasizes the necessity for context-responsive interventions that address the heterogeneous needs of individuals in school and workplace settings. Through models such as the Health Stigma and Discrimination Framework, stakeholders can appreciate and disentangle the barriers to individuals with substance use disorders and enhance their education and labor outcomes (Stangl et al., 2019). The incorporation of healthy-environment promotion programs in schools and workplaces is crucial to prevent substance use and encourage recovery among victims. Stress management programs and mental health services can be employed in schools in efforts to curb pressures leading to educational stress, which could then limit the inclination towards substance use. Similarly, workplaces can also benefit from initiatives to promote mental health awareness and provision of resources for employees who have addiction problems. Through the exchange of ideas among educators, employers, and healthcare professionals, support networks can be built so that individuals can access the resources they need to succeed academically and professionally. Lastly, addressing the twinned problems of work and learning through the prism of drug addiction also secures individual recovery as well as the broader social fabric of society (Pascoe et al., 2019) (Figure 2.17).

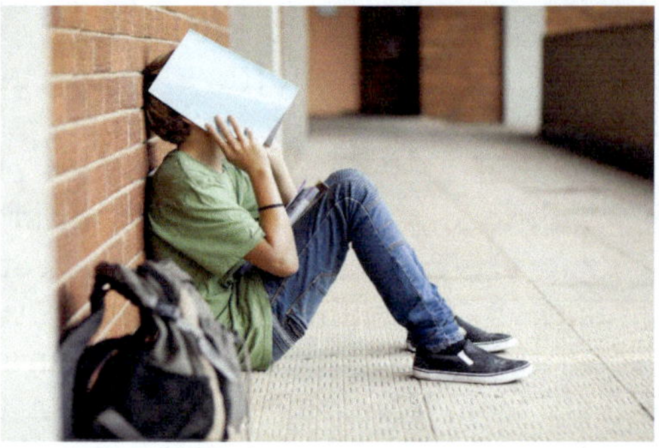

Figure 2.17. Impact of substance abuse on education.

Source: https://www.justthinktwice.gov/sites/justthinktwice.com/files/images/iStock_000020631102_Large.jpg.

2.4.3. Financial Consequences

The economic effects of addiction and substance abuse extend far beyond the user and affect families and society as a whole. For most addicted persons, the short-term economic costs are borne in the form of the runaway costs of acquiring substances. These costs can engender severe economic hardship and often result in job loss, further debt, and depletion of personal and family resources. Besides, the impact on family life can be shocking, as financial insecurity brought about by addiction has a way of breeding tension, family conflict, and even the possibility of domestic violence. As addiction progresses, families will end up spending enormous sums of money on treatment interventions, legal fees, and even child protective services in some cases, projecting costs exponentially as they are incurred over this challenging period (Forțu et al., 2025). In addition to the financial burden at the family and individual level, drug abuse has overall societal costs. The society bears the costs of increased crime that is both drug and alcohol-related, and the consequent higher law enforcement and judicial expenses. The National Center for Drug Abuse Statistics highlights how drug abuse among young people not only affects their own well-being and health but also involves long-term economic burdens to the community through lower productivity and medical costs (Gomes et al., 2024). Moreover, utilization of public funds for combating substance abuse – prevention efforts, treatment centers, and centers for rehabilitation – is an expensive financial undertaking. Such costs and burdens at the community level underscore the imperative need for prevention and treatment intervention measures that cut the economic burden caused to the communities under the influence of substance addiction. Reducing the economic burden of drug and alcohol use requires structural reform at policy and practice levels. Stakeholders need to give a very high priority to strategic investment in early intervention programs and support systems that can halt the tide of development of addiction among high-risk groups, particularly young people. By reducing the incidence of drug abuse at the source, communities can prevent the economic burden of lost productivity and healthcare expenses. Moreover, encouraging education and awareness campaigns can give the appropriate tools to potential users and their families so that they can make responsible decisions about substance use, thereby reducing future costs. As evidenced by research, the emphasis on community-based practices emphasizing prevention, screening, and treatment creates an environment where one is not as likely to turn to substances, thereby reducing the economic ripple effect on families and society at large (Forțu et al., 2025) (Figure 2.18).

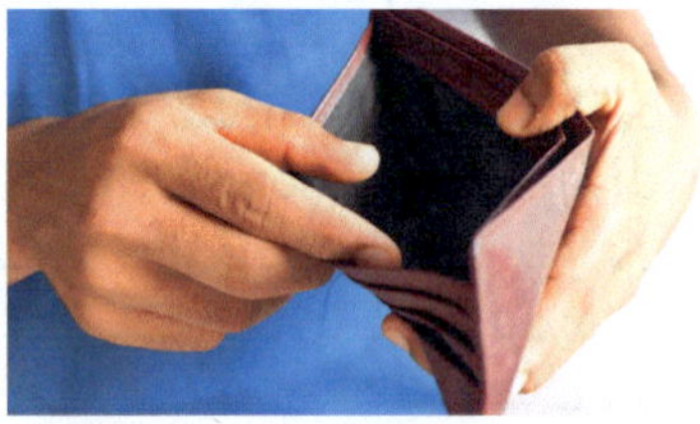

Figure 2.18. Financial effects of drug abuse.

Source: https://www.aspenridgerecoverycenters.com/wp-content/uploads/2022/02/addiction-and-drug-abuse.png.

Test Your Knowledge

1. How does drug abuse affect personal relationships?
2. What are the financial consequences of substance abuse?

2.5. Societal Implications

Learning Outcome

1. Describe the healthcare costs associated with substance abuse and addiction
2. Understand the crime and legal issues
3. Know the impact of substance abuse and addiction on families and communities

The social effects of addiction and drug abuse extend far beyond individual consequences to families, communities, and public health systems. Communities such as Cookeville, Tennessee, illustrate the subtle reach of addiction within which individuals with potential for productive lives are engulfed in cycles of dependency. This not only affects individual well-being and health but also significantly contributes to the loss of community cohesion and social fabric. Families are usually scattered as addiction surrounds members, leading to strained relationships and high stress levels among non-addict family members. These dynamics give rise to a perpetual cycle of dysfunction, which can reinforce the stigma surrounding addiction, thereby hindering proper support networks and mechanisms of rehabilitation in society (Simpson et al., 2022). Consequently, the common burden of addiction resonates through several levels of society, manifesting as increasing healthcare costs, crime rates, and rates of demand for rehabilitation treatment. Furthermore, conversation about drug abuse has a tendency to neglect salient details of developmental stages, particularly for adolescents. Adolescents are particularly susceptible to the effects of drugs due to ongoing brain development, which causes irreversible cognitive and behavioral impairments. Studies have determined that teenagers are more susceptible to addiction due to their neurobiological vulnerabilities, yet the public discourse tends to overlook this fundamental reality. Without a fundamental understanding of how drug use affects this population, prevention education may be deficient. Lack of adequately confronting teenage drug use in the public sphere leaves room for intervention and assistance to be overlooked, which underscores the requirement for more informed conversation regarding recovery strategies and addiction. This knowledge gap undermines policy development in efficient areas that account for the unique requirements of younger populations. Socio-economic expenditure of drug abuse is yet another key aspect of achieving its implications. The societies that are hit by out-of-control addiction generally suffer economically in the form of a dwindling workforce, increased healthcare expenses, and growth in criminal justice involvement through substance-related offenses. Such settings are stifled of economic progress, creating cycles of poverty that are often inextricably linked to addiction. Moreover, pressure on communal resources, including law enforcement and healthcare workers, is increased as they contend with the effects of drug use. This strain can contribute to reduced service efficacy and accessibility, pushing those who need assistance further toward society's periphery. The demand for comprehensive community-based recovery and educational programs is evoked in the immediate call for a collective responsibility in addressing the system problems underlying substance misuse and its resonant echoes throughout society (Simpson et al., 2022) (Figure 2.19).

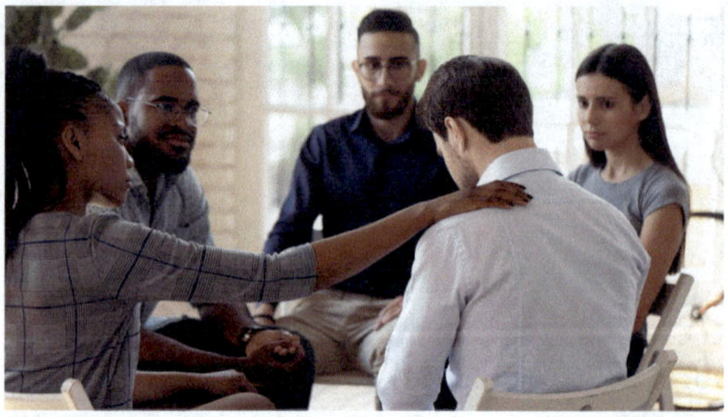

Figure 2.19. Social effects of drug abuse on society.

Source: https://www.humanservicesedu.org/wp-content/uploads/2022/08/social-effects-drug-abuse-society.jpg.

2.5.1. Healthcare Costs

The rising healthcare costs associated with addiction and substance abuse pose a serious issue to society and the individual. Substance-addicted patients spend an enormous amount of time in medical care, including hospitalization, rehabilitative treatments, and ongoing psychological therapy. The costs to the healthcare system are also elevated by the comorbidities that typically present with substance abuse, such as mental disorders and chronic illnesses. As noted by other research, drug-abusing families suffer the most additional financial burdens, which further cause a chain reaction of adverse effects such as loss of income and higher healthcare needs on the part of the abuser as well as his or her dependents (Manurung, 2024). The economic costs of treating addiction and related medical conditions are thus far greater than individual costs, impacting public health expenditure as well as community resources. The societal cost of drug addiction also translates into enormous economic losses driven by the burden imposed on healthcare systems due to the systemic nature. Once an individual consumes substances, their productivity declines, leading to increased absenteeism in workplaces and reduced job performance. This decline is the cause of the total loss of workforce efficiency, and companies are confronted with employee turnover expenses and the costs of training new employees. In addition, as the health system copes with the consequences of drug addiction, the economic burden increases. Much of the money flows towards emergency treatment and long-term treatment facilities, thereby draining funds that could be applied to prevention and other priority health programs (Kouhnavardi et al., 2022). The cycle of dependency with the relapse and continuing healthcare needs also contributes to the richness of the financial situation, necessitating multifaceted and goal-driven strategies to reduce these pervasive expenditures. The excessive healthcare expenses related to drug use require a multidisciplinary approach focusing on prevention, education, and rehabilitation. Effective intervention programs that identify and treat at an early stage can substantially reduce the cost to healthcare systems. Evidence shows that targeted interventions, like family support and outreach programs, can diminish the load on health resources while promoting recovery and social reintegration for addicts (Manurung, 2024). Additionally, treatments with fewer side effects and reduced risks of dependency are critical since they can play a role in more effective management of addiction without adding to existing health costs (Kouhnavardi et al., 2022). By investing in prevention and recovery-oriented models, society can contribute to the reduction of the economic burden of substance abuse, ultimately leading to healthier communities and more sustainable health systems.

2.5.2. Crime and Legal Issues

Addiction and substance abuse have long-reaching implications for crime and the law since they often make appearances in offenses against the law. Most frequently, addicts are driven into crimes such as robbery or drug possession as a means of sustaining their addictions. This overlap of drug abuse and crime suggests the necessity of a legal system that deals with underlying causes rather than punishing crime. Most states are realizing that mass incarceration for nonviolent drug offenses is not only costly but frequently self-defeating. Legal options, such as court-ordered treatment programs, can serve the individual and society equally well by providing better outcomes and reducing recidivism, thus promoting a more rehabilitative system of justice (McKean et al., 2004). Furthermore, the social reaction to drug offenses has changed, illustrating heightened sensitivity to issues involved. Traditional law enforcement approaches often resulted in overcrowded jails, and a recidivism cycle might. Consequently, reform is being driven by other communities in support of treatment rather than prison. For instance, community-based interventions foster a collective dialogue on substance abuse in society, as addressed in various issue guides (Aguiniga et al., 2015). This movement prioritizes learning about one's own experience with substance use, which may shed light on the broader societal impact and help create well-informed policies that are more beneficial to individuals and communities. In discussing crime, legal issues, and substance abuse, it must be pointed out how overall policy reform affects these areas. The other options—comparing community governance, collaborative care, and preventative measures—hold tremendous benefits. By opening up discussion on these issues, the stakeholders can find a common ground, supplying the vehicle by which people can develop tailored solutions that address the concerned parties and their communities. Engaging different voices in this dialogue, as observed through the work of diverse organizations, ensures that responses to substance abuse transcend punitive measures, upholding a fairer system of justice that emphasizes rehabilitation, public health, and social reintegration of victims of substance abuse (Aguiniga et al., 2015) (Figure 2.20).

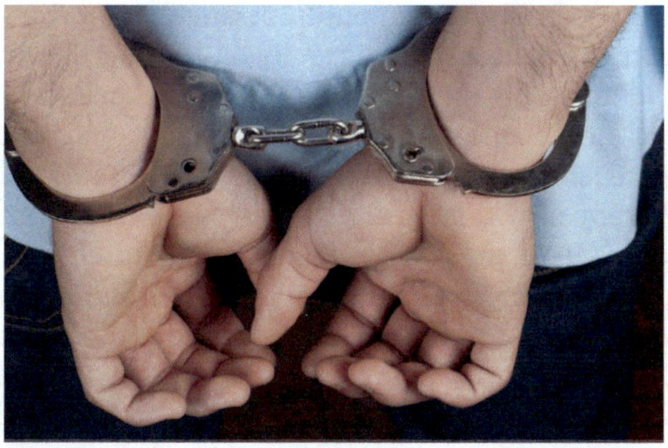

Figure 2.20. Legal consequences of addiction.

Source: https://www.drugrehab.us/wp-content/uploads/2011/09/legal-consequences-of-addiction-1024x679.jpg.

2.5.3. Impact on Families and Communities

The impact of addiction and drug use extends far beyond the perpetrator, radically affecting communities and families. Families are usually subject to the emotional and financial destruction provoked by the addiction of a loved one. The strain on the psyche can cause family relationships to deteriorate, establishing an environment of distrust and resentment. Children in these families are prone to being abused and neglected, with continuous emotional and behavioral issues that result in addictive and traumatic patterns within the family. Addiction needs to be acknowledged as a family disease that not only treats the patient but also provides help to family members suffering from this crisis. Thus, family therapy-based recovery programs play an important role in reconciliation and healing, helping families restore relationships that have been damaged because of drug addiction. Communities are also greatly affected because of widespread drug abuse and addiction. The social fabric of a community disintegrates as general problems of addiction lead to increased crime rates, homelessness, and societal unrest. Substance-using populations are likely to be sources of public strain on resources, from healthcare services to law enforcement and social services. These strains create a cycle of perpetuation where citizens become increasingly disenfranchised and marginalized. Moreover, the stigma regarding addiction also serves to further isolate families and individuals, lessening their chances to seek assistance or services. This public health epidemic emphasizes the need for community intervention programs that promote awareness, prevention, and recovery, ultimately developing an environment conducive rather than stigmatizing individuals with substance abuse disorders. The interface between addiction and public health crises, such as the COVID-19 outbreak, has contributed to the problem for families and communities. The at-risk populations, including individuals with substance use disorders, are worse off during these crises because of the lack of access to healthcare, increased social isolation, and inaccessibility of social support services. In recent conversations, it has been mentioned that individuals with substance use disorders experience compounding health threats, leading to further exacerbated psychosocial trajectories and overdose rates during times of increased stress and uncertainty. The need for adaptive treatment and policy strategies has emerged in earnest to focus on increasing access to and support for victims and their families. New approaches, such as telehealth for substance use treatment, have emerged as necessary instruments at such moments, reminding us that substance abuse treatment involves both local and systemic response with an emphasis on family and community health and well-being (Becker et al., 2020; Volkow, 2020) (Figure 2.21).

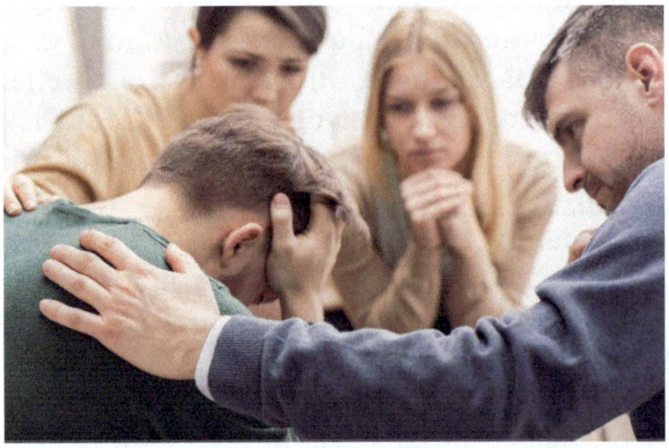

Figure 2.21. The impact of substance abuse and addiction on families.

Source: https://bhoperehab.com/wp-content/uploads/2022/07/substance-abuse-families-scaled.jpeg.

Test Your Knowledge

1. What is the economic burden on healthcare systems?
2. What is the impact of substance abuse and addiction on families and communities?

2.6. Treatment and Recovery Options

Learning Outcome

1. Understand the role of behavioral therapies in addressing substance abuse and addiction
2. Describe the medication-assisted treatment of substance abuse and addiction
3. Understand the role of support groups and community resources in addressing substance abuse and addiction

Effective treatment and recovery plans for addiction and drug abuse are multidisciplinary, just as the disorders are. Treatment must consist of medical, psychological, and social support systems individually tailored to meet the particular needs of the patients. The normal treatment approaches usually include detoxification followed by subsequent rehabilitation, which can either be inpatient or outpatient, depending on the severity of the addiction. Surprisingly, the incorporation of behavioral therapy has been promising to ensure long-term recovery through the elimination of the underlying psychological aspects of substance use disorders. Through strategies such as cognitive-behavioral therapy and motivational interviewing, clients can learn coping skills, enhance self-efficacy, and work toward long-term recovery, underscoring the need for individualized care in any treatment plan. Perhaps the most relevant area of treatment is co-occurring disorder treatment, a common condition among addiction patients. These disorders are psychological in nature, such as depression, anxiety, or PTSD, which complicate recovery. Succeeding interventions, thus, must address mental health and substance abuse concurrently to decrease the risk of relapse and improve overall outcomes. Implementing integrative treatment modalities will enhance efficacy, as research indicates that dual-diagnosis clients function significantly better in programs that offer comprehensive care. These complete approaches recognize the co-dependent situation of drug addiction and mental illness, validating the concept that recovery is a multifaceted process that must be addressed by a balanced and holistic approach. In the face of such complexities, innovative funding methods and policy reform are needed to improve treatment access and outcomes. Charity giving is crucial to respond to the urgent needs of individuals with substance use disorders, as emphasized in recent guidance to funders. By focusing on life-saving strategies and increasing access to treatment, stakeholders can address the reduction of the overall prevalence of abuse as well as its societal effects. These strategies can involve investing in evidence-based interventions and designing systems that make care more effective. As seen, philanthropy has the ability to create sweeping change but needs to be paired with a commitment towards creative solutioning, particularly to the nuances of recovery from alcoholism, which is vital towards guaranteeing successful treatment and ensuring long-term recovery in afflicted individuals (Wallman-Stokes et al., 2015; Anderson et al., 2018) (Figure 2.22).

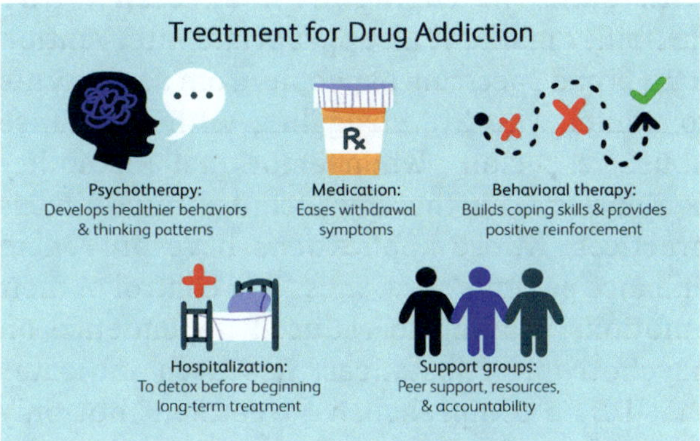
Treatment for Drug Addiction
Rx
Psychotherapy:
Develops healthier behaviors & thinking patterns
Medication:
Eases withdrawal symptoms
Behavioral therapy:
Builds coping skills & provides positive reinforcement
Hospitalization:
To detox before beginning long-term treatment
Support groups:
Peer support, resources, & accountability

Figure 2.22. Treatment for drug addiction.

Source: https://www.verywellhealth.com/thmb/s-1nwHWIhWGGa41GOmxVUHVaDA4=/1500x0/filters:no_upscale():max_bytes(150000):strip_icc()/the-effects-of-drug-addiction-5214343-Final-63ee57687f0a4daa90b104897ad6579e.jpg.

2.6.1. Behavioral Therapies

Behavioral therapies play a significant role in the treatment of drug addiction and drug abuse, particularly in their ability to modify risky behavior associated with drug use. Behavioral therapy is founded on the premise that behavior, such as drug use, can be modified by learning and reinforcement. Other therapies, such as Cognitive Behavioral Therapy (CBT), have been effective in helping individuals to realize the causative determinants of their drug and alcohol use, as well as learning coping skills to deflect cravings and stressors. With the high cost of healthcare as well as detrimental health implications surrounding substance use disorders, these treatments play a key role in long-term recovery. The flexibility of behavioral therapies allows them to be integrated with pharmacotherapy, which can significantly enhance treatment response and reduce relapse and dropout rates of standard interventions. One of the most successful behavioral therapies for addiction is Dialectical Behavioral Therapy (DBT). This multimodal treatment addresses emotional dysregulation and behavior issues that often follow addiction by equipping patients with skills in coping with adversity. DBT flexibility makes it an appropriate intervention for a broad spectrum of people, from adolescents to adults who are struggling with substance abuse, especially when emotional instability is a factor. The therapy includes mindfulness practices, whose applications have proven to enhance patients' awareness and control of their emotions, leading to reduced dependence on psychotropic substances. Research indicates that DBT's comprehensive treatment not only treats drug abuse but also provides emotional regulation strategies, which enhance the probability of long-term addiction recovery, as indicated in various evaluations of the therapy's effectiveness (Herrera-Palacios, 2024). Due to the co-occurring patterns of mental illness and addiction disorders, concomitant treatment systems combining behavioral therapies have become significant. Research shows that co-occurring disorder treatments administered at the same time, such as mood disorders along with substance abuse, lead to more effective results than sequential treatment (Madu et al., 2021). It is an integrated treatment that combines approaches from various behavioral therapies, such as CBT and DBT, to create a customized treatment plan tailored to the individual's needs. Evidence suggests that these interventions increase treatment uptake and decrease relapse rates, offering a comprehensive approach that addresses both the psychological and the behavioral aspects of addiction. Ultimately, integrating behavioral therapies into more complete treatment programs has the potential to enhance not just individual prospects for recovery, but also more general public health outcomes in terms of substance abuse and addiction (Figure 2.23).

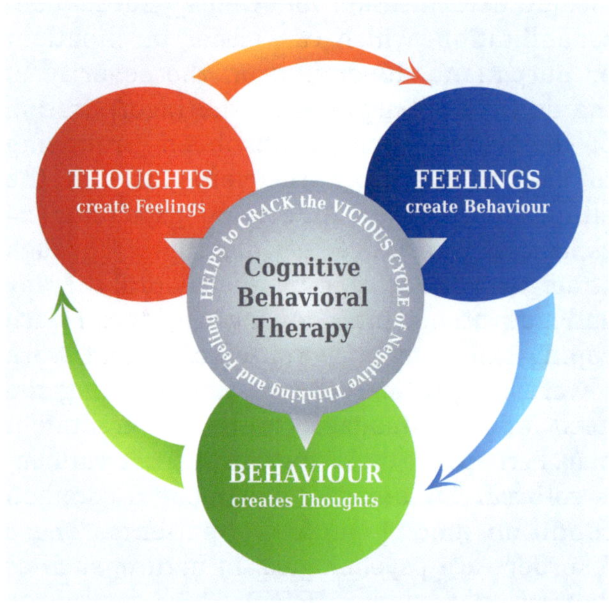
THOUGHTS
create Feelings
FEELINGS
create Behaviour
BEHAVIOUR
creates Thoughts
HELPS to CRACK the VICIOUS CYCLE of Negative Thinking and Feeling
Cognitive
Behavioral
Therapy

Figure 2.23. Cognitive behavioral therapy for addiction.

Source: https://sbdetox.com/wp-content/uploads/2023/02/Cognitive-Behavioral-Therapy-for-Addiction-1024x1024.png.

2.6.2. Medication-Assisted Treatment

Addiction and substance abuse treatment has evolved over the years, and medication-assisted treatment (MAT) is a prominent and effective approach. MAT refers to the use of medications combined with behavior therapies in the treatment of substance use disorders, particularly in alcohol and opioids. Research indicates that medications such as methadone, buprenorphine, and naltrexone can significantly reduce withdrawal syndrome, craving, and relapse rate and hence contribute to improved patient outcomes. By stabilizing patients with substance use disorders, MAT allows for more comprehensive treatment that incorporates counseling and support services and leads to long-term recovery in the long run. Importantly, MAT not only raises the recovery rate of an individual but also reduces the cost of substance abuse within the healthcare system, thereby becoming an essential intervention within public health efforts towards addiction (Wairimu, 2024). Despite the obvious benefits of MAT, access and implementation are plagued with problems. Stigma against drug abuse in the treatment of addiction deters individuals from undergoing it or taking prescribed drugs. In addition, healthcare providers lack adequate training in dispensing MAT, leading to inadequate access. Laws can similarly be barriers to MAT's availability in certain areas, particularly rural and resource-deficient ones. To combat these problems, policymakers and healthcare systems need to promote a better vision of MAT among providers and patients. Policies to reduce stigmatization, more training for professionals, and the extension of treatment access can significantly enhance the efficacy of MAT, making it a better-received addiction treatment (Çınaroğlu, 2024). In the broader treatment context of substance abuse, integrating MAT within an overall model of care is required to address the multifaceted aspects of addiction. This is not merely considering the biological aspects of substance use disorders, but also the psychological and social aspects leading to addiction. Through comprehension of the relationship between drug use and mental health, healthcare professionals can modify treatments to meet the unique needs of recovering patients. Furthermore, combining mental health treatments with MAT has synergistic effects and results in a more stable treatment environment. New strategies, such as digital health interventions and community-based interventions, are gaining increased attention, providing new avenues for assistance throughout treatment. On the whole, a unified strategy toward the use of MAT within an integrated overall system can reverse the lives of victims of substance abuse and addiction (Wairimu, 2024) (Figure 2.24).

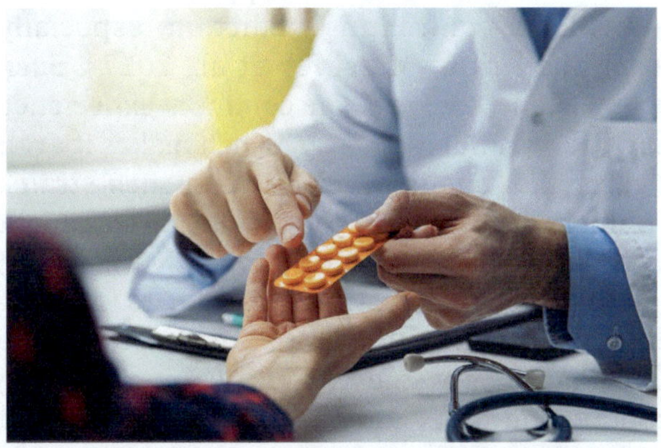

Figure 2.24. Medication-assisted treatment.

Source: https://magnoliaranchrecovery.com/wp-content/uploads/2024/09/Medication-Assisted-Treatment-in-Tennessee.jpg.

2.6.3. Support Groups and Community Resources

Community support and resources are central to the management of addiction and substance abuse, offering the services necessary to help individuals recover and sustain long-term sobriety. This establishment of such support systems is also important in areas with low access to healthcare, as evidenced by the demands in Franklin County. Neighborhood peer support groups, recovery houses, and clinics are lifelines for individuals undergoing addiction, providing not only moral support but practical guidance on overcoming drug addiction (Nilo et al., 2019). Through the establishment of community bonds, they provide individuals with the opportunity to share experiences and methods, which can positively impact a person in recovery on a profound level. The co-participant status of these groups also reduces the social stigma of addiction, facilitating higher levels of participation by individuals who feel isolated. Support groups also gain validity for their effectiveness by successfully raising retention in recovery programs. Research indicates that self-help groups are one of the most accessible modes of support available to individuals confronting addiction, especially in primary care (Meservey et al., 2017). Such groups tend to focus on common experience and shared understanding, which makes it even clearer that one is never alone in such straits. For most people, the entry into formal treatment is intimidating, but with supportive settings, this can become easy. In addition to offering emotional support, the groups may also provide information on safe withdrawal techniques, coping, and other key resources for sustained recovery and hence serve as the backbone of community response to drug addiction and alcoholism. As a last note, awareness about readily available community resources is paramount to healthcare professionals who may be the first point of contact for the addicted. A majority of such patients do not receive aid since healthcare providers are still uninformed about available local services for treating substance use because they have limited access to information (Meservey et al., 2017). Interventions that increase providers' awareness of support groups and resources can significantly improve patient outcomes by providing timely referrals and exposure to appropriate interventions. Additionally, the integration of community resource education into practice increases the likelihood that patients will be open to available support systems. Generally, all the above programs not only help in the recovery of single patients but also in the fight against substance abuse and addiction in society and healthier communities as a whole (Figure 2.25).

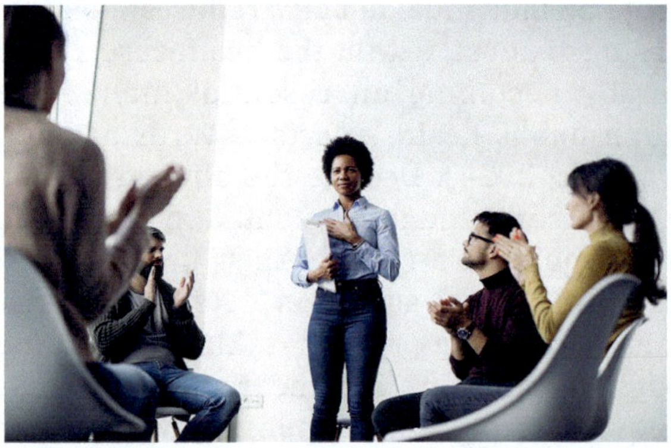

Figure 2.25. Support group for drug addiction.

Source: https://freebythesea.com/wp-content/uploads/2023/04/Benefits-of-Support-Groups-for-Substance-Abuse.jpeg.

Test Your Knowledge

1. What type of behavioral therapy is used for substance abuse?
2. What is medication-assisted treatment for substance abuse?

SUMMARY

In synthesizing the research on addiction and drug abuse, it is important to recognize the multifaceted character of the issue and its widespread consequences for both the individual and society as a whole. The statistics offered in this chapter illustrate that addiction is not only a personal failure but also a complex interplay of social, psychological, and physiological factors. For instance, studies have unveiled significant correlations between drug abuse and variables such as gender, religious values, and genetic history among university students. These findings underscore the importance of general health education programs, with particular attention to prevention and intervention, especially in school settings where susceptibility to experimentation is at its peak. Moreover, the stigma of drug abuse presents additional treatment and recovery difficulties. According to the literature, individuals suffering from substance use and mental illness disorders experience stigmatization differently, in that drug abuse is more socially discrediting than mental illness (Byrne et al., 2016). Stigma discourages individuals from seeking help by slamming the door shut on a successful recovery through the cycle of addiction. Therefore, challenging these social beliefs through targeted anti-stigma interventions is necessary because it can assist in generating a more helpful context for those in recovery and engender acceptance of addicted people. Finally, the conclusions drawn from reviewing existing literature highlight the importance of joint action on the part of health professionals, educators, and legislators if they are to successfully manage substance abuse. Intersecting community resources and educational approaches might prove beneficial for prevention as well as recovery. For instance, having drug awareness programs in high school that continue into university can be effective in preventing early drug use. Lastly, through the development of a culture of education, support, and understanding, society can make its initial step toward reducing the extent of substance misuse and associated harm, toward healthier communities and a better future for those affected by addiction. This is the predominant focus of this thesis.

The biology of drug abuse and addiction emphasizes the interplay of biological, psychological, and environmental processes that result in this multifaceted issue. The understanding of how drugs hijack the brain's reward systems is vital for addressing addiction. Scientists have learned that drugs of abuse hijack these reward mechanisms, ultimately deranging normal reward processes associated with basic needs like hunger and thirst. This alteration is at the cellular level, specifically in the nucleus accumbens, revealing a key molecular substrate—Rheb—that regulates neural responses to natural rewards and drug cues. All this informs us of the mechanistic basics of addiction and underscores the importance of integrative prevention and treatment strategies. Identification of such neural dynamics is crucial in developing evidence-based interventions for substance use disorders, which places the neurobiological foundations of addiction in focus (Tan et al., 2024). Coupled with the biological aspects of addiction, lifestyle medicine offers practical strategies for addressing substance abuse and recovery. The third edition of the book Lifestyle Medicine highlights the importance of lifestyle modification in treatment plans for substance use disorders. Within its paradigm, the Substance Abuse and Addiction segment identifies the focal point of behavioral change in achieving successful outcomes. Notably, the book incorporates evidence-based methods that address nutrition, exercise, and behavior therapy as core elements of recovery. These interventions, as well as addressing substance use disorder, also have benefits that extend to overall well-being. By emphasizing lifestyle change as the linchpin of substance abuse treatment, clinicians can promote long-term recovery and improved quality of life, and highlight the significance of lifestyle medicine principles (Dysinger, 2020). Further, the comprehensive approach to addiction illustrated in **Substance Abuse and Addiction** emphasizes addressing co-occurring disorders and the broader social environment of substance abuse. Addiction is not a standalone issue; rather, it is most commonly a consequence of mental illnesses, social issues, and environmental conditions. Treatment must address these underlying issues in addition to providing overall therapy. With the inclusion of behavioral health, community assistance, and lifestyle change, an even more holistic method emerges that has the capacity for long-term recovery. A multidisciplinary approach not only benefits those suffering from addiction but also supports larger public health policy efforts toward preventing substance abuse and promoting healthier communities. Finally, there should be an integrated approach that melds the biological, psychological, and social dimensions to address the prevalent issue of drug abuse (Dysinger, 2020;Tan et al., 2024).

KEY TERMS FROM THIS CHAPTER

Addiction	Alcohol
Benzodiazepines	Biology
Detoxification	Genetic predispositions
Illicit drugs	Marijuana
Peer pressure	Psychological flexibility
Psychological inflexibility	Psychology
Rehabilitation	Sleep disturbances

CRITICAL THINKING QUESTIONS

1. **Which neurotransmitter is primarily involved in the reward pathway affected by substance abuse?**
   a. Serotonin
   b. Dopamine
   c. Glutamate
   d. GABA
2. **Which of the following is the most commonly abused substance worldwide?**
   a. Cocaine
   b. Alcohol
   c. Cannabis
   d. Tobacco
3. **What is the hallmark symptom of opioid withdrawal?**
   a. Hallucinations
   b. Bradycardia
   c. Severe muscle aches and restlessness
   d. Seizures
4. **What is the most effective pharmacological treatment for nicotine dependence?**
   a. Methadone
   b. Bupropion or varenicline
   c. Naltrexone
   d. Disulfiram
5. **Which medication is used in the treatment of alcohol dependence to discourage drinking by causing unpleasant effects when alcohol is consumed?**
   a. Methadone
   b. Disulfiram
   c. Naltrexone
   d. Acamprosate

Short Answer Questions

1. What is meant by substance abuse?
2. What is addiction?
3. List the types of substances abused.
4. What are the causes of substance abuse?
5. What are the symptoms of addiction?

Answer to Critical Thinking Questions

1. (b); 2. (d); 3. (c); 4. (b); 5. (b).

REFERENCES

1. Hines, L. A., Morley, K. I., Rijsdijk, F., Strang, J., Agrawal, A., Nelson, E. C., Statham, D., Martin, N. G., & Lynskey, M. T. (2018). Overlap of heritable influences between cannabis use disorder, frequency of use and opportunity to use cannabis: trivariate twin modelling and implications for genetic design. *Psychological Medicine, 48*(16), 2786–2793. https://doi.org/10.1017/s0033291718000478Aguiniga, D., Pratt, J., Shelby, K., Cox, M., & Thompson, M. (2015). Over the edge: What should we do when alcohol and drug use become a problem to society? https://core.ac.uk/download/75781210.pdf (accessed on 14th July 2025).
2. Ali, M. O. (2023). Exploring drug & substance abuse implications 2023. *Scholars Academic Journal of Pharmacy*. https://www.semanticscholar.org/paper/a41ef3f9e290adb0e4e00702d009c0f639581872 (accessed on 14th July 2025).
3. Anderson, A. D. (2018). Quitting together: Formative research to develop a social marketing plan for smoking cessation among women in a residential treatment facility for substance abuse recovery. https://core.ac.uk/download/232584031.pdf (accessed on 14th July 2025).
4. Barrado-Moreno, V., Serrano-Ibáñez, E., Esteve, R., Ramírez-Maestre, C., & Sánchez-Meca, J. (2025). The role of psychological flexibility and inflexibility in substance addiction, abuse, or misuse: A systematic review and meta-analysis. *International Journal of Mental Health and Addiction*. https://www.semanticscholar.org/paper/5f2482982ac72498a8fe41d08763964924309368 (accessed on 14th July 2025).
5. Baysinger, A. N., & Gianessi, C. A. (2015). Addiction. *The Yale Journal of Biology and Medicine, 88*, 203–204. https://www.semanticscholar.org/paper/2e77056157def53ae8745930e3b29d8e8e2762e6 (accessed on 14th July 2025).
6. Becker, W. C., & Fiellin, D. A. (2020). When epidemics collide: Coronavirus disease 2019 (COVID-19) and the opioid crisis. *Annals of Internal Medicine, 173*, 59–60. https://doi.org/10.7326/m20-1210 (accessed on 14th July 2025).
7. Bozzola, E., Spina, G., Agostiniani, R., Barni, S., Russo, R., Scarpato, E., Di Mauro, A., et al. (2022). The use of social media in children and adolescents: Scoping review on the potential risks. *International Journal of Environmental Research and Public Health, 19*, 9960–9960. https://doi.org/10.3390/ijerph19169960 (accessed on 14th July 2025).
8. Brand, M., Young, K., Laier, C., Wölfling, K., & Potenza, M. N. (2016). Integrating psychological and neurobiological considerations regarding the development and maintenance of specific Internet-use disorders: An Interaction of Person-Affect-Cognition-Execution (I-PACE) model. *Neuroscience & Biobehavioral Reviews, 71*, 252–266. https://doi.org/10.1016/j.neubiorev.2016.08.033 (accessed on 14th July 2025).
9. Byrne, T. H., Corrigan, P., Harnish, A., et al. (2016). A comparison of substance use stigma and health stigma in a population of veterans with co-occurring mental health and substance use disorders. https://open.bu.edu/bitstream/2144/22787/1/FINAL%20DRAFT%20AH%20edits%208%201%202016_TB.pdf (accessed on 14th July 2025).
10. Cannon, Y. (2019). The kids are not alright: Leveraging existing health law to attack the opioid crisis upstream. https://core.ac.uk/download/225012727.pdf (accessed on 14th July 2025).
11. Cansız, A., & Koçhan, M. E. (2024). The impact of sexual abuse on addiction: A case study on food addiction. *Journal of Awareness*. https://www.semanticscholar.org/paper/a2b84c5ae096913bd4eb745cc0d86b46d0a89adb (accessed on 14th July 2025).

12. Chandler, A., Cooper, S., Cunningham-Burley, S., et al. (2018). Problematization and regulation: Bodies, risk, and recovery within the context of neonatal abstinence syndrome. https://core.ac.uk/download/293885458.pdf (accessed on 14th July 2025).

13. Charuni, T. (2024). Narrative review on the spectrum of diseases prevalent among substance-addicted populations and their interconnected health dynamics. *Journal of Science of the University of Kelaniya*. https://www.semanticscholar.org/paper/5541757f1920a7f9c40eb755728a1f51bfebef9b (accessed on 14th July 2025).

14. Çınaroğlu, M. (2024). Intersecting realities: Body dysmorphic disorder and substance abuse in women–A holistic treatment approach. *Sakarya Üniversitesi Kadın Araştırmaları Dergisi*. https://www.semanticscholar.org/paper/fefaf0c94bf5a5ea7eacfd7aaf5dc68156e74573 (accessed on 14th July 2025).

15. Clarke, D. E., González, M., Pereira, A., Boyce-Gaudreau, K., Waldman, C., & Demczuk, L. (2015). The impact of knowledge on attitudes of emergency department staff towards patients with substance related presentations: A quantitative systematic review protocol. *The JBI Database of Systematic Reviews and Implementation Reports, 13*, 133–145. https://doi.org/10.11124/jbisrir-2015-2203 (accessed on 14th July 2025).

16. Crnić, K., & Kovačević, M. (2020). New psychoactive substances: Challenges. *Hospital Pharmacology – International Multidisciplinary Journal*. https://www.semanticscholar.org/paper/191aa6fc3f07ca454cd038b7cc20203da7ea26a6 (accessed on 14th July 2025).

17. Cruz Valiño, J. M., Delgado-Lobete, L., Gándara Gafo, B., et al. (2020). Individual and environmental factors associated with tobacco smoking, alcohol abuse and illegal drug consumption in university students: A mediating analysis. https://core.ac.uk/download/323288158.pdf (accessed on 14th July 2025).

18. De Pauw, S., Meulewaeter, F., & Vanderplasschen, W. (2019). Mothering, substance use disorders and intergenerational trauma transmission: An attachment-based perspective. https://core.ac.uk/download/237011860.pdf (accessed on 14th July 2025).

19. Döring, N., & Walter, R. (2022). Alcohol portrayals on social media. *DOCA–Database of Variables for Content Analysis*. https://www.semanticscholar.org/paper/3ec3419afe9e7cfb3090a187390e9fc3082335bc (accessed on 14th July 2025).

20. Dwivedi, Y. K., Hughes, L., Baabdullah, A. M., Ribeiro-Navarrete, S., Giannakis, M., Al-Debei, M. M., Dennehy, D., et al. (2022). Metaverse beyond the hype: Multidisciplinary perspectives on emerging challenges, opportunities, and agenda for research, practice and policy. *International Journal of Information Management, 66*, 102542–102542. https://doi.org/10.1016/j.ijinfomgt.2022.102542 (accessed on 14th July 2025).

21. Dysinger, W. (2020). Lifestyle medicine (3rd ed.). *American Journal of Lifestyle Medicine, 14*, 107–108. https://www.semanticscholar.org/paper/7a4028f0e9aa6232850d2502e33a20527e2c4f13 (accessed on 14th July 2025).

22. El-Olaimy El-Shiekh, H., Farouk, H., Abd-Elmaksoud, S., & ElNawasany, A. M. (2024). The role of parenting attitudes towards adolescents with substance use disorder: A study of an Egyptian sample. *Benha Journal of Applied Sciences*. https://www.semanticscholar.org/paper/e588d418011eb9591f9b6e03cced056ccecab23e (accessed on 14th July 2025).

23. Ferraguti, G., Lucarelli, M., & Pascale, E. (2015). Alcohol addiction: A molecular biology perspective. https://core.ac.uk/download/54518723.pdf (accessed on 14th July 2025).

24. Forțu, A. C., & Rada, C. (2025). Drug use and alcohol abuse among inmates–Causes, consequences, prevention. *Anthropological Researches and Studies*. https://www.semanticscholar.org/paper/0bd422bdca019a080057fec05efa06775af0782f (accessed on 14th July 2025).

25. Gomes, N., & Paccione-Dyszlewski, M. (2024). Decoding youth substance use: Insights and strategies. *The Brown University Child and Adolescent Behavior Letter*. https://www.semanticscholar.org/paper/94436648370eec014bb4862da7e90848d947ff1f (accessed on 14th July 2025).

26. Herrera-Palacios, A. (2024). Intervention based on dialectical behavioral therapy for the treatment of problems related to substance use. *Mexican Journal of Medical Research ICSA*. https://www.semanticscholar.org/paper/99af14e10a78c8cc3054853142fd54dc5c9f1387 (accessed on 14th July 2025).

27. Holmes, R., Patel, A., & Desai, A. P. (2022). Psychiatric disorders and their treatment: Impact of outcomes in patients with chronic liver disease. *Clinical Liver Disease, 20*, 32–37. https://doi.org/10.1002/cld.1204 (accessed on 14th July 2025).

28. Karki, P. (2024). Dynamics of drug addiction and abuse in India: Socio-economic profiles of individuals in treatment for drug addiction in northwest India. *South Asian Journal of Social Studies and Economics*. https://www.semanticscholar.org/paper/e09b4a35d312e4f733f111c5bee46aba7162aa30 (accessed on 14th July 2025).

29. Kouhnavardi, S., Ecevitoglu, A., Dragačević, V., Sanna, F., Arias-Sandoval, E., Kalaba, P., Kirchhofer, M., et al. (2022). A novel and selective dopamine transporter inhibitor, (S)-MK-26, promotes hippocampal synaptic plasticity and restores effort-related motivational dysfunctions. *Biomolecules, 12*. https://www.semanticscholar.org/paper/b487489fb32a9ce4182d24e15541df002df6a772 (accessed on 14th July 2025).

30. Madu, L. U., Sharp, J., & Bellflower, B. (2021). Efficacy of integrating CBT for mental health care into substance abuse treatment in patients with comorbid disorders of substance abuse and mental illness. https://www.semanticscholar.org/paper/80bb555c8554eb4d46593b0cc3330921adaf11f0 (accessed on 14th July 2025).

31. Manurung, L. (2024). The impact of drug abuse on families and society (Literature review). *MSJ: Majority Science Journal*. https://www.semanticscholar.org/paper/17451b0294cfc58c6b6c2aabd2e6e725df388582 (accessed on 14th July 2025).

32. McKean, L., & Shapiro, S. K. (2004). Sentencing reform for nonviolent offenses: Benefits and estimated savings for Illinois. https://core.ac.uk/download/71339201.pdf (accessed on 14th July 2025).

33. Meservey, A. J. (2017). Addiction recovery support: Connecting primary care providers and community resources. https://core.ac.uk/download/84397660.pdf (accessed on 14th July 2025).

34. Mohammed Nawi, A., Ismail, R., Ibrahim, F., Hassan, M. R., Abdul Manaf, M. R., Amit, N., Ibrahim, N., et al. (2021). Risk and protective factors of drug abuse among adolescents: A systematic review. *BMC Public Health, 21*. https://doi.org/10.1186/s12889-021-11906-2 (accessed on 14th July 2025).

35. Morse, S. J. (2006). Addiction, genetics, and criminal responsibility. https://core.ac.uk/download/62553458.pdf (accessed on 14th July 2025).

36. Newton, D. E. (2016). *Youth Substance Abuse.* https://www.semanticscholar.org/paper/8c2ffb3e3dcccbda8dc5deb06d56c52a8dcf5d28 (accessed on 14th July 2025).

37. Nilo, M. (2019). Social support groups focused on substance abuse and addiction available to patients in Franklin County, Vermont. https://core.ac.uk/download/223071499.pdf (accessed on 14th July 2025).

38. Parolin, M., & Simonelli, A. (2016). Attachment theory and maternal drug addiction: The contribution to parenting interventions. https://core.ac.uk/download/53531260.pdf (accessed on 14th July 2025).

39. Pascoe, M. C., Hetrick, S., & Parker, A. (2019). The impact of stress on students in secondary school and higher education. *International Journal of Adolescence and Youth, 25*, 104–112. https://doi.org/10.1080/02673843.2019.1596823 (accessed on 14th July 2025).

40. Reeves, C. (2019). Medical rhetoric and the sympathetic "inebriet": 1870–1930. https://core.ac.uk/download/286537046.pdf (accessed on 14th July 2025).

41. Siddiqui, J., Eldous, A. M., Qureshi, S., Alotaibi, H. M., Hamdan, S., & Almahruqi, A. A. (2025). The prevalence of sleep disorders among substance abusers admitted to drug de-addiction unit at Eradah and Mental Health Complex, Taif, Saudi Arabia. *Journal of Psychiatry Psychology and Behavioral Research.* https://www.semanticscholar.org/paper/b5a927b6f5c42952de494bf87aa2bd3c0593081f (accessed on 14th July 2025).

42. Simpson, J. B. (2022). Using intentional relationship building and community presence to minister to an addicted population in Cookeville, Tennessee. https://core.ac.uk/download/516439676.pdf (accessed on 14th July 2025).

43. Sivaprakash, G., Vasudevan, V. M. K., Rajendran, S., Marudhan, A., Lakshmanan, J., Anthonysamy, C., & Muthuchamy, P. (2025). Breaking the chains–A descriptive study on how substance abuse affects daily functioning and mental well-being. *International Journal on Science and Technology.* https://www.semanticscholar.org/paper/512d8b69dc7d6e5a410dc050348e007c8c64d6c3 (accessed on 14th July 2025).

44. Sohn, S. Y., Rees, P., Wildridge, B., Kalk, N. J., & Carter, B. (2019). Prevalence of problematic smartphone usage and associated mental health outcomes amongst children and young people: A systematic review, meta-analysis and GRADE of the evidence. *BMC Psychiatry, 19.* https://doi.org/10.1186/s12888-019-2350-x (accessed on 14th July 2025).

45. Soltaninejad, M., Naderi, Y., Rouhi, L., & Banazadeh, M. (2024). Substance abuse and sexual functioning: An overview of mechanisms. *Addiction & Health, 16*, 286–296. https://www.semanticscholar.org/paper/e93d60f1a6efd3d4a8a129999727ac7db537a66a (accessed on 14th July 2025).

46. Stangl, A., Earnshaw, V. A., Logie, C. H., van Brakel, W. H., Simbayi, L. C., Barré, I., & Dovidio, J. F. (2019). The Health Stigma and Discrimination Framework: A global, crosscutting framework to inform research, intervention development, and policy on health-related stigmas. *BMC Medicine, 17.* https://doi.org/10.1186/s12916-019-1271-3 (accessed on 14th July 2025).

47. Taha, S. I., & Hadi, S. A. (2024). The phenomenon of drug and psychotropic substance abuse–Traditional and digital–Causes, effects, solutions. *European Journal of Contemporary Business Law & Technology: Cyber Law, Blockchain, and Legal Innovations.* https://www.semanticscholar.org/paper/793330861ff075e0c5f5cc5f82de4b8da4b08214 (accessed on 14th July 2025).

48. Tan, B., Browne, C. J., Nöbauer, T., Vaziri, A., Friedman, J. M., & Nestler, E. (2024). Drugs of abuse hijack a mesolimbic pathway that processes homeostatic need. *Science (New York, N.Y.), 384*, eadk6742–eadk6742. https://www.semanticscholar.org/paper/5c21c456aff5bb4a6287f3df1508c5b097c04f5d (accessed on 14th July 2025).

49. Tarantino, G., Cataldi, M., & Citro, V. (2022). Could alcohol abuse and dependence on junk foods inducing obesity and/or illicit drug use represent danger to liver in young people with altered psychological/relational spheres or emotional problems? *International Journal of Molecular Sciences, 23*. https://www.semanticscholar.org/paper/315e5c1f62144d61e3131333caaf20ccff63a770 (accessed on 14th July 2025).

50. Turchick, A., Lacy, M., & Horien, C. (2016). The aging brain. *The Yale Journal of Biology and Medicine, 89*, 1–2. https://www.semanticscholar.org/paper/8433fb456c8ac13dccb87b8dd721c1a348932ddf (accessed on 14th July 2025).

51. Volkow, N. D. (2020). Collision of the COVID-19 and addiction epidemics. *Annals of Internal Medicine, 173*, 61–62. https://doi.org/10.7326/m20-1212 (accessed on 14th July 2025).

52. Wairimu, M. G. (2024). Addressing the dual challenges of substance abuse and HIV/AIDS in Uganda via innovative approaches. *Research Output Journal of Biological and Applied Science*. https://www.semanticscholar.org/paper/cc250c594ef5aa24f04a5132dc045ffbe1ca36e4 (accessed on 14th July 2025).

53. Wallman-Stokes, C., Bechtolsheimer, G., Appel, J., Gable, J., Chiu, J., Rosqueta, K., & Hobble, R. (2015). Lifting the burden of addiction: Philanthropic opportunities to address substance use disorders in the United States. https://core.ac.uk/download/75783859.pdf (accessed on 14th July 2025).

54. Wen, L. S., & Sadeghi, N. B. (2020). The opioid crisis and the 2020 US election: Crossroads for a national epidemic. *The Lancet, 396*, 1316–1318. https://doi.org/10.1016/s0140-6736(20)32113-9 (accessed on 14th July 2025).

55. Wooton, N. (2021). The opioid epidemic: How our society is contributing to the stigma. https://core.ac.uk/download/520100780.pdf (accessed on 14th July 2025).

GERIATRIC CARE

3

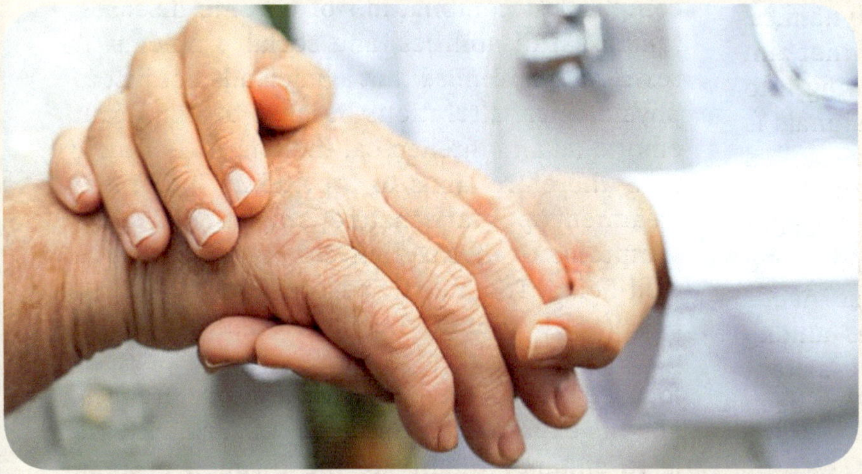

LEARNING OBJECTIVES

After studying this chapter, you will be able to:

1. Describe the aging population
2. Describe the common health issues in the elderly
3. Understand the geriatric assessment
4. Describe ethe care models for the elderly
5. Understand the role of healthcare professionals
6. Understand the role of family and caregiver support in geriatric care

Introduction

With an ageing population, the demand for an efficient framework in geriatric care is all the more apparent. The rise of the geriatric population in the United States has significant implications for healthcare services, most notably in specialty sectors such as oncology. Because the diagnosis of cancer is largely a concern for the elderly, there is a particular surgical management that is needed, which effectively addresses the unique needs of this age group. A comprehensive pre-surgical geriatric assessment is a critical component in optimizing care in patients who are oncogeriatric. Despite being recognized by medical professionals as an essential step, it remains underutilized, indicating a significant gap in the provision of quality geriatric care. This is both a challenge and an opportunity for healthcare practitioners to rethink how they work, so that older people are accorded the dignity and specialized care they require (Lampugnane et al., 2017). The barriers to the use of comprehensive geriatric assessment are multifactorial, yet time is the most significant. Doctors, particularly those in surgical fields, have busy timetables that limit their capacity to conduct comprehensive assessments. This deficit not only undermines the ability to adequately stratify risk among geriatric patients but also jeopardizes the quality of care being provided. Current research indicates that certain domains within these assessments, such as the Frailty Index and the Social Support Survey, are most predictive of surgical outcomes. Understanding these measures is essential for geriatric clinicians who must navigate complex health dynamics. Hence, creating educational programs that aim to integrate geriatric assessment training into curricula for future healthcare professionals is vital so that they can ultimately be more skilled in elderly care (Lampugnane et al., 2017). In addition to clinical assessments, the broader context of eldercare, especially for those who require home healthcare services, also needs to be considered. High turnover rates among home care caregivers have been a persistent issue, most notably because there has not been proper training and support.

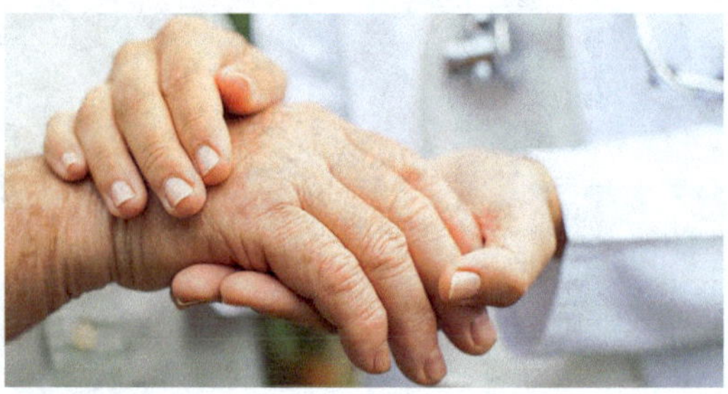

Figure 3.1. Geriatric care.

Source: https://papayacare.com/wp-content/uploads/2023/09/Geriatric-Care-Papayacare.jpg.

The Institute of Medicine's 2008 report recommendations speak to the necessity of improving caregiver education and training. This initiative is intended to address the numerous challenges caregivers face when serving geriatric clients, with emphasis on developing a sustainable workforce. By investing in the education and care of these professionals, we may be able to enhance the quality of geriatric care, consistent with the broader goal of developing a superior system of geriatric care (Figure 3.1).

Definition of Geriatric Care

Geriatric medicine is a specialty of medicine that takes on the unique health issues of older adults, generally characterized by their complicated combination of chronic diseases, functional disabilities, and social problems. It rests on the premise that aging leads not just to physiological alterations but also to significant emotional and intellectual challenges. Geriatric care, therefore, aims to provide an integrated treatment approach that not only attends to the symptoms of disease but also to psychosocial well-being. The holistic perspective is required because it honors the individuality of each patient and makes the intervention person-focused, respecting their values, preferences, and life experiences. The spirit of geriatric care is to enhance quality of life through optimal interventions, ranging from disease prevention and chronic disease management to palliative care, to ensure a dignified and fulfilling life for the elderly. A key element of successful geriatric care is the employment of integrated assessment to direct clinical decision-making. These assessments consider various fields, including physical health, mental health, social environment, and functional ability, allowing medical physicians to formulate a general treatment plan. Evidence indicates that older individuals are not properly represented in standard diagnostic criteria, and as such, the geriatric assessment plays a key role in illuminating their specific health needs. Despite the recognized utility of thorough pre-surgical testing, studies suggest that fewer than a quarter of oncogeriatric patients receive it, underscoring the need for systemic changes in healthcare processes. Increasing awareness and education among clinicians about these tests is of prime importance, as it can help optimize care planning tailored specifically to older individuals, with the ultimate implication of better health outcomes and greater patient satisfaction (Lampugnani et al., 2017). Allows. Also, geriatric care heightens the focus on the complexities entailed in the increased complexity of health needs in older populations. The confluence of age, chronic disease, and vulnerability can significantly impact both costs and the quality of health care provision. By reviewing the elements of care management, the potential to enhance service quality and effectiveness emerges as a central focus. Successful geriatric models of care integrate interdisciplinary approaches that involve not only healthcare professionals but also family and community networks. As research unfolds, it is evident that maximized management of care can limit healthcare costs while concurrently improving patient outcomes. Thus, geriatric care not only has the immediate purpose of treating the latter's direct health ailments but also acts as a model for systemic change within the healthcare community and is hence a vital area for ongoing research and practice (Berry-Millett et al., 2009) (Figure 3.2).

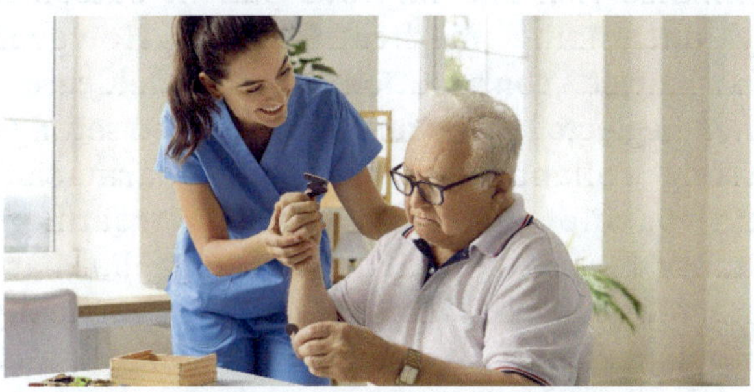

Figure 3.2. Definition of geriatric care.

Source: https://slchc.edu/wp-content/uploads/2023/10/geriatric-care-SLCHC-scaled-2560x1280.jpeg.

Importance of Geriatric Care in Modern Society

With society entering an era characterized by an expanding aging population, geriatric care is not emphasized enough. The population profile is characterized by a sharp increase in the number of individuals aged 65 and older, who currently account for the vast majority of the population. The unique health issues of this set of individuals and the prevalence of chronic diseases among elderly people require that there be special emphasis on healthcare. Older patients are often perceived through past stereotypes associating aging and weakness with dependency. Such fallacies have the potential to produce substandard care and treatment, particularly in oncology, when, as suggested, two-thirds of cancer diagnoses fall into this patient group, putting a high premium on specialist geriatric care (Swaminathan et al., 2015). It is crucial to correct such problems to ensure elderly individuals receive proper medical care that is a reflection of their depth and uniqueness. Incorporating holistic-oriented practices into the assessment of geriatric patients is essential for addressing the intricate needs of older adults. Traditional medical assessments fail to account for central elements of a patient's life experiences, particularly emotional and spiritual ones. The comprehensive geriatric assessment (CGA) is a powerful tool for developing tailored treatment plans; however, it typically fails to incorporate factors such as religious and spiritual beliefs, which play an influential role in outcomes. Ellingson's review points out that this model of assessment must transform to better understand the old patient's situation and needs (Ellingson et al., 2009). By incorporating these key dimensions into the CGA framework, doctors can develop a more compassionate and effective model of geriatric care, thereby enhancing the well-being of older persons. In addition, social implications of effective geriatric care extend far beyond the individual's well-being. With the increasing percentage of the population entering old age, the sustainability of healthcare systems is in greater jeopardy. Good geriatric care can help ease the strain on healthcare resources by preventing complications from chronic diseases and reducing hospital stays. By formulating multi-disciplinary care plans that include both health and quality of life, health systems can improve health outcomes while simultaneously containing overall costs. Policymakers ought to be cognizant of the economic and ethical dimensions involved in elderly care. Encouraging innovations in geriatric health care will not merely serve the elderly but also strengthen society as a whole and ensure that the needs of an aging and diverse population are recognized proactively and with consideration (Figure 3.3).

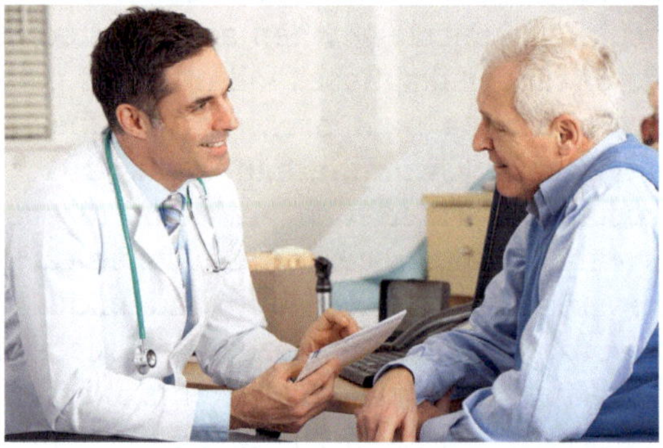

Figure 3.3. Importance of geriatric care.

Source: https://sa1s3optim.patientpop.com/assets/images/provider/photos/2394779.jpg.

3.1. The Aging Population

Learning Outcome

1. Understand the demographic trends in aging
2. Know the impact of aging on healthcare systems
3. Describe the challenges faced by the elderly

The aging population is one of the enduring demographic shifts that challenges healthcare systems worldwide. As life expectancy increases, the proportion of elderly individuals in the population is rising rapidly. The transition calls for a reframing of health care services, particularly geriatric care, as the elderly have complex health issues. One of the pressing problems in geriatric health care is the prevalence of oral disorders among older adults, as indicated in the reports of the Ministry of Health Malaysia. The prevalence of dental caries and periodontal diseases is high and presents a tremendous challenge to dentists serving the elderly. For dentists to effectively treat these conditions, it is vital that dental students are taught geriatric dentistry. This advanced learning not only enhances students' understanding of the unique needs of geriatric patients but also equips them to provide comprehensive care, thereby improving overall health in this population (Husna et al., 2009). Another vital aspect of care for the elderly is treating polypharmacy in aging populations, particularly those with cancer. Polypharmacy, or concurrent use of numerous drugs, is risky in the potential for drug-drug interactions and side effects, particularly in these patients with numerous comorbid disorders. Among many elderly cancer patients, treatment regimens consist of multiple neoplastic medications, so their pharmaceutical care is even more complicated. It has been noted that the involvement of clinical pharmacists in the management of polypharmacy would minimize risk and improve patient outcomes by optimizing medication use. However, pharmacists' contribution to older adult care is often neglected in resource-constrained settings. Strong collaboration between pharmacists and oncologists can enhance treatment quality for older patients, making pharmacy interventions critical to address the complexity of polypharmacy in older populations (Khanal et al., 2019). Furthermore, the increasing number of older individuals has broader social implications that should not be disregarded. As older individuals increasingly require specialty care, social systems must transform to meet their diverse needs. Community program participation, availability of transport, and social networks are necessary to enable older persons to reach health facilities effectively. Also, the growing population of older persons living independently necessitates integrated home care plans and policies that support them in maintaining their independence without jeopardizing their welfare. With increasingly aware health providers, older patients can be served more effectively to address both medical and non-medical problems. It requires a multidisciplinary approach involving different sectors of services, such as healthcare, social services, and community organizations, to create an enabling environment that supports the aging population in maintaining their quality of life and good health (Figure 3.4).

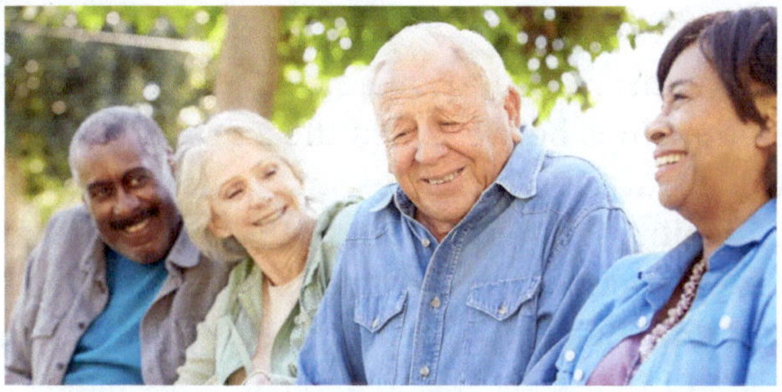

Figure 3.4. The aging population.

Source: https://harvestportfolios.com/wp-content/uploads/2023/08/How-Aging-Population-Affect-Healthcare-Sector.webp.

3.1.1. Demographic Trends in Aging

With the world's aging population, demographic trends are showing dramatic changes with significant implications for geriatric services. One of the most striking changes is longer life expectancy with declining fertility rates, a phenomenon not seen only in industrially developed nations but also in nations like Malta. The transition from a traditional pyramidal age structure to a block structure reflects a growing older-to-younger proportion of the population. The implications of these population changes are widespread, as populations must adapt to support an increasing number of older persons. With declining numbers of working-age adults, governments face the challenge of ensuring resources and services are adequate to support the needs of an aging population, and therefore there is a need for integrated geriatric care strategies that promote healthy aging and community engagement (Formosa et al., 2013). With demographic changes, the evolving view of cognitive health among the elderly has created pressing issues about geriatric assessment. Recent inter-organizational conferences, such as the one hosted by the National Academy of Neuropsychology, highlight the necessity for standardized screening for cognitive impairment in the medical environment. These issues highlight the multidimensionality of aging since cognitive impairments contribute importantly to an older individual's overall management of health. Participants at the summit not only discussed who should be screened but also underscored the importance of using validated screening tools appropriate to the individual cultural and educational levels of the target populations.

This approach highlights an essential aspect of care for older adults: the need for high-order, culturally appropriate methods to assess and address the characteristic problems they face in maintaining cognitive status (Adler et al., 2018). Also, the role of older people in the workplace and society is shifting, as observed through an active aging and engagement model. Malta's demographic trends show how older people increasingly make a positive contribution to society in a range of roles, such as caregiving, volunteering, and even employment. This process not only allows older people to feel a sense of contribution but also allows society as a whole to address complex social needs. The social policy of active aging emphasizes settings that enable older persons to live independently while receiving appropriate health and social care. As populations age, geriatric care models must shift to enable older people to remain vibrant, engaged, and valued contributors to society (Formosa et al., 2013).

3.1.2. Impact of Aging on Healthcare Systems

As the population ages, healthcare systems face overwhelming challenges that require broad reforms to meet the evolving needs of older adults. The increasing number of elderly individuals suffering from chronic conditions and functional impairments not only overwhelms healthcare resources but also necessitates new patterns of care that put prevention and management at the center. Evidence-based policies that promote care coordination and facilitate patient self-management have become central strategies for enhancing geriatric care. In addition to improving health outcomes, these strategies enable more efficient use of healthcare resources, which, in turn, benefits both providers and patients within a beleaguered system. Also, setting a priority on the palliative care options for elderly patients can significantly enhance the quality of life, reflecting the urgent need for healthcare systems to adapt to the complexities involved in an aging population (Morton et al., 2015). The urgent need for cognitive health screening in the aging population further underscores the significance of aging in healthcare systems. With rising cognitive impairments such as Alzheimer's disease and other forms of dementia, health care professionals have a responsibility to prioritize early detection and intervention strategies. Recent discussions, including the one held during the National Academy of Neuropsychology's Summit, highlighted the importance of creating standard screening protocols for cognitive impairment in clinical care.

The screenings will help detect individuals at risk and provide appropriate attention and management of associated morbidity. Because cognitive impairment tends to complicate treatment for chronic conditions, robust screening and ongoing evaluation are essential to the delivery of effective, tailored geriatric care, thereby relieving pressure on the healthcare system from the demands of aging (Adler et al., 2018). Better geriatric care is not only the responsibility of healthcare providers; involvement by policymakers, families, and caregivers is also essential. Addressing the multifaceted challenges posed by an aging population requires a collaborative approach that includes long-term care financing and workforce development strategies. Properly supporting family caregivers, who may be able to fill important roles in caring for elderly relatives, is critical to preserving home care choices and alleviating pressure on healthcare systems.

Furthermore, developing collaborative relationships between healthcare organizations and local communities may improve the availability, continuity, and quality of care for older persons. Collaborative approaches are key to building a comprehensive healthcare system that addresses the varied and changing needs of the elderly population, thereby providing them with the respectful and effective care that they deserve (Morton et al., 2015) (Figure 3.5).

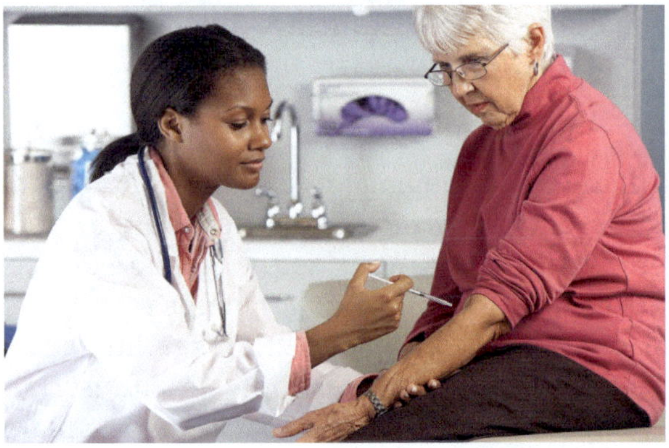

Figure 3.5. The impact of the aging population on healthcare.

Source: https://images.squarespace-cdn.com/content/v1/53023f77e4b0f0275ec6224a/1504144875073-H78EQ8APUME87B5CCC32/Depositphotos_24655247_m.jpg?format=1500w.

3.1.3. Challenges Faced by the Elderly

The older population faces multifaceted problems that affect their health-related quality of life, most of which are related to healthcare. As one ages, they tend to face a myriad of long-term chronic diseases like heart disease, diabetes, and arthritis that should be treated in an integrated manner. The complexity of care introduces an enormous burden on the elderly, caregivers, and the healthcare system. Moreover, the lack of preventative policies and appropriate interventions exacerbates these problems. According to a systematic review, evidence-based policies for prioritizing prevention and care coordination are crucial but are not adequately implemented to address these populations' healthcare needs. Such interventions may help build capacity, enabling older individuals to manage their own health, ultimately resulting in better health and greater independence in old age (Morton et al., 2015). Social isolation is another critical concern for the elderly, beyond health issues. Many of the elderly are plagued by the loss of social networks as a result of retirement, the death of peers, or mobility limitations, precipitating depression and isolation. These social problems further interrupt their mobility to engage in community activities or access requisite services, engendering a vicious cycle that worsens their overall health. To counteract this, health professionals must ensure that social interaction is a core component of geriatric care interventions. More robust community activities and initiatives that promote connectivity and interaction can be a useful solution. By establishing socialization settings, the significant psychological load that accompanies isolation may be reduced, ultimately improving mental wellness and overall quality of life for the elderly (Morton et al., 2015). Another serious issue affecting the elderly is the sustainability of caregiver support, which is essential to their care continuum. Turnover among home care aides seriously jeopardizes the quality of care the elderly individuals receive. It is caused by issues such as low pay, stressful working conditions, and limited opportunities for career advancement that discourage specialists from remaining in the field. The shocking statistics underscore the need for more training and compensation for caregivers to drive up retention levels and ensure continuity of care for older Americans. Initiatives such as the Community College Caregiver Training Initiative align with recommendations from prominent organizations, such as the Institute of Medicine, that focus on improving education and support for caregivers. By solving these workforce-related problems, a more stable and productive caregiving environment can be established that will directly impact the elderly (Figure 3.6).

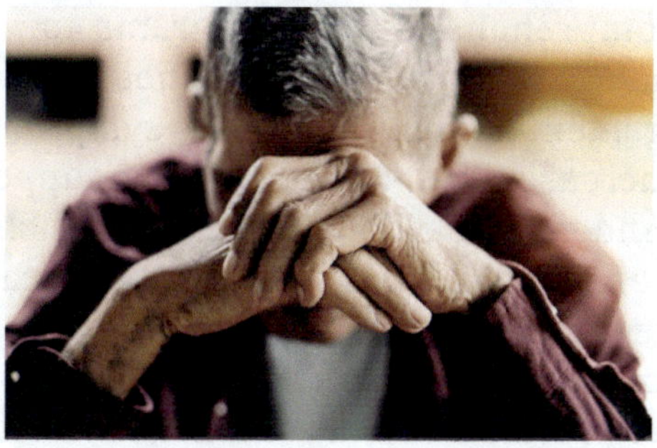

Figure 3.6. Challenges facing the elderly.

Source: https://www.griswoldcare.com/wp-content/uploads/2024/04/shutterstock_701935606-1.jpg.

Test Your Knowledge

1. What are the demographic trends in aging?
2. What is the impact of aging on healthcare systems?

3.2. Common Health Issues in the Elderly

Learning Outcome

1. Describe the chronic diseases and conditions in the geriatric population
2. Understand the mental health concerns
3. Describe the mobility and physical limitations of older adults

The elderly are faced with a high incidence of health issues, and chronic diseases are more common because they are brought about by the process of aging. Diseases such as arthritis, diabetes, and hypertension significantly affect the well-being of the elderly. These diseases are likely to require long-term management and may lead to complications if not closely monitored. For instance, arthritis can restrict movement, and consequently, the physical activity is reduced, whereas diabetes necessitates tight dietary control and regular monitoring of blood glucose levels. The high prevalence of these conditions underscores the need for targeted interventions and comprehensive care programs for these patients, tailored to their unique needs. Effective management not only minimizes symptoms but also increases well-being, thereby supporting independence in older people. Hence, chronic disease management is a constant, critical part of care for the geriatric population to ensure an acceptable quality of life. Polypharmacy is another prevalent health condition in the elderly, particularly those who have several chronic diseases. As elderly individuals are given a number of medications for the treatment of their chronic conditions, the polypharmacy-related risks are higher. Adverse drug reaction, drug-drug interaction, and medication nonadherence can complicate the treatment regimen and lead to severe health consequences. A critical in-depth analysis reveals that polypharmacy is underemphasized in clinical practice but carries severe risks among high-risk elderly patients. Current research highlights the critical role of clinical pharmacists in mitigating these risks by reviewing medication regimens and providing individualized pharmaceutical care. As Khanal et al. (2019) note, it is important to identify and manage the consequences of polypharmacy through a multi-disciplinary process in which clinical pharmacists take an active role on the healthcare team to ensure elderly patients receive safe and effective medication management. Finally, mental illness, such as depression and anxiety, is more and more common among the elderly, frequently complicated by physical health issues and social isolation. Emotional disturbances in older people can have serious consequences for their overall health outcomes, including limiting the management of existing chronic conditions. Even though the problems are acknowledged by health professionals, geriatric assessments that cover mental health assessment are underutilized. Literature review highlights that such assessments are important in estimating morbidity and mortality among elderly patients and identifying areas such as the Geriatric Depression Screening that are sensitive to change among this group. This clinical practice gap highlights the importance of integrating mental health assessment into geriatric practice, as efforts on the psychological dimension are core to ensuring quality of life and treatment benefits for oncogeriatric patients, as hypothesized by Lampugnani et al. (2017) (Figure 3.7).

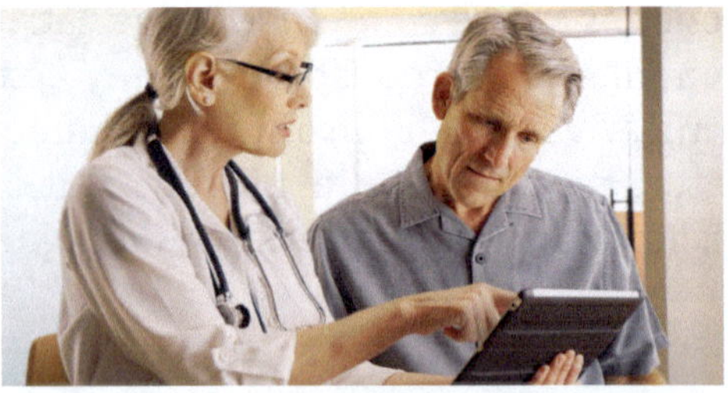

Figure 3.7. Most common senior health problems.

Source: https://s11727.pcdn.co/wp-content/uploads/2018/06/what-are-the-most-common-health-problems-of-older-adults.jpg.

3.2.1. Chronic Diseases and Conditions

The burden of diseases and chronic conditions among the elderly population presents an actual challenge to health facilities around the globe. Aging comes with the occurrence of ailments such as hypertension, diabetes, and cardiovascular disease that are likely to have an incapacitating effect on individuals and lower the quality of life. Evidence indicates that close to 80% of older individuals have one or more chronic illnesses, with most finding it difficult to cope with more than one condition simultaneously. The management of these diseases requires a comprehensive approach that incorporates early detection, patient education, and interdisciplinary treatment. Integration of these elements is able to enhance cure rates as well as allow older patients to be active collaborators in the process of treatment, potentially decreasing the burden on healthcare services and families, too. The management of chronic diseases is one of the problems that is made more difficult by the existence of unrecognized depression in geriatric individuals. Up to 40% of older people who have a chronic disease may remain undiagnosed with depression, significantly influencing their ability to retain important healthcare information and comply with treatment instructions (Wynn-Grundy et al., 2016). Depression is viewed to take place via cognitive disruption, which undermines the elderly's ability to concentrate and acquire information related to their healthcare. Furthermore, the convergence of chronic disease and mental illness calls for an integrated care model that treats both physiological and psychological elements simultaneously. Promoting depression detection and treatment can immensely assist healthcare providers in chronic disease management and enhance elderly patients' well-being, leading to improved health outcomes. Policy initiatives aimed at improving elderly care often target the implementation of research-based programs that support the management of chronic disease and facilitate patient self-management (Morton et al., 2015). Studies have shown that intervention programs focused on overall care coordination and preventive health services lead to better health outcomes for older adults. Despite strong evidence for such interventions, the gap persists in translating this evidence into large-scale policy action. Measures that aim to empower patients through self-management strategies and provide robust support systems for caregivers and healthcare providers are of paramount importance. With the increasing population of older adults, it is imperative that health policies evolve to encompass these vital areas so that the geriatric population receives proper care that addresses their complex health needs (Figure 3.8).

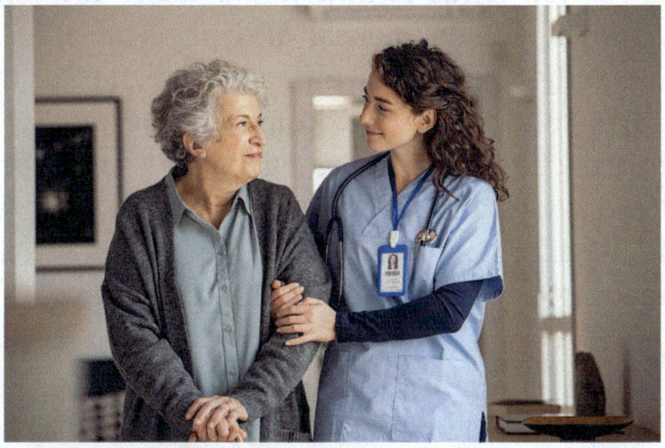

Figure 3.8. Common chronic diseases in elderly people.

Source: https://www.toplinemd.com/carreras-medical-center/wp-content/uploads/sites/12/2023/10/Young-Caregiver-Helping-Senior-Woman-Walking.jpg.

3.2.2. Mental Health Concerns

The intersection of geriatric medicine and mental health presents a primary area for concern, particularly with undiagnosed depression among the elderly. It has been discovered that a significant percentage of elderly patients with chronic illness may be undiagnosed, and up to

40% of them have depression (Wynn-Grundy et al., 2016). This inability to recognize always has the consequence of poor retention of health training, as depression symptoms, such as impaired concentration, get in the way of the older adults' capacity to acquire important information. Because of this, mental health care is necessary not only to improve individual well-being but also to encourage engagement with health practices. Because the aging population will only continue to grow, the overall need for high-quality mental health assessments in medical practices cannot be overstressed. The overall practices employed in geriatric assessments can also overlook important aspects of the older adult's religious and spiritual life experiences. Ellingson's criticism identifies the limitations of the comprehensive geriatric assessment (CGA) model in acknowledging these rich, multifaceted aspects of aging (Ellingson et al., 2009).

By omitting spirituality, healthcare providers risk losing valuable information that can be applied to further patient-centered interventions, ultimately affecting treatment plans and overall mental health management. Integration of these variables into geriatric assessments can lead to more balanced models of care that address the elderly's not only physical conditions but also their psychological and emotional needs. Such an approach is crucial in ensuring resiliency and improving mental health outcomes among the elderly. Mental health emphasis in geriatric care extends beyond mere screening; it also influences the efficacy of treatment interventions. Because depression tends to impair judgment and limit participation in therapeutic programs, awareness of its impact on mental and physical well-being is accorded the highest importance. This is especially relevant as undiagnosed mental health disorders have the potential to worsen other health conditions, compromising the quality of life. Mental health disorders, therefore, need to be proactively incorporated into geriatric practice, and healthcare professionals should turn to alternative solutions for screening and intervention. Empirical data, including research illustrating the need for depression screening, will play a key role in guiding practice that engages older patients meaningfully throughout their care pathway to support recovery and well-being (Figure 3.9).

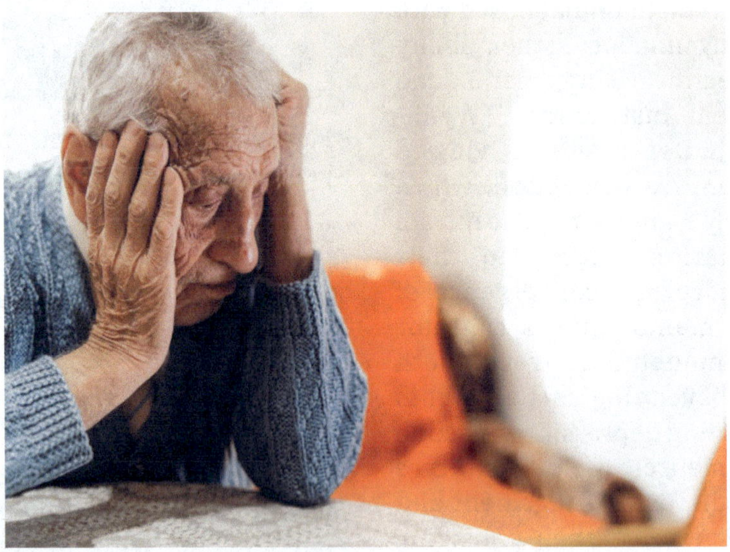

Figure 3.9. Mental health issues in old age.

Source: https://thearborsassistedliving.com/wp-content/uploads/2019/09/9.26-arbors.jpg.

3.2.3. Mobility and Physical Limitations

Mobility among the elderly is an important aspect of their overall health and quality of life. As one ages, they will often experience different physical restrictions, which can be attributed to a variety of causes, including chronic diseases, muscle weakness, and diseases like arthritis. These may severely undermine their autonomy and ability to conduct everyday functions. For instance, mobility impairments tend to reduce the likelihood that elderly persons are socially active or access necessary health care. Thus, these mobility impairments become a priority in geriatric practice and call for individualized care aimed at maintaining or optimizing functional capacity through rehabilitation, physical exercise, and assistive technology. Further, the mobility environment among older adults cannot be divorced from the rising trend of chronic disease, which makes physical status complex. As has been argued in current literature, a comprehensive assessment involving physical function is called for, particularly in the setting of geriatric oncology clinics, where patients may present with concomitant mobility issues resulting from both aging and disease processes. Geriatric assessment tools that assess physical impairment, such as the Frailty Index and Mini-Nutritional Assessment, are particularly valuable because they inform treatment selection and surgical risk stratification (Lampugnale et al., 2017).

By prioritizing these measurements, health practitioners will be better positioned to individualize interventions to improve mobility, so that older adults can maintain functional independence for as long as possible. Lastly, new models such as rabblement programs have a holistic approach to facilitating mobility and physical capacity among older persons, especially those with cognitive impairments such as dementia. They focus on the utilization of assessment and intervention in most domains, including physical functioning, support systems, and caregiver involvement, thereby enriching the broader view of geriatric care. The objective is to facilitate older adults not merely to maintain mobility but also to adapt when recovery from physical disability is not feasible (Adelman et al., 2017). The integration of rabblement interventions into routine care highlights the importance of addressing mobility holistically, so that older individuals can move around their environments safely while enhancing their independence and wellness (Figure 3.10).

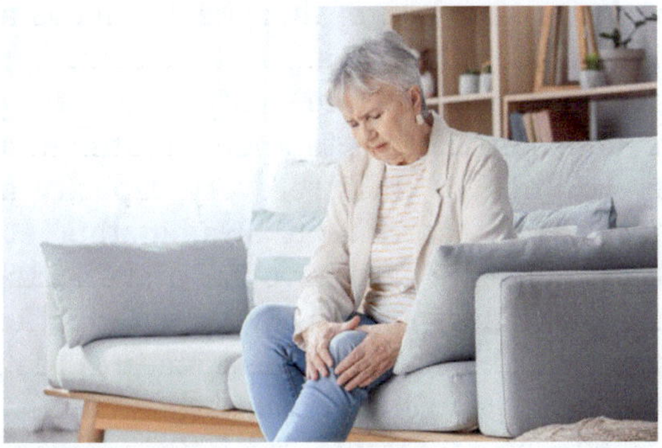

Figure 3.10. Conditions that lead to mobility limitations in seniors.

Source: https://www.homecareassistanceamarillo.com/wp-content/uploads/2020/03/Senior-Woman-Suffering-from-Pain-in-Knee.jpg.

Test Your Knowledge

1. What are chronic diseases and conditions?
2. Why is mobility important for older adults?

3.3. Geriatric Assessment

Learning Outcome

1. Know the purpose of geriatric assessment
2. Describe the components of a comprehensive assessment
3. Understand the tools and techniques used in geriatric assessment

The geriatric assessment is a key element in geriatric care, especially given the population's aging. As age advances, the patient usually presents with more than one comorbid condition, making diagnosis and treatment difficult. The geriatric assessment is used to fully assess the medical, functional, psychological, and social conditions of the elderly patient's health. This holistic approach not only identifies individual problems of health but also assesses the patient's capacity to take care of their health needs and be independent. Above all, societal stereotypes about aging eclipse the complexity of aged care, which often leads to under-treatment and misperception of their recovery capacity and quality of life. According to Swaminathan et al. (2015), such care gaps have harmful effects on health outcomes, particularly for older patients with serious illnesses such as cancer. In reality, the inclusion of geriatric assessment must be a priority in addressing the individual needs of older individuals, specifically in oncology. Older patients with cancer can sometimes have special physiological difficulties and reactions to treatment due to being extremely old. The effectiveness of individually tailored treatment regimens can be significantly improved when informed by an extensive geriatric evaluation that incorporates factors such as frailty, social support, and nutritional status. Literature highlights evidence that when these evaluations are used, they not only enhance patient treatment but also inform clinical decisions that lead to improved surgical outcomes (Lampugnale et al., 2017). Given the reality that time constraints are a problem for health care professionals, integrating such assessments into routine practice is essential for efficient management of geriatric patients and thereby evolving a more responsive health care system. Training programs on geriatric assessments for health care professionals can also help bridge the gap between the theoretical importance of these evaluations and their practical application in clinical practice. Developing curricula that emphasize frailty, psychological health, and social interactions in patient care will prepare future clinicians to prioritize geriatric care. This training imperative is critical, given that the demographics of older patients are set to soar, necessitating physicians trained in geriatric oncology to handle complex cases (Lampugnane et al., 2017). By establishing confidence and competence in geriatric assessments, healthcare providers are better positioned to improve the overall quality of care for aging patients and to preserve their dignity and independence in their healthcare (Figure 3.11).

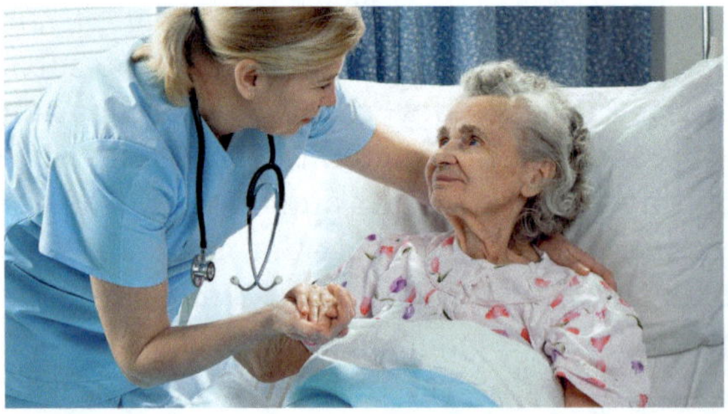

Figure 3.11. Geriatric assessment

Source: https://c.files.bbci.co.uk/89A1/production/_108233253_gettyimages-120672387.jpg.

3.3.1. Purpose of Geriatric Assessment

The objective of geriatric assessment is actually to enhance the overall management of elderly patients through a holistic appraisal that considers numerous diverse physiological, psychological, and social factors. As the population of older adults continues to grow, estimated to reach the level where in 2029 20% of the United States will be above age 65, there is an increasing need for healthcare professionals to be aware of the unique challenges this population poses (Wynn-Grundy et al., 2016). Geriatric assessment involves a multidimensional evaluation of the health of an older adult, including physical function, mental health, and social support systems. The multidimensional approach allows health practitioners to identify areas of possible concern, such as cognitive impairments or unexpected depression, that may undermine effective health care management and learning about care in the vulnerable population (Wynn-Grundy et al., 2016). Also, geriatric assessment plays a critical role in guiding personalized treatment interventions that meet the needs of older adults. Using standardized measures like the Geriatric Depression Scale, practitioners can quantify mental health problems and ensure that any underlying psychological problems are addressed in addition to physical disorders (Wynn-Grundy et al., 2016). The process of evaluation prioritizes the interaction between different domains of health, such as when geriatricians and clinical care providers assess functional capacity, they are actually able to assess the appropriateness of specific interventions or surgical options. Holistic pre-surgical geriatric assessment has been found critical to oncogeriatric risk stratification because it identifies frailty and other biomarkers associated with morbidity and mortality. Interestingly, the application of geriatric assessments has broader implications for optimizing health results and quality of life among older people. The majority of health systems still face challenges integrating these assessments into routine care, largely due to time pressures on caregivers. Therefore, new medical and physician assistant educational interventions would prepare future clinicians more effectively to conduct effective geriatric assessment with a stronger focus on the needs of older patients. Merging competency-based education with clinical practice enables future healthcare professionals to develop competence and self-confidence in assessing geriatric patients, ultimately improving clinical decision-making. By designing a setting in which integrated geriatric assessment is paramount, healthcare providers can facilitate a more effective and compassionate approach to geriatric care.

3.3.2. Components of a Comprehensive Assessment

Comprehensive assessment lies at the heart of geriatric practice, encompassing a variety of elements particularly well adapted to the needs of the elderly. Prior to this assessment is a physical health assessment that takes into account chronic disease, drug therapy, and disability. All such assessments are typically comprehensive in nature to ascertain patients' capacity to perform activities of daily living and thus establish any physical disabilities that can affect independence. In addition, the test checks for the presence of geriatric syndromes—multifactorial diseases prevalent in older persons, such as cognitive dysfunction and mobility disorders. Detection of these syndromes through a comprehensive geriatric assessment is important because it enables healthcare providers to manage symptoms effectively without risking complications, thereby enhancing the quality of life among older adults (Reuben et al., 2016). Alongside physical well-being, overall assessment also needs to address psychological well-being, equally essential in geriatric practice. Mental illnesses, like depression and anxiety, may be underdiagnosed in the elderly at times, but exert a significant impact on their health and life quality. Psychological status is evaluated using standardized screening tools and intensive interviews to determine emotional resilience and social support systems. Also, there needs to be a cognitive ability review to establish problems like dementia or delirium, which have the ability to hamper effective decision-making and self-care functions. Treatment of such psychological issues enables health professionals to apply intervention strategies tailored to each patient's psychological and emotional concerns, thereby promoting improved holism in geriatric care (Reuben et al., 2016). It is vital to incorporate social elements of a patient's life into a comprehensive assessment, especially given that determinants of social origin play a greater role in shaping health outcomes. Housing issues, social support systems, and economic factors can highly determine the course of an older adult's health. A geriatric assessment needs to investigate these aspects so that an enabling care plan may be established that promotes maximum independence for patients and enables well-being. More recent arguments establish that religion and spiritual behaviors must be integrated into this assessment framework because they can influence health and coping. By including these other elements in their consideration, healthcare professionals can gain a more comprehensive understanding of their patients, enabling them to make interventions more attuned to the complex interplay of physical, psychological, and social forces in geriatric care (Figure 3.12).

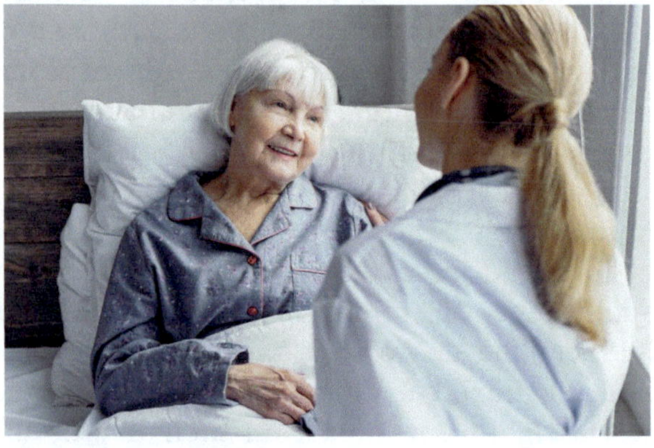

Figure 3.12. Comprehensive geriatric assessment.

Source: https://www.mna-elderly.com/sites/default/files/styles/960px_width/public/2021-09/mini-nutritional-assessment.jpg?itok=_Y_XFb36.

3.3.3. Tools and Techniques Used in Assessment

In geriatric care, high-quality assessment tools and processes are needed to enhance patient outcomes and appropriate interventions. Tools for assessing medications that reduce the risk of adverse drug events are among the factors used to evaluate older patients. Medication assessment tools belong under two broad categories: implicit and explicit inappropriate prescribing criteria. Implicit criteria involve individualized factors, such as adequate dosing and adherence, whereas explicit criteria involve standards developed through consensus, such as a medication list to be excluded in older individuals. The application of a logical drug review process can significantly improve the safety and efficacy of drug therapy in older patients, as outlined by Corsonello et al. (2016). Therefore, the utilization of such assessment tools becomes paramount in the process of personalizing drugs to the specific needs of older individuals. The other most important aspect of assessing geriatric patients is their cognitive function, which generally impacts their global status and care. Screening tools such as the Ottawa 3DY (O3DY) and the Short Blessed Test (SBT) have been researched to determine their effectiveness in detecting cognitive dysfunction (CD) in elderly patients. A study comparing these tests in an emergency room found that the SBT had high sensitivity and specificity for detecting CD and is a valuable addition to clinical assessments (Barbic et al., 2018). Both the O3DY and SBT were also found to have good inter-rater reliability, ensuring a uniform application by healthcare professionals. With the use of reliable cognitive screening tools, geriatric care professionals can identify cognitive impairments early and address them, thereby enhancing the quality of care for older adults. The teamwork involved in geriatric care, above all, through interprofessional working, optimizes the efficiency of assessment techniques. Health care providers, including clinical pharmacists, nurses, and physicians, work together to conduct detailed medication reviews, using unfettered access to patients' medical records and laboratory test results. Interdisciplinary communication is critical to the implementation of educational interventions and decision support systems that help curb inappropriate prescribing. As demonstrated by the practices in Corsonello et al. (2016), such inter-professional collaboration not only improves medication management but also enables tailored care plans to be developed based on diverse healthcare perspectives. Subsequently, the use of diverse assessment tools as well as multi-professional collaboration serves to improve the quality of care and safety for geriatric patients, ultimately resulting in better health outcomes.

Test Your Knowledge

1. What is the purpose of geriatric assessment?
2. What are the components of a comprehensive assessment?

3.4. Care Models for the Elderly

Learning Outcome

1. Describe the home-based care
2. Understand the assisted living facilities
3. Describe the nursing homes and long-term care

Care model development for the elderly has become more prominent in successful geriatric care. With demographic changes and a growing population of older individuals, there has been a need for robust collaborative networks within health systems. This is particularly relevant in aging societies such as Germany, where integrated care has become more prominent. The coordination between rehabilitation care centers and acute hospitals lies at the heart of addressing the complex needs of elderly patients. By developing an interagency platform focused on early intervention, seamless communication, and standardized procedures, medical professionals can maximize the quality of care while minimizing hospital stays. Emphasis on integrated services and networking is vital to ensuring that the elderly receive care tailored to their unique needs, which ultimately leads to improved health outcomes and increased patient satisfaction in their remaining years (Heribert et al., 2025). Moreover, care coordination is of paramount concern when dealing with elderly patient care, as it bridges gaps between various healthcare services as well as settings. The paradigm shift towards person-centered care models requires a proactive role for patients and family members, recognizing the instrumental role they play in the care cycle. Policy based on evidence that aims at prevention and patient self-management speaks to the emphasis on the development of autonomy for older adults to cope with their health, enhance independence, and improve overall well-being. Also, incorporating palliative care into such models provides comprehensive care for patients with long-term illness or at the end of life. By addressing not only medical but also emotional and social care needs of older individuals, the healthcare system can promote dignity and quality of life in later life (Morton et al., 2015). Lastly, the ongoing advancement of models for the care of the elderly calls for a changing strategy that addresses the complex challenges of an aging population. This means not only ensuring the full potential in care through improved coordination across various healthcare sectors, but also advocating policy interventions that favor long-term good health of the elderly. Although research demonstrates the benefits of care coordination and coordinated services for enhancing patient outcomes, it is important to translate these results into policy action. Financing for long-term care, the healthcare workforce, and the vital role that family caregivers play are similarly pressing concerns. By creating comprehensive strategies that encompass these dimensions, the geriatric care landscape can be transformed, ensuring that elderly populations receive the care they deserve (Morton et al., 2015; Heribert et al., 2025) (Figure 3.13).

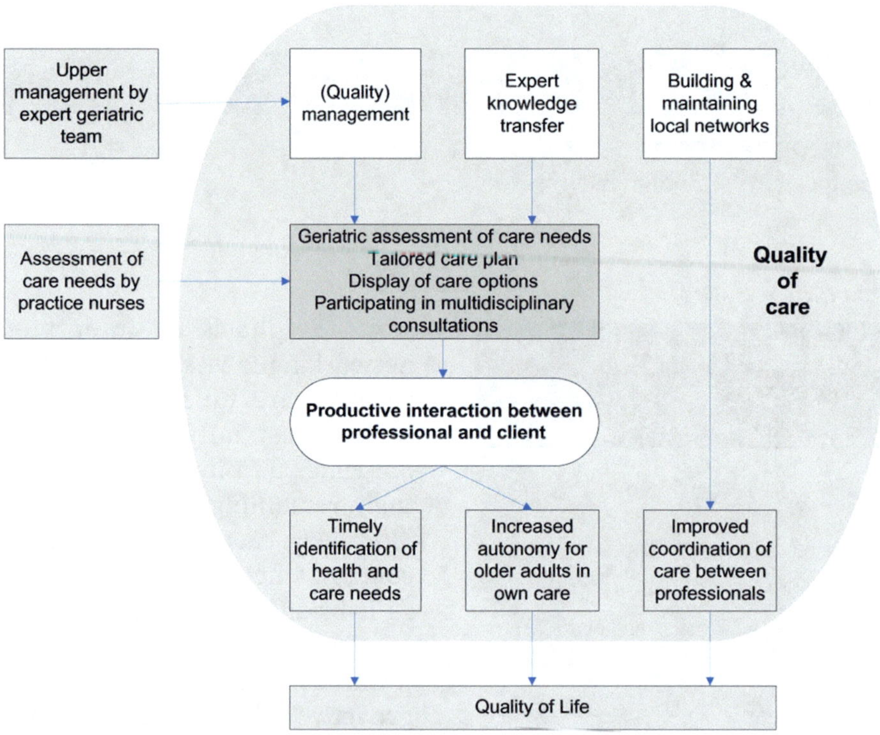

Figure 3.13. Schematic representation of the geriatric care model.

Source: https://www.researchgate.net/profile/Emiel-Hoogendijk/publication/224869488/figure/fig3/AS:669582066978816@1536652213055/Schematic-representation-of-the-geriatric-care-model.png.

3.4.1. Home-Based Care

Home care is an innovative method of caring for the elderly, focused on providing elderly patients with the required health care services within the comfort of their homes. This type of care is specifically designed for the elderly, who experience mobility issues or chronic illness, making it less convenient for them to seek facility-based care. The importance of home care is also highlighted by the growing demand for patient-centered care that focuses on a person's specific conditions and preferences. Evidence has demonstrated that home-based care not only enhances the quality of life for elderly patients but also improves health outcomes and reduces hospital readmission. Also, by providing an environment conducive to recovery, patients will experience fewer levels of stress and anxiety, factors that are crucial for general health among elderly individuals. Another critical component of home care success is coordination among healthcare providers and caregivers, which can also affect the quality of care provided to older adults. This coordination is essential, as elderly patients often present with complex healthcare needs. For instance, effective care management strategies have been shown to reduce costs while enhancing the quality of care, especially for older patients who often have more than one healthcare condition to manage. Consequently, care managers' role comes in handy in regulating communication among caregivers and patient families to ensure religious compliance with care plans and adjustments thereto. Recent findings from studies underscore the efficacy of such interventional measures, which have established coordinated care as significantly enhancing the health status of elderly individuals and satisfaction with the health care system (Berry-Millett et al., 2009). Though its advantages are profound, home-based care also poses problems that need to be addressed and addressed innovatively. The sustainability of the model depends considerably on breaking down system huddles, such as funding and the accessibility of skilled practitioners who can provide home-based services. These issues are best tackled by policymakers through well-designed programs that promote cost-effective, just home care solutions. Of special importance is that families also serve as the main caregivers, which places them under additional pressure as they try to manage their own responsibilities. Therefore, support systems must be established to enable families to handle caregiving duties, particularly to promote preventive care and self-management, as outlined in current policy plans (Morton et al., 2015). By expanding resource availability and caregiver as well as patient support, the effectiveness of home-based care in the geriatric population could be significantly amplified (Figure 3.14).

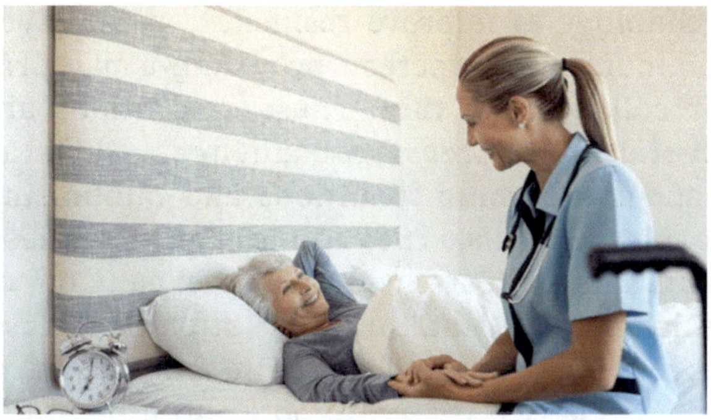

Figure 3.14. Home-based care.

Source: https://samahospital.com/wp-content/uploads/2021/08/Untitled-design-14-1-1-860x500.png.

3.4.2. Assisted Living Facilities

Assisted Living Facilities (ALFs) are a key part of the continuum of care for the elderly, bridging the gap between living independently and skilled nursing. ALFs offer services such as personal care, including assistance with activities of daily living (ADLs) such as bathing, dressing, and medication. Apart from providing required care, ALFs also create a social environment and emotional support that is immensely crucial for elderly care recipients who may feel lonely and isolated. Acute geriatric care in such centers not only maintains physical well-being among residents but also addresses the psychological and social dimensions of care, thus enhancing their quality of life. As there is greater demand for these care facilities due to an expanding older population, it is important to understand their operation and role in geriatric care conversations (Estes et al., 2007). Various models of operations are available in Assisted Living Facilities, depending on the regulatory guidelines and specific needs of their residents. In regions like California, which have the most vulnerable elderly population, policymakers are increasingly compelled to expand current programs and support systems within ALFs to meet growing demand. These can involve incorporating wellness programs and technology to improve resident and caregiver communication, thereby providing a platform for collaborative care. These innovations are pivotal in addressing challenges, such as managing chronic conditions and minimizing hospitalizations. The applications of these programs reflect the ongoing expansion of assisted living, indicating an attempt toward more comprehensive, resident-centered care, which is necessary to promote and protect the health and well-being of older persons residing in them (Estes et al., 2007). Comparative studies investigating various models of care have also made the benefits of alternatives, for example, Green Care Farms (GCFs), evident through the combination of agriculture and nature-based elements with care for people who are dementia patients. It has been established that GCFs offer certain advantages, such as increased physical activity and improved diet, compared to traditional Assisted Living Facilities.

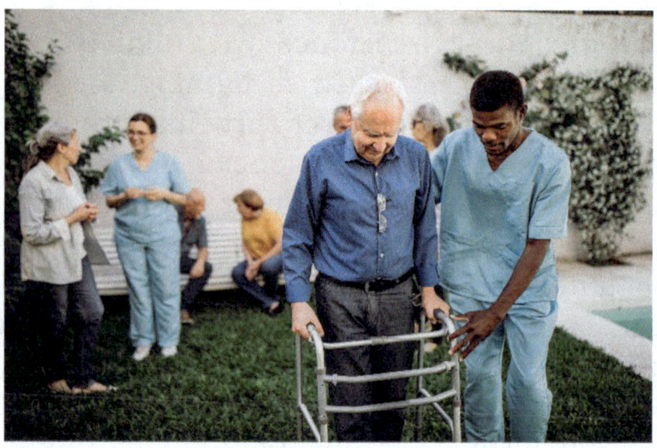

Figure 3.15. Assisted living facility.

Source: https://pro-assets.morningconsult.com/wp-uploads/2020/09/14112050/Assisted-Living-GettyImages-1195963496-scaled.jpg.

These findings validate that different programs and environments can play a significant role in the well-being of older people, particularly those with cognitive impairment. By incorporating environmental factors and arousal activities, GCFs were shown to improve certain health outcomes and maintain caregivers' quality of life. This points to the need for a multi-dimensional approach in geriatric care, expanding current knowledge on successful care modalities beyond conventional ALFs (Figure 3.15).

3.4.3. Nursing Homes and Long-Term Care

The face of long-term care and nursing homes has changed significantly over the last few decades, largely due to increasing pressure driven by the growing demand from an aging population. As the most rapidly growing sector of society, the elderly are imposing new challenges on the health system, calling for the development of more long-term care facilities. During the early 1970s, the underlying deficiencies of nursing homes were laid bare by researchers like Townsend, who brought to light systemic issues through testimony from family and healthcare staff. This backlash generated efforts such as the Department of Health, Education and Welfare's Long Term Care Facility Improvement Campaign, an effort to inspect and improve the quality of care. However, despite these advancements, ongoing monitoring of nursing home quality remains an issue, as it still falls short of meeting expectations for the best care for the elderly, underscoring an acute need for ongoing reform (Cantu et al., 1987). Infection control has remained a potential concern in nursing homes and long-term care facilities, with particular regard to the vulnerability of the aged to infectious disease. Research indicates that staff in nursing homes with unsatisfactory infection-control practices can undermine patient safety and health. In a study conducted by infection control practitioners, effective infection prevention requires a significant number of resources, with an estimated 513 hours per 100 beds to implement infection control practices in a model nursing home. These findings underscore the necessity of implementing explicit standards tailored to long-term care facilities. More emphasis on infection control not only enhances the quality of care but also addresses the challenges from the special clinical settings inherent in such centers. Encouraging improvement in this sector is essential in achieving holistic geriatric care. Integration of quality improvement activities into nursing homes is essential in fostering an environment that respects the dignity and well-being of residents. The issues facing nursing homes go deeper than poor staffing and infection control; they include a broad range of issues, such as caregiver lack of training and lack of individualized care plans, which are essential elements of geriatric care. Policy and healthcare administrators must prioritize training and resources to better prepare staff and enforce adherence to established standards of care. This measure not only enhances patients' quality of life but also reduces the adverse effects of neglect and poor hygiene. Lastly, prioritizing best practices and continuous improvement in nursing homes can significantly influence the delivery of long-term care, both to residents and to the health system overall (Cantu et al., 1987) (Figure 3.16).

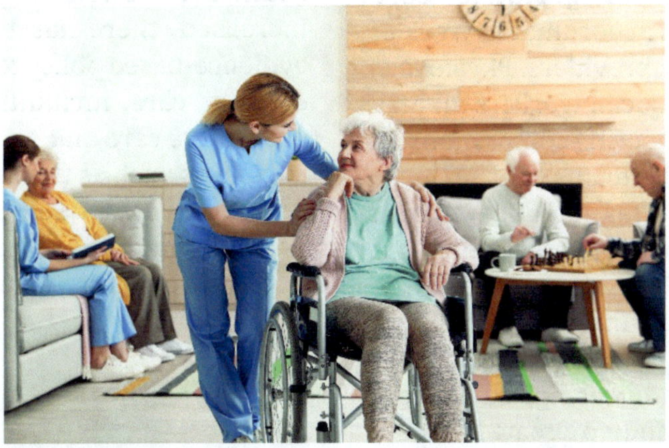

Figure 3.16. Pathway to excellence in long-term care organizations.

Source: https://www.myamericannurse.com/wp-content/uploads/2020/12/shutterstock_1423975322-scaled.jpg.

Test Your Knowledge

1. What do you mean by home-based care?
2. What do most assisted living facilities provide?

3.5. Role of Healthcare Professionals

Learning Outcome

1. Understand the geriatricians and their specialization
2. Understand the importance of multidisciplinary teams
3. Describe the training and education for care providers

The effective delivery of geriatric care necessarily depends on the coordinated work of a wide range of healthcare providers. Physicians, nurses, pharmacists, and social workers all play complementary roles in ensuring comprehensive care for older patients. Physicians bear primary responsibility for the diagnosis of health conditions and the direction of treatment, but their value also lies in ensuring coordination of the entire plan of care across multiple disciplines. Nurses, the patients' first and nearest point of contact, provide vital monitoring, education, and emotional support, and so create a stable background favorable to rehabilitation. Social workers navigate the complex social interactions among elderly patients and assist them in transitioning between care points, advocating for resources to enhance quality of life. This interprofessional approach is necessary to meet the unique and sophisticated demands of the elderly and deliver complete, integrated care. Pharmacists generally have emerged as prime members of the health care team in the care of the elderly, especially with the extensive application of polypharmacy among the elderly. The population is at greater risk for drug-related complications, hence precise medication management. The function of the pharmacist involves carrying out comprehensive medication reviews and identifying potential drug interactions, underdosing, or overdosing conditions that can adversely affect patient health. The application of evidence-based instruments, coupled with specific criteria for detecting inappropriate prescribing, is essential for optimizing therapeutic outcomes among older patients. Perhaps most importantly, coordination among pharmacists with other healthcare professionals provides a systematic strategy towards pharmaceutical care. This teamwork not only ensures medication adherence but also general patient safety, a fundamental aspect of geriatric care as evidenced by literature (Corsonello et al., 2016). Beyond direct patient care, health professionals also play an active role in shaping policies that impact geriatric health services. As the population of seniors has increased, there has been an urgent need for evidence-based policy to address the complexities of elder care, including increased funding for preventive care and care coordination. Research in centers such as the Stern Center highlights the need for patient self-management-supporting policies and the engagement of family caregivers in the caregiving process (Morton et al., 2015).

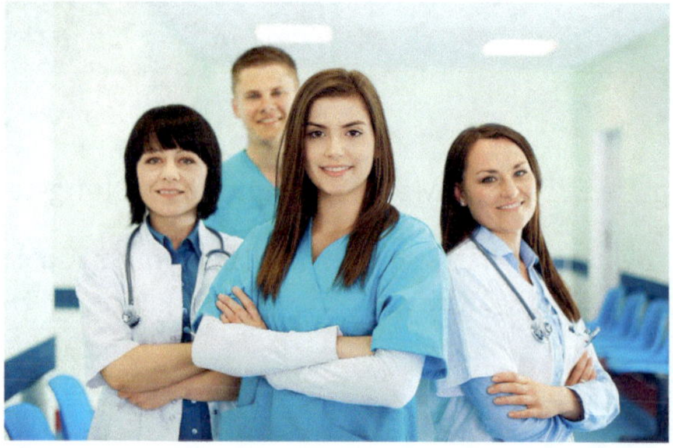

Figure 3.17. Healthcare professionals.

Source: https://medipharm.com.au/wp-content/uploads/2024/02/successful-medical-team.jpg.

Healthcare workers are well-suited to drive such reforms by leveraging their own anecdotal evidence of the issues their patients experience. By highlighting areas where policy intervention is needed despite strong research evidence, such as palliative care, these workers can drive actual changes that improve healthcare for the elderly.

This serves not merely to drive improved patient outcomes but to improve the healthcare system as a whole (Figure 3.17).

3.5.1. Geriatricians and Their Specialization

The geriatrician's expertise is crucial to the evolving picture of healthcare, particularly with the world population aging. Geriatricians are trained to deal with the unique medical issues of elderly patients, who commonly have more than one disease occurring at once and presenting as complicated, multifactorial health issues needing an all-encompassing approach to treatment. Specialist skills are needed because older people often have more than one chronic disease, which requires comprehensive examinations and personalized treatment regimens. The importance of the specialty has grown enormously, as indicated by a steady increase in the number of older adults needing geriatric specialist care to achieve the best health outcomes. As geriatric science progresses, ongoing education and professional development of caregivers remain essential to enhance the quality of care delivered to such populations, including the physical and psychological aspects of aging. In examining collaborative procedures among geriatricians within hospitals and general practitioners, significant inequalities emerge by region of health facilities. Research indicates that regions with an effective network of geriatric care enhance communication and collaboration among professionals, as well as improve patient outcomes. According to the success of collaboration, mutual understanding, respect, and continuous communication about the respective roles and responsibilities of both parties form the cornerstone. Lack of geriatric services in some regions may lead to misconceptions, suspicion, and uncoordinated multidisciplinary working among health care professionals, indirectly influencing the quality of care for patients. Interventions aimed at enhancing multidisciplinary working, for instance, inter-professional education, repeated meetings, and the development of shared care protocols are thus important in promoting the more integrated delivery of geriatric care and optimizing the management of the health outcomes among the elderly patients (Dagneaux et al., 2012). To understand the specialist care needs of the older patients, one must study the holistic model of care that geriatricians follow. The geriatricians do not just assess medical conditions; they also consider functional independence, mental status, and social support systems. This is particularly observed in the setting of increased prevalence of conditions such as dementia among the aging population. In addition, geriatric medicine focuses on preventive care and the preservation of quality of life, not merely on disease management. Studies have shown that integrating principles of geriatric care into broader healthcare practices can substantially improve the well-being of older patients. For instance, interprofessional collaboration between geriatricians and general practitioners has been shown to improve communication of treatment approaches, reduce hospitalization rates, and increase overall awareness of the aging process (Dagneaux et al., 2012). For this reason, there is an acute need for a highly skilled and specialist geriatric workforce to meet the growing demands of an aging population (Figure 3.18).

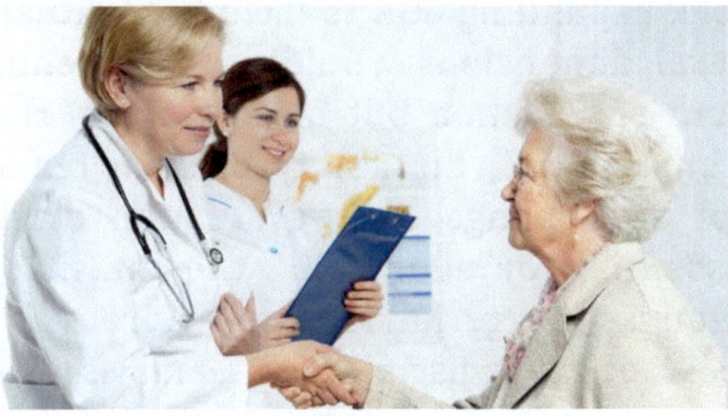

Figure 3.18. Geriatrician.

Source: https://ucmscdn.healthgrades.com/98/fd/08e756ea4c19824bae3b55ad3181/geriatrician-ftb-is-738x399-stk-88515586.jpg.

3.5.2. Importance of Multidisciplinary Teams

The integration of multidisciplinary teams is paramount to maximizing geriatric care, particularly given the complex health status of older patients. Older patients can present with several comorbidities, and the collaborative process among many healthcare workers ensures a comprehensive, individualized approach to care. Each multidisciplinary team player, from physicians to nurses, social workers, and therapists, brings particular expertise that complements the overall treatment plan. This synergy not only aids in the solving of medical issues but also of psychological and social aspects of patient care, which are foremost in ensuring quality of life. An interdisciplinary-friendly environment can, therefore, lead to more effective and holistic interventions for the elderly population. Most important to the success of multidisciplinary teams is the application of holistic geriatric assessment (CGA), a central instrument for understanding and managing the heterogeneity of needs in older patients. In Ellingson's view, the traditional model of CGA has increasingly downplayed core aspects of patients' lives, such as their spirituality and religious practice. With the identification of these dimensions, multidisciplinary teams can develop more tailored intervention strategies that resonate with patients' essential values and beliefs. Expanding CGA to include spiritual and cultural dimensions would not only enhance patient satisfaction but also improve clinical outcomes. Thus, the ability of such teams to adapt and change their evaluation methods is essential for addressing the multifaceted challenges of geriatric care. Moreover, the success of multidisciplinary teams is evident not only in direct patient care but also, significantly, in healthcare expenditures and resource allocation. The multifaceted healthcare needs of elderly patients have been shown to drive increased expenditures, according to evidence (Berry-Millett et al., 2009). Multidisciplinary management of care has been shown to improve care quality and streamline redundant hospitalizations and siloed costs. The multidisciplinary framework facilitates more effective resource allocation and simplified communication, reducing service duplication and enabling timely interventions. Therefore, not only does the multidisciplinary framework improve the quality of care for older patients, but it also has far-reaching implications for the sustainability of healthcare systems that serve an increasingly older population (Figure 3.19).

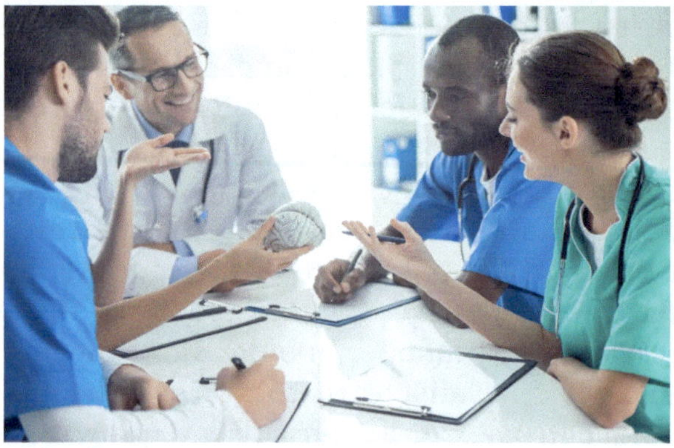

Figure 3.19. The role of multidisciplinary teams in providing coordinated care.

Source: https://uniquecs.co.uk/ogloaroa/2024/04/MDTs.webp.

3.5.3. Training and Education for Care Providers

In geriatric care, proper training and education among caregivers cannot be overstressed. As the population ages, healthcare professionals should be adequately trained in specialized knowledge to address the particular needs of this group. Training curricula can include modules on patient-centered communication, pain control, and chronic disease management, fostering a general understanding of geriatric health. In addition, the programs would need to prioritize evidence-based practices and interprofessional approaches so that providers are equipped to provide optimal care. By prioritizing synchronized collaboration across health sectors, providers would be able to maximize the overall effectiveness of geriatric services. The importance of system training programs is further validated by a more recent study demanding policies to support care coordination and patient self-management with an emphasis on the imperative for robust educational models within geriatric healthcare (Morton et al., 2015). Apart from initial training, ongoing education is obligatory for providers in geriatric care settings. The constantly evolving health environment demands that clinicians stay up to date with the latest studies and developments in aging. Ongoing professional development, such as workshops or specialized certifications in geriatric care, may ensure that caregivers are equipped and knowledgeable about new assessment tools. For example, although comprehensive geriatric assessments are known to be necessary, they are not implemented adequately due to time limitations (Lampugnane et al., 2017). Incorporating this component into educational curricula will allow future healthcare professionals to learn how to implement these assessments effectively. This continuous series of learning environments is not only beneficial for the individual healthcare provider but also contributes to the quality of care delivered to the geriatric population, ultimately translating into better clinical outcomes and patient satisfaction. Furthermore, integrating simulation-based and competency-based training practices into the geriatric training curriculum can significantly enhance care providers' readiness. Through actual situations in simulated environments, students of health care are able to practice fundamental assessment skills and hone clinical capabilities before working with actual patients. The experiential approach fosters confidence and capability in assessing the elderly, which significantly mitigates the anxiety normally linked with coping with older patients. As highlighted by recent research, preparing students for the most predictive fields of geriatric assessment can lead to better surgical outcomes among oncogeriatric patients (Lampugnani et al., 2017). Therefore, including such training in learning programs not only leads to enhanced individual proficiency but also to a general enhancement of geriatric care quality. Thus, adopting new training strategies will pay dividends in the long run, significantly overcoming the obstacles that accompany the provision of geriatric care.

Test Your Knowledge

1. What is the specialization of geriatricians?
2. What is the importance of multidisciplinary teams?

3.6. Family and Caregiver Support

Learning Outcome

1. Understand the role of family in geriatric care
2. Describe the resources for caregivers
3. Know the impact of caregiving on family dynamics

Family and caregiver support within geriatric care is also necessary, as older adults are likely to greatly rely on their immediate social networks for help with activities of daily living. This level of dependence requires family caregivers to possess the requisite knowledge and skills to provide effective care to their older family members. Having available care programs that instruct caregivers on the distinct needs of the elderly can significantly improve the quality of care. Proper training, such as in the management of chronic conditions and understanding age-related complications, is provided to family members by these programs, serving as a buffer against future caregiving stressors. The provision of formal educational pathways for family caregivers enhances the health of older persons and caregivers alike, leading to healthier family relationships (Vaughan-Wrobel et al., 2008). In addition to fostering caregiving skills, family support systems may incorporate respite care services to offer temporary relief to the primary caregiver. Such services are vital in preventing caregiver burnout, a factor that can have serious negative implications for both the caregiver and the elderly individual being cared for. Access to respite care enables family members to recover from exhaustion, allowing them to maintain the capacity to offer the required support without detriment to their own well-being. There is evidence that proves frequent access to caregiver support services correlates with improved emotional and physical health outcomes in caregivers and older adults. Through such support systems facilitated by healthcare professionals, more sustainable caregiving practices are promoted, consequently helping to build a solid support system likely to benefit the elderly (Lampugnane et al., 2017). Further, recognizing the crucial crossroads of family life and geriatric care is essential to the successful implementation of assistance programs. Families are usually the foremost source of information, advocacy, and emotional support for older adults in difficult healthcare situations. As such, efficient communication between healthcare professionals and family members is important in creating individualized care plans that reflect the desires and needs of elderly patients. Initiatives that actively engage families in decision-making will not only empower caregivers but also optimize the efficiency of care. As geriatric care transitions toward a holistic approach, integrating families as care collaborators will be key to improving health outcomes and fostering a sense of community among older adults (Vaughan-Wrobel et al., 2008) (Figure 3.20).

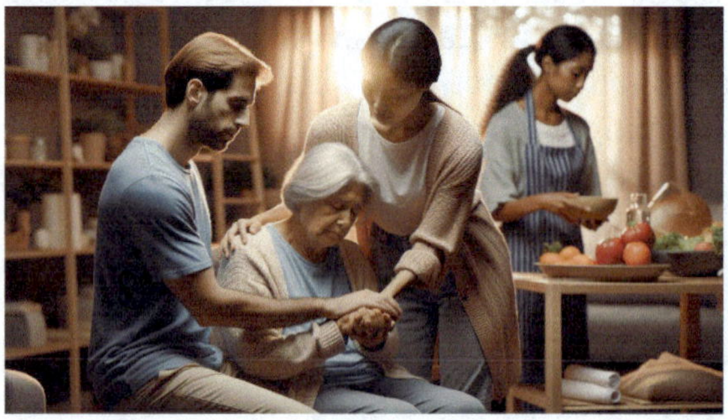

Figure 3.20. Family Support

Source: https://cdn.growtha.dev/6516de5dbcce181d2bd88c56/665c1e42466d2c17a15598d6_1695575082593x234550197059517630-1717311976151x977968634208739100-dalle-TREMR.png.

3.6.1. Role of Family in Geriatric Care

The role of the family in caring for the elderly is an important component of the healthcare system that has profound impacts on both the quality of care and the quality of life of the elderly patient. Family members typically serve as the primary caregivers, providing emotional support, assistance with activities of daily living, and assistance with navigating the complexities of the healthcare system. This family involvement is particularly significant since elderly individuals typically have multifaceted healthcare needs that reflect both chronic illness and social challenges. Evidence indicates that the interaction between quality of care and family involvement is significant, as families can advocate on behalf of their relatives and ensure that their voice and preferences are heard in care arrangements. Emphasizing the importance of such interaction is likely to improve health profiles among older adults and enhance their overall quality of life in residential and nursing homes (Clay et al., 2025). In addition, the demand for integrated geriatric models of care necessitates the integration of family viewpoints, especially given that older individuals in these situations often report feelings of loneliness or isolation within these institutional settings. Involvement of family members not only provides instrumental aid but also a sense of belonging, which is crucial for mental health. Intimate relationships among healthcare providers and relatives can aid communication, leading to patient-oriented care in care facilities. As per the literature, good family involvement is largely associated with improved management practices in care, potentially leading to enhanced quality of care for the elderly in the future. By valuing the family role, geriatric care can better cope with age-related issues, i.e., issues of mental health, chronic diseases, and integration (Berry-Millett et al., 2009). Finally, the families themselves suffer from issues of their own while caring for aging loved ones, highlighting the absolute necessity for support systems in geriatric care. Caregiver burden has been found to induce stress and burnout, affecting both the family member involved and the older individual being cared for. It then becomes important for healthcare systems to provide resources and support mechanisms to address these problems. This includes providing information on caregiving activities, respite care, and opportunities for family members to share their experiences and concerns. The physical and emotional well-being of family caregivers can significantly impact the quality of care for older individuals. In managing the intricacies of geriatric care, a team-based model that recognizes the importance of family participation ensures a more wholesome equilibrium between caregiving duties and the elder individuals' needs, thereby translating into better health outcomes as well as increased quality of life (Clay et al.) (Figure 3.21).

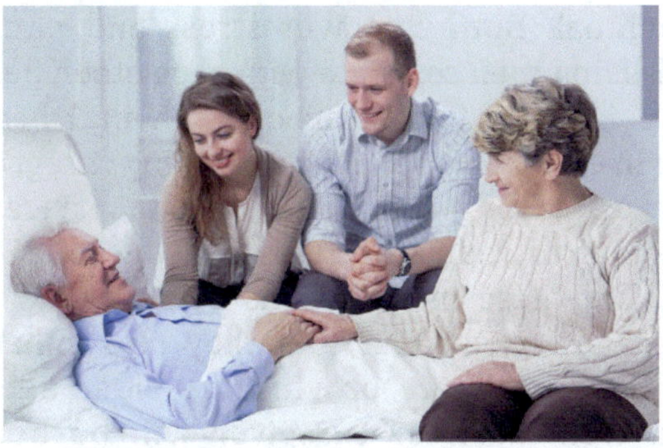

Figure 3.21. Role of family in geriatric care.

Source: https://eldercarehomehealth.com/wp-content/uploads/2019/09/palliative-care.jpeg.

3.6.2. Resources for Caregivers

Among elderly care, caregivers are a significant part in the sufficiency of handling the complex needs of older individuals, particularly when they are chronically ill or disabled. Access to resources created for caregivers can significantly help them provide adequate support. Training programs, for instance, can equip caregivers with the skills and competence required in resolving common problems presented by caregiving. These interventions generally focus on functional areas, such as medication management and mobility assistance, but also address emotional and psychological care. Caregivers are also supported by community resources, such as counseling services and support groups, which provide a forum for sharing experiences and coping strategies. These resources are essential because they contribute to caregivers' resilience and ability to provide high-quality care to their loved ones, which, in turn, affects the well-being of both caregivers and older adults. The caregivers' mental and emotional well-being is a vital consideration that is often overlooked in geriatric care. Epidemiological studies have shown that caregiving stress affects both caregiver and care recipient negatively. For instance, caregivers of hip fracture patients experience a great psychological burden, thereby affecting the psychological state of the elderly individual. Both caregiver stress and patient well-being then correlate with each other, hence there is a need to incorporate mental health care in caregiving services. Providing caregivers with counseling and mental health services is essential to reducing stress and burnout. Not only are these interventions beneficial to the caregivers themselves, but they also enhance the quality of care provided to older adults, as a well-cared-for caregiver will be better able to react favorably to the care recipients' needs and preferences (Bellanti et al., 2016). In addition, geriatric consultations are imperative tools that may actually assist caregivers. Although it is known to be an important step, its use in clinical settings is inconsistent, particularly among oncogeriatric patients. The pre-surgical geriatric consultation can provide key information on a patient's frailty, support system, dietary requirements, and psychological status. These findings are highly correlated with surgical outcomes and can inform caregivers in understanding how to manage expectations and prepare for appropriate care strategies. Initiating educational programs that train caregivers and healthcare providers to perform these assessments can help create a more supportive environment for geriatric patients. This not only optimizes treatment outcomes but also provides caregivers with data to address the complexities of aging care as older citizen populations continue to evolve (Lampugnani et al., 2017) (Figure 3.22).

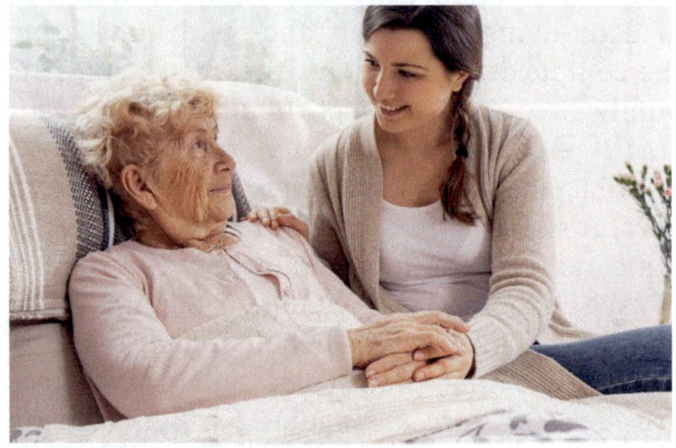

Figure 3.22. Resources for caregivers.

Source: https://www.bassett.org/sites/default/files/hg_features/mercury_image/d4a810656566a3b29fe75467b67cb108.jpg.

3.6.3. Impact of Caregiving on Family Dynamics

Caregiving has a profound effect on family relationships, reshaping roles and relationships in the home. When caregiving responsibilities fall to family members, changes in day-to-day routines and emotional relationships are common. The caregivers role becomes dominant in family life, leading to increased stress and potential conflict between siblings or other relatives who fall behind or feel excluded from the caregiving process. Furthermore, research has indicated that caregiving can redefine caregivers' identities and priorities, creating emotional challenges such as resentment or isolation. This emotional pressure can sweep through the family, creating a cycle of tension that extends beyond the caregiver to the person being cared for and other family members. An extension of understanding these dynamics is crucial for responding to the broader mental health consequences within family units (Henwood et al., 2017). Moreover, every caregiving experience is unique and thus scrutiny is in order regarding the effects of cultural, economic, and demographic factors on them. Different caregivers will respond to their role in varying manners depending on their circumstances or the character of the person in need of care. Research on caregiver burden indicates that experiences can differ significantly along axes of socioeconomic status, ethnicity, and extant family support systems. For example, studies document Caucasian American caregivers reporting increased levels of anxiety and depression regarding caregiving responsibilities, while African American caregivers report increased levels of resourcefulness and mental health (Bekhet et al., 2015). These findings emphasize the need to develop support interventions that are aptly targeted to these diverse experiences, thereby enhancing the resilience of caregivers and their corresponding family systems (Henwood et al., 2017). Further, the effects of caregiving reach beyond the immediate family, with implications for community and societal structures. When care is a family obligation, it tends to generate a mandate for systemic interventions, such as healthcare access, respite, and community education. Families tend to say they are overwhelmed, indicating that in the absence of adequate support mechanisms, the family as an entity cannot be sustained. This strain can have negative health outcomes for not only caregivers but also recipients of care, as declining caregiver health can negatively impact the quality of care. Therefore, awareness building and provision of caregiving resources must be accorded priority at policy and community levels, and within an enabling environment in which the families are able to navigate such problems together and gain access to the assistance they require for their preservation and functioning (Bekhet et al., 2015).

Test Your Knowledge

1. What is the role of family in geriatric care?
2. What is the impact of caregiving on family dynamics?

SUMMARY

Finally, the environment of geriatric care demands sustained efforts to develop models of care that address the unique needs of the aging population. Considering the increasing complexity of healthcare requirements, coupled with the inevitable frailties that arise with age, the call for integrated models of care is clear. Quality care of geriatric patients not only improves health but also potentially reduces total health expenditure. This is particularly crucial since the field is confronted with resource management challenges and care delivery systems amid such demographic change. In addressing these challenges, integrating sophisticated care management practices with patient-centered methodologies will be required, ultimately enhancing the quality of care provided to the elderly (Berry-Millett et al., 2009). Moreover, the use of professional evaluations, such as pre-surgical geriatric evaluation, identifies the interdependent relationship between coordinated care and improved treatment outcomes. While acknowledging the benefits of these evaluations, many healthcare providers fail to utilize them due to time constraints and complexities in geriatric practice. This failure is crucial for determining the ability to develop interventions specifically for elderly patients undergoing surgery. Placing the incorporation of formal geriatric assessment in clinical practice on the agenda enables care professionals to optimize more efficiently on the diverse needs of elderly patients. These interventions not only optimize risk stratification but also optimize the likelihood of successful outcomes in oncogeriatric patients and justify individualized treatment approaches (Lampugnale et al., 2017). Last but not least, geriatric care in the future will rest heavily on the education and training of healthcare providers. As the population ages, it is crucial that future healthcare providers are educated and trained to address the special needs of this population. Educational programs that highlight the importance of geriatric evaluation, particularly in the surgical context, will be invaluable in shaping the next generation of clinicians to manage the complexities of aging patients. By enhancing confidence and skill levels among young professionals, the specialty of geriatric care can look forward to improved patient outcomes and advocate for a healthcare system that fully addresses the needs of its most frail citizens. Where education, assessment, and patient-centered care converge is where the paradigm shift to enable successful geriatric care in the ensuing years will be decided (Berry-Millett et al., 2009).

Regarding geriatric care, it is essential to be aware of the prevalence and impact of mental illnesses such as depression so that interventions and education can be effectively planned. It has been found that a vast majority of the elderly are afflicted with undiagnosed depression, particularly in those with chronic illness, and 40% have been estimated to be unknown and untreated. This undiagnosed illness has the potential to greatly destroy cognitive functions, and it becomes impossible for the aged to remember important healthcare facts. Such a recent study, having utilized the Geriatric Depression Scale (GDS), made this association possible by correlating higher depression scores with lower knowledge retention following a nutrition education session, thus proving the need for more stringent screening practices within geriatric healthcare environments in an effort to improve patient outcomes and educational efficiency (Wynn-Grundy et al., 2016). One significant argument is based on the transforming dynamics of long-term care (LTC) systems among the elderly, particularly in Europe. The ANCIEN project is a classic example of an integrated approach to the complexity of LTC, examining how shifting population structures will impact the future of older persons' care demands. By comparing differences internationally, the study aims to understand demand, supply, and system performance overall in responding to the needs of an aging population. When the results of such studies are published, they can inform policy and practice in aged care, enabling systems to be altered effectively in accordance with projected demographic changes (Palenik et al., 2010). Adding conclusions from mental health assessments to firm LTC system evaluations will significantly improve the quality of care for the elderly. Ensuring that the mental health needs of older adults are thoroughly addressed is important for better health outcomes and overall well-being. Thus, healthcare workers must accord the greatest significance to holistic evaluations that encompass both mental status examinations and knowledge of the functional contrasts in LTC in various societal contexts. By synthesizing these main components into a cohesive whole, the field of geriatric care can better set itself in relation to the unique needs and challenges brought about by a growing elderly population towards a more responsive and cost-effective system of healthcare that promotes the dignity and quality of life in advanced years (Palenik et al., 2010; Wynn-Grundy et al., 2016).

KEY TERMS FROM THIS CHAPTER

- Cancer
- Geriatric assessment
- Healthcare services
- Medication management
- Palliative care
- Polypharmacy
- Social environment
- Community organizations
- Geriatric care
- Home-based care
- Oncology
- Physical health
- Religious beliefs
- Social services

CRITICAL THINKING QUESTIONS

1. **What is the most common cause of disability in older adults?**
   a. Osteoporosis
   b. Dementia
   c. Osteoarthritis
   d. Cardiovascular diseases
2. **Which of the following is considered a normal age-related physiological change?**
   a. Decreased bone density
   b. Increased cardiac output
   c. Enhanced kidney filtration rate
   d. Increased elasticity of blood vessels
3. **Which screening test is recommended for all women over the age of 65?**
   a. Mammography
   b. Bone density testing (DEXA scan)
   c. Colonoscopy
   d. Pap smear
4. **What is the most common type of dementia in older adults?**
   a. Vascular dementia
   b. Alzheimer's disease
   c. Frontotemporal dementia
   d. Lewy body dementia
5. **Which of the following is a validated tool for screening depression in older adults?**
   a. PHQ-9
   b. Geriatric Depression Scale (GDS)
   c. Beck Depression Inventory
   d. CAGE questionnaire

Short Answer Questions

1. What is geriatric care?
2. What is the importance of geriatric care?
3. What are the most common health issues in the elderly?
4. Describe the role of healthcare professionals.
5. What is the role of family and caregiver support in geriatric care?

Answer to Critical Thinking Questions

1. (c); 2. (a); 3. (b); 4. (b); 5. (b).

REFERENCES

1. Poulos, C. J., Bayer, A., Beaupre, L., Clare, L., Poulos, R. G., Wang, R. H., Zuidema, S., & McGilton, K. S. (2017). A comprehensive approach to reablement in dementia. *Alzheimer S & Dementia Translational Research & Clinical Interventions*, *3*(3), 450–458. https://doi.org/10.1016/j.trci.2017.06.005Adler, D., Alban, C., Bondi, M., Braun, T., et al. (2018). Population health solutions for assessing cognitive impairment in geriatric patients. https://core.ac.uk/download/323065242.pdf (accessed on 14th July 2025).
2. Barbic, D., Barbic, S. P., Carpenter, C. R., Kemplin, M., et al. (2018). Diagnostic accuracy of the Ottawa 3DY and Short Blessed Test to detect cognitive dysfunction in geriatric patients presenting to the emergency department. https://core.ac.uk/download/212860802.pdf (accessed on 14th July 2025).
3. Bekhet, A. K. (2015). Resourcefulness in African American and Caucasian American caregivers of persons with dementia: Associations with perceived burden, depression, anxiety, positive cognitions, and psychological well-being. https://core.ac.uk/download/213059018.pdf (accessed on 14th July 2025).
4. Bellanti, G., Eleuteri, S., & Falaschi, P. (2016). Hip fracture: Preliminary results supporting significative correlations between the psychological well-being of patients and their relative caregivers. https://core.ac.uk/download/98343305.pdf (accessed on 14th July 2025).
5. Berry-Millett, R., & Bodenheimer, T. (2009). Care management of patients with complex health care needs. https://core.ac.uk/download/71346306.pdf (accessed on 14th July 2025).
6. Cantu, T. G. (1987). Prescribing of neuroleptics for geriatric nursing home patients: A focus on indications and dosing. https://core.ac.uk/download/276267189.pdf (accessed on 14th July 2025).
7. Clay, D., Hyde, J., Nelson, S., Szczepura, A., et al. (2025). Models for providing improved care in residential care homes: A thematic literature review. https://core.ac.uk/download/49048.pdf (accessed on 14th July 2025).
8. Corsonello, A., Jha, A., Leendertse, A., Somers, A., Somers, A., Somers, A., Spinewine, A., et al. (2016). Geriatric pharmacotherapy: Optimization through integrated approach in the hospital setting. https://core.ac.uk/download/55809733.pdf (accessed on 14th July 2025).
9. Dagneaux, I., De Lepeleire, J., & Gilard, I. (2012). Care of elderly people by the general practitioner and the geriatrician in Belgium: A qualitative study of their relationship. https://core.ac.uk/download/pdf/26905148.pdf (accessed on 14th July 2025).
10. de Bruin, S. R. (2009). *Sowing in the Autumn Season: Exploring Benefits of Green Care Farms for Dementia Patients*. https://core.ac.uk/download/pdf/29250250.pdf (accessed on 14th July 2025).
11. Ellingson, L. L. (2009). Spirituality within the comprehensive geriatric assessment process. https://core.ac.uk/download/215442322.pdf (accessed on 14th July 2025).
12. Estes, C. L., Yeo, G. W., Molina, L. C., Plumb, M., Hernandez, M., Goldberg, S., Wallace, S. P., et al. (2007). Women, health and aging: Building a statewide movement. https://core.ac.uk/download/71355916.pdf (accessed on 14th July 2025).
13. Fastenmeier, H., & Leuca, M. (2025). Problems and chances at the interface between hospital care and geriatric rehabilitation. https://core.ac.uk/download/pdf/6294474.pdf (accessed on 14th July 2025).

14. Formosa, M. (2013). Population trends and ageing policy in Malta. https://core.ac.uk/download/46602372.pdf (accessed on 14th July 2025).
15. Henwood, M., Larkin, M., & Milne, A. (2017). Seeing the wood for the trees: Carer-related research and knowledge–A scoping review. https://core.ac.uk/download/145186527.pdf (accessed on 14th July 2025).
16. Husna, A. A., Robaiyah, K., & Tanti, I. R. (2009). Dental students' knowledge and perception of elderly in relation to geriatric dentistry training. https://core.ac.uk/download/11491051.pdf (accessed on 14th July 2025).
17. Khanal, S., Shrestha, S., & Shrestha, S. (2019). Polypharmacy in elderly cancer patients: Challenges and the way clinical pharmacists can contribute in resource-limited settings. https://core.ac.uk/download/287605655.pdf (accessed on 14th July 2025).
18. Knapp, K. A. (2009). Innovative programs serving diverse populations: The community college caregiver training initiative. https://core.ac.uk/download/71356405.pdf (accessed on 14th July 2025).
19. Lampugnale, C. A. (2017). Surgical assessment of the geriatric oncology patient. https://open.bu.edu/bitstream/2144/26707/5/Lampugnale_bu_0017N_13146.pdf (accessed on 14th July 2025).
20. Morton, S., & Dunn, W. (2015). Addressing the health needs of an aging America: New opportunities for evidence-based policy solutions. https://core.ac.uk/download/75783019.pdf (accessed on 14th July 2025).
21. Palenik, V., & Radvansky, M. (2010). The Slovakian long-term care system. *ENEPRI Research Report No. 86*. https://core.ac.uk/download/5086633.pdf (accessed on 14th July 2025).
22. Reuben, D. B., & Ward, K. T. (2016). Comprehensive geriatric assessment. https://core.ac.uk/download/595556693.pdf (accessed on 14th July 2025).
23. Swaminathan, D., & Swaminathan, V. (2015). Geriatric oncology: Problems with under-treatment within this population. https://core.ac.uk/download/41992493.pdf (accessed on 14th July 2025).
24. Vaughan-Wrobel, B. C., & White, S. (2008). An educational pathway for geriatric home caregivers. https://core.ac.uk/download/71356265.pdf (accessed on 14th July 2025).
25. Wynn-Grundy, N. J. (2016). Undiagnosed depression in the elderly and healthcare education. https://core.ac.uk/download/70426926.pdf (accessed on 14th July 2025).

CHRONIC DISEASE MANAGEMENT

4

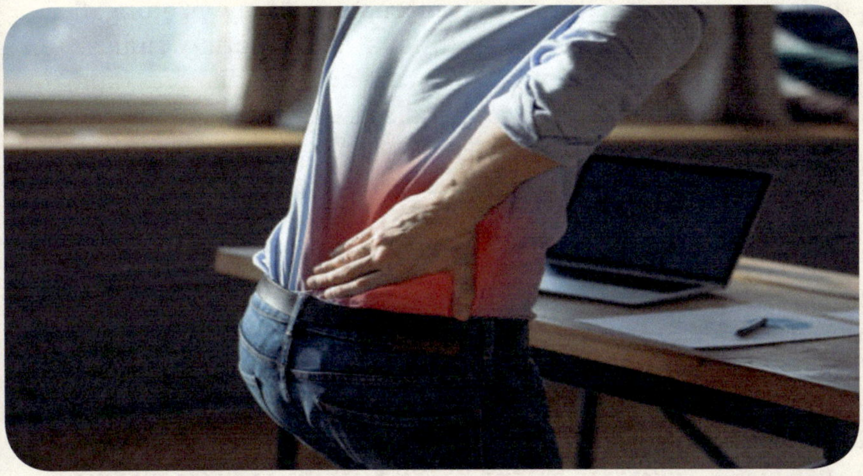

LEARNING OBJECTIVES

After studying this chapter, you will be able to:

1. Describe the types of chronic diseases
2. Explain the risk factors for chronic diseases
3. Know the impact of chronic diseases on individuals
4. Describe the strategies for chronic disease management
5. Understand the role of healthcare providers in chronic disease management
6. Understand the role of community and public health initiatives in the management of chronic diseases

Introduction

Chronic disease is a large-scale threat to public health characterized by consistent illness that is often treated and managed consistently with medical intervention. Hypertension, cardiovascular disease, and diabetes are types of chronic conditions that complicate individuals' health but also weigh down healthcare systems globally. Since they are increasingly becoming widespread among various populations, it is important to delve deeper into the complexities of managing chronic disease in an effort to develop significant interventions. With the alteration in lifestyles in society, risk factors for disease development and disease progression, like sedentary lifestyle and diet, have become more common. This requires an integrated approach to understanding the medical and social determinants of chronic disease trajectories, which provides new leads for improved strategies in healthcare delivery and patient education. Effective control of chronic diseases depends on an interdisciplinary approach that unites healthcare professionals, patients, and community resources.

Coordination across various sectors is reflected in initiatives intended for the betterment of public health. For example, recent discussions regarding the neglected tropical diseases underscore the importance of coordinated advocacy, public health interventions, and research to construct an integrated health policy framework, thereby highlighting the intricacy of addressing health matters at both the grassroots and international levels. (Harries et al., 2013). Such interdisciplinary collaboration is capable of generating new practices that will enable patients to assume more active roles in their own care, thus improving outcomes and quality of life. Management of chronic diseases thus requires not only clinical interventions but also a systemic approach that identifies and addresses root health conditions affecting populations. As we delve deeper into the management of chronic diseases, it is crucial to overcome obstacles in the way of good care. Factors such as socioeconomic status, access to healthcare resources, and beliefs about health can influence disease severity and the success of management. Furthermore, the stigma usually associated with chronic diseases can deter individuals from obtaining timely medical care, contributing further to management difficulties. The debates over chronic diseases must address these intricate issues while formulating viable solutions.

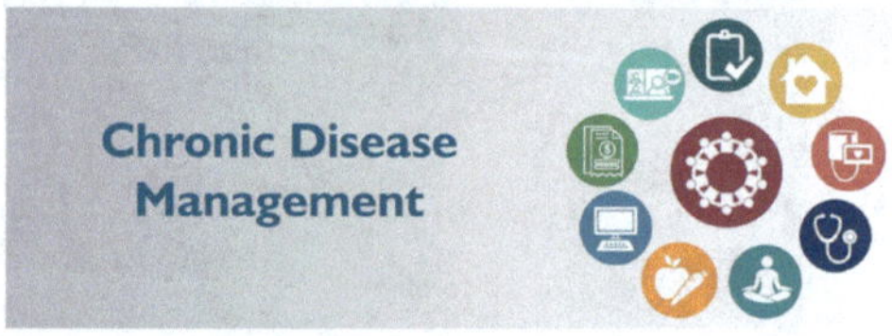

Figure 4.1. Chronic disease management.

Source: https://www.medicoverhospitals.in/images/articles/navigating-path-effective-chronic-disease-management.webp.

Thus, the primary concern remains providing a supportive setting for patients, which can be facilitated through education and community-based programs. This integrative method, besides fostering active health management, also complements best practices of contemporary patient-focused care, which is grounded in facilitating wellness and preventing disease progression through informed decision-making and community-based assistance (Figure 4.1).

Definition of Chronic Diseases

Chronic illnesses are a significant category of health issues characterized by prolonged and ongoing conditions necessitating endless medical attention. Heart disease, diabetes, and chronic respiratory disease emerge among the conditions that outdo acute health issues in terms of duration as well as complexity. Chronic illnesses tend to present multifactorial etiology, for example, resulting from a spectrum of genetic, environmental, and lifestyle factors. For example, diet, stress, and exercise may be related to hypertension; hence, understanding these factors is necessary for effective management programs. Moreover, the impacts of chronic illnesses extend beyond health, as most chronic illnesses lead to psychosocial and psychological issues, showcasing the need for managing chronic diseases through a multidisciplinary approach that takes into account the body as well as the psychosocial dimensions of patient care. An intrinsic characteristic of chronic illness is that it tends to have a gradual progression, with the potential for occasional flare-ups. This often necessitates constant monitoring and reconfiguring of treatment plans in order to maximize symptom management. Chronic illness may require multidisciplinary care teams, including healthcare providers from various specialties, to design integrative care plans tailored to the patient's distinct needs. For example, diabetics will benefit from the collaboration of endocrinologists, dietitians, and diabetes educators to manage their disease in the most optimal way. Without a robust system that integrates these professionals, the likelihood of achieving the desired health outcomes is significantly reduced. Additionally, chronic diseases have the potential to radically alter an individual's quality of life, further highlighting the need for holistic and preventive disease management strategies that include medical, emotional, and social support components. Proper chronic disease management not only involves their definitions and implications but also focuses on patient empowerment and education. Patient education equips patients to take an active role in managing their own health, which is crucial for effective chronic disease management. For instance, education regarding the signs and symptoms of their illness enables patients to recognize when they need medical attention, preventing complications. Education interventions also need to incorporate lifestyle modifications that are healthy for long-term health, such as exercise, diet, and stress management. With shifting models of care, the integration of technology, such as telehealth visits and mobile health applications, becomes a progressively valuable tool for assisting patients. This approach addresses the chronic illness complex and finds it essential to learn continuously and be adaptable in therapies, keeping in mind that each patient's course is unique and requires flexible management regimens (Figure 4.2).

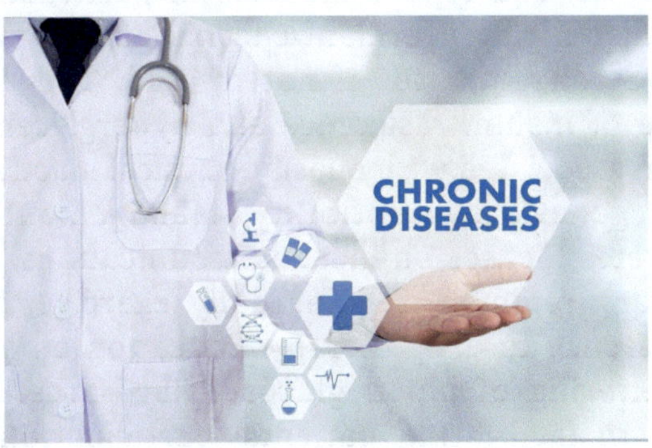

Figure 4.2. Chronic diseases.

Source: https://nutrition.org/wp-content/uploads/2022/08/CHRONIC-DISEASES-Healthcare-concept.jpg.

Importance of Chronic Disease Management

Chronic disease management is not just vital for patient health results, but also affects public health and fiscal stability. Chronic conditions such as diabetes, heart disease, and obesity are increasingly prevalent, so organized management programs are crucial to enhance patients' quality of life and contain healthcare costs. Effective control of chronic disease enables patients to control their condition by promoting self-management interventions that can alleviate symptoms and prevent complications. Effective education and support can enable individuals to make informed lifestyle choices, adhere to treatment regimens, and become active participants in their health care. Therefore, this preventive action is paramount for improving health outcomes and ultimately reducing the economic burden that chronic diseases impose on healthcare systems and society as a whole, according to the discussion of organizational performance and employee wellness (Lawson et al., 2019). In addition, integrating chronic disease care in healthcare systems minimizes the adverse effects of chronic diseases on quality of life and productivity. Chronic patients typically experience not just physical difficulties, but also emotional and psychological burdens that lower their capability for engaging in daily activities. By integrating holistic management systems, medical professionals can address the complex needs of such patients, improving overall physical and psychological well-being. Multifactorial interventions, such as peer support and health coaching, are effective in fostering resilience and promoting mental wellness. Such interventions are especially important for organizations seeking to enhance employee wellness, as research has shown that healthier employees exhibit higher levels of engagement and productivity, thereby enhancing organizational performance (Lawson et al., 2019). Besides, the convergence of climate change and chronic disease management poses new risks and necessitates flexibility in public health policy. As the expanding danger from environmental change worsens, chronic disease might worsen with increased pollution and altered climate trends that affect determinants of health. The CDC's Building Resilience Against Climate Effects (BRACE) model illustrates that developing strategies not only to manage chronic disease but also to strengthen community resilience against the health impacts of climate change is essential. The development of initiatives in resilience, such as addressing the varied social and environmental determinants of health, is most critical for addressing the health impacts of a changing climate. By emphasizing such holistic approaches, health systems are better positioned to meet the needs of chronic disease management amid ongoing environmental changes, thereby ensuring sustainable health gains for future generations.

4.1. Types of Chronic Diseases

Learning Outcome

1. Describe the cardiovascular diseases
2. Understand the management of diabetes mellitus
3. Learn about chronic respiratory diseases

Chronic diseases include a broad category of health conditions that require chronic management and typically significantly impact the quality of life in those with them. The most prevalent categories include cardiovascular diseases, such as hypertension, heart failure, and coronary heart disease. These diseases are caused by a combination of genetic predisposition, behavioral patterns, and environmental factors. Effective management, in most cases, involves lifestyle adjustments such as improved diet, increased exercise, and adherence to medication. The chronic nature of these diseases requires long-term commitment to treatment and follow-up, as such complications may arise if management measures are not adhered to. Also, cardiovascular diseases underscore the importance of an integrated strategy for chronic disease management through ongoing education and patient support systems, so that patients may have control over their conditions in coordination with healthcare staff. Yet another huge category of chronic diseases is respiratory diseases, encompassing chronic obstructive pulmonary disease (COPD) and asthma. These conditions are primarily due to chronic exposure to air pollution, smoking, and allergens, which result in inflammation and airway obstruction. Respiratory chronic disease patients present with a variety of symptoms ranging from mild to severe that interfere with their ability to function on a daily basis. Effective management measures include pharmacologic interventions, such as bronchodilators and corticosteroids, and non-pharmacologic interventions, such as smoking cessation and pulmonary rehabilitation. Continued monitoring of respiratory function and the delivery of tailored treatment plans are central to effective chronic disease management. They not only cure symptoms but also help reduce the rate of exacerbations and hospitalization, as well as ensure improved overall patient health status. Diabetes, and type 2 diabetes in particular, is another highly prevalent chronic disease with grave consequences if not treated. This is a state of insulin resistance and hyperglycemia, often associated with obesity, physical inactivity, and genetic susceptibility. Management of diabetes focuses on lifestyle modifications, i.e., dietary regimen, regular daily exercise, and adherence to drug therapy. Education on self-monitoring of blood glucose plays a central role in facilitating patients' participation in managing their disease. Involving the patient in their care increases feelings of ownership and accountability, which are required for long-term adherence to treatment protocols. Meeting the multidimensional aspects of diabetes care by providers can improve patient outcomes and reduce the risk of diabetes complications such as neuropathy, nephropathy, and cardiovascular disease, underscoring the immediate need for integrative approaches to managing chronic diseases (Figure 4.3).

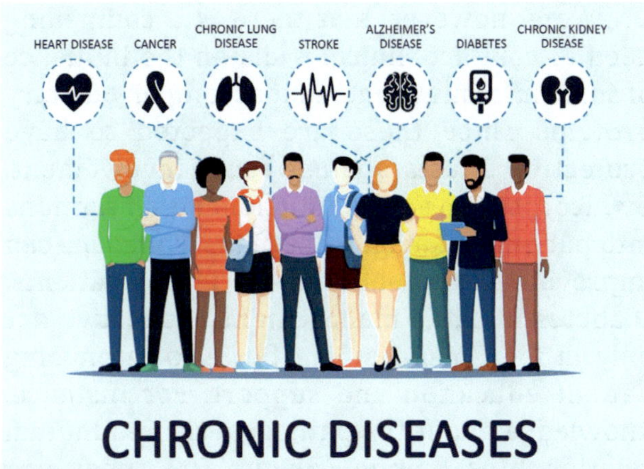

Figure 4.3. Types of chronic diseases.

Source: https://mantracare.org/wp-content/uploads/2021/12/What-Is-Chronic-Illness.jpg.

4.1.1. Cardiovascular Diseases

In the treatment of chronic diseases, cardiovascular diseases (CVDs) are one of the major challenges and are noted for their widespread prevalence and complexity. CVDs are a collection of heart and blood vessel disorders that encompass hypertension, coronary heart disease, and heart failure. The epidemiologic evidence identifies lifestyle factors such as diet, physical inactivity, and smoking as responsible for a high proportion of the risk of CVDs. Furthermore, the intersection of lifestyle and environmental exposures cannot be overlooked. Climate change, an international issue of concern, is increasingly impacting cardiovascular well-being, as documented by the increasing frequency and intensity of heat events and weather-related extremes that exacerbate disease states (Aytur et al., 2014). These shifting dynamics necessitate an integrated appreciation for not only the biological and behavioral determinants that underpin CVDs but also the broader environmental determinants that shape their management. Inflammaging, a clinical description of the chronic low-grade inflammatory state commonly encountered in older age, has become a determinant of the pathogenesis of many chronic diseases, including cardiovascular disease (Elias et al., 2019). This inflammatory response can lead to endothelial dysfunction and increased arterial stiffness, both of which are typical of heart disease. The elderly are at particular risk because the combination of systemic inflammation with other chronic illnesses renders them more challenging to treat. Effective treatment of CVDs in this population requires a multimodal approach that addresses inflammation through lifestyle modifications, including an anti-inflammatory diet, exercise, and, possibly, pharmacological intervention. Second, targeted intervention strategies must account for the distinctive inflammatory patterns of older individuals to maximize benefits and mitigate the impact of cardiovascular disease. Finally, the contribution of social determinants of health to the management of cardiovascular disease cannot be overstated. Determinants, including socioeconomic status, availability, and education, all influence the prevalence and management of CVDs within groups. Community action programs aimed at improving heart health can empower individuals to make sensible lifestyle choices, eventually reducing their risk. Furthermore, overall public health campaigns must include climate adaptation as an integral component, developing resilience against adverse health impacts of environmental change that instigate cardiovascular risks. It requires intersectoral collaboration among policymakers, healthcare practitioners, and communities to support holistic chronic disease management, in which interventions are not merely clinically ideal but also contextually and culturally tailored to various populations (Aytur et al., 2014) (Figure 4.4).

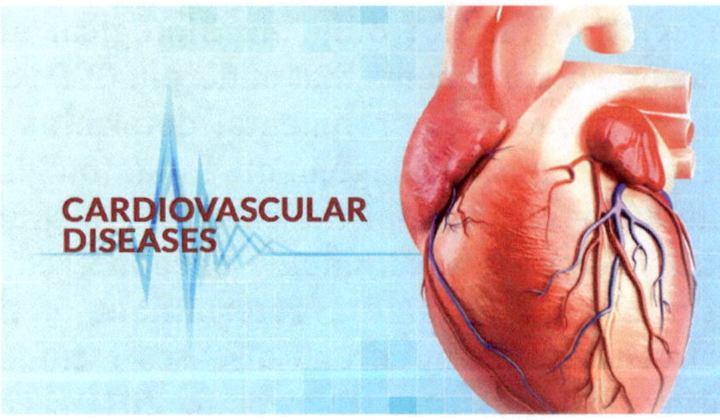

Figure 4.4. Cardiovascular diseases.

Source: https://cardiologybd.com/wp-content/uploads/2023/10/Risk-Reduction-of-Cardiovascular-Disease.jpeg.

4.1.2. Diabetes Mellitus

Management of Diabetes mellitus (DM) is essential in consideration of its position as a chronic disorder with long-term health implications globally. DM is characterized by an excess of blood glucose due to defects in insulin secretion, insulin action, or both. noteworthy is the fact that this polyetiologic diffuse syndrome encompasses various etiologies, as emphasized by the need for accurate diagnosis and classification based on underlying etiology. It is important to distinguish between the two forms of DM—Type 1 and Type 2 —and the other forms, because they have different management plans. Moreover, clinical presentation often represents not only hyperglycemia but also the severity and stage of the disease, which is involved in long-term treatment decision-making. Such multifaceted knowledge allows practitioners to start particular therapeutic regimens that can enhance the outcomes in patients and neutralize the risks of chronic diabetic complications. Dietary management is a cornerstone of effective DM control, reflecting greater recognition of nutrition's important role in the management of chronic disease. New dietary approaches have arisen, particularly with regard to the prevention of diabetic nephropathy (DN) and progression to more severe renal stages. Properly adapted macronutrient intake—balanced with caloric reduction to counteract obesity—has long been advocated. Recent studies emphasize the significance of the source of dietary proteins and their gliotoxin content, as they may play important roles in arresting the progression of DN. Note, however, that there is a compelling need to conduct clinical trials on the influence of some micronutrients that accompany dietary proteins since these are expected to have protective effects against renal involvement. By incorporating such nutritional interventions into patients' management plans, clinicians can improve overall quality of life in DM patients. Diabetes mellitus management is effective not only in food management but also in ongoing patient education and support. For instance, knowledge about the pathogenesis and mutual relationships among various DM types can encourage patients to follow self-management practices tailored to their condition. Education on self-management of medication, exercise, and blood glucose monitoring is a critical component of patient education.

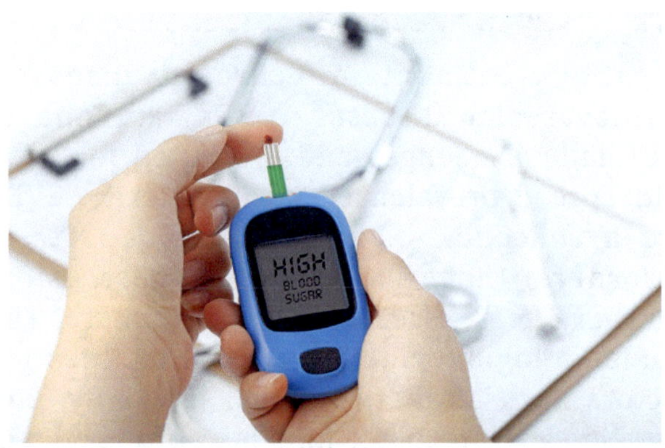

Figure 4.5. Diabetes mellitus.

Source: https://jsshospital.in/wp-content/uploads/2022/03/Blog.jpg.

Clinicians should also consider the psychological dimensions of living with diabetes, including the stress involved in chronic disease management. Embracing a holistic approach to patient care can enable better adherence to maintenance management and ultimately improve health outcomes. The acknowledgement of these diverse factors towards an integrated strategy for the control of DM highlights the imperatives of ongoing research and the modulation of therapeutic modalities that align with both current evidence and patients' lifestyles (Figure 4.5).

4.1.3. Chronic Respiratory Diseases

Chronic respiratory diseases, such as illnesses like chronic obstructive pulmonary disease (COPD), asthma, and pulmonary hypertension, are a serious public health issue globally. Not only do these illnesses reduce the quality of life for affected individuals, but they also have significant economic implications for healthcare systems. COPD, for example, is characterized by irreversible respiratory symptoms and airflow limitation caused primarily by prolonged exposure to injurious particulates or gases, commonly through cigarette smoking. With the growing incidence of such conditions, effective chronic disease management must include comprehensive assessments to tailor interventions to the symptoms and etiology of respiratory issues. Providing programs focused on the elimination of smoking, ventilation, and patient education is crucial to improving health outcomes and reducing hospitalizations for chronic respiratory illnesses. The management of chronic respiratory conditions also requires a multidisciplinary approach, with emphasis on care coordination among health professionals. Coordination is essential during disease monitoring, exacerbation control, and lifetime adherence to treatment regimens. For instance, pulmonary hypertension patients require not only pharmacologic management but also lifestyle modification to minimize symptom exacerbation. Critical strategies include routine follow-ups and the use of telemedicine technologies that enable patients to document symptoms remotely, thereby enabling timely adjustments to therapeutic interventions. Also, managing comorbidities typically associated with chronic respiratory diseases, such as cardiovascular disease, is essential to enhancing patients' general well-being and providing comprehensive health care for complex needs. In understanding the broader meaning of chronic respiratory disease, there is a corresponding necessity to understand the environmental determinants of its worsening.

Climate change, for example, has a strong impact on respiratory outcomes by altering the frequency and magnitude of environmental pollutants and allergens. The Centers for Disease Control and Prevention recommends that building community resilience is an essential step towards countering health disparities fueled by climate effects, which can disproportionately affect those already living with chronic respiratory conditions (Aytur et al., 2014). Thus, integrating environmental health approaches into the management of chronic diseases is necessary to reduce their incidence. Governments and health systems must work together to establish policies that address both clinical and environmental determinants of health, thereby creating sustainable solutions to chronic respiratory diseases and enhancing public health outcomes (Figure 4.6).

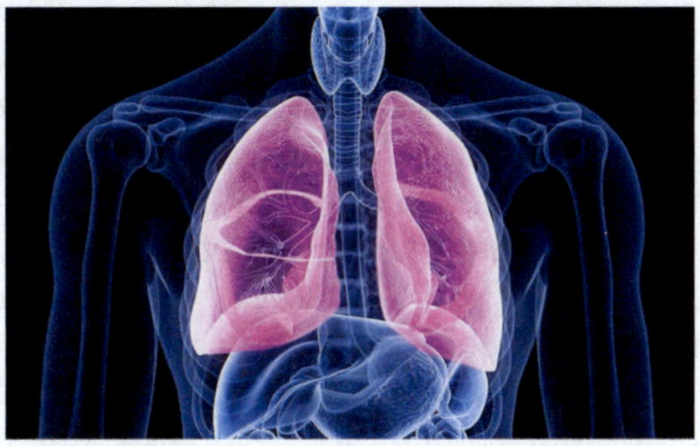

Figure 4.6. Chronic respiratory disease.

Source: https://ebv2e3r5onu.exactdn.com/wp-content/uploads/2020/01/Lung-Diseases.jpg?strip=all&lossy=1&ssl=1.

Test Your Knowledge

1. What is cardiovascular disease?
2. What are the 3 chronic respiratory diseases?

4.2. Risk Factors for Chronic Diseases

Learning Outcome

1. Understands the role of lifestyle choices in the management of chronic diseases
2. Know the concept of genetic predisposition
3. Describe the environmental influences in chronic disease management

Chronic disease risk factors are multivariate and include genetic, environmental, and lifestyle factors. Genetically predetermined susceptibilities can hugely elevate people's vulnerability to such diverse diseases as cardiovascular diseases and diabetes. The contribution of the environment, such as exposure to toxins and health hazards resulting from climate, remains increasingly important. Global climate change poses a major threat through more air pollution and heat illness, which risks exacerbating underlying chronic disease. According to the Centers for Disease Control and Prevention (CDC) in their Building Resilience Against Climate Effects (BRACE) framework, effective handling of these threats requires a combination of measures that integrate public health programs and environmental policy. This structured approach underscores the importance of understanding how to build community resilience and how to minimize the adverse effects of chronic diseases linked to environmental transformation (Aytur et al., 2014). Lifestyle factors are also an important factor in the outcome of chronic diseases. Unhealthy eating habits, lack of physical exercise, and smoking are common risk factors responsible for conditions like obesity, hypertension, and type 2 diabetes. The intersection of these lifestyle variables and social determinants of health underscores a broader context, illustrating how healthcare access and socioeconomic status influence individual choices. For example, individuals residing in food deserts struggle to receive healthy foods, leading to further diet-related disease. Effective chronic disease management, therefore, needs to address these inequities by promoting improved lifestyle options through education and community-based resources and developing a broader worldview that bridges personal health to environmental and socioeconomic determinants (Aytur et al., 2014). Furthermore, the complexity of chronic diseases also lies in their classification and treatment modalities, such as in pulmonary hypertension (PH).

This disorder illustrates how chronic diseases can result from a range of underlying causes and therefore require an individualized management and diagnostic strategy. Dividing PH into categories, such as those associated with left heart disease or pulmonary disorders, helps reinforce the importance of identifying chronic diseases as multifactorial disorders. As is the case in the literature on current consensus statements that dictate comprehensive management and treatment in veterinary medicine, human medicine must similarly adopt a multidisciplinary model for chronic illness management. This involves not only treating the primary disease but also addressing any comorbidities, thereby adopting a more integrated model of care that maximizes overall health and enhances outcomes (Figure 4.7).

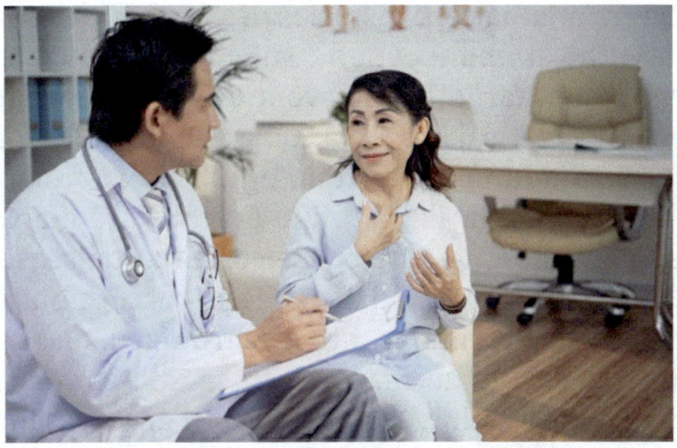

Figure 4.7. Risk factors for chronic diseases.

Source: https://primocare.com/en/wp-content/uploads/sites/3/2023/06/Common-Risk-Factors-1024x683.jpg.

4.2.1. Lifestyle Choices

Lifestyle plays a major role in controlling chronic diseases and in the state and quality of health. Decisions regarding diet, exercise, and stress management form the foundation for the prevention and control of chronic disease. For instance, eating a well-balanced diet rich in fruits, vegetables, and whole grains can lead to dramatic reductions in obesity, diabetes, and cardiovascular disease. Additionally, regular exercise protects not just against weight gain but also enhances cardiovascular health and guards against the effects of stress. With these connections, a holistic strategy emphasizing healthy lifestyle changes is essential to successful management of chronic diseases, enabling individuals to become their own partners in their health narratives. Stress management is yet another indispensable element of lifestyle choices that can play a drastic role in the trajectory of chronic diseases. Evidence highlights that chronic stress may lead to negative health consequences through physiological mechanisms that might be implicated in disease development and exacerbation. Individuals underestimate the powerful role psychological states play in their physical well-being, leading to a lack of integration between psychosocial and physical care. This disconnection between interventions in health care highlights the need for health care models that address both psychosocial and biological aspects. Understanding these connections, health practitioners can better enable patients with stress management techniques and thus improve the outcomes of chronic conditions. The trend toward an integrated understanding of health emphasizes the need for individuals to create room for stress reduction in daily life. Furthermore, socioeconomic and cultural environments surrounding lifestyle need to be included in the conversation regarding managing chronic diseases. Social organization typically constructs barriers that dissuade individuals from practicing healthier behaviors, citing gender and broader public health determinants.

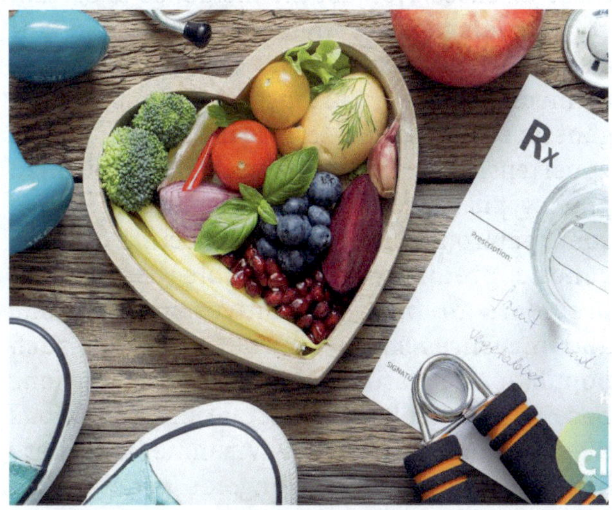

Figure 4.8. Lifestyle changes to reduce chronic disease risk.

Source: https://s3.us-west-2.amazonaws.com/community-health-partners/_rectangle/CHP_lifestyle-changes-blogHeader_1080x1920.jpg.

A case in point is the way gender attitudes dissuade men from accessing preventive care or engaging in healthy practices, lowering their chances of being able to manage chronic disease effectively. The evidence from a recent report indicates the way cultural norms and social attitudes promote unhealthy lifestyles and therefore enhance chronic disease risks. Addressing these cultural barriers through directed interventions can encourage healthier behaviors that ultimately lead to improved health outcomes in diverse groups. By recognizing that lifestyle is shaped by a complex interplay of social factors, healthcare professionals can develop improved plans for chronic disease management across diverse settings and further enhance public health efforts (Figure 4.8).

4.2.2. Genetic Predisposition

The concept of genetic predisposition plays an essential role in the treatment of chronic diseases, as it accounts for the biological processes that make individuals susceptible to these diseases. Not just the incidence of certain chronic diseases, genetic differences might also affect disease severity and the response to medication. For instance, populations with genetic susceptibility to disease states such as hypertension or diabetes may exhibit intensified phenotypic expressions of these diseases upon some environmental stimuli. Detection of these genetic predispositions enables healthcare providers to plan preventive interventions and measures more appropriately for such populations. Awareness of such predispositions becomes particularly important in populations living in industrialized environments, where lifestyle determinants alongside genetics are rapidly adding to the prevalence of chronic diseases. In addition, the genetic basis of chronic disease is evident in most research that assigns heritable etiologic contribution to conditions such as nontuberculous mycobacterial infections and allergic responses. For instance, research indicates that individuals with intrinsic lung pathology, such as bronchiectasis and cystic fibrosis, are at high risk of developing pulmonary infections caused by nontuberculous mycobacteria (NTM) (Adcock et al., 2017). This alignment underscores the complexity of chronic disease management, in which genetic predisposition is intertwined with environmental factors and patient histories. By further peeling back the immunogenetic substrate, clinicians can design targeted interventions that not only treat the clinical presentation of such conditions but also address their etiology. This approach holds the potential to refine overall care plans, reducing the long-term burden of chronic disease. In addition to pulmonary, genetic susceptibility strongly determines other chronic diseases, such as atopic dermatitis, which shares many similarities with its counterpart in dogs, canine atopic dermatitis (CAD). From the research, it is apparent that environmental and lifestyle trends, together with genetic susceptibilities, have led to a surge in allergic diseases among humans (Nødtvedt et al., 2007). It is feasible to recognize individuals at risk and also advise individualized treatment plans based on these genetic influences. These approaches, based on knowledge of genetic susceptibility, can be employed to manage chronic disease more effectively by providing guidance on dietary and lifestyle changes aimed at limiting exposure to allergens or pathogens that trigger exacerbations of such disease. Ultimately, an understanding of genetic predisposition deepens the conversation about chronic disease management, engaging preventive and integrated care approaches in clinical settings.

4.2.3. Environmental Influences

The relationship between chronic disease management and the environment is multifaceted, encompassing physical, social, and built environments that, together, determine the behavior and health outcomes of individuals. An example is the availability of green space and exercise space, which significantly affects an individual's lifestyle, particularly obesity and obesity-related morbidity. This is the case of Mexican American women, who often report low physical activity in their free time. There is evidence that higher levels of partner support are associated with higher levels of physical activity and that networks can be effective at changing health-related behavior. As a result, improving environmental factors—such as making physical activity safe and accessible—can have direct implications for better health and facilitate chronic disease management across various populations (Brecht et al., 2020). Also, the built environment plays a crucial role in shaping the food choices readily available to communities, as a foundation for chronic disease prevention. Access to healthy food shops easily is highly dependent on geographical location. Locally defined areas referred to as food deserts with low access to healthy food stores exacerbate the spread of diseases such as diabetes and cardiovascular disease. Thus, through the inclusion of supportive physical spaces and policies that promote healthy access to food, supportive physical environments are essential to achieving a revolutionary effect on disease management programs. Such programs must be informed by comprehensive early childhood policies that create supportive, consistent environments for young children, thereby laying a foundation for lifelong health and disease prevention. Moreover, environmental intervention must be accomplished by collective interventions involving community members, policymakers, and health professionals. Interventions specifically designed to fit cultural environments and community needs may ensure sustainable outcomes. For instance, participatory community-based research can identify barriers to physical activity and help build strategic partnerships to enhance support systems. Involving family and significant others can form a supportive social network that promotes healthier lifestyle choices. With the emphasis on the interaction between environmental determinants and behavior, it is clear that sustainable chronic disease care must incorporate an ecological approach, which, in the long run, translates into a healthier population and improved public health outcomes (Brecht et al., 2020) (Figure 4.9).

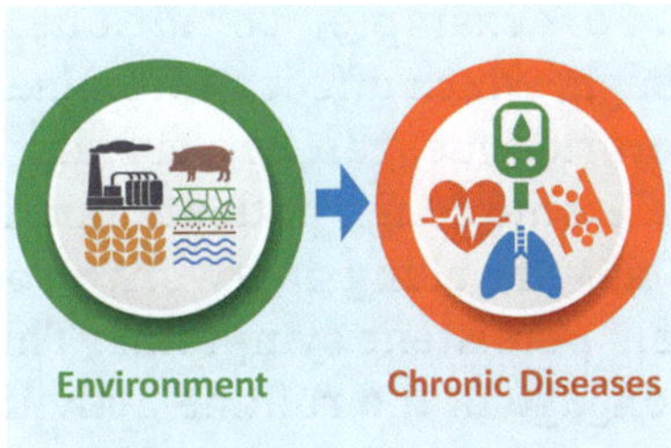

Figure 4.9. Environment strongly influences chronic disease development.

Source: https://factor.niehs.nih.gov/sites/niehs-factor/files/2025/03/feature/environment-predicts-chronic-disease-body1_0.jpg.

Test Your Knowledge

1. What is the role of lifestyle choices in the management of chronic diseases?
2. Explain the environmental influences in chronic disease management.

4.3. Impact of Chronic Diseases on Individuals

Learning Outcome

1. Know the physical health consequences of chronic diseases
2. Describe the psychological effects of chronic diseases
3. Understand the economic burden of chronic diseases

Chronic illnesses can significantly influence individuals' lives, extending beyond physical well-being to encompass emotional and social domains. For example, conditions such as chronic cough, which affect approximately 10% of adults worldwide, can be very disruptive to daily life. Chronic cough patients find it hard to have a social life alongside work productivity due to their persistent symptoms. This lack of ability to engage in the routine activities of life can lead to isolation and anxiety, compounded by the difficulty of their physical status. The psychological impact of chronic diseases typically demands an integrated management process, in which the health practitioner considers both the physical and psychological aspects of the condition to maximize quality of life. It is vital to appreciate the extent of such impacts to guide effective interventions in chronic disease management that address the intricate needs of individuals living with the conditions (Brooks et al., 2023). Of particular significance is the role played by health literacy in chronic disease management. Individuals with the capacity to understand and negotiate health information are well-positioned to effectively manage their condition. Health literacy empowers patients with chronic conditions such as diabetes and hypertension to make informed choices regarding treatment and lifestyle changes necessary for management. Furthermore, adequate health literacy has been found necessary to enhance self-care abilities, which are crucial to the maintenance of health and the avoidance of complications. This association emphasizes the need for health practitioners to facilitate health literacy by making effective communication and educational interventions, so that patients are adequately knowledgeable about their treatment options and their own health needs. By facilitating health literacy, we can bridge the gap between professional advice and patients' interpretation, thereby enhancing the effectiveness of managing chronic diseases (Kadar et al., 2024). In addition to the physical and mental disabilities, chronic diseases also frequently weigh patients and their families financially. Repeated medical charges, pharmacy expenses, and potential loss of income due to illness can drain financial resources. Patients with chronic diseases are often forced to maneuver complex healthcare systems that also work to promote feelings of uncertainty and stress.

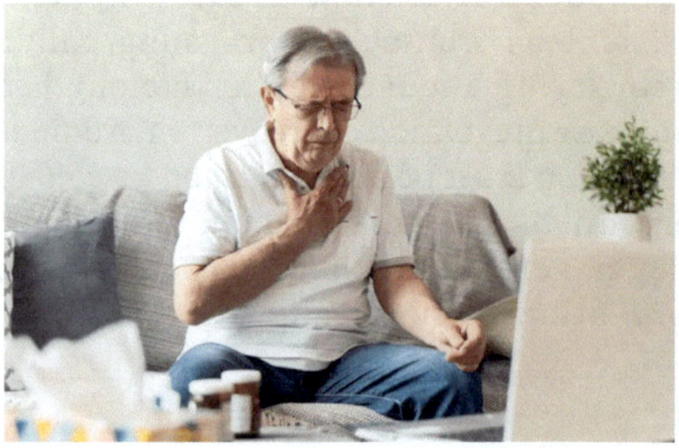

Figure 4.10. Impacts of chronic diseases on health.

Source: https://eghealthcare.net/app/uploads/2023/05/image-8-1024x681.webp.

They may also be discriminated against socially or even in the workplace, making their challenges even greater. Such economic impacts should be remembered by healthcare policymakers when designing programs to better manage chronic disease. It may make care and support systems cheaper and more accessible for individuals with chronic illness. Lastly, an integrated approach that considers the economic, emotional, and social dimensions of chronic diseases is key to effectively managing them and achieving improved health outcomes (Brooks et al., 2023) (Figure 4.10).

4.3.1. Physical Health Consequences

Chronic disease care is highly interrelated with subsequent physical health ramifications of the diseases. Chronic disease often manifests not only by the presenting complaint of the disease, but also by secondary resulting medical complications that make patient management more complex. For instance, patients with chronic diseases will typically present with obesity, diabetes, and cardiovascular diseases that make the underlying condition more difficult to manage. These secondary health conditions can lead to reduced overall physical health, thereby increasing healthcare costs and necessitating an integrated management program that addresses various dimensions of health. Furthermore, the reciprocal relationship between chronic diseases and physical results of chronic diseases supports the significance of monitoring patients on an integrated level to ensure that treatment is not merely focused on the primary condition but also adapted to minimize its complications as well as maximize the overall quality of life, (Aytur et al., 2014). Physical outcomes of patients living with chronic disease are also affected by behavioral health factors. Depression, on the other hand, has been proven to have significant correlations with cardiovascular disease, including ischemic heart disease. Patients with major depressive disorder (MDD) exhibit a number of systemic features that make them susceptible to these conditions and find themselves in a vicious cycle of deteriorating health. The body's response to stress, as embodied by sympathetic overdrive and alterations in the hypothalamic-pituitary-adrenal axis, has the capability to lead to diminished heart function as well as increased morbidity. Addressing the psychological aspects of chronic disease care is thus imperative to improve physical health outcomes. With the application of integrated care practices that unify mental and physical care, healthcare providers are better positioned to care for patients living with the double burden of chronic disease and its psychological factors (Budiono et al., 2017). The physical setting also determines the health effects of chronic disease care. Urban planning, accessibility to green spaces, and transportation all contribute to people's capacity to lead healthy lives. Neighborhoods that incorporate active living through pedestrian walkability and recreational activity proximity reflect lower rates of obesity, diabetes, and other chronic diseases. Social determinants of health, such as socioeconomic status and healthcare access, also significantly contribute to physical health outcomes in individuals with chronic disease. With the increasing influence of chronic disease, it is essential to adopt a holistic strategy that is sensitive to the interplay among environment, behavior, and physical health. Successful chronic disease control is thus a means of synthesizing these in promoting robust communities which foster integrative health (Aytur et al., 2014) (Figure 4.11).

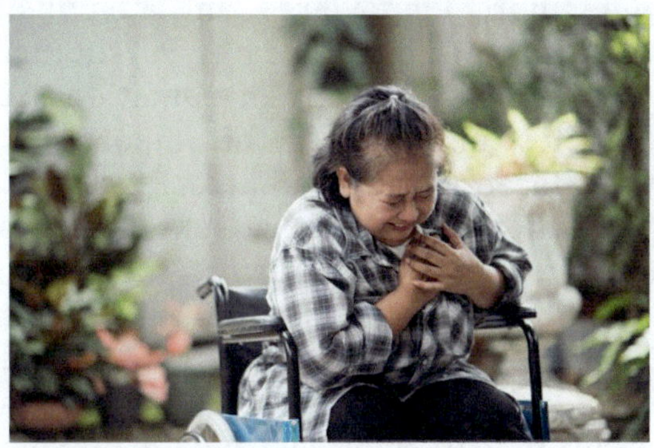

Figure 4.11. Chronic diseases and their adverse influence on physical health.

Source: https://lirp.cdn-website.com/450dd43d/dms3rep/multi/opt/elderly-woman-have-heart-disease-sitting-wheelchair-640w.jpg.

4.3.2. Psychological Effects

The psychological effects of chronic diseases significantly influence patients' overall health and coping mechanisms. Chronic diseases have a great tendency to induce immense psychological distress in the form of depression and anxiety, thus aggravating the physical presentation of the disease. This interaction between psychological and physical well-being is best demonstrated in conditions such as rheumatoid arthritis, where psychological distress adversely affects the response to therapy. The dissatisfactions of managing such chronic illnesses can spark a vicious circle of impaired coping abilities, as patients increasingly become incapable of properly managing both their physical and emotional health. Detection and management of these interconnected psychological factors are essential to improving health outcomes and minimizing the disease burden on patients, underscoring the need for care approaches that integrate medical therapy with psychological intervention (Geenen et al., 2015). In addition to mere tracking of medical information, the role of information technology in managing chronic diseases also significantly contributes to shaping patients' psychological empowerment. Effective communication via IT enables the patient to become more empowered and responsible for his/her own health care. Psychological empowerment, especially in conditions such as diabetes, underscores the importance of proper education and awareness. Psychological empowerment can enhance self-efficacy and motivate patients to adhere to life-changing health interventions. As patients sense they can manage their condition effectively, their overall satisfaction with care significantly rises, leading to improved health outcomes. This connection suggests that establishing an appropriate environment through rich-media communication can bridge the gap between healthcare professionals and patients, enhancing psychological resilience in the management of chronic diseases (Chawla et al., 2014). Treatment of the psychological effect of chronic illness must encompass more than one domain that unites mental health care and physical health care. Identification of the psychological components' role in controlling disease paves the way for coordinated treatment models that address both emotional and physical health demands. Coupled with therapeutic strategies such as cognitive-behavioral therapy, mindfulness, and social support, will counterbalance feelings of isolation and helplessness among patients to adopt healthier coping mechanisms. Secondly, interdisciplinary teams comprising medical personnel, psychologists, and social workers can provide holistic care to individualized needs. By including these psychological variables in chronic illness disease management programs, health systems can improve patients' quality of life and ultimately enhance treatment adherence and recovery outcomes (Geenen et al., 2015) (Figure 4.12).

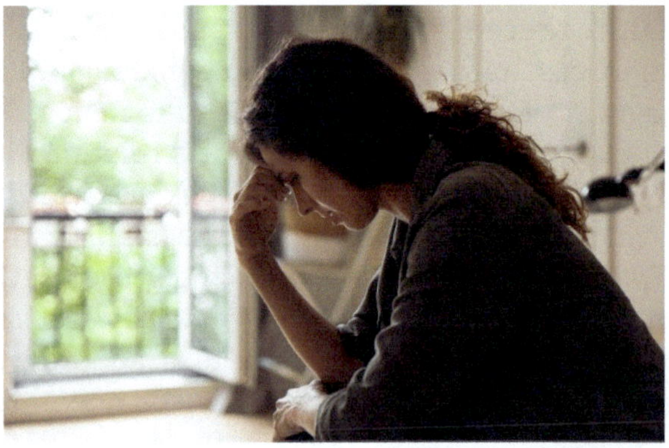

Figure 4.12. Psychological effects of chronic diseases.

Source: https://www.news-medical.net/images/Article_Images/ImageForArticle_23285_16679182446702017.jpg.

4.3.3. Economic Burden

The economic burden of chronic diseases places a huge health cost to health systems worldwide, impacting not only patients but also communities and economies nationally. Chronic diseases such as heart disease, diabetes, and respiratory diseases are highly prevalent and contribute to a vast number of healthcare costs in the form of hospitalization, outpatient visits, and long-term care. The economic impacts extend beyond direct health expenditures; they also include lost productivity and diminished quality of life for individuals. As chronic disease prevalence continues to rise due to the drivers of aging and lifestyle, the imperative for wise chronic disease control strategies only intensifies. Meeting this economic cost requires comprehensive public health interventions, including prevention and education, to mitigate the risks associated with these conditions. One aspect of addressing the economic costs associated with chronic diseases is understanding how they interact with other infectious diseases. One such disease that exemplifies how chronic diseases can create entrenched economic challenges for entire regions or countries is brucellosis. Disease management is more complex when one considers the socioeconomic effects on health systems, particularly in the developing world. The achievement of adopting effective public policy aimed at reducing the economic cost of chronic diseases, for example, chronic diseases resulting from zoonotic infections, can be exceptional. Multidisciplinary approaches, as advocated in the literature, espouse One Health as a framework that balances human, veterinary, and environmental health initiatives to combat the explosive economic burden incurred by communities plagued by chronic and infectious diseases, thereby enhancing societal resilience and growth (Fournier et al., 2018). Chronic diseases also reflect a deep relationship with health disparities, with socioeconomically disadvantaged populations being disproportionately affected. Individuals in such groups are more likely to face barriers to access to healthcare commodities, leading to less effective chronic disease management and increased economic costs. The high prevalence of infection among the vulnerable in soil-transmitted helminths contributes to this association with more distressing burdens in health due to high prevalence. Interventions are indicated but inequitably delivered; in 2016, only a majority of children at risk received the needed interventions (Addiss et al., 2018). Addressing this inequality is crucial to effectively mitigating the economic burdens of these chronic diseases on a large scale. A multi-faceted approach that includes greater healthcare access, improved education, and better public health interventions is essential for ensuring that all people, regardless of socioeconomic status, can effectively manage their chronic diseases and mitigate their economic burdens.

Test Your Knowledge

1. What are the physical effects of chronic disease?
2. What are the physiological effects of chronic illness?

4.4. Strategies for Chronic Disease Management

Learning Outcome

1. Understand the role of lifestyle modifications in the management of chronic diseases
2. Learn about medication adherence of chronic disease management
3. Describe the regular health monitoring of chronic disease management

Effective control of chronic disease requires an interdisciplinary team that includes lifestyle modification, medical treatment, and ongoing patient education. One of the strategies is encouraging healthy behaviors such as good eating, exercise, and drug adherence. Lifestyle modification has been effective in the prevention of increased severity and progression of chronic diseases such as diabetes and hypertension. In addition, self-management education provides patients with knowledge and skills to become actively involved in their care. It is important that healthcare providers customize these methods to suit an individual's needs according to age, socioeconomic status, and comorbidities. Customizing interventions can enable healthcare providers to enhance patient participation, leading to better health outcomes and quality of life. Furthermore, continuous monitoring of patients' progress is imperative, enabling timely adjustment of the treatment plan to address new complications or adherence barriers. The incorporation of technology and data analytics into patient care is another key part of chronic disease management. Telemedicine platforms, mobile health apps, and wearable technology enable real-time health tracking and facilitate improved patient-provider communication. For instance, remote patient monitoring can track changes in vital signs or medication use, providing invaluable information to inform clinical judgments. Further, the use of electronic health records (EHRs) can help coordinate multidisciplinary teams, enabling multiple health professionals to function optimally in managing complex chronic diseases. This network of communications not only optimizes care but also enables innovative strategies, such as predictive analytics, that identify at-risk patients before complications occur. Applying technology to manage chronic disease not only improves patient outcomes but also helps healthcare systems plan resources and reduce the costs of acute interventions. Lastly, investigating the role of the microbiome in chronic disease therapy is a new frontier that holds much promise. Increasing evidence has shown that alterations in the gut microbiota are associated with a range of chronic diseases, from metabolic to cardiovascular disease.

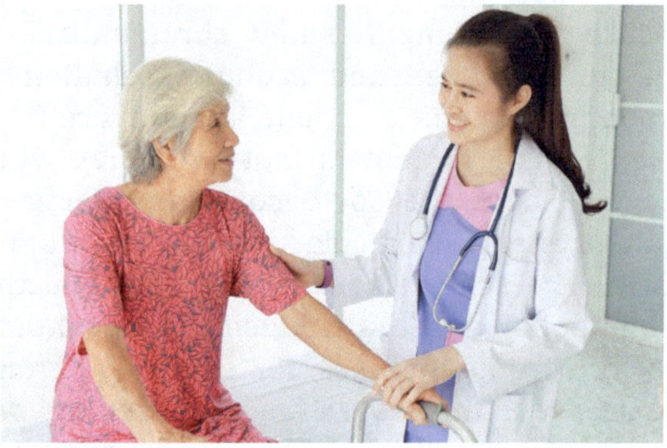

Figure 4.13. Strategies for chronic disease management.

Source: https://www.absclinicalservices.com/wp-content/uploads/2024/01/chronic-disease-strategies-for-effective-management.jpg.

Altering these microbial communities through dietary modification or probiotic supplementation could be a preventive or therapeutic intervention. Interventions aimed at restoring the balance of the microbes can enhance the immune function and overall health of patients. As more is investigated about the relationship between chronic illnesses and microbiome composition, there will be a need to incorporate such findings into patient management regimens. This holistic approach, which considers the complex interplay between microbiome health and chronic disease, reflects evolving strategies for controlling chronic diseases in humans (Abbott et al., 2020; Durack et al., 2019) (Figure 4.13).

4.4.1. Lifestyle Modifications

Lifestyle interventions play a crucial role in the management of chronic diseases, particularly in preventing disease-related complications in conditions such as obesity, diabetes, and cardiovascular disease. The inclusion of lifestyle modifications, such as dietary modification, exercise, and smoking cessation, can significantly benefit patient outcomes. Evidence indicates that interventions such as Health Risk Assessments (HRAs), in combination with supportive programs, have very strong evidence for preventing tobacco and controlling dietary fat intake. Comprehensive interventions like these encourage healthier lifestyles, thereby reducing the incidence of related diseases and improving the quality of life for individuals with chronic diseases. Effective lifestyle modification interventions also yield reduced healthcare costs in the long run, with evidence strong enough to suggest an incremental advantage of $3.20 for every dollar invested in these interventions, thereby underscoring their valuable role in the control of chronic diseases (George et al.). Dietary changes have gained particular popularity for their role in shaping chronic disease epidemiology. Emerging literature suggests that the gut microbiome, its coordination with inflammation and metabolic status, and dietary habits can collectively influence the generation of health-promoting metabolites, such as short-chain fatty acids (SCFAs). Not only do the metabolites ensure gut health, but they are also thought to be involved in improvements in immune function and metabolic control, of notable interest in conditions like cardiovascular disease and diabetes. In spite of the proven benefits of diet therapy, traditional food cultures in patients with chronic illnesses, like high-fat and low-fiber dietary habits, are still prevailing, which may exacerbate their illness. Hence, enhanced adherence to high-fiber and Mediterranean-type diets would be a useful approach to improving health and reducing the risk of these chronic diseases (Cadenhead et al., 2017). Engaging patients in lifestyle modification requires individualized approaches that account for specific circumstances, including socioeconomic status and personal choice. Successful control of chronic disease is often contingent on the ability to inspire and empower patients to adopt and maintain healthier lifestyles. Employer-based wellness programs that combine economic incentives with educational resources, for instance, have proved highly effective at encouraging increased engagement in health promotion practices.

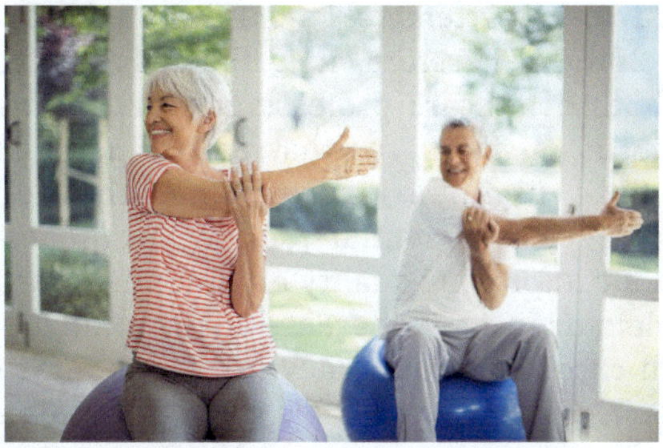

Figure 4.14. Exercise is the key to managing chronic conditions.

Source: https://www.chenmedicalcenters.com/sites/default/files/2023-01/Staying%20Active%20to%20Manage%20Chronic%20Conditions.jpg.

These interventions not only address workers' needs today but also foster a healthy organizational culture. In addition, these interventions have the potential to create long-term behavior change that will sustain health improvement. This evidence supports the importance of multi-level interventions and collaboration among patients, healthcare providers, and community resources to implement lifestyle changes and offer an integrated strategy for the management of chronic disease (Figure 4.14).

4.4.2. Medication Adherence

An essential component of chronic disease management is maintaining drug adherence among patients, with a direct impact on health outcomes. Diabetes and inflammatory bowel disease (IBD) are such chronic diseases requiring patients to stick to regimens of therapeutic treatment to the letter. Non-compliance not only hinders the efficacy of treatments but also encourages complications, relapse, and further problems for health. Indeed, research indicates that more than 40% of IBD patients demonstrate non-adherence, especially at times of remission when they are less aware of the need for maintenance therapies (Lakatos et al., 2009). Therefore, it is the responsibility of both healthcare professionals and patients to focus on measures that ensure adherence to drug regimens, recognizing that drug adherence is essential for long-term health and for improving quality of life. Some reasons explain drug non-adherence among individuals with chronic disease. They include the doctor-patient relationship, complexity of the treatment process, and socioeconomic determinants such as education and family support. In a recent study on diabetes management, variables such as age, level of education, and family involvement significantly influenced adherence (Aladin et al., 2024). Secondly, how health workers communicate with patients also plays an important role in promoting adherence. Misunderstanding of how to use drugs or lack of support can lead to poor levels of adherence. The health systems should therefore employ a patient-oriented approach that is tailored to individual needs, thereby improving patients' knowledge and adherence to treatment regimens. Improving medication adherence involves taking multimodal strategies tailored to the complexities of each chronic disease. To combat non-adherence, medical professionals must engage in adaptive communication with patients to educate them on the importance of ongoing treatment, even when symptoms are absent. Additionally, simplifying drug regimens and ongoing follow-up will enhance levels of adherence. Effectively implemented interventions may additionally include building support interventions aimed at patient education and self-care, specifically designed to break barriers to compliance (Lakatos et al., 2009). Addressing predictors of non-adherence and incorporating adaptive interventions, such as increased family support and patient involvement, will allow healthcare professionals to optimize outcomes in chronic disease control, paving the way for improved population health amid the growing prevalence of chronic disease (Figure 4.15).

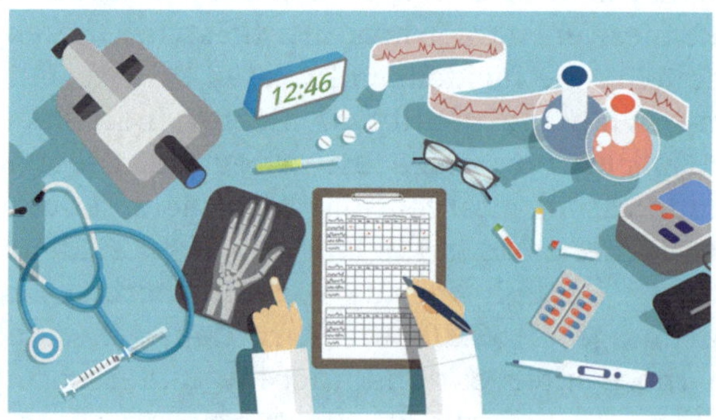

Figure 4.15. Improving medication adherence for chronic disease management.

Source: https://patientengagementhit.com/images/site/features/2017-patient-satisfaction.jpg.

4.4.3. Regular Health Monitoring

Regular health monitoring is an integral component of chronic disease management, going a long way towards improving patient outcomes and quality of life. It is a rational process of continuous monitoring of health parameters so that healthcare providers can institute informed, timely interventions according to individual patient needs. For conditions such as congestive heart failure, which are chronic, continuous monitoring will allow for earlier complication diagnosis without requiring hospital readmission, as well as patient adherence to medication and treatment protocols. Through organized monitoring programs, as the HICMan study illustrates, patients receive comprehensive evaluations aimed at both physical and psychosocial determinants of their health, so emphasizing coordinated models of care in tackling chronic conditions effectively (Steptoe et al., 2007). The integration of telemedicine with care coordination services also increases the effectiveness of periodic health monitoring. The Advancing Care Coordination & Telehealth Deployment (ACT) Program illustrates how these technologies can be utilized to ensure efficient communication and interaction among patients, healthcare professionals, and care staff. Telehealth enables healthcare teams to monitor patients remotely, providing interventions promptly when signs of deterioration are detected using health markers. The intervention illustrates that when patients feel cared for by an allocated contact person and that their health care team is committed to caring for them, they exhibit significant increases in treatment adherence. As such, regular health checks can become more than mere routine practice, fostering a team environment in which patients are enabled to be the facilitators of their own health trajectories without increasing the risk of deteriorated outcomes of their chronic conditions (Baroni et al., 2015). In addition, ongoing health monitoring contributes to the enhancement of general healthcare delivery systems by encouraging a culture of proactive rather than reactive care. It provides critical information to support clinical practice and organizational strategies for optimizing care coordination between healthcare providers. For instance, ACT program results show that patient compliance mutual responsibility is crucial; both patients and healthcare providers must be actively involved in the healthcare process. Increased monitoring and availability of data can foster better resource allocation and usage methods, which in turn increase effective chronic disease management. Through the creation of a uniform routine health monitoring system, healthcare systems can identify care gaps and use targeted interventions to maximize patient outcomes while focusing on the prevention of the complexity of managing chronic diseases (Steptoe et al., 2007; Baroni et al., 2015) (Figure 4.16).

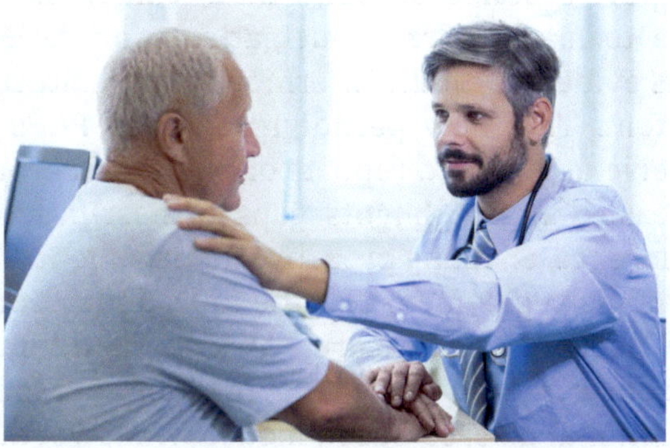

Figure 4.16. Regular health monitoring.

Source: https://creeksidemedical.ca/wp-content/uploads/2025/05/male-doctor-examining-patient-scaled.webp.

Test Your Knowledge

1. What is the role of lifestyle modifications in the management of chronic diseases?
2. What is the importance of regular health monitoring?

4.5. Role of Healthcare Providers

Learning Outcome

1. Understand the role of patient education and support in the management of chronic diseases
2. Describe the multidisciplinary care teams in chronic disease management
3. Describe the use of technology in the management of chronic disease

The role of the physician in chronic disease management remains of utmost importance, particularly given the steady increase in the global incidence of these conditions. The providers, particularly the Primary Care Providers (PCPs), are the initial contact persons for the patients who have been battling chronic diseases such as asthma, diabetes, and depression. Through the use of clinical decision support systems on solid data, clinicians are able to learn more about patient populations as is evident with the Intermountain Healthcare system. This new paradigm enables PCPs to receive aggregated reports on multiple chronic diseases, and highlights gaps in best-practice adherence, enabling proactive management. The strategic deployment of these tools underscores the need for healthcare workers to adopt a patient-centered model, leaving behind a more traditional disease-based model (Wadsworth et al., 2013). In recognizing the multidimensional nature of chronic diseases, healthcare workers also need to take into account a multitude of factors affecting their patients' health. Factors such as resource availability, emotional well-being, and patients' literacy greatly affect how individuals manage diseases. The fact that the disease is chronic underscores the importance of a structured, patient-centered process that encourages patients to become involved in making their own treatment decisions. Nonetheless, there remain obstacles likely to hinder the successful realization of patient-centered care, as evidenced by the literature. It is then crucial that healthcare professionals not only acknowledge such barriers but also shift focus to solutions that encompass guidance and support initiatives, ultimately creating a situation in which patients feel welcomed and guided on the path to health (Gomes et al., 2017). Further, the dynamic nature of healthcare requires providers to keep themselves and their clients informed about chronic disease management. The integration of formal procedures that aim to optimize patient-oriented care can play a crucial role in the effectiveness of interventions as well as in improving the outcomes of patients. It is important to educate health practitioners through these procedures because it will equip them with the required skills to facilitate patients' participation in managing their care. It can also enhance awareness of the emotional and psychological concerns associated with chronic disease, thereby improving the relationship between providers and patients. This collaborative approach not only enhances adherence to treatment regimens but also fosters trust, leading to a more effective experience of chronic disease management for patients (Wadsworth et al., 2013; Gomes et al., 2017) (Figure 4.17).

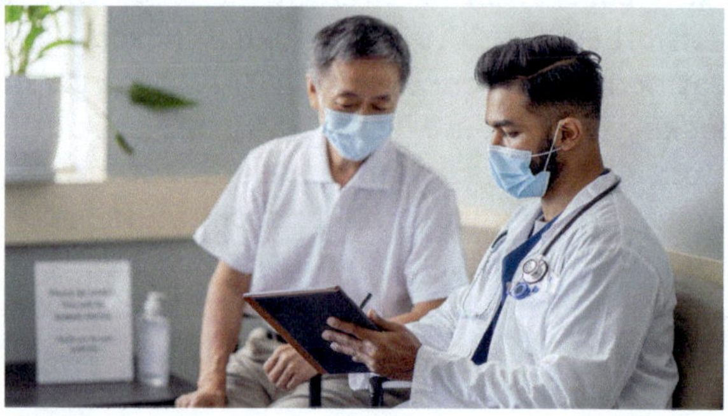

Figure 4.17. Role of healthcare providers.

Source: https://www.cdc.gov/disability-and-health/media/images/doctor-showing-patient-chart-wearing-masks-1200px.jpg.

4.5.1. Patient Education and Support

Patient education and support are at the heart of chronic disease management, enabling people to find out about their condition and make informed decisions about their care. Effective patient education is the imparting of essential information about disease processes, available treatments, and self-management practices. This enables people to become active participants in their care, leading to a sense of autonomy and empowerment. Secondly, studies have shown that well-informed patients tend to adhere to treatment recommendations, which may lead to improved health outcomes. A systematic review observed that patients' decision-making, particularly regarding initiation and termination of dialysis, is multifaceted; patients weigh quality of life against survival, underscoring the imperative of value- and preference-based educational interventions (Flemming et al., 2015). Support systems, including family and healthcare providers, are critical to the effective management of chronic illness. They provide emotional support, instrumental support, and facilitate communication between patients and healthcare teams. Collaborative patient education, where open discussion is invited and collaborative decision-making is engaged, has been shown to enhance patients' understanding and recall. As seen in the review of dialysis decision, patients have often complained of being short of discussion of their treatment choice, yet it is an important lacuna in supportive communication (Flemming et al., 2015). Closing this gap via comprehensive information programs and ongoing supportive dialogue can help empower patients, engaging a collaboration in which the patient is more in control of treatment decisions and overall well-being. Moreover, it is essential in planning successful education programs to understand the affective aspects of chronic disease care. Chronic conditions place patients in a state of anxiety and uncertainty that can constrain their information processing capacity and decision-making ability. Healthcare providers can construct a more conducive environment by incorporating approaches that support both emotional and factual learning. For instance, providing patients with the ability to express their complaints and sentiments can lead to better coping. Among the patients, some listed emotional control in decision-making as their preference, a sign that emotional fulfillment is of equal importance to the clinical details provided. This combined approach aligns with the desire for increased open, honest training among healthcare teams, as proposed by the appeal for more research on shared decision-making between patients with chronic conditions and healthcare professionals (Flemming et al., 2015).

4.5.2. Multidisciplinary Care Teams

The efficacy of multidisciplinary teams in the management of chronic diseases is based on their interdisciplinary approach to care. The convergence of a group of health professionals, including physicians, nurses, social workers, and dieticians, provides comprehensive assessment and individualized treatment plans that address the complexities of chronic disease. This collaboration is particularly significant as chronic diseases often present with multifactorial presentations that require interventions across health dimensions. With these diverse practitioners working together, they apply their abilities to produce comprehensive plans that not only cover the medical aspects of a disease but also the psychological and social concerns. This comprehensive strategy improves the overall quality of care and enables better health outcomes by enabling team members to alert each other and coordinate care, maximizing patients' experiences throughout the healthcare system. Moreover, a well-organized multidisciplinary team facilitates better communication and continuity of care, significant factors in chronic condition management. Shared electronic health records enable such communication and instant access to vital patient data for the entire team. Such transparency between caregivers enables timely interventions and the alteration of treatment plans based on up-to-date data and patient feedback. As discussed in descriptions of successful care delivery models, implementing practices that enable collaboration and information sharing are key to improving patient adherence to treatment plans and augmenting self-management abilities (McCarthy et al., 2009). Lastly, an integrated communication approach among multidisciplinary teams eliminates silos in care delivery, a significant contributor to better chronic disease management. The dynamic model of chronic disease care also indicates the importance of ongoing education and reinvention of multidisciplinary teams. Medical practitioners must be cognizant of current research and best practice and continually improve their teamwork abilities. For instance, studies of Vietnamese healthcare management emphasized the critical role of top management in fostering teamwork-oriented settings to achieve optimal patient outcomes (Hayashi et al., 2012).

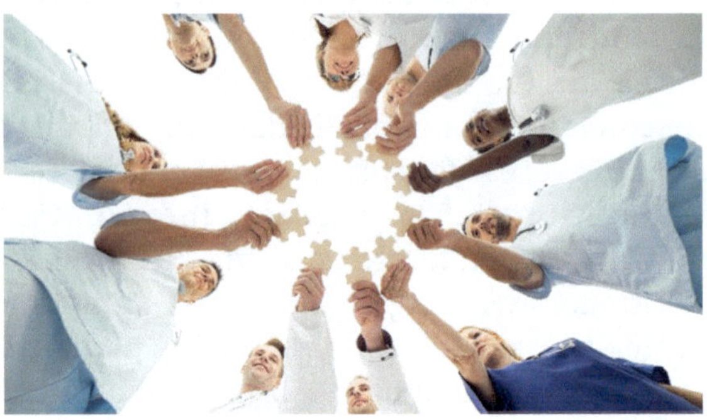

Figure 4.18. Multidisciplinary care teams in diabetes management.

Source: https://nursingeducation.org/wp-content/uploads/2024/01/How-Do-Nurses-Prepare-to-Work-in-a-Multidisciplinary-Team_.jpg.

By empowering team members through training and building a shared vision for patient care, multidisciplinary teams can adapt rapidly to shifting patient needs and healthcare settings. Thus, these teams are not merely a group of specialist providers; rather, they are a collaborative strategy to meet chronic disease with collective responsibility, expertise, and commitment to continuous improvement, finally benefiting patients as well as healthcare systems (Figure 4.18).

4.5.3. Use of Technology in Management

Integration of technology in chronic disease management has become a focal point of interest in healthcare today, mainly due to its potential to improve patient outcomes and streamline care processes. Telehealth, electronic health records (EHRs), and mobile health platforms are among the technologies that have revolutionized how healthcare providers interact with patients, enabling earlier intervention and personalized treatment plans. Telemedicine, for instance, allows patients suffering from chronic illness to make appointments with their health care providers in the convenience of their own homes, removing access barriers and even having the potential to lower the risk of complications from delayed treatment. Technology advances such as these encourage patient engagement, creating an environment in which patients are more effectively able to make decisions about managing their health, which helps ensure better adherence to treatment regimens and better health outcomes. Furthermore, the use of advanced data analytics to manage chronic disease is an example of how technology can optimize healthcare delivery. By analyzing big data gathered from EHRs, health practitioners can identify patterns and trends that indicate prospective intervention windows or the need to alter treatment protocols. This approach complements a more forward-thinking approach to managing chronic disease, moving away from reactive models that address issues only when they arise. The application of artificial intelligence in predictive analytics has the potential to improve the prevention of complications before they progress to advanced stages, thereby facilitating preemptive action at an earlier stage. As emphasized in recent literature, these innovations also encompass the field of neuroticism and neuroimmunology, where comprehension of complex disorders can significantly influence patient care overall (Marder et al., 2008). As much as there is a definite benefit to technology use in chronic disease management, there is also a need to balance the economic considerations of innovation and adoption. The entire healthcare reform will need to confront the cost of adopting new technology, as it is likely to impact coverage, payment to physicians, and general care processes. Determining a balance between cost control and innovation will be required to ensure these technological advances do not exacerbate disparities in access to care. Good and equitable management of these technologies will determine whether their benefit will subsequently bolster chronic disease management strategies. Policymakers should take these issues into account so that the adoption of technology will benefit the sustainability of healthcare systems and the overall health of populations (Emanuel, 2008) (Figure 4.19).

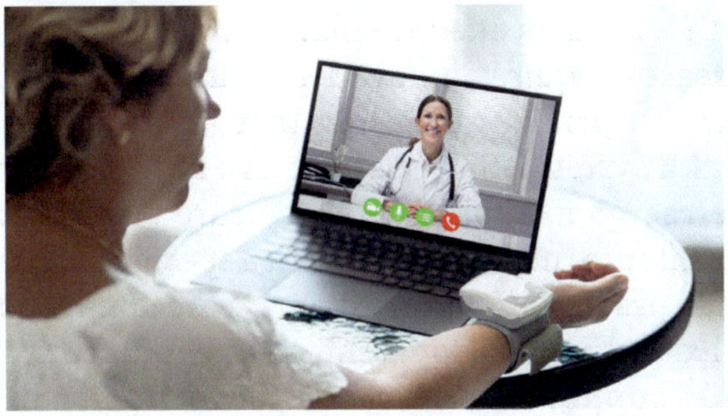

Figure 4.19. Solving chronic disease management problems with telehealth.

Source: https://www.greenwayhealth.com/sites/default/files/styles/webp/public/image/2022-04/chronic%20disease%20management.png.webp?itok=vUSbTEJz.

Test Your Knowledge

1. What is the role of patient education and support in the management of chronic diseases?
2. What is the use of technology in the management of chronic disease?

4.6. Community and Public Health Initiatives

Learning Outcome

1. Understand the role of awareness campaigns in the management of chronic diseases
2. Describe the access to healthcare resources of effective chronic disease management
3. Understand the role of policy changes and advocacy in the effective management of chronic diseases

Public and community health programs are the focal point for controlling chronic diseases because they are the building blocks for encouraging a healthier lifestyle and delivering enhanced care. Such programs tend to involve alliances among different stakeholders, such as healthcare practitioners, community organizations, and policymakers. By bringing together resources and expertise, such programs aim to create an enabling environment in which individuals can effectively manage chronic conditions. For instance, governments have embraced comprehensive models of care, particularly for Medicaid and Children's Health Insurance Programs, which are focused on enhancing the quality of care while containing costs. As presented in most studies, the strategy underscores the imperative of embracing interventions tailored to a specific population and the individualized needs of the local population, thereby improving health outcomes and reducing the economic burden of treating chronic diseases (Takach et al., 2009). Further, effective management of chronic diseases requires innovative solutions directed towards primary care and that reinforce local health systems. State policies are now targeting the reorganization of primary care to enhance chronic care management, with a specific focus on small practices. Policies comprise the application of leadership development, payment incentives, and supporting infrastructure to enable healthcare providers to deliver coordinated care efficiently. Through encouragement of such supportive environments, public and community health programs can enable care plans to be more likely tailored, improve monitoring techniques, and enable timely interventions that are pivotal in the management of long-term illnesses. The experiences gained from such practices demonstrate the benefits of an organized approach that is not just focused on patient care but also on sustainable healthcare systems (Gauthier et al., 2010). Above all, the community's role in such programs cannot be overemphasized. Involving community members directly in health promotion efforts encourages responsibility and ownership for the outcomes of community health. Such programs that promote education on chronic disease risks and management, along with prevention services, substantially enhance health literacy among communities. The more people are aware of their conditions and the resources that are available to them, the better they can manage their health. The more so when communities unite to advocate for policies and resources that support chronic disease management. Thus, the synergy of community involvement and directed public health action is successfully reinvigorating the model for chronic disease control, ultimately yielding healthier communities and reduced demands on healthcare systems (Figure 4.20).

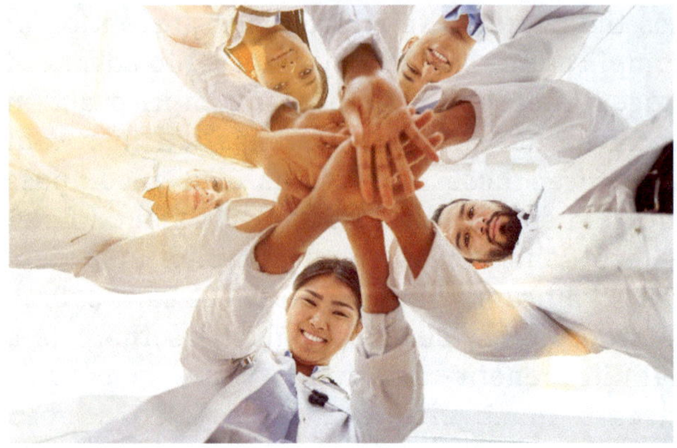

Figure 4.20. Enhancing community health initiatives for better wellness.

Source: https://online-learning-college.com/wp-content/uploads/2024/04/Community-Health-Initiatives-Promoting-Wellness-Locally-scaled.jpg.

4.6.1. Awareness Campaigns

Awareness campaigns are also extremely important in the control of chronic illnesses, as they help develop an understanding of the conditions of ill health and cultivate preventive behavior in the general populace. Awareness campaigns inform individuals about risk factors, signs and symptoms, and the importance of early detection and control of chronic conditions such as diabetes, hypertension, and cardiovascular disease. Through media platforms such as social media, public service announcements, and community outreach programs, awareness campaigns can reach large populations and provide important information. The opioid crisis being most notably emphasized, reports indicate that there is a necessity for combined efforts to alert health care providers and patients to safe prescribing and the danger of addiction (Alexander et al., 2015). Through this, successful awareness campaigns not only enable individuals to take control of their health but also help reduce the overall prevalence of chronic diseases. Awareness campaigns produce impacts beyond individual-level direct health education by encouraging collective action and inducing policy change. As awareness of chronic diseases advances, campaigns can foster public interest and mobilize resources toward better healthcare services and facilities. For instance, the opioid crisis has fueled stakeholder discussion around prescribing habits and addiction treatment that provokes numerous professionals from various fields (Alexander et al., 2015).

Created awareness can manifest as political pressure on policymakers to implement evidence-based practices and support health programs. In addition, campaigns can promote a greater appreciation of the interconnection between chronic diseases and socioeconomic determinants, thereby advocating for health equity. Therefore, awareness campaigns both enhance person-level health literacy and set the stage for systems-level change in healthcare. In addition, the success of awareness campaigns can be gauged on the basis of their ability to alter public understanding and behavior towards chronic diseases. This shift is of utmost significance in ensuring healthy options and a healthy environment for persons suffering from such conditions.

Promotions that emphasize collaboration among stakeholders, including patients, healthcare providers, and community organizations, are particularly effective at conveying that it is everybody's business to control chronic diseases. Additionally, ongoing assessments of these campaigns are necessary to ascertain their scope and effectiveness, enabling the identification of areas for improvement and best practices. By lobbying for policies that prioritize holistic approaches to chronic disease control, awareness campaigns ensure that patients receive the education and support they need to effectively manage their health journeys. In doing so, they significantly contribute to the overall goal of improving health outcomes and quality of life for people with chronic diseases.

4.6.2. Access to Healthcare Resources

Access to healthcare resources is a bedrock of successful chronic disease management, as it determines the quality of care delivered and aggregate health outcomes for patients. Unequal access to healthcare can widen health inequities, depriving vulnerable populations of required medical care. The United Nations Sustainable Development Goals recognize that providing equal access to quality healthcare is key to enhancing well-being for everyone at every age. The third SDG emphasizes the provision of health resources to the most vulnerable, and this is much needed for those with chronic diseases, who require continuous care and management. In the absence of timely access to healthcare services, the patients' condition will get even worse, and the rates of morbidity and mortality will rise. Improvements in technology, primarily the introduction of 5G and related future technologies, hold the ability to revolutionize access to healthcare. Technologies such as the Internet of Things (IoT), big data, and artificial intelligence lay the groundwork for remote patient monitoring and telemedicine, in which patients can receive care outside traditional healthcare centers. These technologies can enhance chronic disease management through real-time health monitoring, treatment tailored to specific needs, and improved patient-caregiver communication. The integration of 5G technology into healthcare systems also answers the classic limitations that have hindered equal access. As healthcare conditions change, leveraging such technologies helps overcome barriers to ensure high-quality care for all, regardless of geographic or socioeconomic factors (Farooq et al., 2017). Further, the socioeconomic implications of inadequate access to healthcare resources are clearly evident among populations suffering from chronic diseases. The brucellosis case is an example of such a problem; it imposes a high cost on public health systems and stifles economic growth in affected areas. Resolving such diseases requires an integrated public policy intervention that addresses the interrelated impacts on animal and human health. One Health encourages improved disease surveillance infrastructure, public education campaigns, and utilization of targeted disease control measures in livestock and wildlife. By focusing on joint solutions that encompass healthcare, economic growth, and disease management, society can expand access to needed healthcare facilities and mitigate the adverse effects of chronic disease (Fournier et al., 2018) (Figure 4.21).

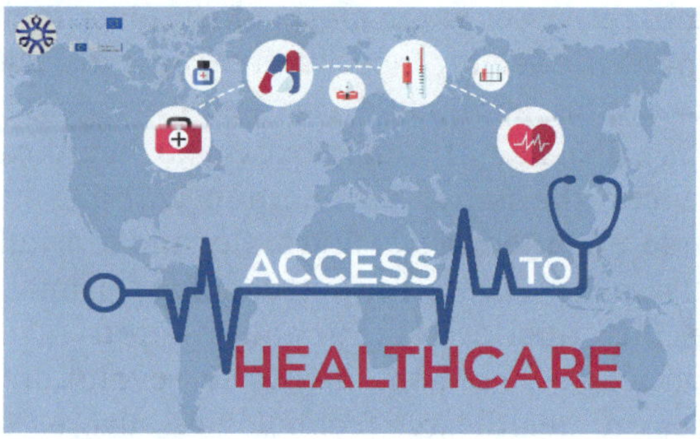

Figure 4.21. Access to healthcare.

Source: https://epsa-online.org/LLeaP/wp-content/uploads/2019/04/access_banner.png.

4.6.3. Policy Changes and Advocacy

The intersection of policy changes and advocacy is pivotal in the effective management of chronic conditions throughout human populations. Advocacy is essential in bringing to policymakers' attention the individualized needs of individuals with chronic conditions, most of which include the intricate matters of healthcare access, drug affordability, and the call for comprehensive care models. By highlighting these concerns, stakeholders can foster a climate that facilitates the implementation of solutions to improve patient outcomes. Research highlights that evidence-based policy proposals can have a lasting impact on chronic disease management, as evidenced by gains achieved through prevention initiatives and care coordination activities identified in earlier studies. Such programs not only prioritize patient health but also optimize the utilization of resources, with long-term benefits accruing to the healthcare system and, by extension, society, thereby validating the role of advocacy in shaping major policy reforms (Morton et al., 2015). Moreover, policy changes related to chronic disease management have historically been reactive, with legislatures more likely to act after the fact, that is, post-crisis, rather than in advance through proactive preventive measures. This reactive nature has left voids in healthcare provision that now strike marginalized groups. These voids can be filled by advocacy groups through active advocacy for legislative bills that enhance health equity, particularly for low-income and marginalized groups. The 2007 proposal to enhance primary care outcomes in Medicaid and State Children's Health Insurance Programs is just one illustration of how advocacy can lead to favorable policy environments, here targeted at primary, preventive, and developmental health care (Plaza et al., 2008). By focusing efforts on building these regions, policies can be designed not just to treat chronic disease more effectively but also to prevent it, demonstrating the pivotal role of ongoing advocacy at the policy level. Aside from reorienting attention toward preventive methods, successful advocacy in addressing chronic diseases requires lifelong dedication to policymakers and the public. This ongoing dialogue provokes a realization about chronic disease and calls for much-needed reform. Education plays a critical role, since informed communities are well-placed to articulate their health interests and insist that the system be altered. Advocacy groups can use evidence-based research to reveal the social determinants that affect chronic disease rates and health outcomes. By laying out such evidence before policy makers, the supporters are in a position to clearly specify the requirements for sweeping health reforms that address the multifaceted determinants of chronic illness. This methodology not only requests the resources needed but also promotes policies that are specific to boost patient self-management and palliative care options, highlighting the comprehensive nature of chronic disease management policy (Morton et al., 2015) (Figure 4.22).

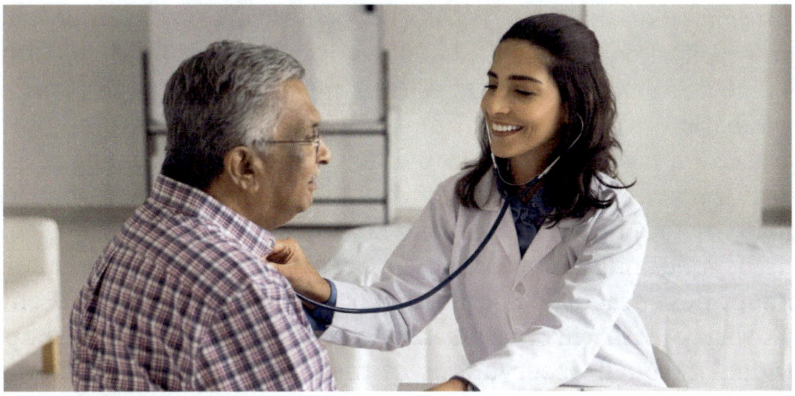

Figure 4.22. Advancing advocacy for chronic disease prevention & management.

Source: https://nationalhealthcouncil.org/wp-content/uploads/2025/01/shutterstock_2546335017-e1738359797733.jpg.

Test Your Knowledge

1. Why are awareness campaigns important?
2. What is the role of policy changes and advocacy in the effective management of chronic diseases?

SUMMARY

In generalizing the complexities of managing chronic disease in humans, there must be contextualization of disparity between various health challenges, such as novel diseases like COVID-19 and traditional diseases like HIV. As the literature points out, the identification of distinct virological and clinical characteristics of such diseases aids public health interventions and treatment protocols. The acute nature of SARS-CoV-2 infections stands in contrast to the long-term development of HIV infections, thus highlighting the need for targeted intervention protocols. It is through such an appreciation that healthcare providers can effectively manage resources and design targeted interventions that achieve optimal outcomes for patients, stressing the need for ongoing research and adaptability within public health systems (Olebo et al., 2025). Moreover, chronic disease management extends beyond individual health concerns to broader systemic impact. Integration of resource management best practices is crucial, particularly for water and environmental health concerns that often overlap with chronic disease. Holistic measures that emphasize sustainable practices become evident through observations of the relationship between clean environmental conditions and public health outcomes. Such a correlation validates the assumption that the management of chronic diseases is not only a medical issue but should also be handled through the reduction of environmental determinants, which increase health inequities (Elmadani et al., 2024). Therefore, an integrative approach with intersectoral action will eventually foster chronic disease management. In all, chronic disease control requires an interdisciplinary approach that recognizes the natural complexity of individual disease processes and the interdependence of environmental determinants. Policymakers, clinicians, and community partners need to work together to develop solutions that not only address issues comprehensively but are culturally and contextually tailored to the diverse groups they serve. In addition, continuous evaluation and adjustment of management strategies are important to remain sensitive to emerging public health issues. By embracing an integrated strategy for chronic disease management, the health care system can better position itself to confront the evolving nature of human health with evidence-based, effective interventions (Elmadani et al., 2024 Olebo et al., 2025).

Management of chronic disease in man requires an integrated approach that accounts for the interplay among genetic, environmental, and microbial contributors. Researching metagenomics, the examination of the overall microbial genomes found in human ecosystems, is a focal point of research. It is a new area of investigation that diverges from the discovery of the dominant pathogen to a comprehension of the large-scale microbial contributions to disease. Based on Izard et al. (2015), it is possible to identify novel biomarkers by understanding these microbial interactions, which could potentially prevent chronic disease. Understanding the human body as a super-organism enables researchers to develop approaches that affect the microbiome, potentially maximizing health benefits and reducing healthcare spending on chronic disease maintenance. In addition to microbial interactions, management of chronic conditions would frequently necessitate innovative strategies to address gaps in current care. Current therapies for numerous kinetoplastid diseases, such as African trypanosomiasis and Chagas disease, underscore the need for effective, safe, and cost-effective therapeutics. While recent advances have led to the release of new combinations and drugs, the treatment landscape remains controversial, particularly for diseases such as cutaneous leishmaniasis, which remain underdeveloped (Alsford et al., 2012). With these opportunities arising, there is an increased demand for end-to-end solutions that bring together new pharmacological advancements and enhanced diagnostic approaches in a bid to facilitate successful management strategies. Finally, ongoing research is key to advancing chronic disease care through the discovery and validation of novel biomarkers and therapeutic agents. The chronic nature of diseases necessitates adaptable models that can respond to shifting clinical needs. From discussions in Izard et al. (2015), integrating metagenomics results presents avenues for investigating the root causes of chronic disorders and for prevention. With that said, the requirement for new oral therapies and improved diagnostic technology underscores the call for an integrative approach through clinical research to public health programs. Joint action will not only enhance the quality of care for chronic disease sufferers but might also reduce the broader public health burden of these pervasive conditions.

KEY TERMS FROM THIS CHAPTER

- Air pollutants
- Allergens
- Blood glucose
- Chronic diseases
- Coronary artery disease
- Diabetes mellitus
- Dietary choices
- Exercise
- Heart failure
- Nutrition
- Obesity
- Patient-centered care
- Respiratory illnesses
- Smoking

CRITICAL THINKING QUESTIONS

1. **Which of the following is a key component of chronic disease management?**
   a. Focus on acute symptoms
   b. Patient-centered care and education
   c. Avoidance of multidisciplinary teams
   d. Single-visit treatment strategies
2. **What is the first-line treatment for hypertension in most patients with no contraindications?**
   a. Beta-blockers
   b. Calcium channel blockers
   c. Thiazide diuretics
   d. ACE inhibitors
3. **Which of the following is the hallmark of chronic obstructive pulmonary disease (COPD)?**
   a. Reversible airflow obstruction
   b. Persistent airflow limitation
   c. Reduced cardiac output
   d. Hyperactive airway response
4. **Which screening tool is commonly used to monitor blood glucose control in patients with diabetes?**
   a. Fasting blood glucose
   b. HbA1c
   c. Random blood sugar
   d. Oral glucose tolerance test
5. **Which lifestyle modification is most effective in managing type 2 diabetes?**
   a. High-fat diet
   b. Physical activity and weight loss
   c. Elimination of all carbohydrates
   d. Smoking cessation

Short Answer Questions

1. What are chronic diseases?
2. Why is chronic disease management important?
3. List the types of chronic diseases.
4. What are risk factors for chronic disease?
5. What are the effects of chronic disease on individuals?

Answer to Critical Thinking Questions

1. (b); 2. (c); 3. (b); 4. (b); 5. (b).

REFERENCES

1. Dar, O. A., Hasan, R., Schlundt, J., Harbarth, S., Caleo, G., Dar, F. K., Littmann, J., Rweyemamu, M., Buckley, E. J., Shahid, M., Kock, R., Li, H. L., Giha, H., Khan, M., So, A. D., Bindayna, K. M., Kessel, A., Pedersen, H. B., Permanand, G., . . . Heymann, D. L. (2015e). Exploring the evidence base for national and regional policy interventions to combat resistance. *The Lancet, 387*(10015), 285–295. https://doi.org/10.1016/s0140-6736(15)00520-6Abbott, J., Borgarelli, M., Clercx, C., Kellihan, H., et al. (2020). ACVIM consensus statement guidelines for the diagnosis, classification, treatment, and monitoring of pulmonary hypertension in dogs. https://core.ac.uk/download/323070279.pdf (accessed on 14th July 2025).
2. Abdul-Rasoul, M., Agarwal, A., Ahlgren, K., Alejandro, R., American Diabetes Association, Anderson, R., Appleton, J., et al. (2016). What's in a name? Classification of diabetes mellitus in veterinary medicine and why it matters. https://core.ac.uk/download/76980783.pdf (accessed on 14th July 2025).
3. Abramson, C. I., Almunia, J., Dudzinski, K. M., Feucht, K., et al. (2020). Distinguishing personal belief from scientific knowledge for the betterment of killer whale welfare–A commentary. https://core.ac.uk/download/305124363.pdf (accessed on 14th July 2025).
4. Adcock, I. M., Garssen, J., Kazempour Dizagie, M., Mirsaeidi, M., et al. (2017). What immunological defects predispose to non-tuberculosis mycobacterial infections? https://core.ac.uk/download/157859147.pdf (accessed on 14th July 2025).
5. Addiss, D. G., Fenwick, A., Jourdan, P. M., Lamberton, P. H. L., et al. (2018). Soil-transmitted helminth infections. https://core.ac.uk/download/96884381.pdf (accessed on 14th July 2025).
6. Aladin, A., Gustina, E., & Zaman, C. (2024). Medication adherence in diabetes mellitus patients. https://core.ac.uk/download/631324822.pdf (accessed on 14th July 2025).
7. Alexander, G. C., & Frattaroli, S. (2015). The prescription opioid epidemic: An evidence-based approach. https://core.ac.uk/download/75783788.pdf (accessed on 14th July 2025).
8. Alsford, S., Alvar, J., Barrett, M. P., Ben Salah, A., Berman, J., et al. (2012). Management of trypanosomiasis and leishmaniasis. https://core.ac.uk/download/9652405.pdf (accessed on 14th July 2025).
9. Angelos, J. A., Arens, A. L., Cadriel, J. L., Johnson, R., et al. (2017). One Health in food safety and security education: Subject matter outline for a curricular framework. https://core.ac.uk/download/323068605.pdf (accessed on 14th July 2025).
10. Aytur, S., Bucci, J., & Wake, C. P. (2014). An assessment of the impact of climate change on human health in New Hampshire. https://core.ac.uk/download/84123597.pdf (accessed on 14th July 2025).
11. Baroni, I., Barrett, D., Bescos, C., Buskens, E., et al. (2015). What does it take to make integrated care work? A 'cookbook' for large-scale deployment of coordinated care and telehealth. https://core.ac.uk/download/155776181.pdf (accessed on 14th July 2025).
12. Brecht, M. L., Congello, N. C., Hays, R. D., Heilemann, M. V., et al. (2020). Associations of partner support and acculturation with physical activity in Mexican American women. https://core.ac.uk/download/286729008.pdf (accessed on 14th July 2025).
13. Brooks, D., Grave, A. S., Oliveira, A., Satia, J., et al. (2023). Impact of chronic cough on quality of life. https://core.ac.uk/download/610603214.pdf (accessed on 14th July 2025).

14. Budiono, B. P., Headrick, J. P., Neumann, D. L., & Peart, J. N. (2017). The heartbreak of depression: 'Psycho-cardiac' coupling in myocardial infarction. https://core.ac.uk/download/196605092.pdf (accessed on 14th July 2025).

15. Cadenhead, K. S., Depp, C., Joseph, J., Schmid-Schönbein, G., et al. (2017). Modified Mediterranean diet for enrichment of short chain fatty acids: Potential adjunctive therapeutic to target immune and metabolic dysfunction in schizophrenia? https://core.ac.uk/download/287622216.pdf (accessed on 14th July 2025).

16. Chawla, S., Deng, X., Ghosh, K., Khuntia, J., et al. (2014). Media reinforcement for psychological empowerment in chronic disease management. https://core.ac.uk/download/301377482.pdf (accessed on 14th July 2025).

17. Durack, J., & Lynch, S. V. (2019). The gut microbiome: Relationships with disease and opportunities for therapy. https://core.ac.uk/download/323062877.pdf (accessed on 14th July 2025).

18. Elias, P. M., & Man, M. Q. (2019). Could inflammaging and its sequelae be prevented or mitigated? https://core.ac.uk/download/323062598.pdf (accessed on 14th July 2025).

19. Elmadani, M., Kiptulon, E. K., Simon, K., & Orsolya, M. (2024). Systematic review of the impact of natural resource management on public health outcomes: Focus on water quality. *Resources*. https://www.semanticscholar.org/paper/b01c1455f01d739cf1de01d67d4012549a8bf5b6 (accessed on 14th July 2025).

20. Emanuel, E. J. (2008). Comprehensive health care reform and biomedical innovation. https://core.ac.uk/download/71346438.pdf (accessed on 14th July 2025).

21. Estrine, J., & DeLisle, L. (2006). Stress: Putting the brain back into medicine. https://core.ac.uk/download/71356692.pdf (accessed on 14th July 2025).

22. Farooq, S., Imran, M. A., Latif, S., Qadir, J., et al. (2017). How 5G wireless (and concomitant technologies) will revolutionize healthcare? https://core.ac.uk/download/143476480.pdf (accessed on 14th July 2025).

23. Flemming, K., Hussain, J. A., Hussain, M., et al. (2015). Patient and health care professional decision-making to commence and withdraw from renal dialysis: A systematic review of qualitative research. https://core.ac.uk/download/151157328.pdf (accessed on 14th July 2025).

24. Fournier, A., Gregoire, A., Arenas-Gamboa, A. M., Al-Talafhah, A. H., Arenas-Gamboa, A. M., Dean, A. S., Dean, A. S., et al. (2018). Brucellosis remains a neglected disease in the developing world: A call for interdisciplinary action. https://core.ac.uk/download/146489704.pdf (accessed on 14th July 2025).

25. Gauthier, A. K., Sims-Kastelein, K., Takach, M., & Kaye, N. (2010). Strengthening primary and chronic care: State innovations to transform and link small practices. https://core.ac.uk/download/71355266.pdf (accessed on 14th July 2025).

26. Geenen, R., Jacobs, J. W., Pereira da Silva, J. A., Santiago, M. B., et al. (2015). Psychological factors associated with response to treatment in rheumatoid arthritis. https://core.ac.uk/download/75985969.pdf (accessed on 14th July 2025).

27. Gomes, A. I., Grilo, A. M., Rita, J., Santos, J., et al. (2017). Promoting patient-centered care in chronic disease. https://core.ac.uk/download/322430061.pdf (accessed on 14th July 2025).

28. Harries, A. D., Bode, A. V., Restrepo, B. I., Restrepo, B. I., Lee, B. Y., Lee, B. Y., Lee, B. Y., et al. (2013). Ears of the armadillo: Global health research and neglected diseases in Texas. https://core.ac.uk/download/12215483.pdf (accessed on 14th July 2025).

29. Hayashi, Y. (2012). Research on awareness of hospital managers about chronic diseases and the care by multidisciplinary teams towards sustainable health care services in Vietnam. https://core.ac.uk/download/16515345.pdf (accessed on 14th July 2025).

30. Iacobini, C., Menini, S., Pesce, C., Pugliese, G., et al. (2017). Dietary interventions to contrast the onset and progression of diabetic nephropathy: A critical survey of new data. https://core.ac.uk/download/80314820.pdf (accessed on 14th July 2025).

31. Izard, J. (2015). Steps in metagenomics: Let's avoid garbage in and garbage out. https://core.ac.uk/download/286028026.pdf (accessed on 14th July 2025).

32. Kadar, K. (2024). Enhancing health literacy and self-care abilities among individuals with chronic diseases. https://core.ac.uk/download/617747067.pdf (accessed on 14th July 2025).

33. Lakatos, P. L. (2009). Prevalence, predictors, and clinical consequences of medical adherence in IBD: How to improve it? https://core.ac.uk/download/20381498.pdf (accessed on 14th July 2025).

34. Lawson, K., Yocum, S., et al. (2019). Health coaching case report: Optimizing employee health and wellbeing in organizations. https://core.ac.uk/download/223117465.pdf (accessed on 14th July 2025).

35. Marder, E., DeLong, M. R., Gazzaniga, M. S., & Wichmann, T. (2008). *2008 Progress Report on Brain Research*. https://core.ac.uk/download/71349141.pdf (accessed on 14th July 2025).

36. McCarthy, D., Wrenn, J., & Mueller, K. (2009). Mayo Clinic: Multidisciplinary teamwork, physician-led governance, and patient-centered culture drive world-class health care. https://core.ac.uk/download/71352991.pdf (accessed on 14th July 2025).

37. McHugh, B., Estrine, J., & Moran, R. (2004). Promoting men's health: Addressing barriers to healthy lifestyle and preventive health care. https://core.ac.uk/download/71356600.pdf (accessed on 14th July 2025).

38. Morton, S., & Dunn, W. (2015). Addressing the health needs of an aging America: New opportunities for evidence-based policy solutions. https://core.ac.uk/download/75783019.pdf (accessed on 14th July 2025).

39. Nødtvedt, A. (2007). Epidemiology of canine atopic dermatitis. https://core.ac.uk/download/11695161.pdf (accessed on 14th July 2025).

40. Olebo, D. F., & Igwe, M. C. (2025). Comparative analysis of virology and pathogenesis of SARS-CoV-2 and HIV infections: Implications for public health and treatment strategies. *Infection and Drug Resistance, 18*, 269–283. https://www.semanticscholar.org/paper/f30820e06415bf4589dfc64e55689c18df6e370a (accessed on 14th July 2025).

41. Pisani, S. (2010). The nurse of the Mediterranean. https://core.ac.uk/download/46602269.pdf (accessed on 14th July 2025).

42. Plaza, C., Fitzgerald, C., & Bruner, C. (2008). Improving child health care through federal policy: An emerging opportunity. https://core.ac.uk/download/71352190.pdf (accessed on 14th July 2025).

43. St George, A., Bellew, B., & King, L. (2025). Workplace screening programs for chronic disease

prevention: A rapid review. https://core.ac.uk/download/pdf/30678020.pdf (accessed on 14th July 2025).

44. Steptoe, A., Löwe, B., Ruo, B., Mathe, C., Opasich, C., Muth, C., Green, C. P., et al. (2007). Rationale, design and conduct of a randomized controlled trial evaluating a primary care-based complex intervention to improve the quality of life of heart failure patients: HICMan (Heidelberg Integrated Case Management): Study protocol. https://core.ac.uk/download/14500332.pdf (accessed on 14th July 2025).
45. Takach, M., & Kaye, N. (2009). Building medical homes in state Medicaid and CHIP programs. https://core.ac.uk/download/71349689.pdf (accessed on 14th July 2025).
46. Wadsworth, J. C. (2013). *Master of Science.* https://core.ac.uk/download/276264265.pdf (accessed on 14th July 2025).

GERIATRIC MENTAL HEALTH

5

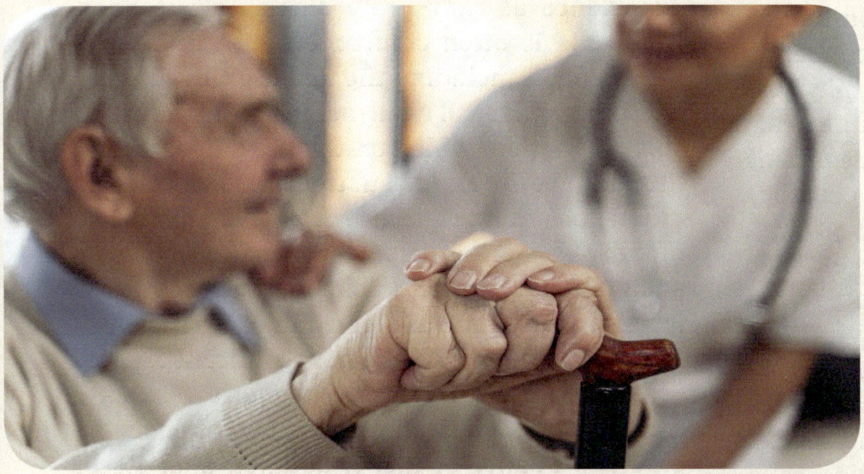

Introduction

A geriatric mental health study is essential for the psychological well-being of an increasingly aging population. With age, individuals are prone to various physical disorders, social isolation, and midlife change, which have a direct effect on their mental condition. The research indicates a rising prevalence of disorders of the mental kind among the elderly, particularly depression and anxiety, hence necessitating an integrated treatment and care strategy. The challenge of diagnosing and treating these disorders is compounded by the stigma associated with mental illness, which can deter older individuals from seeking assistance. Thus, it is of great importance to investigate the various factors that influence geriatric mental health, including socioeconomic status, marital status, and life satisfaction, to enhance the detection and treatment of vulnerable individuals and improve their quality of life (Mayhew et al., 1989). Additionally, the implications of geriatric mental health consequences are not just on the individual but also on families and the healthcare system. Cognitive impairment

LEARNING OBJECTIVES

After studying this chapter, you will be able to:

1. Describe the common mental health disorders in the elderly
2. Understand the risk factors for mental health issues
3. Describe the impact of mental health on quality of life
4. Describe the barriers to mental health care
5. Know the treatment options for geriatric mental health
6. Understand the role of caregivers and family support

in older persons is usually accompanied by increased levels of healthcare use and long-term care placement, which imposes economic strains on families and society as a whole. Effective management of psychiatric disorders in older persons can lead to improved overall health outcomes, decongesting the healthcare facilities. As researchers and healthcare providers recognize the unique needs of older people, more emphasis has been placed on geriatric assessments with individualized strategies. The assessments were modified to address multifaceted mental health concerns, enabling holistic care responsive to physical and psychological demands (Lampugnane et al., 2017). The development of specific interventions for mental health in older adults is necessary since the demographic trend continues to shift. Prioritizing geriatric mental health enables practitioners to implement a more integrated model of care that supports longevity and quality of life in older adults. Educational initiatives that equip health professionals with training in geriatric assessment and the special mental health challenges faced by this group are paramount.

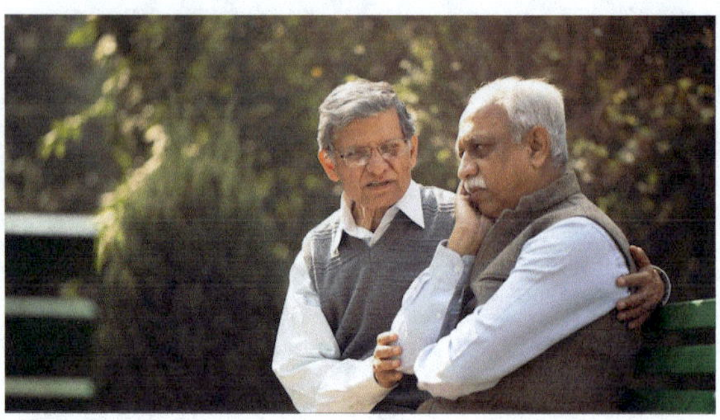

Figure 5.1. Geriatric mental health.

Source: https://akm-img-a-in.tosshub.com/indiatoday/images/story/202402/health-073030369-16x9_0.jpg?VersionId=SDjpO53AOZF8TMyopzuCTMz3YeQU1XKL&size=690:388.

These interventions are able to empower practitioners to effectively diagnose and treat mental illnesses with regard to the complexity of aging. Ultimately, the future of geriatric mental health relies on ongoing studies, policy changes, and a commitment to removing barriers to treatment so that older adults have the care they deserve (Mayhew et al., 1989) (Figure 5.1).

Definition of Geriatric Mental Health

The concept of geriatric mental health is the psychological welfare of the elderly that emphasizes the specific challenges they experience as they grow older. As one ages, he or she is often confronted with numerous life changes, including the death of loved ones, declining physical well-being, and increased social isolation, which tend to negatively affect mental well-being. Furthermore, geriatric mental health must acknowledge the prevalence of various mental diseases in this population, such as depression, anxiety, and cognitive impairments, such as dementia. These are not mere byproducts of aging but significant aspects of comprehensive care that require adequate assessment and management to enhance the elderly's quality of life. A detailed analysis of these factors is crucial as it assists in formulating appropriate treatment plans and facilitating mental well-being in older patients. In geriatric mental health, the function of assessment tools cannot be ignored, and they are employed to establish needs in older adults. Comprehensive questionnaires and diagnostic assessments, such as the Geriatric Depression Scale and cognitive function assessment, provide good information about the mental health status of elderly persons. Their implementation has been hampered by time constraints experienced by professionals in practice, leading to poor assessment of mental illness among the aged. This lack of thorough assessment can result in undertreatment and underdiagnosis of significant mental health conditions. An attempt to bridge these barriers through educational and institutional change is required so that healthcare providers can conduct competent assessments. Barriers to successful geriatric mental health assessment identification will be crucial to intervening and ultimately improving care quality for older adults. Further, the co-existence of physical and mental health in older adults is a key part of geriatric mental health. Older adults can have chronic physical diseases, which can exacerbate or contribute to mental illness, creating a fine line between physical and psychological well-being. For instance, patients with chronic disease can feel powerless or depressed because they are struggling with their medical conditions. Furthermore, the older person's self-neglect, as reported in today's literature, can also limit the use of healthcare services. Self-neglect is often a consequence of wanting to live independently and be in control of one's life, something that could be misinterpreted by caregivers, hence it becomes challenging to tackle mental illness among this group (Braye et al., 2011). Thus, responding to geriatric mental health needs requires a comprehensive understanding of physical and mental health concerns, necessitating convergent models of care that are best suited to treating the intersecting needs of older adults.

Importance of Mental Health in Older Adults

Mental well-being has a key contribution to make in the overall health of older individuals, with considerable effects on their quality of life and physical outcomes of illness. With increasing age, there are many problems that arise, including chronic illness, loss, and loneliness, and all have adverse consequences for mental well-being. Symptoms of depression are particularly prevalent in older individuals and, therefore, are likely to exacerbate other illnesses that they might experience. Where physical health and mental well-being intersect is best illustrated through studies that highlight the interplay between arthritis and depression. Depressive screening of older adults with diagnosed arthritis by medical professionals helps to identify those at higher risk for future morbidity and take corresponding interventions. Prioritization of mental health in geriatric care is therefore fundamental to ensuring resilience and maximizing health outcomes among such a vulnerable group. Research has increasingly demonstrated the intersection of cognitive decline and mental illness among elderly populations. Dementia disorders, often associated with aging, not only lead to mental disability but also considerably compromise emotional and psychological well-being. Anxiety, depression, or hopelessness may afflict older persons who battle cognitive changes and a projected loss of independence. Treatment of such mental illness is necessary, as it may progress into a cycle of social isolation and further cognitive decline. It becomes important for mental health professionals to create holistic plans involving cognitive rehabilitation in addition to psychological counseling. By doing so, treatments can address the multifaceted needs of older adults more effectively and enhance cognitive resilience and emotional stability in the face of aging-related issues. The importance of adopting a holistic approach to the mental health of elderly individuals is followed by the necessity of social connections and support systems. Loneliness and social isolation are both prevalent issues for elderly individuals, with consequential negative effects on mental and physical health. Studies show that older adults with healthy social networks have fewer symptoms of depression as well as better overall health outcomes. Mental health practitioners, in this case, must recognize the importance of fostering community engagement and implementing programs that promote social interaction among older adults. Minimizing loneliness through activities in communities not only improves emotional well-being but also serves as a protective factor against other mental illness challenges, like those related to chronic illnesses. As the number of the elderly population increases, integrating mental health services with social support programs will be crucial to providing a healthier and happier life to older people, and emphasizing the significance of targeted policies and programs in geriatric mental health (Figure 5.2).

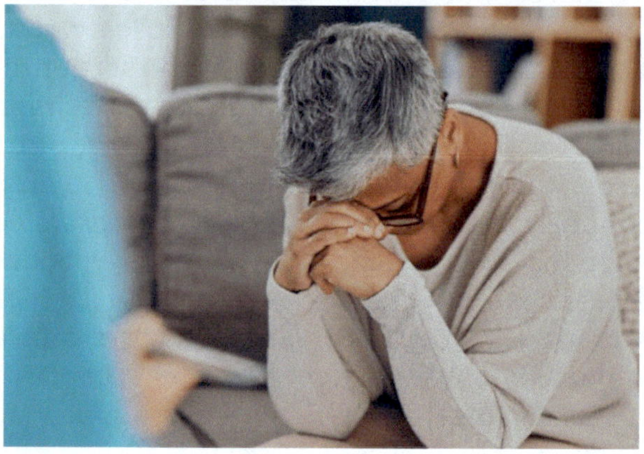

Figure 5.2. Importance of mental health of elders.

Source: https://www.inhousemedicare.com/wp-content/uploads/2024/08/importance-of-elderly-mental-health.png.

5.1. Common Mental Health Disorders in the Elderly

Learning Outcome

1. Understand the depression and its prevalence
2. Describe the anxiety disorders among older adults
3. Describe the dementia and cognitive decline

Among the elderly, the prevalence of active mental illnesses such as depression and anxiety is very high. Research has found that in some populations, depression is experienced by approximately 21.9% of older individuals, demonstrating the severity to which this mental health crisis must be addressed. The complexities of aging, including the death of loved ones, declining health, and loneliness, often exacerbate the feelings of hopelessness and despair. In a study conducted in rural India, it was found that a staggering 33.9% of the elderly had come out positive for mental illness, and thus, there is a call for active mental health care specifically tailored for the elderly. This is vital, as depression, if left unmanaged, can lead to more deteriorating health and reduced quality of life among the elderly, making proper screening and treatment efforts all the more necessary (Nair et al., 2015). Anxiety disorders are common among the elderly as well, impacting around 10.7% of the elderly population according to recent reports. These can include persistent worry, restlessness, and body symptoms such as increased heart rate. Anxiety is often found together with other disorders such as depression, further complicating diagnosis and treatment. It is crucial for physicians to recognize such co-occurring issues to deliver holistic care. Studies that compared psychiatric morbidity across different living conditions show that older individuals in old age homes are possible to have higher levels of depression compared to community elders, for instance, 36% of the inmates at old age homes presented depressive symptoms, while the community presented 22%. This discord points towards a complex interaction between mental health and conditions of living, with supportive environments required in order to minimize anxiety and maximize mental well-being (Majgi et al., 2012). Cognitive impairment in the form of dementia, along with other forms of cognitive impairment, is also a challenge faced by the elderly. One study has identified cognitive impairment in 16.3% of the elderly and an even greater percentage in persons aged more than 80 years. This deterioration of cognitive impairment typically accompanies behavioral issues and may actually significantly compromise the autonomy and quality of life of the elderly. As cognitive disorders may lead to confusion, mood changes, and loss of memory, effective intervention activities like cognitive therapies and social support become essential components of geriatric mental health interventions. The coordinated operation of cognitive functions and mental well-being necessitates a coordinated approach in which psychiatric interventions are embedded within more universal geriatric care, with older adults being offered the appropriate management to prevent the problems of old age while maintaining their dignity and well-being (Nair et al., 2015) (Figure 5.3).

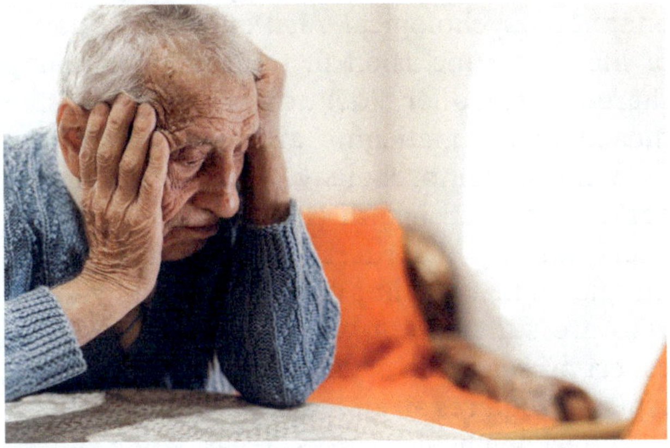

Figure 5.3. Mental health issues in old age.

Source: https://thearborsassistedliving.com/wp-content/uploads/2019/09/9.26-arbors.jpg.

5.1.1. Depression and Its Prevalence

Depression among the elderly has emerged as a critical concern. With the expansion of the geriatric population, it becomes increasingly important to realize the etiology of depression so that effective intervention can be made and support can be rendered. Existing research indicates that depression among this age group is attributable to various determinants such as health perception, life satisfaction, and social loneliness. One such research study that probed these intercorrelations in a group of older adults found strong intercorrelations between depression and lifestyle factors such as marital status and bereavement experiences. Involving 44 individuals aged between 51 and 79 years, the study points to the complexities of geriatric depression and the requirement of multi-modal approaches in order to detect and treat the disorder at an early point of its occurrence (Mayhew et al., 1989). Besides, the global prevalence of depression among the elderly is staggering, with new figures stating that about 30% of elderly individuals possess depressive symptoms. A cross-sectional study in Selangor, Malaysia, used a validated scale, the Geriatric Depression Scale-15, to screen for mental status in its elderly participants. Findings showed an elevated rate of prevalence and a disturbing correlation between mental health literacy and depression in older individuals. Individuals who possessed higher educational levels were discovered to have more depression, indicating that factors other than simply the level of education, including social support and previous life experiences, play an important role in deciding mental health outcomes (Khaiyom et al., 2024).

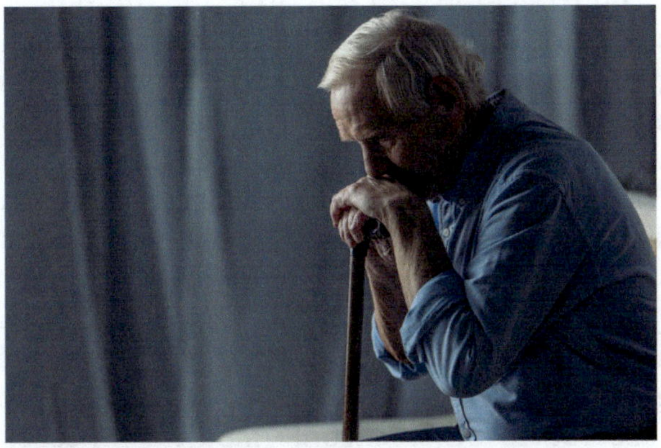

Figure 5.4. Depression in older adults.

Source: https://homecare-aid.com/wp-content/uploads/2024/04/Dipression.jpg.

The complexity of the aforesaid relationships calls for expert research in order to develop effective screening and intervention approaches. Based on these findings, bolstering mental health literacy appears to be a significant intervention approach to the prevention of depression among the elderly. Stronger mental health literacy is discovered by the aforesaid study to lead to better understanding, identification, and treatment of depressive disorders, hence promoting well-being among the elderly. It emphasizes the importance of programs that raise mental health awareness in a collaborative effort between learning institutions and the government. By raising awareness of mental health among this age group, stakeholders can ensure that older people receive the support they require. Lastly, prioritizing mental health literacy not only promotes the welfare of individuals but also helps address the broader social costs of depression among an ageing population (Khaiyom et al., 2024) (Figure 5.4).

5.1.2. Anxiety Disorders Among Older Adults

Anxiety disorders are among the most prevalent mental disorders of the elderly, constituting a multifaceted interaction of biological, psychological, and social processes. As people grow older, they are likely to encounter increasing experiences of loss, chronic illness, and cognitive decline that provoke anxiety. The expression of anxiety disorders in older patients is not the same as in younger patients, manifested in somatic symptoms rather than typical anxiety symptoms. This complicates diagnosis and leads to under-recognition and undertreatment of such patients. Anxiety also exacerbates other chronic medical illnesses, and thus, overall health and quality of life are compromised. Management of these disorders among older adults requires an understanding that is sensitive to the specific needs and challenges of this population, with priority given to effective screening and intervention methods tailored to their needs (오병훈, 2017). Treatment of anxiety disorders among older adults needs an interdisciplinary treatment plan that addresses both pharmacological and non-pharmacological interventions. Even though medications like selective serotonin reuptake inhibitors (SSRIs) are helpful, they must be prescribed cautiously due to the potential for polypharmacy and heightened sensitivity to their side effects in aging individuals. Complementary and alternative therapies, including Tai Chi and Qi Gong, have also been shown to act as good adjuvants to traditional therapies, with the potential to reduce symptoms of anxiety and improve mental health in the elderly. A 2013 review by Abbot and Lavretsky supports these practices, suggesting they can enhance psychological resilience and quality of life. Their inclusion in treatment planning, therefore, can offer older adults comprehensive measures for managing anxiety, culminating in a more comprehensive understanding of geriatric mental health (Price et al., 2017). In short, anxiety disorders in older adults pose unique challenges not only for the individuals who are suffering but also for clinicians. The covert presentation of anxiety in this population typically requires an awareness of and sensitivity to underlying health issues. Treatment requires a balance of scientifically based treatments, both pharmacologic and adjunctive, that address both emotional and physical health. There needs to be a multidisciplinary model that allows interaction among healthcare providers to create and implement individualized treatment plans. By focusing on global care for older individuals with anxiety disorders, we can improve their mental health status and quality of life, laying the groundwork for healthier aging in this at-risk population (Figure 5.5).

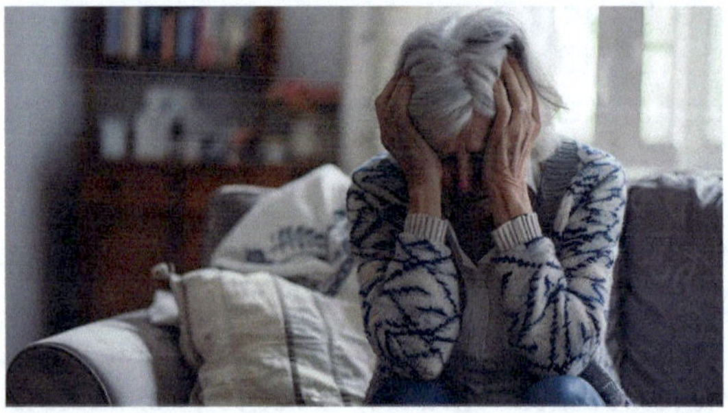

Figure 5.5. Anxiety disorders in elderly.

Source: https://images.onlymyhealth.com/imported/images/2024/August/26_Aug_2024/mn-anxiety-disorder-in-seniors.jpg.

5.1.3. Dementia and Cognitive Decline

Cognitive decline, or dementia as it is called in geriatric mental health, is an underlying challenge that refers to a decline in cognitive functioning that adversely affects reasoning, memory, and daily functioning. The course of dementia alters the day-to-day experiences of older adults so as to cause frequent emotional distress and exacerbation of pre-existing mental disorders. Familiarity with the psychological consequences of cognitive decline is necessary to create proper interventions. Recent research highlights the complex nature of resilience, noting that weakening cognitive functions and associative mental health problems may be mitigated by developing internal and external strengths. Concepts such as self-efficacy and social support have been identified as significant in fostering resilience in older adults with dementia-related problems, reducing depressive symptoms, and improving overall well-being (Funes et al., 2019). Behavioral disturbances are prevalent in dementia and help add complexity to aged care interactions. The symptoms, including aggression and agitation, can be extremely distressing for the residents and staff. Treating these behavior issues using individualized psychosocial interventions has been a promising strategy for geriatric mental health. In an influential study, it was found that there was a modest yet significant decrease in the severity of disruptive behavior with the use of non-pharmacological, individualized interventions. Importantly, this reduction not only reduced caregivers' perceived burden but also maintained residents' placement in mainstream aged care facilities amid cognitive function decline (Buchanan et al., 2007). This represents the potential of such interventions to enhance residents' quality of life and reduce the stressors on caregivers.

Dementia-induced cognitive decline requires a strategy that encompasses many aspects beyond pharmacological approaches. While medication can potentially bring some symptom relief, ensuring psychosocial well-being has a role to play equally in checking dementia's expansive outcome. Incorporating interventions targeting cognitive resilience and behavioral symptoms enables an inclusive treatment plan. Having the capacity to provide a sense of purpose and introducing strategies that facilitate healthy coping mechanisms can have a lasting impact on residents' emotional states. In addition, as set forth in recent research, an understanding of psychosocial resilience dynamics and neurobiological constructs provides a lens for individualized treatment planning for aging dementia patients. The blended format, in addition to enhancing mental health maintenance, optimizes care environments for residents and staff, thereby improving outcomes in geriatric mental health (Funes et al., 2019) (Figure 5.6).

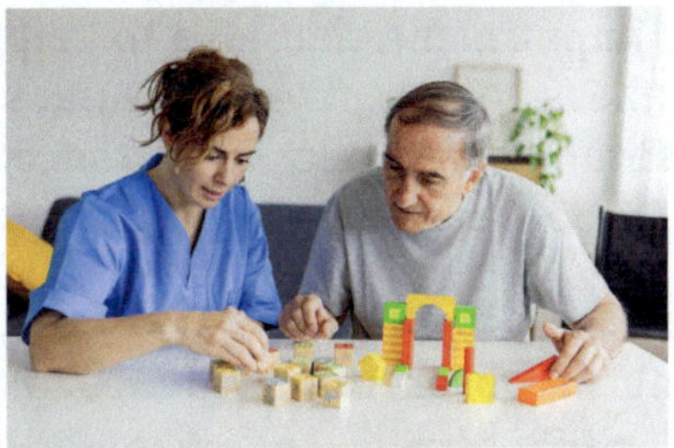

Figure 5.6. Cognitive decline in older adults.

Source: https://standrews1.com/wp-content/uploads/2024/07/Cognative-Decline.jpg.

Test Your Knowledge

1. What is the prevalence of depression?
2. What is the most common anxiety disorder in older adults?

5.2. Risk Factors for Mental Health Issues

Learning Outcome

1. Understand hotel maintenance management and its impact
2. Perform preventive maintenance
3. Discuss about breakdown maintenance

- Understand the biological factors affecting mental health
- Know the social isolation and its impact
- Describe the chronic physical health conditions

It is important to comprehend the multifactorial risk factors for geriatric mental illness in a bid to offer effective intervention and care. Of all the dominant factors for the onset of mental health illnesses, such as late-life depression (LLD), the presence of physical illnesses stands out as the most crucial one. Older adults are likely to have a co-occurrence of health conditions, such as cardiovascular disease, diabetes, and cognitive impairment, that lead to helplessness and loneliness. Where physical health struggles meet mental health, the importance of care addressing both becomes apparent.

General practitioners are therefore important in observing evidence of mental health decline because many older patients might complain somatically rather than openly expressing their emotional despair. Increased monitoring and the use of screening measures can greatly boost detection and treatment of LLD, which aligns with the results underscoring complexities in the diagnosis of mental illness among older adults (Declercq et al., 2018). Moreover, psychosocial influences exert a significant influence on the mental health setting for older individuals. Challenges such as social isolation, loss, and life change are able to significantly influence mental health so that one is more susceptible to depression. Studies have highlighted loneliness and perceived poor health among the elderly and asserted that those who perceive themselves as socially isolated are more susceptible to depression. Marital status, financial security, and the availability of social support systems emerge as vital variables affecting mental health outcomes in older persons. Dependent on successful social connections, studies place adequate social connections as a buffer against depression, and thus, it is imperative to understand the value of establishing community and familial connections. Exploring such psychosocial factors adds depth to the consideration of mental health risk factors in the geriatric population and raises the prospect for targeted preventative intervention (Mayhew et al., 1989).

Finally, life satisfaction and mental health must not be overemphasized when considering the geriatric population. Life satisfaction is often undermined by causes of financial hardship, loss, and loss of autonomy, which contribute to the risk of developing mental illness. Sensitivity of health professionals to these issues enables them to deliver more targeted interventions to build resilience and improve overall quality of life. By assisting in enhancing life satisfaction through consequential involvement and support services, practitioners can mitigate some of the psychological vulnerabilities inherent within the aging process. Mental health interventions using leisure activities, counseling, and community involvement have the ability to empower older adults across all socioeconomic statuses to maintain their mental health, potentially reducing the occurrence of illnesses such as LLD or associated anxiety disorders within the population (Mayhew et al., 1989) (Figure 5.7).

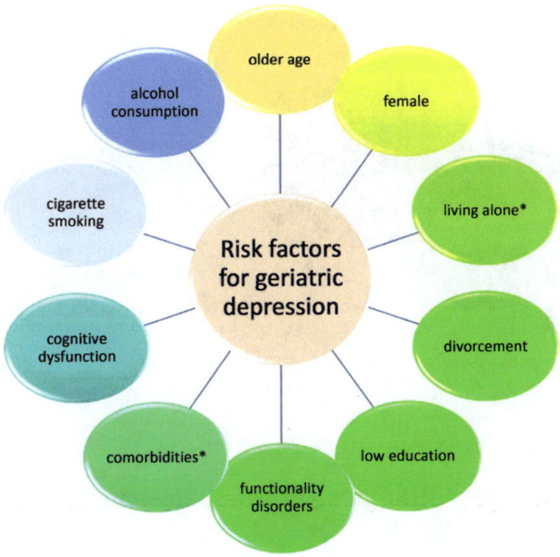

Figure 5.7. Risk factors for geriatric depression.

Source: https://ars.els-cdn.com/content/image/3-s2.0-B9780128179901000445-f44-01-9780128179901.jpg.

5.2.1. Biological Factors Affecting Mental Health

The knowledge of the biological factors that influence mental health is crucial, especially in geriatric mental health. As a person grows older, there are significant changes in neurobiological processes, e.g., diminished neuroplasticity and changes in neurotransmitter functions, and these can impact mood and cognition. Lack of neurotransmitters like serotonin and dopamine, e.g., has been widely linked to increased depression levels in older persons. Also, disease conditions that are common in the elderly, such as cardiovascular disease and diabetes, have been known to exacerbate mental health by introducing body stress as well as chronic inflammation. It is therefore important that biological health be addressed together with psychological and social health to prevent the onset of mental disorders in the elderly. New research has identified resilience as a central factor in the treatment of late-life depression (LLD), capturing the complex confluence of biological and psychosocial mechanisms. Resilience is not a static trait; rather, it is an active process driven by neurobiological and psychosocial factors that shape the capacity to withstand stressors associated with aging. For example, certain psychobiological factors, including genetic predisposition and inflammatory responses, can significantly impact a person's susceptibility to developing LLD and guide the course of illness. Additionally, psychosocial characteristics—such as coping skills, purpose, and support—have been found to be promising in enhancing resilience. Interventions of the psychosocial and biological causes can provide greater support for elderly individuals with mental illness, proposing that the multi-aspect intervention can provide better results in LLD prevention and treatment (Funes et al., 2019).

Geriatric mental health also needs a critical examination of accessible care frameworks and procedures. Current studies reveal substantial variations in the quality of care provided in residential and nursing homes, in which aging populations typically reside. Due to the lack of distinction between nursing and residential care facilities, it is important to develop care strategies that meet the distinct needs of these populations. Evidence indicates multidisciplinary interventions, such as pharmacist medication reviews, are effective for managing mental health medications but are typically limited to nursing homes and never penetrate residential care environments. To address the mental health needs of older populations, healthcare systems must place priority on proactive and preventive interventions, specifically targeted at enhancing quality of life and mental health outcomes. Continued learning and practice refinement, in particular on the application of mental health management, will prove vital for enhancing mental health in aging populations (Clay et al., 2025) (Figure 5.8).

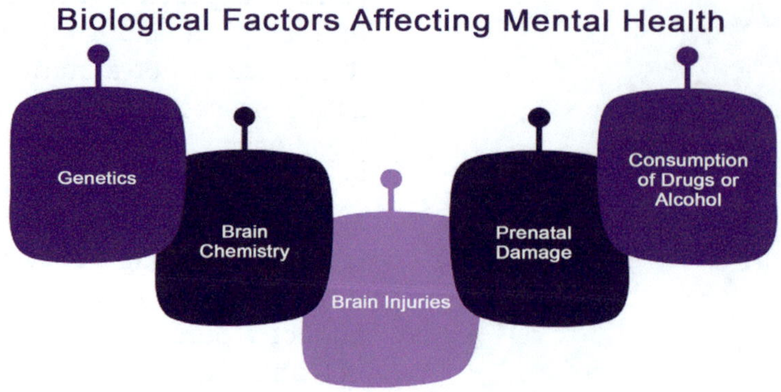

Figure 5.8. Biological factors affecting mental health.

Source: https://www.theknowledgeacademy.com/_files/images/Biological_Factors_Affecting_Mental_Health%281%29.png.

5.2.2. Social Isolation and Its Impact

Social isolation is an emerging problem in geriatric mental health because it directly reflects on the psychological well-being of older adults. The majority of older adults are isolated due to factors like loss of mobility, bereavement, and loss of social relationships. These changes bring about intense emotional pain marked by depression and loneliness. Social isolation has also been known to exacerbate already existing mental illnesses and bring about new ones, a condition that significantly impacts the quality of life among older adults. Such emotional burden often spreads beyond this group to their caregivers, at times subjecting the supportive caregivers to heavy stress and burden. Thus, the fight against social isolation is crucial for enhancing the psychological quality of life among elderly populations, demanding interventions that facilitate social interaction and develop social networks. The implications of social isolation extend beyond the emotional pain; they have a significant bearing on physical health outcomes as well. For instance, studies have shown that socially isolated older adults tend to develop chronic illnesses, and the interplay between physical and mental health acquires a special intensity. The relationship between social networks and health is two-way—while poor mental health will result in people being isolated, isolation can exclude the use of health care and make a person more susceptible to loss of autonomy and cognitive decline. Moreover, social isolation is linked with a host of adverse outcomes, including higher mortality in older adults. This interconnectedness also underlines the necessity of an integrated approach to geriatric mental illness that addresses psychological and physical elements and enables interventions not only promoting mental health but also enhancing health. Because of the intricate interaction between social isolation, mental illness, and caregiver burden, it is recommended to involve both caregivers and patients in planning for mental health. Current studies highlight the relationship between older adults and their caregivers' psychological well-being. For instance, caregivers have reported higher levels of stress, which correlate with their recipients' psychological distress, indicating that the burden of caregiving has also been shown to affect caregivers' mental well-being (Bellanti et al., 2016). Additionally, family members taking care of dementia patients also have unique challenges, such as increased risk of physical and mental disease, and an additional increase in burden if the care recipients deteriorate, such as falling (McIntyre et al., 2011). Addressing the needs of the older adults and their caregivers based on a bio-psychosocial approach would alleviate some of the ill effects of social isolation, thus giving them enough support and resources for coping with their problems.

5.2.3. Chronic Physical Health Conditions

Chronic physical health conditions are an important determinant of the health and well-being of older adults and directly influence their mental health status. Increasing age is associated with an increase in the incidence of such conditions, including diabetes, heart disease, and arthritis, and these often involve complicated interactions between physical and mental health. Chronic disease stress can exacerbate depression and anxiety in older adults, possibly perpetuating a cycle that is difficult to break. Moreover, limitations due to these illnesses can lead to limited socialization and mobility, further isolating elderly individuals and making them more vulnerable to mental illness. It is important that healthcare professionals to understand the need for care practices that incorporate consideration of physical and mental health concerns among older persons. Social determinants such as income and living circumstances significantly influence the psychological well-being of older adults with chronic physical illness. Low incomes can lead to feelings of frustration or worthlessness, particularly when health-related limitations keep them from engaging in productive activities. As an illustration, aging single adults or bereaved individuals may find that their plight is exacerbated by illness-related problems, with a heightened risk for depressive symptomatology. (Mayhew et al., 1989) puts forward these connections through the observation of depressive states to be associated with subjective self-evaluations of health, life satisfaction, and the experience of loneliness. The impact of such determinants underscores the need for interventions that not only attend to older people's health but also to their social and economic environment, thereby promoting paradigms of integrated care that promote mental health in addition to physical health. In the field of geriatric mental health, one has to adopt an aggressive strategy for the management of the effects of chronic physical illness. This includes universal screening for depression in older patients with chronic diseases, as their psychological condition is overlooked with a focus on somatic complaints.

Early identification and appropriate interventions can avert the adverse effects of comorbid depression, which, if left unmanaged, will result in declining mental as well as physical well-being. Through holistic assessment that considers physical health status and mental health, practitioners can devise individually tailored treatment plans that address the unique needs of older adults. With the subject ever-changing, there needs to be ongoing research to understand these intricate relationships and improve the lives of older adults who are faced with the double trouble of long-term physical disease and mental illness, as suggested by Khezrian et al. (2017) (Figure 5.9).

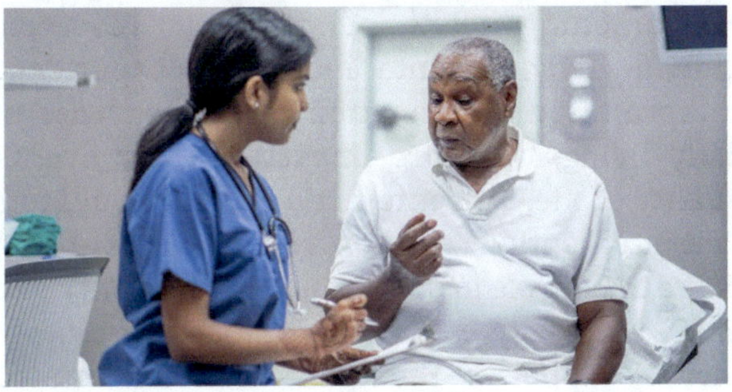

Figure 5.9. The intersection of mental health and chronic disease.

Source: https://publichealth.jhu.edu/sites/default/files/styles/social_image/public/2021-12/mental-health-and-chronic-illness-gettyimages-1212821220.jpeg?itok=SvjAUx3u.

Test Your Knowledge

1. What are the biological factors affecting mental health?
2. What is a chronic physical health condition?

5.3. Impact of Mental Health on Quality of Life

Learning Outcome

1. Describe the effects of mental health on daily functioning
2. Know the influence of mental health on physical health
3. Understand the importance of family and social networks in geriatric mental health

Mental illness has a direct effect on the quality of life of the geriatric individual, influencing not just his or her emotional state but also physical health and functioning in everyday life. Chronic disease, common in the elderly, typically accompanies mental illness such as depression and anxiety. The presence of disease often contributes to physical disability among the elderly. It leads to a self-reinforcing cycle of worsening health. As noted in research, individuals with mental illness may experience compromised participation in the activities of daily living, therefore impacting their overall quality of life. This interaction further suggests that interventions to improve mental well-being play a major role in promoting independence and improving daily experience among the elderly, thereby supporting the significance of integrated interventions in geriatric care (Au-Yeung et al., 2020). Involvement in therapeutic activities can be a significant intervention for enhancing the psychological health of older adults and thus their quality of life. Visual art therapy, for example, is being shown to be effective, with a positive relationship to affective and cognitive change in older adults. Some studies indicate that art therapy may reduce self-reports of bereavement and depression and enhance social contact and cognitive stimulation. As aging populations worldwide increasingly confront the burdens of old age, the inclusion of art-based therapy within traditional rehabilitative regimens is likely to improve not only emotional well-being but also overall life satisfaction. Physical therapy and creative activities enable older patients to benefit immensely through improvements in their activities of daily living (ADLs) and sense of well-being, underscoring the transformative impact of mental health interventions on the lives of older individuals (Mayhew et al., 1989).

Moreover, understanding the relationship between mental health and various socio-economic determinants is critical in addressing the needs of the aged. Studies have shown that loneliness, subjective perceived state of health, and quality-of-life satisfaction are related to mental well-being. Loss, income status, and social support are critical components to reflect on; for instance, isolated elderly citizens are prone to report more depression, which further reduces the quality of life. Thus, continued studies of these interactions are required, particularly with the growing number of the elderly. Treatments for psychiatric enhancements should also address the socio-economic conditions of the elderly. With an integrated strategy that addresses social, economic, and psychological considerations, caregivers and medical professionals can enhance the quality of life for the elderly (Mayhew et al., 1989) (Figure 5.10).

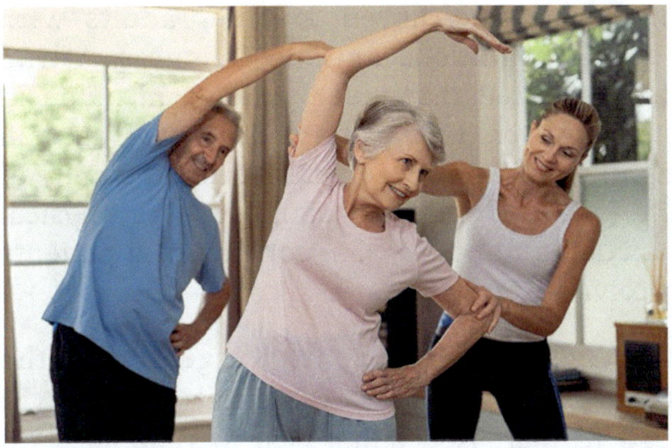

Figure 5.10. Improve the quality of life for seniors.

Source: https://bethesdahealth.org/wp-content/uploads/2019/06/iStock-1029344612-1-e1560808653328.jpg.

5.3.1. Effects on Daily Functioning

The daily functioning of elderly individuals is significantly influenced by their mental illness, and various psychological illnesses impair basic activities. Depression, anxiety, and intellectual disabilities can severely limit the individual from performing daily activities, from the everyday activities of self-care to adapting to domestic chores. With deteriorating mental health, older individuals lose motivation and are less energetic and slip into an inactive routine, which exacerbates their mental illness issues even further. The significance of interventions designed to enhance mental health cannot be exaggerated since successful programs can improve the quality of life of an individual and enable daily functioning. For instance, studies show that rehabilitative programs designed to enhance physical and mental health lead to significant improvements in essential activities of daily living, thereby allowing older people to extend their period of living independently and raising the quality of life as a whole (Adunsky et al., 2010). Furthermore, environmental conditions might strongly determine mental health and performance in everyday activities among older individuals. Supportive environmental conditions can facilitate more environmental mastery, which is associated with fewer symptoms of depression. It was concluded in a study of residents in assisted living that residents perceiving a greater sense of control over their environments had significantly lower depression rates (Akin et al., 2011). This finding underscores the importance of creating environments that enhance older people's autonomy and enable active involvement. Interventions such as encouraging activity participation in the community or providing opportunities for home environment personalization can enhance mental health and, therefore, increase daily functioning and social integration. Hence, addressing environmental issues is central to the overall plan of geriatric mental health. Lastly, the relationship between physical health and mental functioning cannot be neglected in the measurement of effects on daily activities among older adults.

Physical conditions, such as chronic pain or limitations in mobility, overlap with mental illness and have an additive effect on the ability of a person to engage in daily activities. Multimodal treatment approaches that address physical and psychological needs have been shown to improve overall well-being and functioning in geriatric populations. For example, a multicomponent intervention program for older patients recovering from hip fracture demonstrated improved mental health outcomes, including better pain management and physical functioning, indicating that whole-person care improves functioning on a daily basis (Adunsky et al., 2010). These findings are crucial for caregiving and health care professionals advocating for a multi-dimensional geriatric mental health approach, affirming that meeting the full spectrum of needs is necessary to preserve independence in activities of daily living and improve quality of life (Figure 5.11).

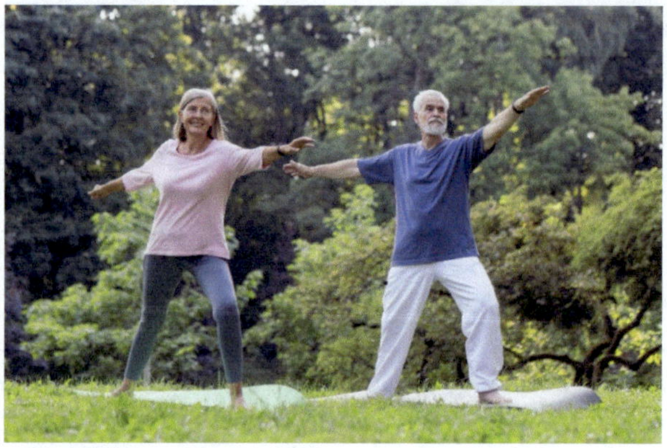

Figure 5.11. Daily routines improve mental health for seniors.

Source: https://bluemoonseniorcounseling.com/wp-content/uploads/2024/06/How-Daily-Routines-Improve-Mental-Health-for-Seniors.jpg.

5.3.2. Influence on Physical Health

The intersection of physical and mental health in geriatrics is a central area of study since mental status directly influences physical health outcomes. For instance, depression and anxiety are common psychiatric disorders among this patient population, leading to diminished motivation to engage in physical activity, which is vital for maintaining strength and mobility. There has been evidence to suggest that older adults who place emphasis on maintaining mental wellness by undergoing therapeutic treatment tend to show improved physical well-being. This is especially noteworthy among older patients who are recovering from incidents like hip fractures, where mental health care can facilitate active participation in recovery programs, ultimately leading to enhanced functional outcomes and quality of life. The potential benefits of such interdisciplinarity cannot be overstated, providing an integrated model of treatment for the aged of factors that consider both physical and mental health. The interrelationship between physical rehabilitation and mental health is illustrated in treatment interventions tailored to older adults with specific conditions like hip fractures. A trial demonstrated that older patients included in an interdisciplinary intervention program had significantly improved health-related quality of life (HRQOL) on dimensions such as physical function and bodily pain compared to patients receiving standard care.

These improvements suggest that the active management of mental health will lead to increased adherence to rehabilitation regimes, which ultimately affects the outcome of recovery. These findings emphasize the importance of putting in place comprehensive health interventions that include mental health assessments and interventions for elderly people after recovering from somatic illness. Clinicians are then in a position to develop settings conducive to both physical and mental rehabilitation, illustrating the interconnected nature of these dimensions of health among older people (Adunsky et al., 2010). Further, an understanding of how mental health impacts physical health is imperative when creating efficient treatment plans for older adults. More so, there is a growing appreciation for the importance of social interaction and engagement in society to facilitate mental resilience, which may possibly enable better physical health outcomes. Interventions that get older adults to participate in group work or social support groups not only help address loneliness but also provide physical activity, which is beneficial for cardiovascular health and overall mobility. Health systems that take a whole-brain approach to mental health interventions can therefore address both psychological and physiological issues in the elderly in advance. Finally, these integrative approaches can potentially maximize health outcomes and quality of life, underscoring the necessity of a complex perspective on health in geriatric medicine (Khezrian et al., 2017) (Figure 5.12).

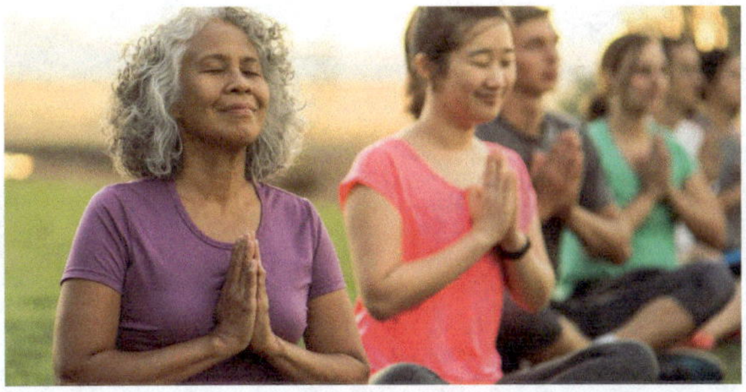

Figure 5.12. The importance of mental and physical health in senior citizens.

Source: https://www.createabilityinc.com/wp-content/uploads/2018/09/Physical-and-mental-wellbeing-of-elderly--870x450.jpg.

5.3.3. Relationship with Family and Social Networks

The role of family and social relationships in mental health in old age cannot be overemphasized, as these interactions significantly affect the emotional and psychological well-being of the elderly. The aging process has usually been linked to significant life transitions, such as retirement, loss of intimate friends, and death of relatives, all of which can deteriorate the quality of social interaction. Intimate family relationships and cohesive social relationships can help neutralize loneliness and isolation, which are prevalent among older people.

Research indicates that those who remain attached to their families and engaged in social networks have better mental health measurements, including lower levels of depression and anxiety. Understanding the dynamics of such relationships, particularly in the context of diversity, has the potential to guide specific interventions aimed at enhancing geriatric mental health and highlight the importance of empowering caregivers whose roles are at the heart of these family structures (Henwood et al., 2017). Specific needs of older individuals, such as caregiving, also underscore the importance of family and social networks. Care for older adults often involves complex emotional and physical demands that may affect caregivers and recipients alike. The diversity in caregiving situations requires consideration of various care settings, with a focus not only on the emotional strength but also on the impact of economic and employment stress. As revealed in most studies, older carers are likely to experience increased stress and potential mental health decline, emphasizing the importance of robust social support structures. Social networks can access the required resources, both providing pragmatic and emotional assistance, thereby maximizing the caregiving process. Good family relations and social relations within the community should therefore take precedence over policy and practice (Henwood et al., 2017). Also working on the dynamic between social relationships and mental health in late life are variables such as loneliness and perceived support, which can exert particularly strong influences on general life satisfaction. Research on these dynamics illustrates that older adults with active social lives will score themselves as more satisfied with their lives and less depressed. For example, the support an individual receives from family and peers most significantly alleviates loneliness, underscoring the importance of emotional support at this stage of life. Aside from this, sociodemographic factors such as marital status, income, and household composition strongly influence these social networks. Charting and understanding these intricate layers of social connectedness can guide intervention programs aimed at promoting mental health among older adults. Overall, enhancing social relationships among older adults lies at the heart of enhancing their mental health and ensuring a holistic approach towards geriatric mental health treatment (Figure 5.13).

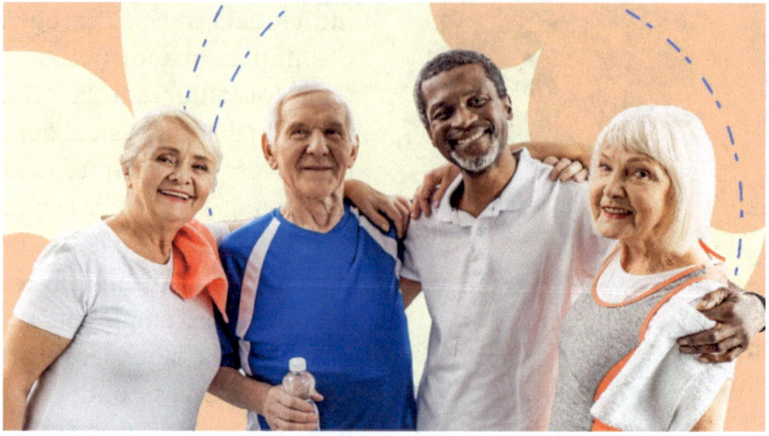

Figure 5.13. The importance of social connections for seniors.

Source: https://www.fivegoodfriends.com.au/user/pages/06.blog/03.posts/157.the-importance-of-social-connections-for-seniors/FGF%20-%20Blog%20-%20The%20importance%20of%20social%20connection%20for%20seniors.jpg.

Test Your Knowledge

1. What are the effects of mental health on daily functioning?
2. What is the importance of family and social networks in geriatric mental health?

5.4. Barriers to Mental Health Care

Learning Outcome

1. Understand the stigma surrounding mental health
2. Understand the lack of access to mental health services for the geriatric population
3. Describe the misdiagnosis and underdiagnosis in geriatric mental health

Mental health care barriers to the elderly population often result from systemic shortfalls in healthcare systems. Most contemporary health care models, based on acute care traditions, are poorly suited to meeting the needs of older patients. As highlighted in research across Europe, these systems place a central focus on specialization and efficiency, ignoring continuity of care that is vital for older patients with chronic illness and often multiple comorbidities. Ineffective coordinated treatment plans can lead to broken care, which is particularly detrimental to older patients who require holistic support beyond medicine's traditional silos (Wait, 2005). This systematic breakdown is not alleviated just by mental health care but adds to the broader health disparities that beset the older population. Another serious hindrance to the accessibility of mental health care among older adults is the prevalence of undiagnosed mental health illnesses, especially depression. Studies indicate that nearly 40% of older adults with chronic illness remain undiagnosed for depression, a situation with a ripple effect on health outcomes and the maintenance of related healthcare learning. For instance, as discussed in a study in which the Geriatric Depression Scale was utilized, those with depressive symptoms demonstrated impaired retention of health content, which is crucial in their ability to optimally manage their conditions. This interdependence means that untreated mental disorder is capable of affecting not only psychological well-being but also the functional ability to engage in and understand healthcare programs aimed at improving their overall health (Wynn-Grundy et al., 2016). Social stigma associated with mental illness among older adults also renders access to necessary care even more challenging. The majority of the elderly may perceive acknowledgment of mental distress as a failing, hence being reluctant to face the problem. Mental health stigma deters some patients from reporting symptoms to healthcare providers, hence robbing them of an opportunity for early intervention and adequate treatment. Moreover, the lack of culturally aware care, mindful of the unique history and experience of the elderly, can increase perceptions of exclusion and confusion, deterring them from utilizing mental health services. Thus, the imperative to break down barriers to mental health care involves a multifaceted process, addressing both deficits at the systemic and societal levels in order to cultivate a more integrated and tolerant sphere for the elderly.

5.4.1. Stigma Surrounding Mental Health

The stigma of mental illness, particularly among the old, is responsible for contributing the most to undertreatment and underdiagnosis of mental illness among the old. The stigma largely arises from the belief of society that equates mental illness with individual failure or weakness. As such, the vast majority of older adults may not seek help or acknowledge the symptoms for fear of being judged or stigmatized. The misguided perception that mental illness is only applicable to youth can also be to blame for exacerbating this situation. This makes older individuals even lonelier and less willing to share their thoughts. By breaking down and addressing the stigmas, it becomes easier to create a more open environment so that older individuals feel comfortable seeking the assistance they need, enabling them to promote overall mental development and resilience in the face of the challenges of aging. Aside from personal stigma, systemic factors also contribute to the common misperception of geriatric mental illnesses. Healthcare providers may not be trained sufficiently in the topic of mental illness among the elderly and consequently misdiagnose or oversimplify disorders such as depression and anxiety. As emphasized in substance-related disorders research, a clear need exists for advanced medical training that explores the unique aspects of addiction and mental illness late in life (Broers et al., 2016). Otherwise, practitioners unintentionally stigmatize by assuming symptoms because of mere characteristics of aging, without regard for the complex tapestry of psychosocial and biological aspects of these diseases. This neglect not only compounds the quality of care but also continues to fuel common myths surrounding mental health, so it becomes a debilitating cycle that isolates older individuals further. In order to tackle stigma effectively, a coordinated strategy is required, with both psychosocial and neurobiological interventions working in concert to enhance resilience and foster mental health among the older population. Interventions that enhance self-efficacy, meaning, and social support can help individuals navigate the nuances of late-life depression as well as other mental disorders (Funes et al., 2019). Additionally, the inclusion of movement-based therapies, such as yoga or tai chi, alongside traditional therapy offers holistic pathways to improved mental well-being. By institutionalizing conversations about mental health and emphasizing the development of resilience strategies, society can establish a culture in which older adults view seeking help as a desirable quality rather than something negative. In the end, reducing stigma and implementing evidence-based interventions will lead to better mental health outcomes for the geriatric population, allowing individuals to live well in their golden years (Figure 5.14).

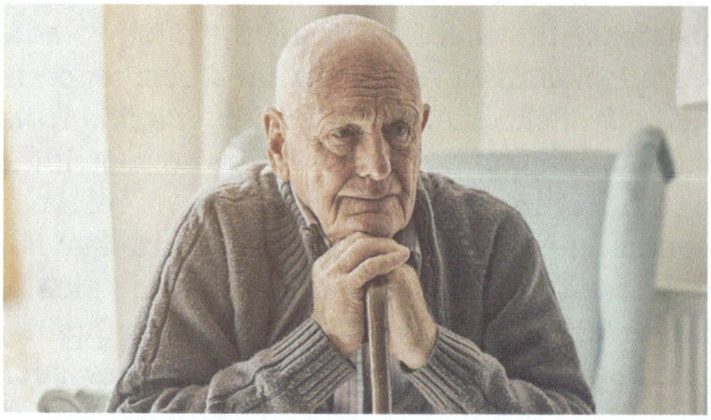

Figure 5.14. Stigma impacts older adults with mental illness.

Source: https://letstalkstigma.org/wp-content/uploads/2019/05/HeaderImage_June.jpg.

5.4.2. Lack of Access to Mental Health Services

The challenge of access to mental health care among the elderly has become increasingly pressing, especially given that demographic projections show an increasing percentage of individuals over the age of 65 requiring psychological care. With the forecast being that one out of four Canadians will be aged 65 or older by 2031, the demand for quality mental health care specific to this age group is more urgent than ever. Sadly, existing models tend to focus more on physical health requirements, creating a void in mental health services targeted toward older adults. Such a lack of focus stems from several barriers, including stigma against mental illness, ageism, and geographical disparities affecting delivery. Limited literature addressing geriatric mental health in regions like Windsor-Essex again highlights the imperative of targeted interventions and advocacy efforts aimed at increasing accessibility for this already compromised population (Nadeem et al., 2018). Compounding the issue is the built-in challenge of the rural-urban divide that further increases the accessibility of mental health services among older adults. Rural older adults can face inordinate travel distances to obtain care, leading to disengagement from essential treatment. Even though collaborative care efforts, such as those designed to merge primary and specialty care in rural settings, show promise, many geriatric patients remain underserved due to low awareness and outreach. For example, early trials of shared mental health care demonstrate the potential for improving geriatric mental health outcomes through collaboration among family doctors and mental health experts. However, such innovations need to be scaled up in various geographic areas, which is a complex problem requiring comprehensive approaches tailored to the circumstances of older populations (Dolansky et al., 2007). The implications of limited access to mental health treatment are broader than individual pain; they also unevenly overburden healthcare systems and communities. Without access to timely and appropriate mental health treatment, older adults are likely to have multiple health complications and increased hospitalization, leading to increased healthcare costs. Further, an uninformed society regarding geriatric mental health may result in poor policy and resource planning, perpetuating the cycle of neglect. All corrections to disparities in the availability of mental health services require collective efforts, such as revising policies, community-level education, and the allocation of targeted funds. Collaboration with health stakeholders, community organizations, and social service agencies is essential for bridging these gaps and ensuring access to the mental health care they are entitled to (Nadeem et al., 2018).

5.4.3. Misdiagnosis and Underdiagnosis

Geriatric mental health misdiagnosis and underdiagnosis are significant issues with the potential to harm the care and quality of life of older adults. Older adults present overlapping or mimicking typical medical conditions symptoms, and these symptoms may lead medical practitioners to attribute them to natural aging processes rather than mental health illnesses. For instance, cognitive impairment, also often mixed up with Alzheimer's disease, may be caused by potentially reversible conditions like depression, which in turn can lead to extreme impairments if not detected. This is compounded by the fact that there is inadequate training in geriatric medicine, as various medical professionals may not correctly diagnose presentations of mental disorders within the elderly patient, and therefore, greater educational systems are needed within the treatment of geriatric populations (Freter et al., 2003). Underdiagnosis is also a pressing concern, where mental illness may be underdiagnosed and left untreated, further compromising the health of older individuals. Contributing factors to underdiagnosis are ageist assumptions that mental decline is an inherent component of aging. Furthermore, communication problems, such as sensory impairment, may limit effective discussion of symptoms between older patients and clinicians. Clinicians do fail to notice marked changes in behavior or emotional distress that, in the older individual, present differently. Consequently, illnesses such as depression and anxiety disorders do go undetected, manifesting in disability and exacerbation of co-morbid medical illnesses. This then brings to the fore the necessity of integrative assessment strategies that prioritize mental health in geriatric practice to avert late detection and intervention. Moreover, the complexity of comorbidities in older adults further complicates diagnosis. Since most older patients have multiple health conditions, doctors prefer to treat physical complaints before evaluating mental well-being. This subsequently produces fragmented care, where mental health becomes shortchanged or becomes misdiagnosed as physical illnesses. For example, a symptom of breathlessness can only be explained by respiratory conditions and fails to explore potential anxiety conditions as the reason for these complaints, like in situations relating to the management of asthmatic patients among elderly groups (Battaglia et al., 2016). Overcoming these challenges to effective diagnosis is not solely about increased clinical training but also about embracing an all-around approach to healthcare, one that puts mental health at the forefront as a critical component of integrative geriatric care. This wide-ranging attention could greatly improve results for this at-risk population (Figure 5.15).

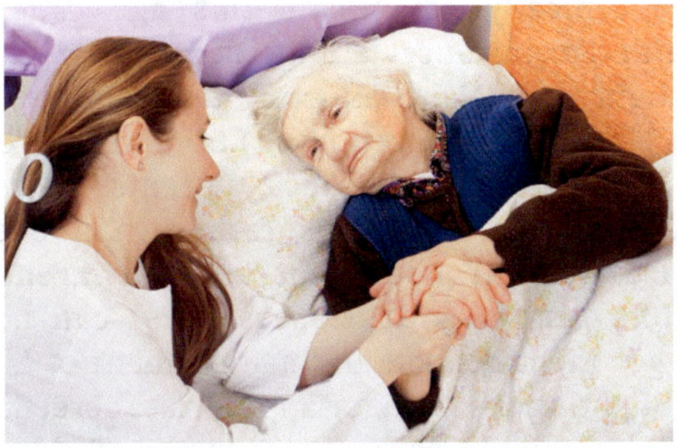

Figure 5.15. Dementia misdiagnosis.

Source: https://www.queensu.ca/gazette/sites/default/files/assets/TVN2.jpg.

Test Your Knowledge

1. What are the barriers to mental health care for elderly people?
2. What are the stigmas surrounding mental health?

5.5. Treatment Options for Geriatric Mental Health

Learning Outcome

1. Understand the importance of psychotherapy and counseling approaches in geriatric mental health
2. Understand the role of pharmacological treatments in managing mental health disorders;
3. Describe the alternative therapies and holistic approaches in geriatric mental health

Treatment for geriatric mental health is also multifaceted, encompassing the various needs of elderly people who can present with a variety of symptoms of mental illness. Treatment for geriatric mental health must take into consideration the interaction of medical, psychological, and social elements that typically complicate this age group's health. For instance, late-life depression (LLD) is highly prevalent, affecting up to 13.3% of the elderly. Identification of LLD can turn out to be challenging because patients present with somatic symptoms rather than overt depression. As noted, increased awareness among general practitioners (GPs) can help trigger identification and management of LLD, highlighting the need for appropriate screening tools to enable early intervention. Tailoring treatment plans to account for the heterogeneity of geriatric patients is central to achieving effective outcomes in mental health (Declercq et al., 2018). Geriatric mental health interventions also need to include pharmacological and non-pharmacological methods. Antidepressants, which are effective, have a side effect risk that is increased by polypharmacy—a not uncommon problem in geriatric practice. Hence, it is important to monitor and modify these therapies according to response in individual patients. Concurrently, non-pharmacological interventions such as cognitive behavior therapy (CBT) and supportive counseling also became effective interventions because they have the capability to treat cognitive decline as well as emotional distress without introducing the risk factor of medication. Additionally, active engagement of elderly people in therapeutic interventions such as group therapy can increase social interactions, which can bridge loneliness that is usually experienced by older adults who have mental illness. Such an integrated method of therapy not only cures symptoms but also ensures overall well-being (Declercq et al., 2018). Policy measures are most crucial for enabling treatment modalities for elderly mental health because they connect research and practice. There is a need for evidence-based policies promoting prevention and care coordination in order to meet the specific needs of older adults, such as insufficient access to mental health services. For example, investing in patient self-management and palliative care can be of vital importance to better the mental health outcomes of elderly people, yet these are underdeveloped in most regions. By shining a light on the importance of incorporating geriatric-focused mental health policies into overall health care systems, one can improve care provision. Syncing treatment alternatives for individuals with a focus on systematically incorporating research findings into patient care will ultimately improve mental health services rendered to the elderly.

5.5.1. Psychotherapy and Counseling Approaches

Recognition of the worth of psychotherapy and counseling interventions in aging mental health necessitates recognition of their high effectiveness in the treatment of a variety of psychological conditions among older people. A systematic review by the British Association for Counselling and Psychotherapy emphasized that various forms of counseling are extremely effective in enhancing symptom improvements for depression and anxiety in older people. Among the 47 reviewed studies, reminiscence therapy and cognitive behavioral therapy were found to be particularly effective, and their outcomes are found to be comparable to those in younger populations. This is especially significant as it dispels the myth that elderly people respond less to therapy. By adapting these interventions to be sensitive to the unique life situations and challenges of older adults, mental health professionals can create a setting that supports recovery and emotional well-being, thereby maximizing overall geriatric mental health status (Brettle et al., 2005). Incorporating a number of different therapeutic methods into the care of the elderly can also enhance the counseling resource base of older adults. One of the most promising treatments is music therapy, which has gained attention for its dramatic effects on individuals with various types of dementia. Research has shown that music therapy helps to preserve memory and even reverse the mental decline that accompanies Alzheimer's disease and other types of dementia. This type of therapy enables patients to remember forgotten memories and enhances communication skills, resulting in a more fulfilling life despite their mental disabilities. Furthermore, when used with established pharmaceutical interventions, music therapy can offer improved treatment efficacy through a holistic means of approaching dementia complications. The multi-faceted strategy highlights the importance of integrating creative therapies and traditional psychotherapy to provide an integrative system for improving geriatric mental health (Shotts et al., 2018). The integration of psychotherapy and counseling within geriatric care addresses not only the mental illness but also the significance of relationship-oriented care among the aged. With the aged battling the psychological and emotional effects of aging, social isolation, loss of autonomy, and grief can then become severe complications of existing mental illness. Therapeutic techniques that are open to free talking and bridge-building create a favorable setting for older adults' disclosure of their experiences and affect. Comforting caregivers or family members during therapy sessions enables practitioners to optimize support systems, creating a sense of community, which is essential to the emotional well-being of older people. The applicability of these counseling modalities is that they foster resilience and adaptive coping, ultimately leading to a higher level of agency and purpose in the geriatric population. As mentioned, with the further development of the field, the uptake of these new therapeutic strategies will be essential to improving mental health outcomes in older people (Brettle et al., 2005) (Figure 5.16).

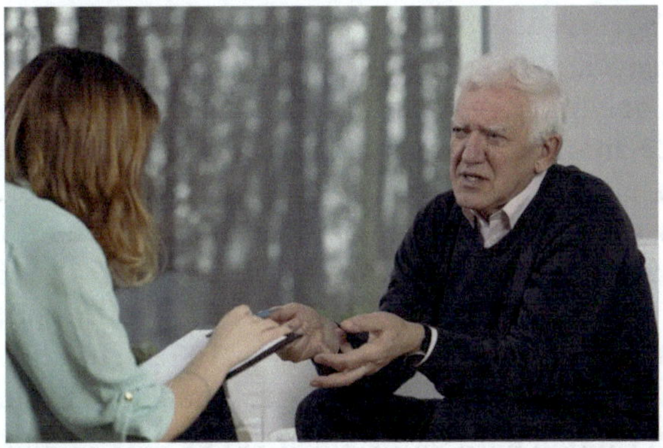

Figure 5.16. Supportive psychotherapy geriatric counseling.

Source: https://mantracare.org/wp-content/uploads/2021/12/Supportive-Psychotherapy-Geriatric-Counseling.jpg.webp.

5.5.2. Pharmacological Treatments

Pharmacologic interventions play a central role in the treatment of mental illness conditions in the aged, particularly in the management of the complexities of late-life depression (LLD). With an occurrence rate of up to 13.3% among older adults, LLD is a significant challenge for healthcare providers owing to the fact that typically imprecise symptoms may be inaccurately misinterpreted as somatic instead of psychological. The importance of identifying and diagnosing LLD cannot be overstressed because untreated depression has catastrophic effects, including increased morbidity and mortality. Pharmacologic management with antidepressants like selective serotonin reuptake inhibitors (SSRIs) and serotonin-norepinephrine reuptake inhibitors (SNRIs) is usually advised for the alleviation of depressive symptoms and improvement of the overall quality of life in elderly patients with this disorder (Le et al., 2009). In addition to SSRIs and SNRIs, the pharmacological treatment of older patients also includes a range of adjunct therapies. Electroconvulsive therapy (ECT) may be provided for patients with treatment resistance to conventional antidepressants or a severe depressive episode. Additionally, the physician often has to cope with the problem of polypharmacy because older patients usually use more than one medication for numerous chronic conditions. This necessitates a careful assessment of potential drug interactions and side effects, which are more serious among elderly patients. Education of clinicians regarding pharmacological care, particularly tailored for geriatric mental health, is thus very important. Clinicians must be able to make logical decisions about medication regimens that minimize risks while maximizing therapeutic responses (Le et al., 2009). In addition to the pharmacological advances made in the treatment of mental health conditions in the elderly population, there still exists an important need for continued education and enhanced screening among healthcare providers. Numerous nurse practitioners (NPs) and general practitioners might feel unsure about their capacity to accurately diagnose between unhappiness that is a part of normal aging and clinical depressive disorders. As proposed in recent research, education programs that improve knowledge of geriatric mental health have the potential to enable professionals to screen more effectively and treat their patients better. Such professional education is important in bridging the care gap, ensuring that older patients receive appropriate and timely pharmacologic intervention. By enhancing overall awareness of LLD and pharmacological interventions, healthcare professionals will be in a position to significantly improve mental health outcomes for older adults, thereby addressing a central realm of geriatric well-being (Declercq et al., 2018) (Figure 5.17).

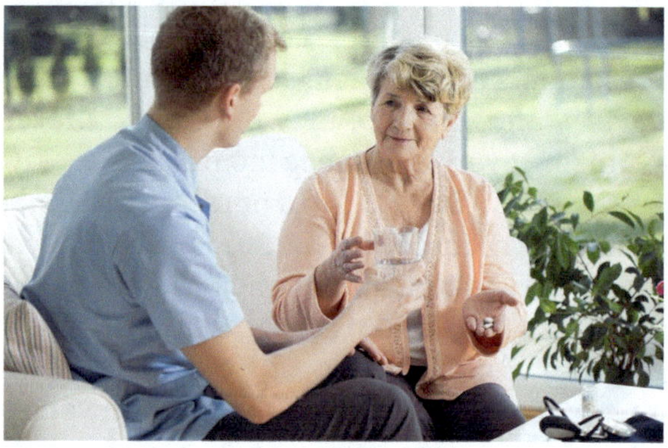

Figure 5.17. Mental health medication.

Source: https://www.ezrahomecare.com/hubfs/Stock%20images/making_sure_your_elderly_parent_is_taking_their_medication_for_mental_health%7C_issues_mental_disorder_tips_how_Home_Care_can_help_Ezra_Home_Care_Massachusetts.jpeg.

5.5.3. Alternative Therapies and Holistic Approaches

Inclusion of alternative care and holistic interventions in geriatric mental health is increasingly recognized as having the potential to optimize well-being among older adults. Although traditional pharmacotherapeutic interventions tend to dominate treatment protocols, a growing consensus among healthcare providers exists concerning the benefits derived from non-pharmacological interventions. These interventions, such as mindfulness, art therapy, and guided imagery, are designed to address the general well-being of older adults rather than just symptoms. A literature review of elderly management of pain indicates that while pharmacological intervention is prevalent within nursing homes, other approaches are emerging as possible alternatives, which require further research (Reid et al., 2006). This trend towards integrative care is bolstered by a set of patient-centered values and a concern for individual experience and the importance of psychological and emotional factors in achieving the best mental health outcomes. The integration of complementary therapies into geriatric care benefits not just psychological conditions, like depression and anxiety, but also results in a sense of community and belonging in elderly patients. Interventions that incorporate these therapies hold the promise of stimulating social interaction, often lacking in the lives of older adults, and thereby decreasing isolation. Community-based music and art therapy programs, for instance, have been shown to enhance cognitive function and facilitate emotional expression. Further, accepting holistic models is synergistic with emerging models of healthcare reform that aim to improve infrastructure and care delivery for older adults. The commitment to incorporating alternative modalities into practice across mental health can lead to innovative payment systems that compensate for the provision of holistic care that is sensitive to individual patient needs, thereby counteracting fragmentation often reported among geriatric health services. Although promising results are associated with alternative therapies, significant barriers lie in their across-the-board adoption. Providers have traditionally viewed pharmacologic treatments as the central therapeutic strategy for mental disorders in the aged, complicating the integration of holistic practices into standard practice. Cultural beliefs, misconstructions of the efficacy of alternative treatments, and organizational inertia are significant barriers that must be resolved. However, the collective evidence supporting the effectiveness of complementary therapies continues to grow, and healthcare professionals are increasingly calling for a more open-minded approach to treatment. Continuing education and training with a focus on the strengths of holistic approaches are critical to eliminating myths and fostering a more integrative care model that actively incorporates alternative therapies into geriatric mental health programs, ultimately enhancing the quality of life for the elderly (Reid et al., 2006) (Figure 5.18).

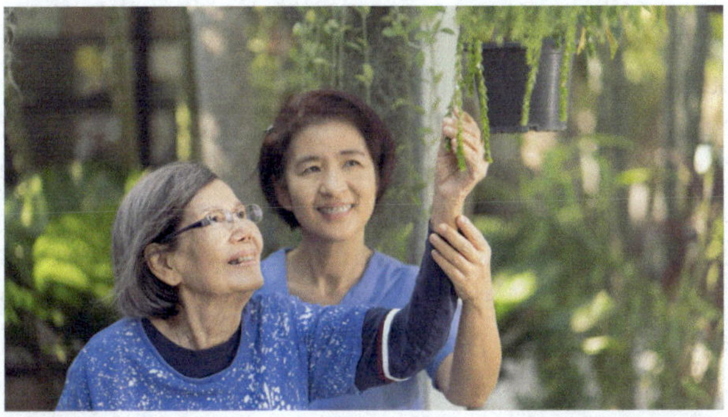

Figure 5.18. Promoting well-being in the elderly: A holistic guide for caregivers on geriatric mental health.

Source: https://static.toiimg.com/thumb/msid-110617341,width-1280,height-720,resizemode-4/110617341.jpg.

Test Your Knowledge

1. What is the importance of psychotherapy and counseling approaches?
2. What is the pharmacological treatment for mental disorders?

5.6. Role of Caregivers and Family Support

Learning Outcome

1. Understand the importance of the education of caregivers
2. Know the strategies for effective communication
3. Describe the role of support systems for caregivers

The intricate relationship between the caregivers and the psychological status of older individuals is most important in geriatric care. As family members are performing the role of caregivers, their own physical and mental status determines the quality of care for older individuals directly. Caregiving can cause stress, anxiety, and depression, not only for the caregiver but also for the mental health of the recipient. It is essential to be aware of the specific caregiving challenges so they can be utilized in creating particular support systems that enhance caregiving resilience and coping ability. Literature calls for the recognition of diverse caregiver populations, particularly those belonging to hard-to-reach groups, including older caregivers who can be marginalized in both policy and research contexts (Henwood et al., 2017). There is a need for an integrated approach to support caregivers appropriately, which will subsequently lead to improved outcomes for the elderly they care for. Also, caregiving relationships completely alter the psychological landscape for each of the actors involved—the caregiver as well as the elderly person. Research indicates that the mental health of elderly patients strongly corresponds with the psychological well-being of their caregivers. For instance, the study indicates that higher caregiver stress correlates with lower psychological well-being in the patient, suggesting a mutual relationship between their mental statuses (Bellanti et al., 2016). Caregivers' emotional status will contaminate the caregiving environment and, in so doing, detract from the elderly individuals' sense of security and well-being. Thus, caregiver burden intervention is beneficial not just for the caregivers themselves but also has very important implications for maximizing patients' mental health outcomes. Additionally, maximizing family support is essential for both older adults and caregivers. Encouraging family relationships can provide the caregivers with much-needed emotional support, eliminate loneliness, and enhance coping skills during the worst times. An extensive geriatric mental well-being outlook recognizes the importance of social support in sustaining caregivers and thereby improving the quality of caregiving. Communication and interfamily, team-oriented interventions that facilitate understanding of caregivers' lives and foster mutual caregiving duties can help enhance caregiving knowledge. Studies have shown that when family support is present, the overall health of the elderly improves, highlighting the need for holistic approaches to treating geriatric mental health (Henwood et al., 2017). Prioritizing family support systems will ultimately help us develop a healthier setting that benefits caregivers and the elderly, resulting in better mental health outcomes among the geriatric population (Figure 5.19).

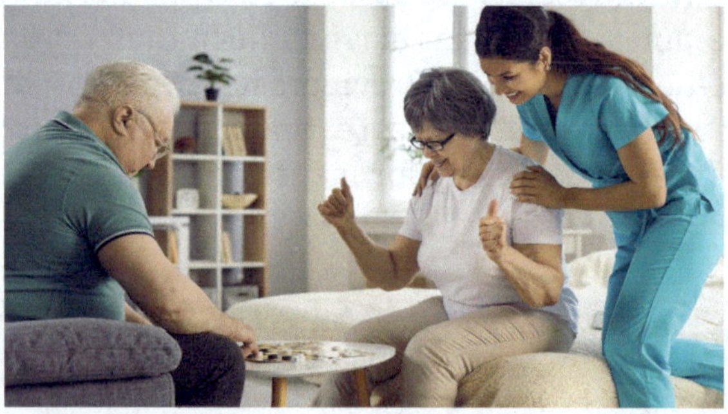

Figure 5.19. Support family caregivers of adults with mental health problems and illnesses.

Source: https://mentalhealthcommission.ca/wp-content/uploads/2013/07/Support-Family-Caregivers-of-Adul.jpg.

5.6.1. Importance of Caregiver Education

Caregiver education is a focal point for enhancing the mental health status of older patients. In the context of an aging population, there is a massive demand for well-educated, compassionate caregivers. Educated caregivers possess the essential information and skills to recognize the mental health issues of elderly patients, for instance, depression and cognitive impairment. Understanding these conditions enables caregivers to provide targeted support, which is essential for ensuring the psychological well-being of their patients. Moreover, if caregivers learn to communicate and intervene appropriately, they can help ward off feelings of loneliness and agitation that are prevalent among many older adults. This forward-looking action not only enhances the quality of treatment but also generates a more therapeutic atmosphere befitting mental health, where the patient receives the comprehensive care they are entitled to in their advanced age. Moreover, caregiver education directly influences the dynamic balance of the caregiver-patient interaction. For complicated health conditions, like cancer in older patients, both caregivers and patients are confronted with a series of unique challenges. Integrated caregiver education, with modules such as the geriatric assessment, can be a key player in reimagining care delivery. For instance, specific educational interventions can equip caregivers with knowledge about the psychosocial aspects of cancer treatment, enabling them to better support patients throughout their medical course. As suggested by recent literature, proper caregiver training may not only improve patient outcomes but also enhance caregivers' well-being, as they gain confidence in their work (Lampugnane et al., 2017). This connection underscores the need to incorporate caregiver education into the healthcare system to ensure strong support mechanisms for the elderly. Moreover, the psychological distress which the caregivers experience is often entangled with the psychological well-being of patients. The literature indicates a critical correlation between the levels of stress being endured by caregivers and the mental health status of their patients, particularly in cases of chronic illness like hip fractures (Bellanti et al., 2016). Educating caregivers about these aspects should help them develop strategies to manage their stress while remaining empathetic to their patients. Recognizing the bi-directional nature of care enables caregivers to keep their own mental health in mind, which is very important for maintaining effective caregiving interventions. Prioritizing the education of caregivers can not only improve the quality of life in older patients but also create a healthier and supportive setting for caregivers, leading to improved psychological outcomes for both parties in the long run.

5.6.2. Strategies for Effective Communication

Effective communication is important in addressing the geriatric population's mental health needs. Older people often face cognitive impairment, sensory loss, and complex medical issues; thus, the methods used to communicate with them must be responsive and adaptive to these challenges. The use of plain, straightforward language, free of jargon, is required to ease understanding. In addition, nonverbal actions such as eye contact, nodding, and appropriate body language are critical to understanding and showing empathy. Researchers find that engaged listening healthcare providers who validate older patients' emotions can establish a conducive environment for open-ended communication. Therefore, implementing training sessions that focus on effective communication among healthcare providers can significantly enhance the quality of care provided to this vulnerable group and ensure that their mental health care is addressed holistically. Collaboration between primary care physicians and mental health professionals is another imperative strategy for efficient communication about geriatric mental health. A pilot shared mental health care scheme developed a framework that complemented the capacity of primary care systems to address the mental health of older adults. The scheme used shared-care strategies that combined education with clinical advice, demonstrating the potential to enhance communication among stakeholders in patient care.

With the integration of both specialty and primary care services, the project also highlighted how the collaborative approach not only improves the quality of mental health care but also leads to a better comprehension of the needs of the patients. Such coordination is critical in developing effective intervention approaches and acquiring resources in order to support ongoing mental health programs for the elderly, thereby bridging gaps in the provision of geriatric mental health care (Dolansky et al., 2007).

Moreover, a systematic review of policy recommendations allows one to analyze current communication practices in geriatric mental health institutions. Research has shown the success of prevention and care coordination strategies that emphasize effective communication. For instance, patient self-management, supported by appropriate communication, could help older people become increasingly involved in their care. In addition, family caregivers must be included in the communication process, as they traditionally play a significant role in supporting the mental well-being of older patients.

By emphasizing policies that promote open communication, clinicians can ensure enhanced coordination and planning for the future, ultimately improving overall mental health outcomes for geriatric patients (Morton et al., 2015). The combination of these methods is important to ensure that the communication not only addresses the short-term needs of older adults but also lays a long-term blueprint for future mental health interventions (Figure 5.20).

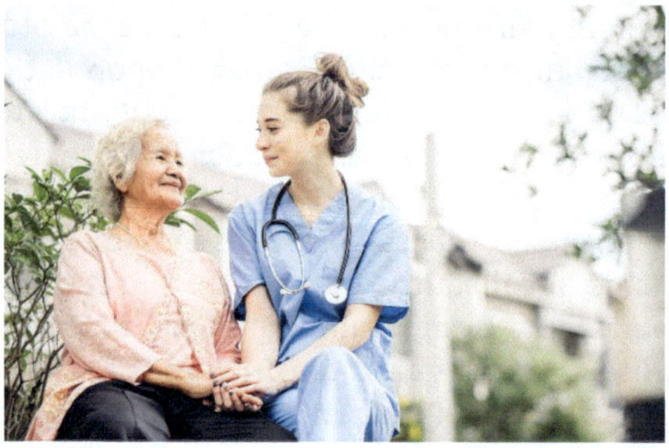

Figure 5.20. Communicating with elderly patients.

Source: https://www.intelycare.com/wp-content/uploads/2024/01/effective-communication-with-elderly-patients.jpg.

5.6.3. Support Systems for Caregivers

In the field of geriatric mental health, the role of caregiving support cannot be overstated. With an aging population, an increasing number of people are taking care of their aging relatives, most of whom will require extensive physical as well as emotional care because of chronic illness or dementia. Caregiving often leads to severe mental illness, including stress, anxiety, and depression, if caregivers become lonely or overwhelmed. Access to supportive systems—family, friends, neighborhood organizations, and social services—can substantially lighten these loads. Support systems can provide emotional support, respite care, and practical assistance to help caregivers recharge and maintain their own health. Research shows that systematic support structures are critical to improving well-being in both caregivers and care recipients, and, by extension, to general geriatric mental health outcomes. Policy initiatives aimed at building caregiving supports also play an important role in guiding effective caregiving environments. Current studies emphasize the need for prevention and care-coordination policies, particularly among older individuals with a number of conditions, for instance, cancer or dementia. While jurisdictions recognize the imperative of caregivers' needs, there is a notable imbalance between research and workable policy that ensures appropriate support for family caregivers. For instance, programs that provide assistance with financial aid, training, and mental health support for caregivers can completely change their lives. It is crucial that laws are formulated to account for these requirements, as they not only build on the noteworthy efforts of caregivers but also improve the mental health of geriatric patients overall by fostering more sustainable caregiving relationships (Morton et al., 2015). Further, successful support systems must also consider the specific health care needs of the receiving individuals. Older people tend to have complex medical conditions that require thorough assessments and tailored care management. This would necessitate the expertise of healthcare professionals, including geriatricians and mental health practitioners, who can guide caregivers in addressing the complexities of care provision. Today, many caregivers are unaware of available resources or are not provided with complete geriatric assessments that define their loved ones' specific needs, leading to potential deficits of optimal care (Lampugnani et al., 2017). By integrating caregiver support with comprehensive geriatric assessment and ongoing educational strategies, we provide caregivers with the information they need to address the challenges they face. Lastly, enhancing the caregiving support system will not only improve the elderly's mental health but also improve care outcomes.

Test Your Knowledge

1. What is the importance of caregiver education?
2. What is role of support systems for caregivers?

SUMMARY

In the research on geriatric mental health complexity, it is evident that respecting the experience of life of older mentally ill persons is essential in ensuring the success of intervention. The lives of OMIOs, as recent studies have shown, present a stark contrast between institutionalized environments and living independently. OMIOs enjoyed better experiences within prison environments than in mental health facilities, suggesting that rehabilitation environments play a considerable role in their outcomes. This indicates that establishing an environment within which older persons can exercise personal control and form connections with the outside world could profoundly affect their well-being. Thus, ongoing research into supportive ideologies and individualized care interventions is essential to improving the mental health climate for this at-risk group (Broekaert et al., 2015). In addition, the singular aspect of the challenges facing older members of the LGBTQ+ community complicates the broader geriatric mental health conversation. Many LGBT elders have to endure extensive difficulties in receiving health care, typically stemming from fear of being unsafe in a disclosure process to healthcare workers in the past. The above reality underscores the need to ensure a safe, welcoming atmosphere in healthcare settings that specifically addresses the needs of this population. Providers must be educated to offer such in-depth care that is sensitive to the subtleties of identity and history, which significantly influence mental health outcomes. According to exploratory research, awareness of such subtleties can help health practitioners provide better care when dealing with older LGBT individuals, thereby enhancing their overall experience within the healthcare system (Burton et al., 2020). Finally, the intersection of mental health, age, and identity necessitates that geriatric health care be multifaceted. Considering aspects such as institutional histories, individuals' identities, and the need to foster caring communities, the delivery of health care can be more efficient by embracing strategies tailored to the needs of the elderly. Care needs to be holistic in nature and combine risk assessment with enhanced overall well-being, especially for those who have to struggle with the intersection of mental health difficulties and marginalized identities. As science advances, stakeholders must ensure that investment is directed toward new models and programs of care that enhance outcomes among older adults, thereby ensuring they are accorded the respect and support they need as they grow old (Broekaert et al., 2015; Burton et al., 2020).

The study of geriatric mental health unpacks the complex dynamics of psychological health and aging. The principal findings point to the prevalence of undiagnosed mental disorders in elderly populations, among which depression ranks among the most overlooked in medical practice. For instance, a significant percentage of elderly patients with chronic conditions is said to be burdened with undiagnosed depression, with studies estimating up to 40% (Chaoyang et al., 2009). This unaddressed depression can lead to decreased quality of life and poor health outcomes, and, therefore, systematic screenings to identify populations at risk are needed. Interventions to increase awareness of geriatric mental health are necessary since they form a foundation to maximize health care delivery and patient outcomes in this population at risk. A critical component of addressing geriatric mental health is the effectiveness of various tools in screening depression. More recent meta-reviews indicated the robustness of some assessment measures, some of which, like the Hospital Anxiety and Depression Scale (HADS), possess moderate screening utility but less utility in some settings, e.g., for the treatment of advanced cancer (Andersen et al., 2015). The Beck Depression Inventory is, however, more versatile for use across different stages of cancer and cancer types. The findings emphasize the importance of health professionals selecting screening instruments appropriate to the unique context of geriatric patients. Such diligent examination of screening tools will help more effectively identify depression and provide timely interventions, enhancing the overall mental health context for the aged. Beyond specific health, the impact of undiagnosed depression reaches broader public health initiatives, particularly in schools. A study found correlation between higher scores on the Geriatric Depression Scale (GDS) and lower retention in medical education among older individuals (Wynn-Grundy et al., 2016). That would mean that mental problems caused by depression could impede individuals' ability to learn crucial information about their health. With an aging population, it is increasingly necessary that healthcare systems integrate mental health screening in medical education. By improving the cognitive health of elderly individuals, providers can enhance educational experiences, enable patients to make informed choices about their health, and contribute to better overall well-being in this population.

KEY TERMS FROM THIS CHAPTER

- Arthritis
- Chronic illness
- Cognitive disorders
- Cognitive rehabilitation
- Geriatric assessments
- Late-life depression
- Marital status
- Autonomy
- Cognitive decline
- Cognitive impairments
- Dementia
- Geriatric mental health
- Life satisfaction
- Social support

CRITICAL THINKING QUESTIONS

1. **Which of the following is the most common mental health disorder in older adults?**
   a. Anxiety disorders
   b. Dementia
   c. Depression
   d. Schizophrenia
2. **What is the hallmark symptom of delirium in geriatric patients?**
   a. Gradual onset of memory loss
   b. Rapid onset of confusion and fluctuating attention
   c. Persistent sadness and low energy
   d. Impaired judgment over years
3. **Which of the following medications is most likely to worsen confusion in elderly patients with dementia?**
   a. Acetaminophen
   b. Anticholinergic drugs
   c. Beta-blockers
   d. SSRIs
4. **What is the most appropriate first-line treatment for late-life depression?**
   a. Electroconvulsive therapy (ECT)
   b. Psychotherapy
   c. SSRI medications
   d. Benzodiazepines
5. **Which of the following is a validated screening tool for depression in the elderly?**
   a. PHQ-9
   b. CAGE Questionnaire
   c. Geriatric Depression Scale (GDS)
   d. Hamilton Anxiety Rating Scale

Short Answer Questions

1. What is geriatric mental health?
2. Why is mental health important in the elderly?
3. What are the common mental health disorders in the elderly?
4. What are the risk factors for mental health?
5. What is the impact of mental health on quality of life?

Answer to Critical Thinking Questions

1. (c); 2. (b); 3. (b); 4. (c); 5. (c).

REFERENCES

1. Abdul Khaiyom, J., Hanum, J., Hisham, B., Qamelia, A., Tohit, M., Faiza, N., Rusli, M., et al. (2024). The relationship between mental health literacy and depression among older adults in Selangor. https://core.ac.uk/download/616550771.pdf (accessed on 14th July 2025).
2. Shyu, Y. L., Liang, J., Wu, C., Cheng, H., & Chen, M. (2010). An interdisciplinary intervention for older Taiwanese patients after surgery for hip fracture improves health-related quality of life. *BMC Musculoskeletal Disorders, 11*(1), 225. https://doi.org/10.1186/1471-2474-11-225Akin, A., Mellor, D., Diener, E., Mahoney, K., McCabe, M. P., Molloy, C., Qualls, S. H., et al. (2011). Environmental mastery and depression in older adults in residential care. http://hdl.handle.net/10536/DRO/DU:30033219 (accessed on 14th July 2025).
3. Andersen, B. L., Becker, M. H., Carey, M. P., Carlson, L. E., Cella, D., et al. (2015). Patient-reported depression measures in cancer: A meta-review. https://core.ac.uk/download/42138163.pdf (accessed on 14th July 2025).
4. Au-Yeung, M., Avila, A., Bandong, J., Ia, J., et al. (2020). The health benefits of visual art activities in the geriatric population. https://core.ac.uk/download/326757894.pdf (accessed on 14th July 2025).
5. Bartels, S. J., Batsis, J. A., Brooks, J. L., Carrington Reid, M., et al. (2018). Prevalence rates of arthritis among US older adults with varying degrees of depression: Findings from the 2011 to 2014 National Health and Nutrition Examination Survey. https://core.ac.uk/download/231135051.pdf (accessed on 14th July 2025).
6. Battaglia, S., Benfante, A., Scichilone, N. A., Spatafora, M., et al. (2016). Asthma in the elderly: A different disease? https://core.ac.uk/download/53305142.pdf (accessed on 14th July 2025).
7. Bellanti, G., Eleuteri, S., & Falaschi, P. (2016). Hip fracture: Preliminary results supporting significative correlations between the psychological wellbeing of patients and their relative caregivers. https://core.ac.uk/download/98343305.pdf (accessed on 14th July 2025).
8. Braye, S., Orr, D., & Preston-Shoot, M. (2011). Self-neglect and adult safeguarding: Findings from research. https://core.ac.uk/download/2721774.pdf (accessed on 14th July 2025).
9. Brettle, A., & Hill, A. (2005). The effectiveness of counselling with older people: Results of a systematic review. https://core.ac.uk/download/104573.pdf (accessed on 14th July 2025).
10. Broekaert, E., De Smet, S., Ryan, D., Van Hecke, N., et al. (2015). Treatment and control: A qualitative study of older mentally ill offenders' perceptions on their detention and care trajectory. https://core.ac.uk/download/55807198.pdf (accessed on 14th July 2025).
11. Broers, B., Crome, I., De Jong, C. A. J., Dom, G., et al. (2016). Substance misuse education for physicians: Why older people are important. https://core.ac.uk/download/288436392.pdf (accessed on 14th July 2025).
12. Brooks, J. L., Titus, A. J., Polenick, C. A., Orzechowski, N. M., et al. (1985). Prevalence rates of arthritis among US older adults with varying degrees of depression: Findings from the 2011 to 2014 National Health and Nutrition Examination Survey. https://core.ac.uk/download/231135051.pdf (accessed on 14th July 2025).
13. Buchanan, G., Davison, T., George, K., Kuruvilla, G., Hudgson, C., et al. (2007). An individualized psychosocial approach for "treatment resistant" behavioral symptoms of dementia among

aged care residents. http://hdl.handle.net/10536/DRO/DU:30007583 (accessed on 14th July 2025).

14. Burton, C. W., Gibbs, L. M., Lee, J. A., Waalen, J., et al. (2020). "Things are different now but": Older LGBT adults' experiences and unmet needs in health care. https://core.ac.uk/download/323082975.pdf (accessed on 14th July 2025).
15. Clay, D., Hyde, J., Nelson, S., Szczepura, A., et al. (2025). Models for providing improved care in residential care homes: A thematic literature review. https://core.ac.uk/download/49048.pdf (accessed on 14th July 2025).
16. Declercq, T., Lemey, L., Petrovic, M., Tandt, H., et al. (2018). Late-life depression: Issues for the general practitioner. https://core.ac.uk/download/154408401.pdf (accessed on 14th July 2025).
17. Dolansky, D., Le Clair, J. K., Leon, S., Parenteau, N., et al. (2007). Shared geriatric mental health care in a rural community. https://core.ac.uk/download/29140872.pdf (accessed on 14th July 2025).
18. Freter, S., Gordon, M., et al. (2003). A 3-week geriatric education program for 4th year medical students at Dalhousie University. https://core.ac.uk/download/pdf/85567.pdf (accessed on 14th July 2025).
19. Funes, C., Krause, B., Laird, K. T., Lavretsky, H., et al. (2019). Psychobiological factors of resilience and depression in late life. https://core.ac.uk/download/323076847.pdf (accessed on 14th July 2025).
20. Henwood, M., Larkin, M., & Milne, A. (2017). Seeing the wood for the trees. Carer related research and knowledge: A scoping review. https://core.ac.uk/download/145186527.pdf (accessed on 14th July 2025).
21. Khezrian, M., McNeil, C. J., Murray, A. D., Myint, P. K., et al. (2017). A review of frailty syndrome and its physical, cognitive and emotional domains in the elderly. https://core.ac.uk/download/131025041.pdf (accessed on 14th July 2025).
22. Lampugnale, C. A. (2017). Surgical assessment of the geriatric oncology patient. https://open.bu.edu/bitstream/2144/26707/5/Lampugnale_bu_0017N_13146.pdf (accessed on 14th July 2025).
23. Le, G. (2009). Depression among the elderly: Screening practices and attitudes among nurse practitioners. https://core.ac.uk/download/223074313.pdf (accessed on 14th July 2025).
24. Majgi, S. M., Mathew, J., Nagaraj, A. K. M., Nanjegowda, R. B., et al. (2012). Psychiatric morbidity among elderly people living in old age homes and in the community: A comparative study. https://core.ac.uk/download/pdf/13598710.pdf (accessed on 14th July 2025).
25. Mayhew, K. M. (1989). An investigation of factors associated with depression in older adults. https://digitalscholarship.unlv.edu/cgi/viewcontent.cgi?article=1079&context=rtds (accessed on 14th July 2025).
26. McIntyre, A. E., & Reynolds, F. (2011). There's no apprenticeship for Alzheimer's: The caring relationship when an older person experiencing dementia falls. https://core.ac.uk/download/18488637.pdf (accessed on 14th July 2025).
27. Morton, S., & Dunn, W. (2015). Addressing the health needs of an aging America: New opportunities for evidence-based policy solutions. https://core.ac.uk/download/75783019.pdf (accessed on 14th July 2025).

28. Nadeem, F., & Nguyen, K. (2018). Investigating geriatric mental health initiatives and treatment plans in the Windsor-Essex region. https://core.ac.uk/download/215510144.pdf (accessed on 14th July 2025).

29. Nair, S. S., Nair, S. S., & Raghunath, P. (2015). Prevalence of psychiatric disorders among the rural geriatric population: A pilot study in Karnataka, India. https://core.ac.uk/download/613044762.pdf (accessed on 14th July 2025).

30. Price, C. A. (2017). *Tai Chi/Qi Gong in Mental Health Treatment and Prevention: A Review of Meta-Analytic Evidence and An Analysis of Evidence Congruence with Training Practices.* https://core.ac.uk/download/84397718.pdf (accessed on 14th July 2025).

31. Reid, D. M., & Schofield, P. (2006). The assessment and management of pain in older people: A systematic review of the literature. https://core.ac.uk/download/177013.pdf (accessed on 14th July 2025).

32. Shotts, A. (2018). Music therapy techniques for memory stabilization in diverse dementias. https://core.ac.uk/download/213462310.pdf (accessed on 14th July 2025).

33. Wait, S. (2005). Promoting age equality in the delivery of health care. https://core.ac.uk/download/71356596.pdf (accessed on 14th July 2025).

34. Wynn-Grundy, N. J. (2016). Undiagnosed depression in the elderly and healthcare education. https://core.ac.uk/download/70426926.pdf (accessed on 14th July 2025).

PALLIATIVE AND END-OF-LIFE CARE

6

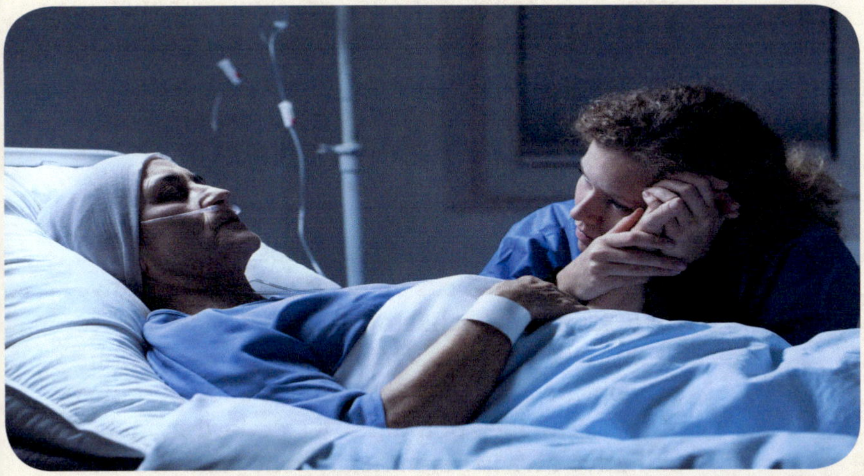

LEARNING OBJECTIVES

After studying this chapter, you will be able to:

1. Understand the principles of palliative care
2. Describe the types of palliative care services
3. Understand the pain management in palliative care
4. Describe the communication of end-of-life care
5. Describe the ethical considerations of palliative and end-of-life care

Introduction

Palliative and end-of-life care is a vital field of practice in the health sector that focuses on the multidimensional needs of patients living with life-threatening conditions. The model of care highlights an integrated management strategy that addresses physical, emotional, social, and spiritual needs across the illness trajectory, rather than curative treatment in isolation. Growing acknowledgment of the part that palliative care plays emphasizes its role in enhancing the welfare of patients and their families in challenging situations. Healthcare systems evolve, requiring standardized systems that support safe, therapeutic, patient-centered, and equitable care to be adopted to achieve the highest returns in palliative settings, according to guidelines intended to ensure high-quality services for populations with diverse needs. The intersection between palliative care and interprofessional education also warrants examination, particularly in how it educates future healthcare professionals. A recent article cited the significant impact of clinical observation sessions on graduate-degree nursing students involved in an interprofessional palliative care program. In these sessions, students engaged with interprofessional personnel, enhancing their awareness of communication patterns between patients, families, and healthcare professionals. Qualitative exploration of students' narratives revealed the nuanced complexities of providing empathetic care and having challenging conversations about end-of-life (Breakwell et al., 2012). Such educational models not only enhance healthcare professionals' abilities but also ensure the effective integration of palliative practice at the healthcare education level. Furthermore, the growing body of literature affirming the need for upgraded palliative care training underscores the need to prioritize interdisciplinary collaboration and training opportunities for medical facilities. Such a method allows healthcare systems to establish a workforce prepared to address the multidimensional needs of end-of-life patients, thereby transforming the patient experience into one that is marked by respect and dignity.

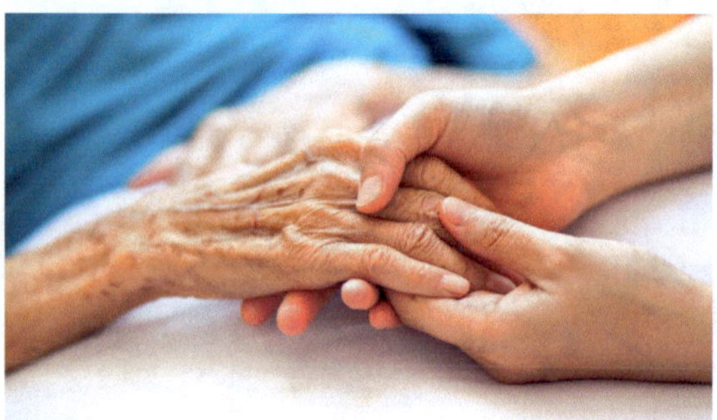

Figure 6.1. Palliative and end-of-life care.

Source: https://franklinstraining.co.uk/wp-content/uploads/2024/02/Palliative-Care-vs-End-of-Life-Care-Whats-the-Difference-Blog-Franklins-e1708357600620.png.

With evolving palliative and end-of-life care, there must be the development of a culture of empathy, continuity, and team-based care with the patient and families at the center. Contrary to such ideals is not just the facilitation of the transition toward holistic models of care, but also the reaffirmation of a commitment to offering compassionate, individualized practices essential for successful end-of-life management (Figure 6.1).

Definition of Palliative Care

The palliative care principle is integral to the global conceptual framework of terminal care, yet it remains widely misconceived. Palliative care has been defined as comprehensive, multidisciplinary medical management with the main aim of symptom control and quality-of-life enhancement for patients with malignant and other debilitating diseases, regardless of disease stage or treatment regimen. Contrary to curative care, symptom management, emotional support, and treatment of patients' psychosocial problems are the primary focus of palliative care. Palliative care is an interdisciplinary practice where healthcare providers from various professions collaborate to formulate patient-specific plans of care. The lack of a unitary standard model of palliative care has significant policy and practice implications, given that care must be tailored to the specific needs of each patient and to cultural variations that inform their disease experience (Gilmore et al., 2010). The fluidity here explains the necessity for an excessive debate about the specifics of palliative care delivery. One of the most significant features of palliative care is its patient- and family-centered nature. This aspect recognizes that the patient is not alone; his or her experience is deeply interwoven with the family and community environments. Palliative care should therefore ensure effective open communication among patients, their families, and medical professionals so that treatment aligns with patients' own values and decisions. This support is not only provided to patients but also to their families, with particular emphasis on addressing family and relational issues in the context of serious illness. Involving families in making care decisions increases the sense of agency and control for patients and reduces the feelings of helplessness that often follow terminal illness. Nevertheless, decision-making is complex without a clear understanding of futile care, and misunderstandings and differences might emerge if treatment options are not explained clearly (Fulp et al., 2007). Therefore, it is advisable to explain palliative care principles to facilitate effective communication and mutual decision-making among all parties involved. In addition, the integration of palliative care into everyday practice in healthcare is becoming increasingly regarded as central to optimizing patient outcomes. With healthcare systems evolving further, the emphasis on providing holistic care, including emotional, spiritual, and psychological needs, increases its popularity. Palliative care is not limited to dying patients; it might be beneficial at earlier stages of advanced illness, often leading to better outcomes and patient satisfaction. By putting focus on symptom control and quality of life, palliative care can, at the same time, increase patient engagement with their treatment regimen and reduce healthcare costs for more aggressive end-of-life treatment. However, a deficiency in an integrative, widely accepted model of palliative care can lead to inconsistencies in delivery and availability (Gilmore et al., 2010). Filling these gaps is essential to creating effective support structures that can be applied universally throughout palliative and end-of-life care settings (Figure 6.2).

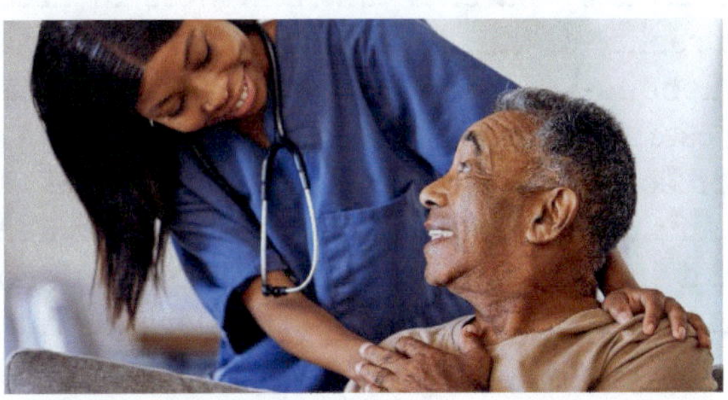

Figure 6.2. Palliative care.

Source: https://tischbraintumorcenter.duke.edu/sites/default/files/styles/social_media_card/public/2023-12/hero-palliative-care.jpg?h=c74750f6&itok=CBDoPODl.

Importance of End-of-Life Care

The importance of end-of-life care is underscored by its role in enhancing quality of life during a patient's terminal stage, a time characterized by pain, uncertainty, and emotional distress. Effective end-of-life care not only addresses the physical pain but also the psychological, social, and spiritual needs of the patients. Proper care would possibly require multi-disciplinary management dealing with pain management, emotional support, and decision-making counseling, so that patients receive care respecting their values and preferences. Without the provision of end-of-life care, unnecessary suffering is imposed on patients, highlighting the greatest importance of healthcare systems to prioritize this aspect of palliative care for ensuring dignity and comfort in the dying. Furthermore, the training and preparedness of healthcare providers also have an influence on the quality of care during end-of-life. It has been observed that a considerable proportion of general practitioners receive no specialized training in palliative medicine, which may undermine their ability to provide comprehensive care (Abela et al., 2015). These gaps in training have the potential to create anxiety among providers when faced with end-of-life decisions, undermining their capacity to engage meaningfully with patients and families in discussions of shared goals of care. The ethical subtleties surrounding patient autonomy and the sustaining of life are also bound to raise doubts among healthcare providers. This underscores the importance of ongoing education and legal advice to ensure healthcare teams are assured they can handle the multitude of issues in end-of-life scenarios, ultimately leading to improved patient outcomes. Lastly, the emotional and spiritual components of end-of-life care must not be disregarded, as they play a very critical role in the overall experience for families and patients. Research emphasizes that spirituality tends to become a comforting and supportive factor during this difficult period (Zogheib et al., 2015). It is important to understand each patient's individual beliefs and values to provide effective communication and emotional support. Physicians should be trained to discuss these factors with sensitivity in order to create an environment where families will feel empowered to share in decision-making. As doctors navigate through end-of-life care concerns, the balance between supportive care and medical interventions is essential in determining patients' sense of peace and acceptance. Hence, equipping providers with the right skills to discuss these is important in seeking holistic end-of-life care (Figure 6.3).

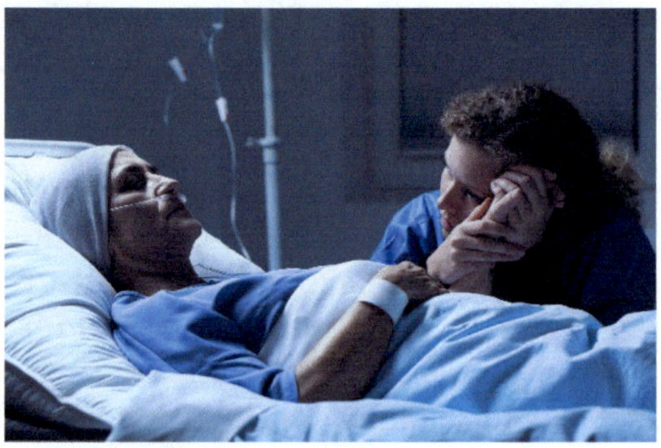

Figure 6.3. Importance of end-of-life care.

Source: https://www.rn.com/siteassets/blog/end-of-life-care.jpg.

6.1. Principles of Palliative Care

Learning Outcome

1. Focus on quality of life in palliative and end-of-life care
2. Emphasize the holistic approach to patient care in palliative and end-of-life settings
3. Understand the interdisciplinary team involvement in effective palliative and end-of-life care

The tenets of palliative care constitute a system meant to enhance the well-being of people with serious illness. Comprehensive symptom management is one of the guiding principles that addresses physical, emotional, and spiritual domains. Since suffering is complex, the providers of palliative care have a primary concern to alleviate symptom distress in the form of pain, anxiety, and depression. This process of integration not only addresses the obvious symptoms of dis-ease in patients but also provides essential support to families struggling with the challenges of serious illness. Research such as the National Consensus Project for Quality Palliative Care emphasizes the relevance of such fundamentals, mandating greater access to quality palliative care, particularly in response to technological developments that bring complex ethical dilemmas into care settings (Breakwell et al., 2014). Through an integrated approach that considers the whole person, parallel care facilitates a respectful illness and end-of-life trajectory. One of the key aspects of palliative care is effective communication and decision-making between the patients, families, and clinicians. Transparent discussions about treatment options, prognosis, and patient preferences are essential in developing a shared knowledge base around care aims. In the pediatric case, for example, the challenge most often encounters early recognition and referral to specialist palliative care. The literature reveals that health workers may frequently be hindered by parents' unwillingness to accept the reality of illness, which can delay referrals (Bluebond-Langner et al., 2014). This delay calls for establishing a culture capable of allowing for open communication about palliative care with an aim to de-mystify its association with death and dying. Educating healthcare providers about these principles can result in earlier integration of palliative care, ultimately making care planning more compatible with patients' needs and preferences throughout the trajectory of the illness. Additionally, principles of palliative care are translated into ethical principles that inform healthcare interventions. These ethical principles are most vital as healthcare providers navigate the complexities of chronic disease management and end-of-life care. Issues of informed consent, patient autonomy, and equitable access to resources require balanced consideration. The ethical issues are compounded by progressive medical technology that prolongs life, pitting the appropriateness of coercive intervention against the value of palliative intervention. For instance, the integration of palliative care can enable patients to make informed decisions aligned with their values and preferences, fostering a sense of empowerment despite disabling illnesses (Breakwell et al., 2014). By emphasizing ethical values as well as clinical competence, palliative care contributes to physical symptom control, upholds the ethical expectations of medicine, and ensures that the patient is treated humanely and with dignity throughout the illness experience (Figure 6.4).

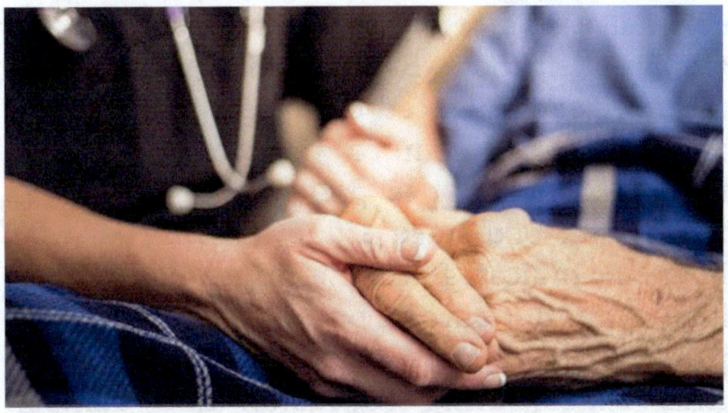

Figure 6.4. Principles of palliative care.

Source: https://hollycare.ie/wp-content/uploads/2024/04/principles-of-palliative-care.jpg.

6.1.1. Focus on Quality of Life

Quality of life continues to be the focus in end-of-life and palliative care, moving beyond symptom relief to the general health and well-being of patients with severe illness. Quality palliative care addresses not only physical comfort but emotional, social, and spiritual care as well, understanding that each individual's illness experience is distinct and multifaceted. By addressing these dimensions, palliative care aims to enhance patients' quality of life so they can experience some form of dignity and independence in their care decision-making. This is an important tactic, particularly in healthcare systems where access to quality palliative care remains inadequate. Hence, policies focused on integrated care models are urgently required to enable the provision of comprehensive palliative care services and improve quality of life, as indicated by findings from the analysis of national health policies (Anderson et al., 2021). Moreover, the actions of healthcare providers, particularly Physician Assistants (PAs), are crucial to closing the gap between patients and high-quality palliative care. PAs most commonly serve as the entry point within the healthcare system, and their identification of the necessity for palliative interventions can significantly contribute to patient outcomes. However, barriers in the form of inadequate training and low perception of the concepts of palliative care discourage many PAs from making timely and proper referrals. This case is a reminder of the importance of educational programs that equip clinicians with the competencies to speak with patients about quality of life and end-of-life care. Greater knowledge and confidence among PAs will facilitate prompt referrals to palliative care, thereby enhancing the quality of care and patient satisfaction at a critical juncture in patients' lives (Petersen et al., 2024). In the overall framework of health care policy, emphasis on quality of life must be reflected not only in the practice of individual clinicians but also in system changes that allow access to end-of-life and palliative care. Priorities for policy must be to promote integrated and individualized care that allows patients and families to participate actively in treatment decision-making. Second, caregivers need support, as it also acknowledges the vital role they play in maintaining patients' quality of life. Together with these connected issues—integrated care, individualized care, and care support for caregivers—health policy can create a more integrated approach to palliative care. Prioritizing these will better align clinical practice with them, enhancing patient experiences and outcomes and ultimately promoting the aim of dignified and compassionate end-of-life care (Anderson et al., 2021) (Figure 6.5).

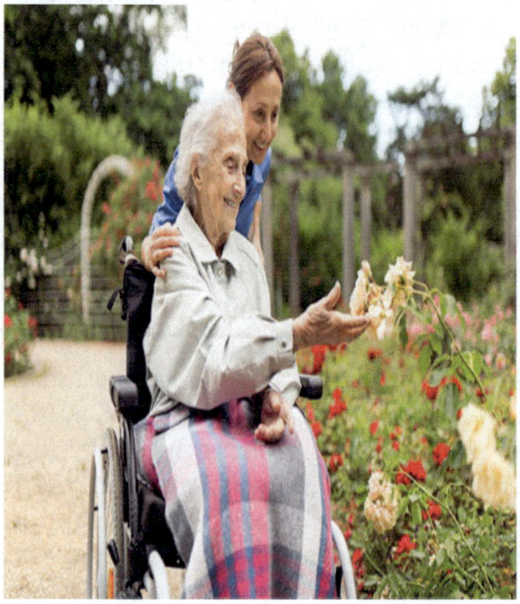

Figure 6.5. Maintaining the best quality of life for palliative care patients.

Source: https://wentwest.com.au/wp-content/uploads/2023/05/Issue18_PalliativeCare_website.png.

6.1.2. Holistic Approach to Patient Care

The integrative model of hospice and end-of-life patient care emphasizes care of the whole person rather than the illness. This model recognizes that patients are not merely biological entities but human beings with particular emotional, social, spiritual, and psychological needs. In this case, healthcare providers strive to understand patients' values, beliefs, and life activities that largely determine their healthcare decisions. Incorporating these aspects into care planning enables more focused interventions that respect patients' preferences and ultimately enhance their quality of life at this critical juncture. Such a patient-focused philosophy fosters stronger relationships among patients, families, and caregivers, so that all aspects of suffering are addressed rather than the medical condition at hand. Moreover, spiritual care is central to the holistic model, offering the patient a means of expressing his or her beliefs and how these affect his or her understanding of illness and death. Spiritual conversation can enrich patients, families, and caregivers' relationships, ultimately informing more compassionate care that is a pillar of palliative practice. For. example. healthcare providers routinely confront. patients. of. different. religions, e.g., Muslim and Jewish patients, without sufficient cultural competence to manage. these interactions (Baddarni et al., 2012). In the face of life's final challenges, closing these gaps via education and awareness will enhance the emotional and spiritual care provided and increase patient and family satisfaction (Baddarni et al., 2012). Also, the need for advanced care planning becomes acutely evident under the comprehensive model, particularly in patient groups such as those with end-stage kidney disease (ESKD). Evidence indicates that this population reports high symptom burden but does not engage in prompt future care preference discussions, thus exacerbating confusion and anxiety. An advance care planning strategy that is proactive and goal-oriented can equip patients with the tools needed to clarify their values and preferences, which will result in better communication and preparedness for changing health conditions. Despite various challenges in the implementation of advance care planning, taking a comprehensive approach opens up windows of improved patient engagement and fills the gap in this population's palliative care needs (Adenwalla et al., 2024). Focusing on the whole patient experience enables the healthcare community to create an even more supportive environment for patients grappling with the complexity of end-of-life care (Figure 6.6).

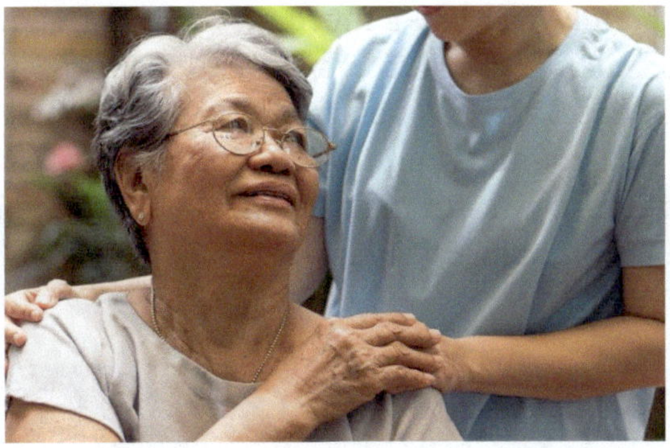

Figure 6.6. The importance of holistic care at the end of life.

Source: https://soulistichospice.org/view/images/blog/uploads/thisis.jpg.

6.1.3. Interdisciplinary Team Involvement

Interdisciplinary collaboration is characteristic of good end-of-life and palliative care, as it fosters inclusive approaches to addressing the multifaceted needs of patients. Palliative care's interdisciplinary profile requires cooperation among various health professions, such as medicine, nursing, social work, and spiritual care. For instance, in a study of students in an interdisciplinary palliative care course, it was noted that their clinical observation sessions significantly enhanced their knowledge of patient-centered communication and teamwork. Through these interactions, students gained valuable lessons regarding teamwork in managing difficult conversations in patients and families and the integration of palliative care principles in clinical practice (Breakwell et al., 2012). This team model not only improves outcomes for patients but also enriches the educational experience for health students, equipping them with the readiness for the realities of practice in high-complexity care environments. Furthermore, interdisciplinary collaboration facilitates holistic care approaches to managing patients, beyond physical symptomology, incorporating emotional, social, and spiritual requirements. The development of formally organized interdisciplinary teams will promote more harmonized care and enhanced communication between the healthcare professionals, patients, and families. Against the backdrop of diverse cultural settings, as evidenced by Estonia's hospitals, there is a need to create flexible models of care responsive to local factors. These models emphasize the role of practitioner collaboration between many different disciplines and, as a result, address the huge demand for integrated care strategies that draw upon the complexity of end-of-life care (Lehtsaar et al., 2017). By establishing environments that foster interdisciplinary collaboration, health organizations can enhance their ability to tailor services to meet the distinct needs of complex patient populations. Finally, the impact of interdisciplinary team involvement extends beyond patient care, as it also drives policy and educational change within healthcare. Embedding interdisciplinary practice in education programs ensures future healthcare practitioners are equipped to operate at their best within multidisciplinary settings.

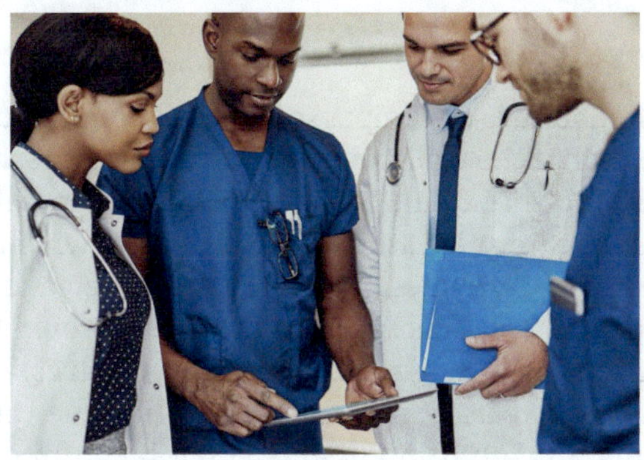

Figure 6.7. The interdisciplinary palliative care team.

Source: https://hospicevalley.com/wp-content/uploads/2021/09/hospice-interdisciplinary-team.jpg.

Not only does this enhance teamwork ability, but it also increases knowledge of multidimensional roles available within care teams, ultimately creating a more integrated model of healthcare. The research shows that learning processes, such as in palliative care interdisciplinary courses, can instill appreciation for cooperation to alleviate distress related to critical illnesses (Breakwell et al., 2012). Thus, the development of robust interdisciplinary models is vital to improving palliative and end-of-life care practice and equipping health professionals with the skills needed to tackle the challenges presented in these delicate settings (Figure 6.7).

Test Your Knowledge

1. What are the aims of palliative care?
2. What is the holistic approach to treating patients?

6.2. Types of Palliative Care Services

Learning Outcome

1. Describe the inpatient palliative care units
2. Describe the outpatient palliative care programs
3. Understand the home-based palliative care options

Palliative care encompasses a variety of services to enhance the well-being of individuals suffering from life-threatening, critical illnesses. A vital form of care is inpatient palliative care, which is commonly provided in hospitals or specialized care facilities. This service focuses on providing comprehensive symptom control, addressing issues such as pain, nausea, and fatigue, and furnishing emotional and spiritual support. Inpatient palliative care teams, occasionally comprising interdisciplinary practitioners, work with primary care teams to offer an integrated approach to care. This interprofessional practice not only improves patient outcomes but also improves communication with the family regarding treatment options and care goals. In this manner, inpatient palliative care is a key resource for patients requiring intense management of complex symptoms and distress from severe illness. Outpatient or community-based palliative care is another crucial component of palliative care services. This model allows patients to be treated within their own homes or within the local community, providing a caring environment that is appropriate for many patients' preferences. Home-based palliative care often consists of regular visits to patients by highly specialized palliative care teams consisting of doctors, nurses, and social workers, and addressing both medical and psychological problems. Such care is particularly beneficial in the case of chronically or progressively ill patients, as continuity and more individualized interventions are emphasized. According to studies, community-based models have been proven to be cost-effective compared to hospital-based models, with higher patient satisfaction and quality of life, and that facilitate the serious role of outpatient services in the whole system of palliative care (Brick et al., 2013). Finally, hospice care is a form of specialized palliative care that is aimed squarely at patients who are near the end of life. Unlike standard palliative care, which can be integrated at any point along the trajectory of illness, hospice care is typically initiated when a patient has been diagnosed with a terminal condition and no longer requires curative treatment. Hospice care emphasizes comfort, dignity, and support for families, offering intensive services such as pain and symptom management, emotional and spiritual counseling, and family bereavement support. Frequent services are provided in the patient's home or at hospice centers so that patients can spend their remaining days in a comfortable atmosphere. As underscored in studies, hospice care models not only improve the quality of life for the dying individual but can also reduce the financial burden of health services, thereby demonstrating its value among palliative care modalities (Haslam et al., 2014) (Figure 6.8).

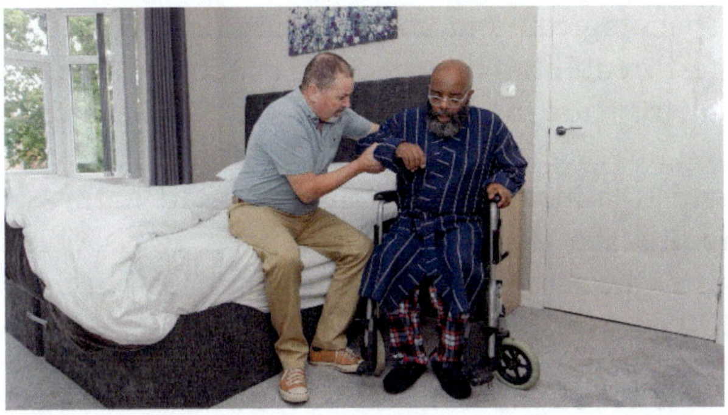

Figure 6.8. Types of palliative care.

Source: https://www.helpinghandshomecare.co.uk/wp-content/uploads/male-carer-green-polo-top-helping-man-in-wheelchair-holding-arm-blue-gown_16x9.jpg.webp.

6.2.1. Inpatient Palliative Care Units

Inpatient palliative care units are high-intensity units dedicated to addressing the complex problems of life-limiting illness patients. In these units, healthcare professionals deliver comprehensive care aimed at controlling symptoms, providing psychosocial support, and optimizing the quality of life. As suggested by Norton Women's and Children's Hospital research, there is significant demand for palliative care in a wide range of settings, with a particular emphasis on intensive care and oncology units, suggesting that a large number of patients would substantially benefit from the high-level services available in these units (Myers et al., 2019). The model of care in the inpatient palliative units is interdisciplinary, incorporating physicians, nurses, social workers, and chaplains to create an integrated support system. Teamwork enables the delivery of care appropriate to each patient's needs, creating an atmosphere in which patients and families feel cared for during times of need. Among the essential activities of inpatient palliative care units is symptom control of acute symptoms most frequently associated with chronic illness, such as pain and delirium. Symptom control to the best degree is important to maximizing quality of life in patients who will experience significant distress during hospitalization. Delirium, on the other hand, is a frequent occurrence in these units in a significant percentage of patients. Evidence indicates that delirium incidence could be 26% to 62% on admission, but increases drastically when patients are nearing the end of life (Hosie et al., 2015). It emphasizes the urgent need for palliative care nurses to be fully equipped with relevant assessment tools and education. Through enhanced recognition and management of delirium, inpatient palliative care units can prevent significant patient and family distress and help fill a significant care gap. Education and training of inpatient palliative care unit caregivers are also crucial to optimal outcomes for the patients. Studies found that education would improve the identification and detection of delirium, which remains undetected in palliative care settings. Through the implementation of evidence-based guidelines and interdisciplinary team practices, institutions can build a more responsive healthcare setting. For instance, integrating the use of instruments such as the Nursing Delirium Screening Scale would enable nurses to identify patients at risk of delirium (Hosie et al., 2015). Concurrently, establishing rapport with patients and integrating families into the care process can enhance communication and understanding of patients' needs. Most importantly, reinforcing healthcare professionals' skill set in these settings is imperative to delivering compassionate, high-quality end-of-life care and enabling patients to have the dignity and support they want for their ultimate journeys (Figure 6.9).

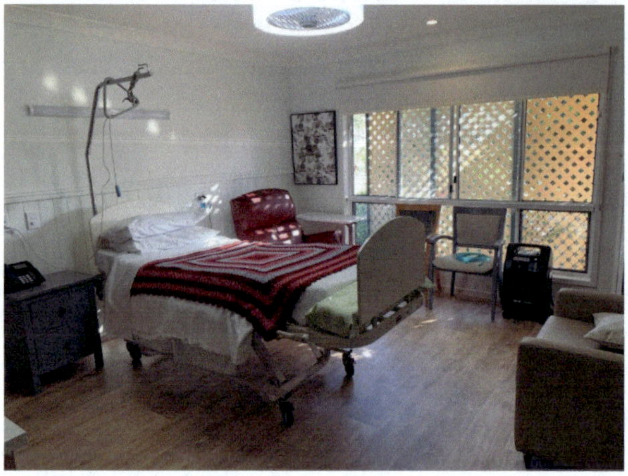

Figure 6.9. Inpatient palliative care units.

Source: https://www.ipswichhospice.org.au/wp-content/uploads/2021/07/Rm-1-1024x768.jpg.

6.2.2. Outpatient Palliative Care Programs

Outpatient palliative care services represent a significant advancement in the evolution of palliative and end-of-life care, as they offer greater support to patients while maintaining their autonomy in their home environments. By focusing on comprehensive symptom management, including pain relief, psychological and spiritual consolation, the services aim to enhance the quality of life for persons with serious illness. Notably, outpatient environments can provide timely interventions that are suited to patients' individual needs to ensure not only that care is patient-centered but also responsive and tailored. With a growing population, ageing, and the occurrence of chronic diseases, the function of such outpatient programs becomes increasingly important because they provide vital support for efficient symptom management and care coordination, bridging the gaps among hospitals, outpatient clinics, and home care (Bekelman et al., 2017). The outpatient palliative care practice has been fostered by collaboration among health care providers and community agencies to enhance the quality of integrated management of severe disease. Initiatives like the Community-Oriented Palliative Care Initiative (COPCI) demonstrate the necessity of collaboration among hospitals, hospices, social services, and other community resources for the coordinated delivery of care. Such networks rely on local knowledge to ascertain each patient's specific needs, thereby ensuring that services address the complex interplay among medical, psychological, and social elements involved in life-threatening illness. Such collaborations not only provide for earlier access to palliative care, as underscored by COPCI evidence, but also help to address the often disjointed nature of healthcare delivery experienced by patients throughout their disease trajectories (Hopper, 2003).

The expansion of outpatient palliative care programs also underscores the critical necessity for ongoing research and evaluation. With improvements in the provision of care continuously emerging, there remains a large gap in knowledge regarding the implications of outpatient palliative intervention. Valid assessment methods and evidence-based practice are crucial to ensure maximum efficiency in such programs. For instance, growing interest in tailoring palliative care approaches to unique populations, e.g., patients with Parkinson's disease, has emerged, highlighting the opportunities and limitations of the current methodology (Bekelman et al., 2017). These results form the basis for future research, not only to meet the diverse needs of patients, but also to guide best practices in delivering outpatient palliative care with the ultimate goal of increasing patient satisfaction and health outcomes alongside serious illness (Figure 6.10).

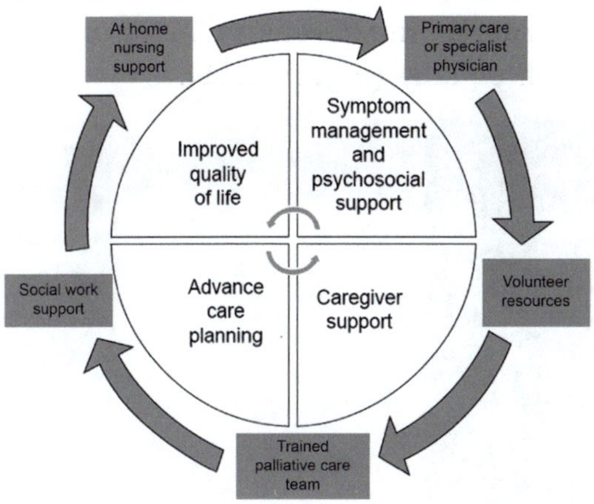

Figure 6.10. Structure and goals of outpatient palliative care services.

Source: https://www.researchgate.net/publication/281605214/figure/fig1/AS:11431281256230247@1719517285590/Structure-and-goals-of-outpatient-palliative-care-services.jpg.

6.2.3. Home-Based Palliative Care Options

With healthcare increasingly recognizing the importance of patient-centered care in palliative therapies, home-based options have emerged as a critical alternative to traditional inpatient therapy. Home-based palliative care allows patients with advanced or terminal illnesses to receive extensive treatment from within the comfort of their own homes. Not only does this enhance the patients' quality of life, but it also assists families in actively participating in the care. Families often face emotional and practical challenges when making end-of-life decisions, so interventions should provide education to inform them about home-based care options. Interventions, such as the FamPALcare model, can empower family members to manage advanced heart failure care at home, thereby reducing hospitalizations and enabling critical conversations about end-of-life decisions (Morrissey et al., 2019). Ultimately, these home-based solutions address the unique needs of both patients and caregivers, providing an improved, more personal, and more compassionate healthcare experience. The introduction of at-home palliative care is part of a broader trend towards filling gaps in access to end-of-life care. Classic inpatient hospice options are not always feasible or desirable for all patients, making it essential to open up at-home services. Evidently, for most families, it is preferred that hospice care be conducted at home, where they can treat their loved ones in comfort (Jawed, 2022). Yet, systemic barriers usually impede access to such critical care. Prioritizing home-based palliative care means healthcare providers can offer flexible, patient-tailored solutions that align with the family's values, goals, and preferences. Such initiatives are particularly crucial in disadvantaged communities, where access and availability of resources and professional services are limited. Drawing attention to home-based palliative care can immediately tackle minimizing disparities and ensure all patients are getting respectful, dignified, and appropriate care towards the end of their lives.

In addition to upholding the home-based palliative care model, evidence indicates that it can enhance health outcomes and reduce healthcare costs. Home-based care was noted to enhance the level of satisfaction among the families, whereby they could personalize interventions in a way that is more suitable to their loved one's specific requirements and preferences. Interventions like FamPALcare demonstrate ways in which educational support and coaching can enhance family competencies in disease management at home, reducing reliance on costly hospitalization and emergency care (Morrissey et al., 2019). Furthermore, greater availability of home-based services can enhance financial burdens among families, reducing preventable hospitalization and aligning healthcare expenditure. In the evolving paradigm of end-of-life and palliative care, establishing a solid home-based alternative not only helps to maintain patient dignity but also to construct an improved and more empathetic health system that considers emotional and physical health equally (Figure 6.11).

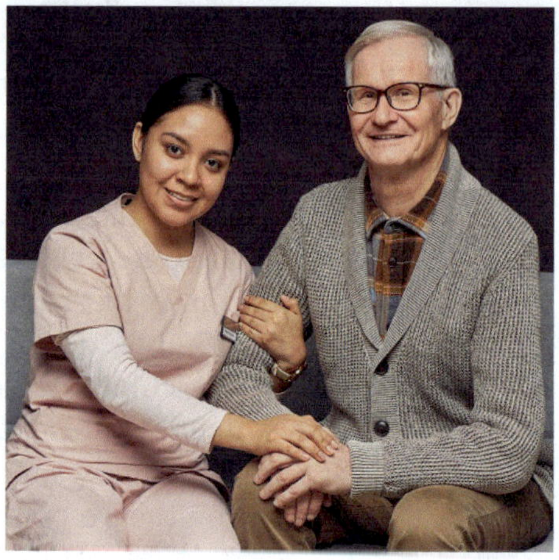

Figure 6.11. Home-based palliative care.

Source: https://www.caremountain.com/wp-content/uploads/2025/04/Home-Based-Palliative-Care-What-It-Is-Who-Needs-It-and-How-It-Works.jpg.

Test Your Knowledge

1. What is inpatient palliative care units?
2. What is outpatient palliative care programs?

6.3. Pain Management in Palliative Care

Learning Outcome

1. Understand the importance of effective pain control in palliative care
2. Describe the role of pharmacological interventions in the management of symptoms for patients engaged in palliative care
3. Understand the role of non-pharmacological approaches in palliative and end-of-life care

Successful pain management is a cornerstone of palliative care and plays a vital role in enhancing the quality of life for individuals with serious illnesses. It is based on individualized treatment, with individualized planning of the treatment specific to the individual's needs and histories of the patient. Multidisciplinary pain management integrates pharmacologic methods, including opioids and adjuvant medications, with non-pharmacologic therapies, including physical therapy, cognitive-behavioral therapy, and adjunctive modalities like acupuncture. This intersectoral strategy is a response to the multidimensional nature of pain, which can be both physical and psychosocial in etiology, and requires an integrative treatment approach that addresses the whole person rather than the disease. Effective pain management, in this manner, not only reduces pain but also enhances patient-physician communication, allowing discussion of goals of care and overall patient satisfaction. In spite of the recognized importance of pain management in palliative care, there are still significant hindrances to pain interventions. Under-treatment of pain affects most patients due to misconceptions regarding the prescription of narcotics, the threat of addiction, and variations in the competence of healthcare professionals in applying measures to manage pain. Socioeconomic factors such as access to health care services and appropriate drugs also hinder the situation of pain management. For example, in a study of sub-Saharan African end-of-life care, 94% of programs reported trouble with pain control issues, such as access to trained providers and legal restrictions related to drug dispensation (Harding et al., 2003).

Such systemic barriers underscore the essential need for intensive training programs for healthcare professionals to create a culture of active pain control in palliative care. To address these obstacles, integration of palliative care within existing healthcare systems is essential. Interventions to bridge gaps in care—particularly in home health settings—have resulted in significant improvement in outcomes. For instance, the integration of palliative care has been linked to better symptom control, improved communication about goals of care, and reduced unnecessary healthcare use (Stober et al., 2018). These findings underscore the importance of education outreach, collaboration among healthcare professionals, and policy development to foster an enabling environment for maximal pain control. In addition, changes in the system to accommodate the financial and regulatory requirements of healthcare professionals may facilitate increased access to basic medications and services, eventually paving the way for more equitable pain management in palliative care for a diverse population (Figure 6.12).

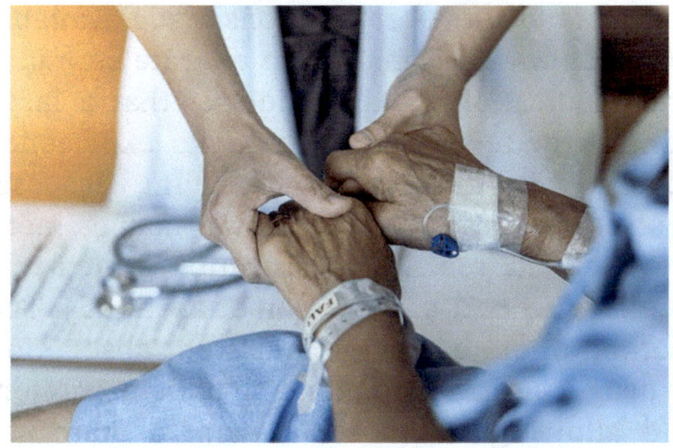

Figure 6.12. Pain management in palliative care.

Source: https://momentuminjury.com/wp-content/uploads/2023/07/Pain-management-in-palliative-care-Momentum-Medical-768x512.png.

6.3.1. Importance of Effective Pain Control

Proper management of pain lies at the center of end-of-life and palliative care, and it profoundly impacts patients' quality of life as they deal with terminal illnesses. The management of pain is not only a professional requirement but an ethical one that imposes dignity on people as they deal with the complexity of death. It is essential to possess an understanding of the complexity of pain and the impact it has on physical as well as psychological well-being. There should be an interdisciplinary strategy, as suggested by experts in the same field, to highlight the need for medical teams to take part in holistic approaches that incorporate pharmacological treatments as well as emotional and psychological support. Holistic care ensures that patients receive a dignified death and are not exposed to unnecessary suffering, which aligns with the fundamental axioms of palliative care outlined by Giaquinta et al. (2015). In the real world, the use of successful pain relief mechanisms can vary widely depending on an individual patient's medical history and circumstances. Recent advances, such as the use of equipment for rectal drug administration, prove state-of-the-art solutions made available to patients who cannot even tolerate standard oral medication. Studies indicate that a large number of terminally ill patients experience severe pain throughout the dying process, prompting the use of other pain management methods like rectal administration, which was found to be cost-saving (Kim et al., 2015). The method offers even and consistent absorption of drugs, ultimately enhancing patient comfort and allowing caregivers to control pain. By prioritizing effective pain management, medical practitioners not only end pain but also validate the patient's sense of control and agency at a critical point in their lives. Further, the consequences of inadequate pain control extend beyond individual patient experience; they have profound effects on families and caregivers as well.

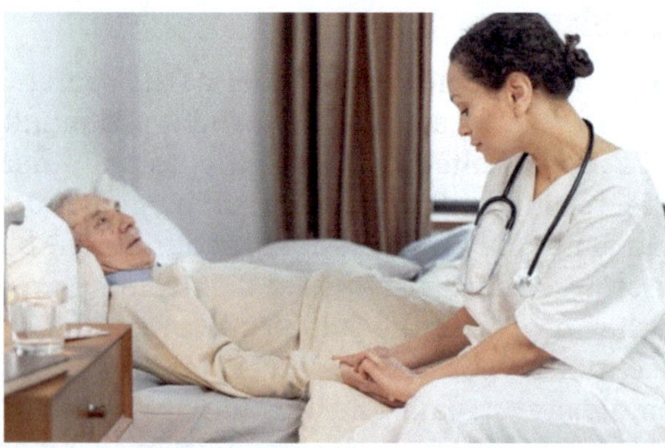

Figure 6.13. Importance of pain control.

Source: https://cdn.prod.website-files.com/5f34e5439213b3ee247b367a/667122baebd18b030d5f51b8_importance%20of%20pain%20management%20in%20palliative%20care.webp.

Chronic pain can amplify stress and emotional distress in patients as well as their families, creating a cycle of suffering that makes mourning harder. Well-managed pain enables families to focus on emotionally meaningful interaction with their loved ones in the dying process. Where pain is well managed, families enjoy improved emotional experiences and an overall sense of closure, attesting to the value of such interventions as fundamental to the palliative care philosophy. Through the choice of good pain control, health care teams not only improve patient outcomes but also provide priceless emotional support to families, thereby making the end-of-life care experience as noted in Giaquinta et al. (2015) (Figure 6.13).

6.3.2. Pharmacological Interventions

Pharmacological management is a fundamental part of symptom management for patients who are under palliative and end-of-life care. Because individuals faced with life-limiting illness often experience enormous physical and emotional distress, drugs aimed at alleviating pain, dyspnea, and other excruciating symptoms are crucial to quality of life improvement. For instance, opioids are routine medications for pain relief, while bronchodilators and corticosteroids can be prescribed to patients with chronic respiratory diseases. These drug approaches allow for a complex balance between life extension and optimizing the entire experience of patients living with end-of-life issues. However, the complexity of drug regimen management demands keen attention to each patient's individual needs, e.g., certain diagnoses and individual preference for modes of treatment, emphasizing the importance of individually tailored interventions in palliative care settings. Besides, the new developments in pharmacological therapies demonstrate the growing demand for ongoing research to establish the best available therapies to manage the new challenges of patients with non-malignant illnesses such as chronic obstructive pulmonary disease, interstitial lung disease, and cystic fibrosis. They are often accompanied by significant psychosocial undertows that can truncate effective symptom control. As highlighted in recent studies, the symptom burden typically carried by such patients—ranging from dyspnea to anxiety—indicates the inadequacy of existing interventions (Boland et al., 2013). This gap in care highlights the need for holistic pharmacological strategies that not only cover symptom control but also psychosocial support. Hence, collaboration among healthcare professionals practicing in the domains of palliative care and respiratory care is the premise for utilizing holistic treatment approaches, thus maximizing patients' overall quality of life. Of special note, the inclusion of pharmaceutical interventions within a broad context of palliative care necessitates thorough evaluation and planning. The majority of patients with progressive fibrotic interstitial lung diseases (ILDs) also have unmet needs that go beyond pharmacological management, and thus it is essential to utilize a multidisciplinary team approach (Adir et al., 2017). Effective care strategies must involve not only medication management but also psychosocial interventions that consider patient and caregiver needs throughout the course of the disease. Misconceptions about palliative care, which is far too frequently limited to terminal situations, can hinder the timely application of beneficial treatments. Bridging this gap in thinking by putting early drug and psychosocial treatments first enables patients to enjoy a better quality of life, even when disease progression is ongoing. Ultimately, effective implementation of these tailored interventions depends upon healthcare providers' combined endeavors to see and respond to patients' all-encompassing care requirements.

6.3.3. Non-Pharmacological Approaches

Non-pharmacological interventions play a crucial role in palliative and end-of-life care by addressing patients' overall needs rather than just symptoms. These interventions often include psychological care, physical therapy, and complementary therapies such as music and art therapy. These interventions play a critical role in enhancing patients' overall quality of life, emotional health, and meaningful interaction with their families. In the case of patients with severe illnesses, such as dementia, the role of non-pharmacologic interventions becomes even more crucial, as traditional pain management could be insufficient. In fact, it has been shown that younger and older people with dementia encounter widespread barriers in receiving quality end-of-life care, which points to the need for holistic, patient-centered approaches that take into consideration dignity and quality of life (Ballard et al., 2006). Not only are non-pharmacological interventions beneficial to the patients, but also to their caregivers, who must deal with crushing emotional and physical burdens. Interventions such as narrative medicine and reminiscence therapy enable improved communication between caregivers and patients on a deeper level, as well as empathizing with the patient's wishes and experiences. Also, mindfulness and stress reduction therapies are increasingly being seen as promising for reducing caregiver fatigue and anxiety and thus improving the caregiving environment overall. By establishing a working health-care provider-patient-family relationship, non-pharmacologic interventions can alleviate some of the existential aspects of end-of-life care. As studies persist to show the psychological and emotional impact of caregiving, the implementation of these strategies is critical in developing lasting care systems for caregivers and patients alike (Aveyard et al., 2007). On the whole, the implementation of non-pharmacologic strategies within palliative and end-of-life care not only enhances the quality of patient comfort but also meets the multidimensional emotional landscape experienced by the caregivers and family members. Engaging patients across multiple treatment modalities can empower them and provide valuable support to their caregivers. Further, demographic shifts that reflect increased prevalence of chronic conditions like dementia will necessitate health systems to prioritize these integrative approaches for planning and implementation. Finally, research expenditure to ascertain and optimize effective non-pharmacological interventions will become increasingly vital to improving care standards and preparing for the future care requirements of an increasingly older population. Not only is such a focus on the delivery of holistic care congruent with respect for patient autonomy, but it also maximizes the collective experience of end-of-life problems (Ballard et al., 2006) (Figure 6.14).

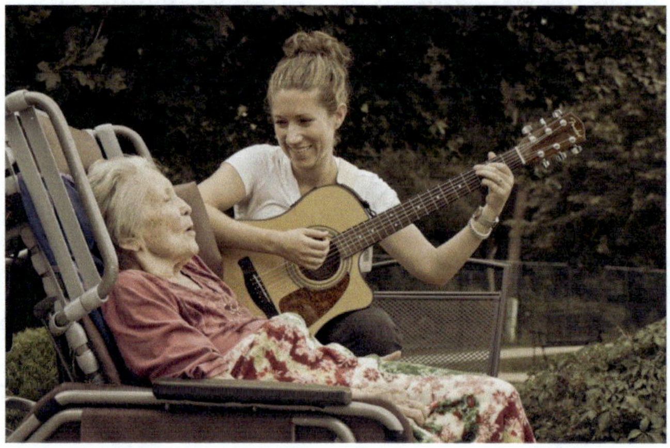

Figure 6.14. Music therapy.

Source: https://cell2soul.typepad.com/.a/6a00d83452a3b369e201b7c9462329970b-pi.

Test Your Knowledge

1. What is the importance of effective pain control in palliative care?
2. What is the pharmacological treatment?

6.4. Communication in End-of-Life Care

Learning Outcome

1. Discuss the prognosis and treatment options
2. Understand the role of advance care planning
3. Support families through the process

Effective communication is at the forefront of the practice of end-of-life care, as it has a profound influence on patients' families and healthcare workers' interactions. The personal nature of end-of-life discussions calls for a compassionate approach, in which the healthcare worker must balance clinical efficacy with empathy. Research indicates that communication conflicts are generally among patients, families, and the multidisciplinary treatment team, creating misunderstandings about treatment plans and patients' wishes. Having open discussions allows for greater patient preferences and values to be recognized on a deeper level, ultimately making the environment a more inclusive one that is able to break down anxiety and enhance satisfaction through these high-stress situations. The success of these discussions extends further than merely informing medical choices, but also as an emotional support source, maintaining the patient's dignity amidst difficult healthcare decisions. Interdisciplinary collaboration allows communication during end-of-life care via synthesis of diverse opinions and know-how, which ensures the patient's care to be comprehensive and patient-focused. It promotes improved communication among the healthcare team and simpler sharing of information about patient preferences and care plans. A study of clinical observation experiences in interdisciplinary palliative care courses recognizes the benefits students perceived in team communications, with respect to the fact that harmonious communication with patients and families is critical in providing empathetic care in difficult conversations. The skills gained through this experience highlight the need for ongoing education in health professionals' communication skills to equip them to deal with emotional and ethical dilemmas in end-of-life care.

This intentional focus on training can build a culture in which interdisciplinary teams work together flawlessly, leading to long-term improvement in palliative patient outcomes. Furthermore, the provision of hospice palliative care services creates a key determinant of the quality of communication with patients dying. While many patients are managed within specialized settings, most also face decisions at home. Awareness of the resources offered, as indicated in hospice palliative home care service reports, is important to patients and families during therapy discussions. Differentiation among settings is important; however, the need for honest and empathetic communication is never compromised, wherever the setting is. As outlined in several studies, hospice-level communication, especially in the context of home care, needs to be addressed through a dual mechanism that addresses both clinical and emotional concerns. Emphasizing strong communication habits in every environment enables better patient and family care through life's final transitions, making dying more dignified and respectful (Figure 6.15).

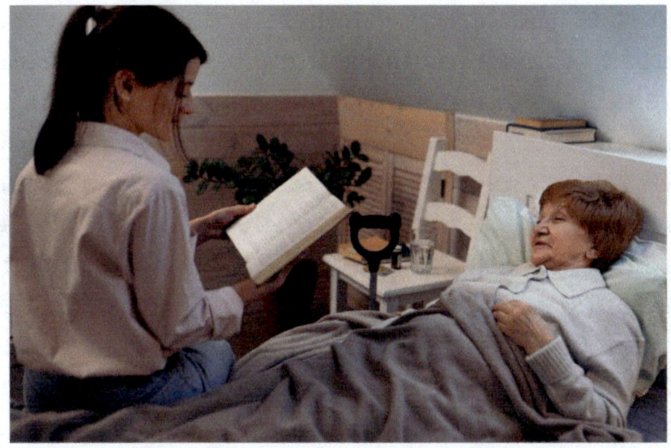

Figure 6.15. The importance of communication in hospice care.

Source: https://inspirehospice.com/wp-content/uploads/2024/08/2150216364.jpg.

6.4.1. Discussing Prognosis and Treatment Options

A key aspect of end-of-life and palliative care is the delicate art of communicating prognosis and treatment to families and patients. Such a conversation is crucial, as it clarifies the decision-making process for both short- and long-term care. Physicians, particularly general practitioners (GPs), often find themselves struggling to find the most effective ways to handle such discussions, which are heavy with emotional intensity and complexity. Evidence highlights that GPs hold varying concepts of advance care planning (ACP), which requires intensive training to prepare them for these conversations. By proactively initiating prognosis discussions, GPs can empower patients to explore their choices and preferences, thereby enhancing their engagement in care decisions and addressing their emotional and practical needs. The intention of these discussions should always be to foster clarity and empathy, providing a platform where patients are not made to feel they are not being heard or judged. Interdisciplinary collaboration in discussions regarding prognosis cannot be overstressed, as it enhances the quality of communication and patient outcomes. Nurses, for example, are at the heart of the transmission of prognosis-related information in pediatric oncology but are often excluded from such discussions. Exclusion not only hinders collaboration but can also erode the quality of care. By recognizing each team member's contribution to the communication process, health care providers can ensure that patients and families receive balanced care. Involvement of nurses in discussions about prognosis and treatment choices enables them to be patient care-oriented. Increased dialogue among physicians and nurses about prognosis can yield better patient experiences and can facilitate a deeper, clearer understanding of treatment. In addition, addressing the nuances of prognosis conversation must consider the psychological and emotional elements inherent in such discussions. The sensitive dynamics of discussing end-of-life care require medical staff to possess not only medical data but also superior communication abilities. These abilities enable them to convey prognostic information effectively while remaining attuned to patients' and families' emotional responses. Studies indicate that when health care teams pay attention to effective communication about prognosis, it results in greater patient and family satisfaction at the end of life (Haglund et al., 2019). Therefore, ongoing training and education of both doctors and nurses are essential to developing a culture in which open, honest, cooperative, and empathetic communication about prognosis and treatment decisions can be created, thereby enhancing palliative and end-of-life care.

6.4.2. The Role of Advance Care Planning

Advance care planning (ACP) is central to palliative and end-of-life care, as it enables patients to express their preferences regarding medical interventions and care as life comes to an end. Through ACP, patients can make their choices and have them respected, thereby enhancing autonomy and minimizing the workload for families and clinicians. This innovative approach to healthcare planning allows patients not just to select the amount of care that they desire, but also where they would like to receive it, either in the home or within clinic settings. Despite the benefits, research reveals a worrisome trend: a greater proportion of the populace fails to complete advance directives or completes them ineffectually, thereby canceling out the advance care planning's possible effectiveness (Hill et al., 2010). Secondly, advance care planning is an essential communication tool between doctors and families. Good ACP promotes goal-of-care conversations and helps families understand their loved one's values and preferences, thereby minimizing the risk of miscommunication at crucial decision-making times. Families, in most instances, are faced with a sense of crisis when a loved one's health changes, usually without being well-prepared for the decisions that come at the end of life. Inadequate advance care planning may lead to unnecessary interventions and emergency department transfers, as families act without definitive knowledge of patients' preferences (Bui et al., 2015). Therefore, enhancing family communication regarding advance care plans is imperative to facilitate smoother transitions of care and respect end-of-life wishes. Advance care planning is not only the effort of individual patients and families but also of healthcare workers and systems. For healthcare professionals, effective ACP can lead to more satisfied patients and improved healthcare outcomes through influencing clinical decisions aligned with the patients' expressed preferences. Furthermore, when clinicians communicate advanced care, they can minimize family members' end-of-life care stress by developing a shared understanding of the options and choices for treatment. As the health care environment evolves, there is increasing demand for systemic improvements in ACP practice to expand its utilization. By focusing on education programs that inform both providers and patients about the necessity of advance care planning, we can enhance the overall quality of palliative and end-of-life care to ensure that patient dignity and autonomy remain priorities (Hill et al., 2010) (Figure 6.16).

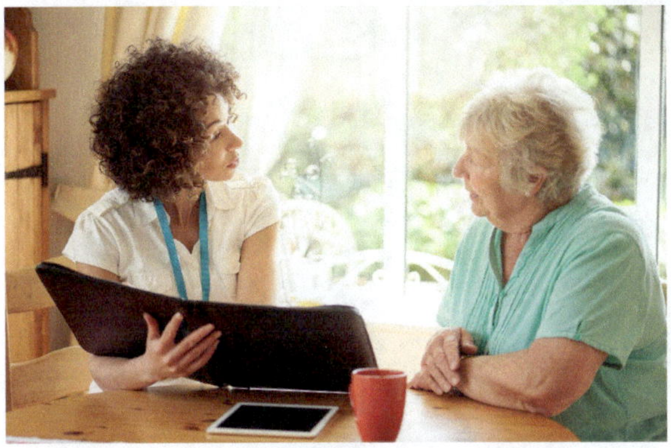

Figure 6.16. The importance of advance care planning in palliative care.

Source: https://contessahealth.com/wp-content/uploads/2024/05/Website-Photos-78.png.

6.4.3. Supporting Families Through the Process

Within the provision of palliative and end-of-life care, engaging with families along the process is essential to ensuring holistic and compassionate care. Families are usually caught up in an overwhelming psychological and emotional load as a result of having a loved one diagnosed with a life-limiting condition. This is further complicated by navigating challenging healthcare systems and making tough choices about where to get care. Good communication between caregivers and families is most important; it can help resolve misunderstandings and build trust. Research has indicated that the inability to communicate openly in most cases fosters disagreements between grieving members of the family and medical professionals, causing unnecessary impediments to the support the families receive in such difficult situations. Therefore, the adoption of effective communication strategies through ongoing education among healthcare professionals is able to significantly enhance the quality of care and family support and eventually improve the end-of-life experience as a dignified and respectful one for patients as well as families, as noted by palliative care study results (Nwaesei et al., 2020). Further, addressing families' emotional needs is essential. Families also express feelings of helplessness and grief during the terminal stage that can spill over into secondary stress and worry. Providing a supportive environment where open discussion and expression of feelings are allowed can be a revolutionary intervention within family relationships at this point. Medical professionals use a variety of interventions, such as support groups and counseling for families, that have been shown to lower emotional distress. These practices not only assist families in their bereavement but also enable them to become active participants in care decisions. For instance, the workshop model employed to enhance healthcare practitioners' capabilities in palliative care emphasizes emotional support as a vital component in mitigating the undesirable effects of caregiving (Nwaesei et al., 2020). This supportive practice, therefore, decreases family segregation and promotes closer familial attachment through the common experience of death. Moreover, the introduction of formal support systems for families who are going through neonatal palliative care proves the worth of targeted interventions in the case of such families. Being the leading cause of mortality in children below the age of five years, neonatal mortality places unique demands that require whole-family based support measures. Involving healthcare professionals and parents in the process of developing core outcome sets for neonatal palliative care can embed practices and standards for ensuring families receive stable and empathetic care. Discussion with essential stakeholders about core outcomes can help healthcare professionals better understand family needs and preferences, thereby enhancing the quality of end-of-life care. This collaborative effort not only empowers healthcare teams with the necessary tools but also fosters a sense of family based on empathy and compassion. Therefore, the development of these models can lead to better family experience and more humane delivery of neonatal palliative care (Figure 6.17).

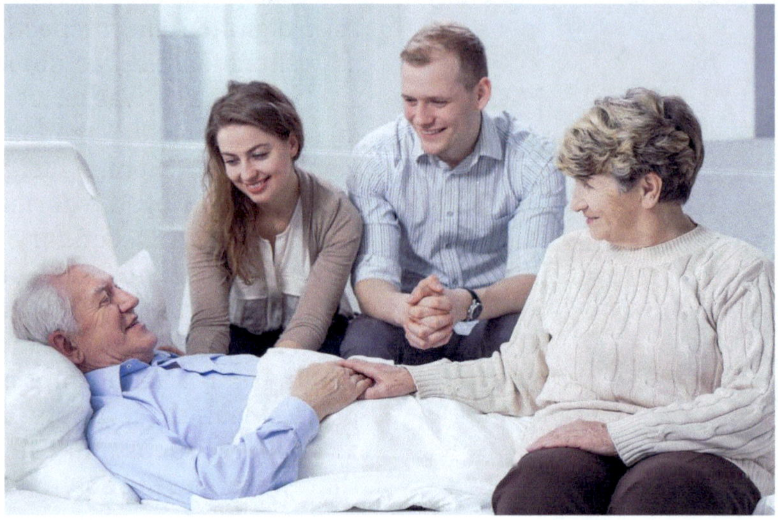

Figure 6.17. Family support

Source: https://www.hlonlinetraining.co.uk/wp-content/uploads/2016/12/what-does-end-of-life-care-involve.jpg.

Test Your Knowledge

1. What is the role of general practitioners?
2. What is advance care planning?

6.5. Ethical Considerations

Learning Outcome

1. Describe the autonomy and patient rights
2. Balance the quality of life and prolonging life
3. Describe the cultural and religious influences on care decisions

The ethical dilemmas in palliative and end-of-life care are multifaceted, typically involving a delicate balance among the principles of beneficence, non-maleficence, autonomy, and justice. Doctors tend to grapple with moral concerns regarding enabling death, particularly among patients who seek to terminate their suffering. Ethical dilemmas tend to center on how much a doctor should legally support requests for assisted dying or euthanasia. The complexities of making such decisions may be compounded by varying religious beliefs, as evidenced by a study showing that 86% of physicians consider their religious beliefs significant in decision-making about end-of-life care. This intersection of religion and medical ethics underscores the importance of having codified ethical schemes within which clinicians can navigate these troubled waters without offending their moral values or patients' rights to autonomy and respectful treatment (Abela et al., 2016). Furthermore, cultural environments have a profound effect on the ethical climate of palliative and end-of-life care. The perspectives of different ethnic groups regarding death can influence how care is perceived and provided. For instance, in the South Asian community, the physical setting of death could be secondary to conformance with cultural and religious customs associated with the process of dying. Older South Asians wish to die at home, viewing it as a place where they can carry out significant rituals that uphold their cultural and family obligations.

The customs illustrate the significance of understanding and valuing the cultural beliefs of the patients as they have explicit effects on ethically providing end-of-life care. Clinicians therefore need to recognize the need for cultural competency to facilitate ethical decision-making in consideration of each patient's values and background (Butt et al., 2014). Palliative care ethics also extend beyond the personal patient interaction to address systemic problems, such as healthcare equity and access. The disparity in palliative care education and resources can lead to differences in end-of-life care experienced by different populations. Implicit biases of healthcare providers also produce differences in pain management techniques and the quality of interventions used, based on a patient's background or perceived quality of life. Sustaining ethical practice within palliative care involves adherence to justice, ensuring that all patients have equal access to quality, compassionate end-of-life care, regardless of socioeconomic status, ethnicity, or cultural beliefs. This integrated concept of ethics within palliative care is pivotal to trust building and improving patient outcomes, and this is due to sustaining ongoing education and sensitivity among all healthcare workers (Abela et al., 2016) (Figure 6.18).

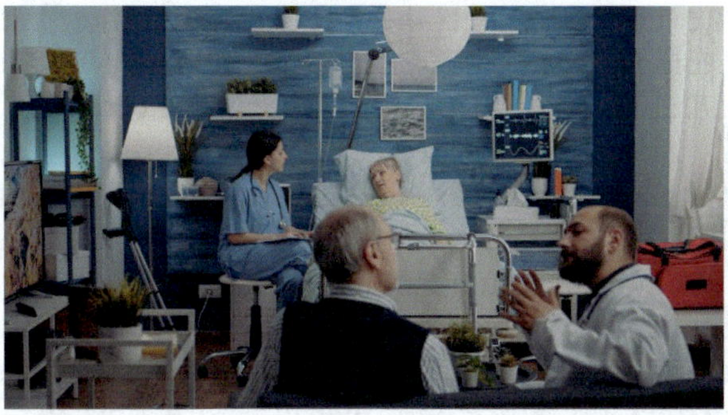

Figure 6.18. Ethical considerations in end-of-life care.

Source: https://cdn.growtha.dev/64f58746ad542d8781e2bab0/6641ae35915df89f7ec51de9_Ethical%20Considerations%20in%20End%20of%20Life%20Care.jpg.

6.5.1. Autonomy and Patient Rights

The concept of autonomy is at the forefront of the patient rights debate, particularly in palliative and end-of-life care. Autonomy allows patients to make decisions regarding their treatment and care, informed, respecting their dignity and individuality. This is most critical in settings where the patients come with life-limiting conditions. The ability to dictate end-of-life care preferences, for example, the possibility of refusing aggressive therapy or the possibility of receiving palliation, is respect for personal values and beliefs. From this point of view, medical professionals must actively engage patients in communicating their desires so their decisions are honored, even if the decisions conflict with prevailing medical protocol. Such practices highlight the importance of having patient-centered care environments in which autonomy not only is recognized but also fostered. The ethical landscape of autonomy also gets complicated with the addition of euthanasia and physician-assisted suicide implications. As the two Dutch and Belgian examples show, discussion has moved on to patients expressing a desire to die not only on the basis of enduring a terminal illness but also existential despair.

The courts' position that irredeemable and intolerable suffering has expanded to include social deterioration is provocative regarding the limits of control in end-of-life choices. The moral stakes involved in assisting patients who claim to be tired of living pose questions to health practitioners and to societies concerning the origins of autonomy. These issues amount to asking basic questions: at what point does respect for autonomy overlap with perceived ethical obligations to preserve life, and how do we interpret suffering in this complex setting? Furthermore, the intersection of autonomy with ethical dilemmas highlights the need for formalized practice codes to guide medical decision-making. Physicians often navigate a landscape fraught with conflicting interests, especially when patients are unable to advocate for themselves. This mandates a response that balances respect for patient rights with attention to broader societal concern, namely the rationing of resources in an increasingly strained health care system. It is therefore necessary for practitioners to embrace a mindset that balances the individual's needs with the professional ethical standards used in medical practice. Having a global code of conduct that everyone can adhere to is crucial in addressing these challenges as it encourages rational and consistent decision-making in patient care without sacrificing autonomy and ensuring the general obligations of the healthcare system (Montalto et al., 2014) (Figure 6.19).

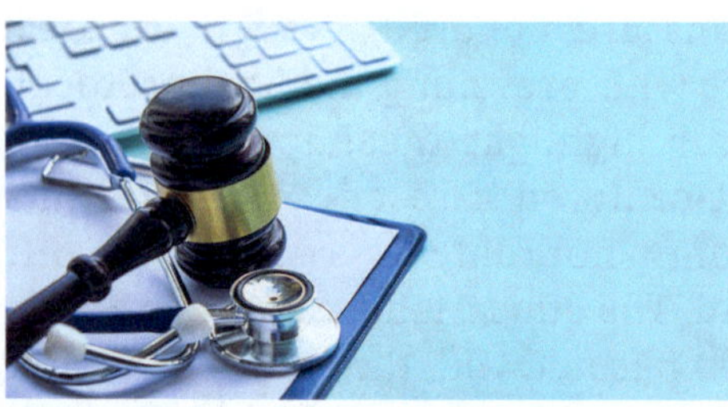

Figure 6.19. Patient rights.

Source: https://www.kimshealth.org/static/kims_nagercoil/images/Patient%20Rights__mobil650x490.jpg.

6.5.2. Balancing Quality of Life and Prolonging Life

In end-of-life and palliative care, the delicate balance between prolonging life and preserving quality of life is a difficult undertaking that healthcare professionals must navigate. While the urge to fight terminal diseases is at the center of medical practice, the experience of living with a disabling disease most of the time requires one to shift emphasis towards maximizing the patients' residual quality of life. This change is particularly apparent when addressing patients' emotional and spiritual needs, which can significantly impact their overall well-being. Research highlights that spiritual care, a core component of palliative care, is frequently overlooked, especially in at-risk populations such as individuals with dementia. Thus, despite the best intentions of medical professionals, inadequate prioritization of these elements can result in poor experiences toward the end of life; hence, there is a greater need for a more thorough approach to palliative care that includes both quality and quantity. Moreover, the ethical aspects of weighing quality of life against prolongation of life cannot be overstated. Health care workers are often presented with situations where life-sustaining treatments will prolong life in exchange for extensive suffering or significantly reduced quality of life. This ethical conflict is also complicated by the financial burden of extended care on health resources, as valuable time and resources can limit the possibilities for improving the distribution of care across patient cohorts. There needs to be an ethical basis to guide these decisions, one that makes the patient's welfare the focus, but does not ignore the consequences for society. That type of framework can facilitate a rational and just decision-making process in end-of-life care that weighs both the patient's wishes and the broader health community's capacity, all in an effort to respect the patient's autonomy and dignity in their dying days. No less important in this discussion, however, is good communication among healthcare providers, patients, and families. The quality of interaction during the patient admission process also plays a considerable role in the course of care, particularly where spirituality is involved. One such illustration is that physician-patient satisfaction has been shown to correlate with the provision of spiritual care, underscoring the need for honest communication about treatment options and dying wishes. Being attuned to patients and their families' diverse beliefs and values is an aspect of providing empathetic and person-centered care. According to research, discussing spiritual concerns openly can help create a more caring environment, leading to greater emotional resilience and satisfaction during the end-of-life journey. This increased communication not only addresses individual needs but also eventually produces a care response that honors the balance between saving lives and supporting quality of life, thus enhancing the overall palliative care experience.

6.5.3. Cultural and Religious Influences on Care Decisions

Religious and cultural factors play a significant role in the making of palliative and end-of-life care decisions. Patients from various cultures hold specific values and beliefs that guide their own perceptions of illness, death, and treatment options. For instance, some cultures view death as a natural phenomenon, with a preference for a holistic approach with an emphasis on spiritual and emotional aspects over maximal medical intervention. Conversely, other cultural paradigms will lean towards maintaining life at any cost, making it tougher to explore palliative care options. In addition, healthcare providers need to walk the thin line of such beliefs, ensuring that care plans honor patients' values while offering intensive and empathetic care. This requirement reflects the necessity for culturally competent care, where healthcare teams are made aware of recognizing and honoring the multifaceted cultural influences on patient decision-making in end-of-life care. The necessity for cultural competency takes on an even larger proportion when applied to the treatment of ethnic minority patients, who might face issues unique in seeking palliative care services. Disparities in language and unfamiliarity with the healthcare system can also interfere with effective communication, reducing the quality of care received. Culturally and linguistically complex patients can struggle to understand intricate medical information, potentially complicating their end-of-life decision-making. Health outcome disparities can also exacerbate these challenges, as they appear to be associated with increased mortality in certain populations. To improve the quality of end-of-life care for such patients, physicians must become more attuned to these barriers and more proficient in managing cultural differences, fostering cooperation and trust. Physicians can ensure that care is not only person-focused but also culturally aware of each patient's environment, fostering an unproblematic and respectful end-of-life experience (Harper et al., 2006). Moreover, the role of family influence in end-of-life care and cultural decision-making cannot be overestimated, given that family members' positions would determine patient care dynamics. Family members in most cultures are the key decision-makers, mirroring values of communalism and interdependence. This can be far removed from Western individualism's emphasis on patient autonomy. Health professionals must be attuned to the importance of involving the family in patient care discussions and decision-making. Attending to families' belief and practice needs may enhance communication and trust development, and ultimately lead to better palliative care outcomes. Also, being aware of migration backgrounds and the resulting family dynamics might prove essential in allowing the professional to strike a balance between ensuring patient safety and comfort originating from family support. By including the family role in care decisions, practitioners can ensure that the delivered palliative care is responsive to the cultural and emotional needs of patients and families (Green et al., 2018) (Figure 6.20).

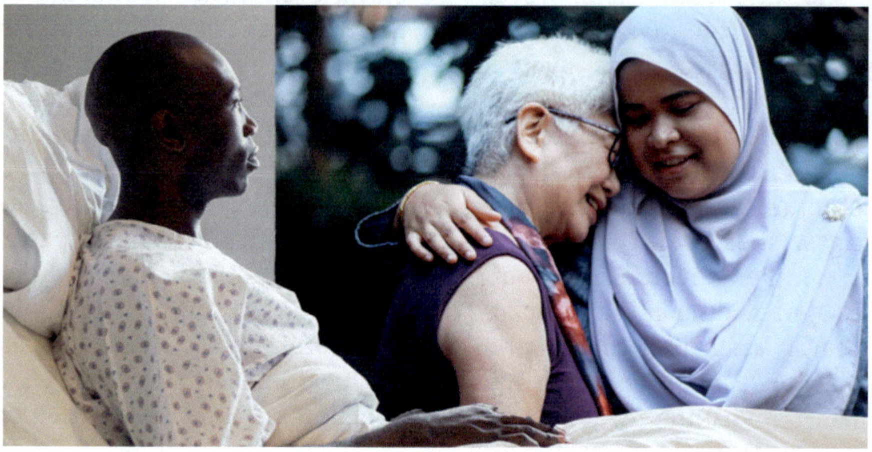

Figure 6.20. Culturally diverse communities and palliative and end-of life care.

Source: https://www.apa.org/images/eol-diversity-title-image_tcm7-244041.jpg.

Test Your Knowledge

1. What is the concept of autonomy?
2. What are cultural and religious influences on care decisions

SUMMARY

The essence of the palliative and end-of-life care debate is the imperative to undertake a transformational approach to managing the complexity of terminal illnesses. It is increasingly evident that terminally ill patients who are struggling with life-limiting illnesses require not just treatment but also psychosocial support that addresses their total needs. As required under the literature, palliative care is necessary for patients struggling with the combined challenges of terminal illness and conditions such as dementia. In particular, Abbey (2006) highlights the requirements for addressing such issues with affected persons, thereby promoting more enlightened, empathetic care protocols. The integration of patient autonomy and family participation in treatment decisions is critical to achieving dignity and respect at the end of life. Additionally, multidisciplinary collaboration is a major determinant in the efficacy of palliative care systems. With the incorporation of health professionals across various specializations, the overall care in symptom management, such as pain, anxiety, and emotional distress, can be achieved. Cachia et al. (2007) identify that excellent palliative care is a coordinated effort aimed at improving the quality of life for patients and their families. The balanced approach acknowledges that treating the physical, psychological, and spiritual aspects of care ensures overall well-being. Besides, while controversy continues to ensue regarding moral issues such as physician-assisted suicide, it is necessary that doctors are equipped with advanced palliative care education in order to deal with these sensitive discussions with sensitivity and refinement. Ultimately, the future of palliative and end-of-life care depends on continuous changes in practices that consider patients' experiences and autonomy as life ends. Training and educating healthcare providers in palliative care skills is a medical priority. It should raise awareness and competence, enabling practitioners to better offer proper and compassionate care in difficult end-of-life scenarios. For this reason, further research and policy development are required to shape a conducive environment that prioritizes palliative care as a core component of the healthcare continuum so that all patients can receive the dignity and respect they deserve in their final days.

In the domain of palliative and end-of-life care, the development of geriatrician-specific specialized competencies is a significant step toward integrated care. Based on a structured review, 35 major palliative care competencies were identified that are directly applicable to geriatricians to further enhance the quality of care in older adults. These competences were the result of a stringent modified Delphi process involving specialists from 12 European countries, which emphasized collaboration to meet diverse healthcare needs across the continent. The European Geriatric Medicine Society (EuGMS) has since embraced an active leadership role in integrating these competences into postgraduate training in geriatric medicine, making them a requirement for geriatricians. This project is critical because it creates a systematic understanding of how palliative care can be effectively implemented within geriatric practice to optimally serve an aging population in their final years of life (Pautex et al., 2021). Furthermore, an awareness of the multifaceted perspectives of patients and family caregivers is critical to the effective use of palliative care interventions. Current reports highlight the importance of addressing the individualized needs of chronic obstructive pulmonary disease (COPD) patients since their end-of-life experience can be distinguishable from those of cancer patients. Patient-caregiver consolidated studies of the themes reveal commonalities that demonstrate overarching concepts in holistic care, illness trajectory, and technology's influence on treatment and support. These results elucidate some of the unmet needs that need to be considered, particularly purposeful and timely conversations about care. Hence, being aware of and acting on such biopsychosocial processes will ensure that care remains aligned with the individual values and experiences of patients with advanced respiratory disease (Johnston et al., 2017). Finally, these arguments emphasize adaptive approaches to palliative and end-of-life care models. Incorporating unique skills in geriatric medicine not only enables practitioners to use the appropriate tools to achieve best practice but also underscores the importance of valuing patient and caregiver perspectives. By fostering an empathetic culture and responsiveness, health systems can significantly enhance the quality of care received by vulnerable populations. With the landscape of palliative care shifting, emphasis on specialist training as well as commitment to patient-focused care ensures an enriched experience of attending to the physical and emotional complexities of end-of-life phenomena, thereby setting the stage for improved health gains and quality of life (Johnston et al., 2017; Pautex et al., 2021).

KEY TERMS FROM THIS CHAPTER

- Continuity
- Empathy
- Healthcare education
- Pain management
- Patient autonomy
- Patient satisfaction
- Spiritual support
- Emotional support
- End-of-life care
- Holistic medical care
- Palliative care
- Patient engagement
- Patient-centered communication
- Team dynamics

CRITICAL THINKING QUESTIONS

1. **What is the primary goal of palliative care?**
   a. To prolong life at all costs
   b. To cure chronic illnesses
   c. To improve quality of life by managing symptoms
   d. To prevent the onset of diseases
2. **Which of the following is a core principle of palliative care?**
   a. Focus solely on the patient's physical symptoms
   b. Provide support only to the patient
   c. Address physical, emotional, social, and spiritual needs
   d. Avoid discussing end-of-life issues
3. **Which of the following conditions is NOT typically managed with palliative care?**
   a. Advanced cancer
   b. Chronic obstructive pulmonary disease (COPD)
   c. Severe heart failure
   d. Acute appendicitis
4. **What is the role of advance directives in palliative care?**
   a. To ensure aggressive treatment is provided
   b. To outline the patient's preferences for medical care
   c. To serve as legal proof of the patient's will
   d. To decide treatment for the patient without their consent
5. **What is the best approach to discussing end-of-life care with patients?**
   a. Avoid discussing sensitive topics
   b. Use clear, empathetic, and patient-centered communication
   c. Focus only on medical facts, ignoring emotional concerns
   d. Make decisions without involving the patient

Short Answer Questions

1. Define the palliative care.
2. What is the importance of end-of-life care?
3. What are the principles of palliative care?
4. List the types of palliative care services.
5. What are the non-pharmacological approaches to care?

Answer to Critical Thinking Questions

1. (c); 2. (c); 3. (d); 4. (b); 5. (b).

REFERENCES

1. Abbey, J. (2006). *Palliative Care and Dementia*. https://core.ac.uk/download/71364855.pdf (accessed on 14th July 2025).
2. Abela, J. (2015). GPs and end of life decisions: Views and experiences. https://core.ac.uk/download/46603092.pdf (accessed on 14th July 2025).
3. Abela, J., & Mallia, P. (2016). Maltese doctors: Views and experiences on end-of-life decisions and care. https://core.ac.uk/download/46604041.pdf (accessed on 14th July 2025).
4. Adenwalla, S. F., O'Halloran, P., Faull, C., Murtagh, F. E. M., & Graham-Brown, M. P. M. (2024). Advance care planning for patients with end-stage kidney disease on dialysis: narrative review of the current evidence, and future considerations. *Journal of Nephrology, 37*(3), 547–560. https://doi.org/10.1007/s40620-023-01841-3Adir, Y., Bajwah, S., Bendstrup, E., et al. (2017). Palliative care in interstitial lung disease: Living well. https://core.ac.uk/download/110623633.pdf (accessed on 14th July 2025).
5. Anderson, J. E., Evans, C. J., Gillam, J., Harding, R., et al. (2021). Priorities and opportunities for palliative and end of life care in United Kingdom health policies: A national documentary analysis. https://core.ac.uk/download/477690172.pdf (accessed on 14th July 2025).
6. Attard Montalto, S. (2014). Ethical principles in pediatric practice. https://core.ac.uk/download/46603075.pdf (accessed on 14th July 2025).
7. Aveyard, B., Schofield, P., & Smith, P. (2007). Developing annotated bibliographies: A tool for education, collaboration and research development. https://core.ac.uk/download/177011.pdf (accessed on 14th July 2025).
8. Bacon, J. (2008). *Hospice Palliative Home Care in Canada: A Progress Report*. https://core.ac.uk/download/71365021.pdf (accessed on 14th July 2025).
9. Baddarni, K., Bar-Sela, G., & Schultz, M. (2012). Reflections on palliative care from the Jewish and Islamic tradition. https://core.ac.uk/download/pdf/8655865.pdf (accessed on 14th July 2025).
10. Ballard, C., Daley, S., Hughes, J., Keady, J., et al. (2006). End-of-life care and dementia. https://core.ac.uk/download/4145979.pdf (accessed on 14th July 2025).
11. Beernaert, K., De Vleminck, A., Deliens, L., Houttekier, D., et al. (2016). How do general practitioners conceptualise advance care planning in their practice? A qualitative study. https://core.ac.uk/download/84044177.pdf (accessed on 14th July 2025).
12. Bekelman, D., Carter, J., Carter, J. H., Fox, E., et al. (2017). Palliative care and Parkinson's disease: Meeting summary and recommendations for clinical research. https://core.ac.uk/download/151161689.pdf (accessed on 14th July 2025).
13. Bluebond-Langner, M., Chant, K., Gallagher, K., Mancini, A., et al. (2023). The NeoPACE study: Study protocol for the development of a core outcome set for neonatal palliative care. https://core.ac.uk/download/595951757.pdf (accessed on 14th July 2025).
14. Bluebond-Langner, M., Craig, F., Hollowell, D. R., Kelly, P., et al. (2014). Underlying barriers to referral to pediatric palliative care services: Knowledge and attitudes of healthcare professionals in a pediatric tertiary care center in the United Kingdom. https://core.ac.uk/download/16251146.pdf (accessed on 14th July 2025).

15. Boland, J., Martin, J., Ross, J. R., Ross, J., et al. (2013). Palliative care for people with non-malignant lung disease: Summary of current evidence and future direction. https://core.ac.uk/download/151156967.pdf (accessed on 14th July 2025).

16. Breakwell, S., Callahan, M. F., Kim, M. J., Phillips, J., et al. (2012). Clinical observation reflections from students in an interdisciplinary palliative care course. https://core.ac.uk/download/213079311.pdf (accessed on 14th July 2025).

17. Breakwell, S., Callahan, M., & Petersen, C. L. (2014). Palliative and end-of-life care: Precepts and ethics for the orthopedic population. https://core.ac.uk/download/213055287.pdf (accessed on 14th July 2025).

18. Brick, A., Normand, C., Smith, S., & O'Hara, S. (2013). *Evidence on the Cost and Cost-Effectiveness of Palliative Care: A Literature Review*. https://core.ac.uk/download/75777777.pdf (accessed on 14th July 2025).

19. Bui, N., Halifax, E., Harrington, C., Lee, M., et al. (2015). Provider perspectives on the influence of family on nursing home resident transfers to the emergency department: Crises at the end of life. https://core.ac.uk/download/323074171.pdf (accessed on 14th July 2025).

20. Butt, J., Charmaz, K., Department of Health (DH), HelpAge International, Office of National Statistics (ONS). (2014). Dying at home: A qualitative study of the perspectives of older South Asians living in East London. https://core.ac.uk/download/9991751.pdf (accessed on 14th July 2025).

21. Cachia, E. (2007). Why palliative care? Encountering challenging issues. https://core.ac.uk/download/46602132.pdf (accessed on 14th July 2025).

22. Cohen-Almagor, R. (2017). Euthanizing people who are 'tired of life.' https://core.ac.uk/download/151161148.pdf (accessed on 14th July 2025).

23. Deliens, L., Gijsberts, M. J. H., Hertogh, C. M. P. M., van der Steen, J. T., et al. (2014). Predictors of spiritual care provision for patients with dementia at the end of life as perceived by physicians: A prospective study. https://core.ac.uk/download/55762597.pdf (accessed on 14th July 2025).

24. Fulp, M. (2007). *Working Toward a Definition of Futile Care in the United States Health Care System*. https://core.ac.uk/download/352871000.pdf (accessed on 14th July 2025).

25. Giaquinta, M. de los A., & Pascucci, J. O. (2015). *Palliative Care: Support And Dignity at The End of Life*. https://core.ac.uk/download/61891223.pdf (accessed on 14th July 2025).

26. Gilmore, A., Hart, B., Mc Namara, B., McNamara, B., McNeil, C., Saunders, C., Seale, C., et al. (2010). What "best practice" could be in palliative care: An analysis of statements on practice and ethics expressed by the main health organizations. https://core.ac.uk/download/pdf/8379500.pdf (accessed on 14th July 2025).

27. Green, A., Green, M., Jerzmanowska, N., Lobb, E. A., et al. (2018). 'Death is difficult in any language': A qualitative study of palliative care professionals' experiences when providing end-of-life care to patients from culturally and linguistically diverse backgrounds. https://core.ac.uk/download/213607752.pdf (accessed on 14th July 2025).

28. Haglund, K., Newman, A. R., & Rodgers, C. C. (2019). Pediatric oncology nurses' perceptions of prognosis-related communication. https://core.ac.uk/download/228028413.pdf (accessed on 14th July 2025).

29. Harding, R., Higginson, I. J., Marconi, K., O'Neill, J. F., et al. (2003). Current HIV/AIDS end-of-life care in sub-Saharan Africa: A survey of models, services, challenges and priorities. https://core.ac.uk/download/pdf/3358127.pdf (accessed on 14th July 2025).
30. Harper, B., Johnson, B., Hudson, C., Deese, D., Burrs, F., Ramsey, G., London, G., et al. (2006). *Key Topics on End-of-Life Care for African Americans.* https://core.ac.uk/download/71364899.pdf (accessed on 14th July 2025).
31. Haslam, C., Theodosopoulos, G., & Tsitsianis, N. (2014). Business models in health care: Accounting for the sustainability of palliative and end of life care provision by voluntary hospices in England. https://core.ac.uk/download/29140428.pdf (accessed on 14th July 2025).
32. Hill, B. C., Lebredo, N., & Shafer, C. R. (2010). Health care reform's proposed end-of-life provisions. https://core.ac.uk/download/213906352.pdf (accessed on 14th July 2025).
33. Hopper, S. S. (2003). *Crossing Organizational Boundaries in Palliative Care: The Promise and Reality of Community Partnerships.* https://core.ac.uk/download/71365063.pdf (accessed on 14th July 2025).
34. Hosie, A. (2015). *Delirium Epidemiology, Systems and Nursing Practice in Palliative Care Inpatient Settings: A Descriptive Mixed Methods Project (The DePAC Project).* https://core.ac.uk/download/61305437.pdf (accessed on 14th July 2025).
35. Jawed, A. (2022). Years of life lost: A call to achieve equitable end-of-life care among children. https://core.ac.uk/download/555562301.pdf (accessed on 14th July 2025).
36. Johnston, B., & Mathews, G. (2017). Palliative and end-of-life care for adults with advanced chronic obstructive pulmonary disease: A rapid review focusing on patient and family caregiver perspectives. https://core.ac.uk/download/96885466.pdf (accessed on 14th July 2025).
37. Kim, Y. T. (2015). Managing end-of-life pain using a rectal medication administration device. https://core.ac.uk/download/154560146.pdf (accessed on 14th July 2025).
38. Lehtsaar, T., & Meel, L. (2017). Interdisciplinary team-based pastoral care: A potentially adaptable model for Estonian healthcare. https://digitalcommons.georgefox.edu/cgi/viewcontent.cgi?article=2019&context=ree (accessed on 14th July 2025).
39. Morrissey, E., Moss, A. H., Petitte, T., Piamjariyakul, U., et al. (2019). Study protocol of coaching end-of-life palliative care for advanced heart failure patients and their family caregivers in rural Appalachia: A randomized controlled trial. https://core.ac.uk/download/322556784.pdf (accessed on 14th July 2025).
40. Myers, M. S. (2019). *Development of Unit-Specific Educational Interventions for Inpatient Palliative Care Needs.* https://core.ac.uk/download/270036207.pdf (accessed on 14th July 2025).
41. Nwaesei, C. (2020). Navigating the trajectory of palliative care pedagogy through the relationship of patient, family members, and healthcare professionals. https://core.ac.uk/download/287870585.pdf (accessed on 14th July 2025).
42. Pautex, S., Roller-Wirnsberger, R., Singler, K., et al. (2021). Palliative care competencies for geriatricians across Europe: A Delphi consensus study. https://core.ac.uk/download/395602199.pdf (accessed on 14th July 2025).
43. Petersen, C. (2024). Barriers primary care physician assistants face in referring patients to palliative care services early in the disease process. https://core.ac.uk/download/624274608.pdf (accessed on 14th July 2025).

ACUTE CARE IN FAMILY PRACTICE

7

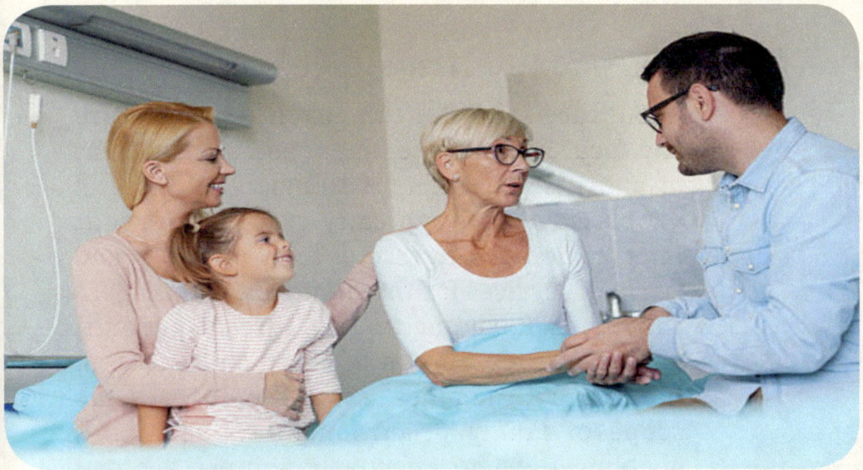

Introduction

In contemporary medical practice, acute care in family practice is an absolute crossroads for addressing rapidly fluctuating patient requirements. Family practice is particularly well-suited to managing acute conditions owing to its patient-centered model of care, based on continuity of care and holistic intervention. Acute complaints among patients vary from respiratory issues to cardiovascular emergencies, and immediate interventions are needed. For instance, acute pulmonary edema—a prevalent emergency department condition—must be evaluated and treated expeditiously to improve health outcomes, underscoring the crucial role of family practitioners in the early detection and stabilization of critically ill patients (Pilgrim, 2023). This emphasis on accelerated action in acute care not only facilitates the easier management of individual cases but also enables an overall prevention strategy by enabling practitioners to offer patient education on risk factors and lifestyle modification. Furthermore, the nuances of managing acute conditions underscore the relevance of evidence-based

LEARNING OBJECTIVES

After studying this chapter, you will be able to:

1. Understand the role of family practitioners in acute care
2. Describe the common acute conditions treated in family practice
3. Know the diagnostic tools and techniques in acute care
4. Understand the treatment protocols in acute care
5. Describe the challenges face in providing acute care
6. Know the impact of technology on acute care

practices and guidelines in family practice. The challenge is not only detecting symptoms but also using appropriate treatment modalities in accordance with accepted medical standards. Hypertension patients, for example, demand meticulous assessment of prescribing practices and adherence to recommended treatment regimens as inappropriate prescribing may lead to side effects and complications (Aydın et al., 2020).

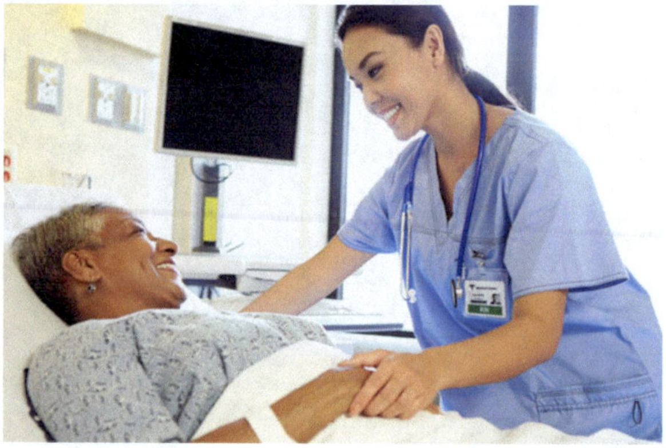

Figure 7.1. Acute care in family practice.

Source: https://thompsonfamilymedicine.com/wp-content/uploads/2021/10/nursing02.jpg.

This requires family practitioners to stay current with revisions to clinical guidelines and to modify approaches to meet the individualized needs of their patient populations. This way, family practice acts both as a front-line defense and a central didactic instrument, informing patients where information is needed while offering front-line, compassionate care. Lastly, integrating acute care into family practice requires a multidisciplinary approach that engages various medical practitioners, thereby enhancing the quality of care provided to patients. The interplay between complementary specialties enables an enhanced approach in the management of acute conditions, whereby specialists, nurses, and allied health professionals can provide their expertise. Such an interdisciplinary methodology not only optimizes clinical performance but also optimizes the learning experience for medical students practicing in family practice settings. By fostering a culture of interdisciplinary collaboration, family physicians can ensure that selected patients receive balanced, effective care at critical moments. Last but not least, acute care in family practice is not merely a response to immediate health crises but also a proactive approach to promoting long-term health and stability for patients and their families (Figure 7.1).

Definition of Acute Care

Acute care is a vital component of healthcare and focuses on the treatment and management of patients presenting with emergent medical problems that typically require urgent intervention. Acute care encompasses a broad range of services for the treatment of emergent conditions, including trauma, surgical patients, and acute presentation of chronic diseases. In practice with families, acute care widens the scope of family practitioners exponentially, enabling them to effectively address a broad spectrum of healthcare scenarios. The idea of acute care, therefore, encapsulates not just the urgency of treatment but also the comprehensive nature that family practice itself embodies, aiming to heal patients while considering their overall health and long-term medical needs. The integration of acute care within family practice emphasizes the importance of continuity of care, ensuring that patients receive holistic care in dynamic healthcare settings. Moreover, the responsiveness of acute care systems can also affect patient outcomes, particularly in family practice, where early intervention prevents subsequent health complications. Family physicians are most likely to provide acute care, ranging from first aid to the management of complicated medical emergencies. Family practice acute care is not only a reflection of the doctors' healthcare abilities but also of the healthcare system's ability to provide medical care to patients at different stages of their healthcare needs. As an example, acute care treatments allow for smoother transitions between several different providers and facilities, in alignment with newer management strategies aimed at enhancing patient care (Sochalski et al., 2010). Transitional care models that foster improved coordination and communication between healthcare teams ultimately lead to enhanced patient recovery and satisfaction.

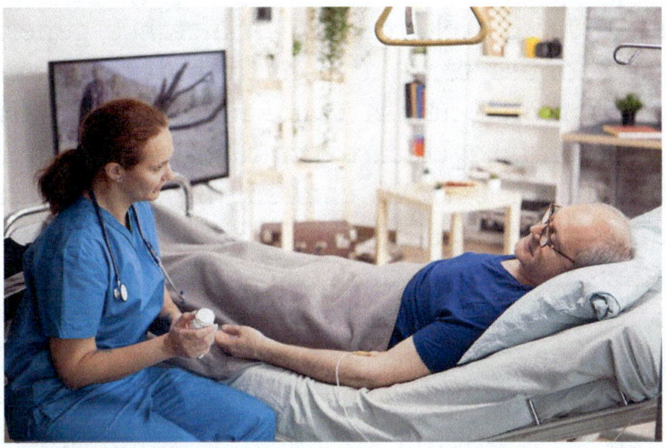

Figure 7.2. Acute care.

Source: https://leafcare.co.uk/alovoocm/uploads/2022/08/Significance-of-Acute-Care-1024x683.jpg.

Within the university setting, the relevance of acute care is further highlighted as health workers respond to the particular needs of student populations. University health facilities play a critical role in responding to acutely developing health problems among students, ranging from emotional disturbances to physical injuries sustained during sports (Gottlieb et al., 1979). These acute care services play a critical role in fostering not only the health of individual students but also the academic environment and social atmosphere of the institution. By situating acute care within family practice, health professionals can provide specialized, responsive care that addresses the health concerns of the student population. This expert care not only addresses the management of acute health concerns but also weaves a preventive health narrative that supports the overall well-being of the students, revealing the profound impact acute care has on broader community health systems (Figure 7.2).

Importance of Acute Care in Family Practice

Acute care is an emergency component of family practice, providing straightforward, efficient treatment for a variety of conditions requiring immediate intervention. Acute care within the context of family medicine defines a wide array of conditions, including infections, trauma, and exacerbations of chronic disease. The ability to meet such emergent medical needs within a family practice environment ensures continuity of care, which is crucial for maintaining multispectral health. Patients prefer to access acute care from their family physicians, as this allows them to remain in a familiar environment where their personal health histories are well understood. This familiarity not only adds to patient comfort but also to quicker diagnosis and treatment, ultimately resulting in improved health outcomes and patient satisfaction. Additionally, the inclusion of acute care in family practice makes the overall healthcare system more efficient. Addressing acute health concerns at the primary care level allows family practices to avoid putting too heavy a demand on emergency departments and specialized facilities. This foresight in the health area has the potential to lower healthcare costs and improve the use of resources, with room for more focused treatment of complex patients' cases. In the process, family doctors also identify early signs of chronic ailments complicated by acute presentation, thereby preventing potential complications arising from delays in treatment. Such intervention is not only essential to the health of individual patients but also essential for promoting public health outcomes in the population as a whole. In addition to the resolution of immediate health issues, acute care in family practice involves elements of dignified and empathetic care that resonate very strongly with practitioners and patients alike. It has also been established that the dignity and quality of care provided to patients are intrinsic to the overall treatment process. Research demonstrates that valuing the "little things" that matter—e.g., patient involvement in decision-making, empathy, and timely communication—builds the therapeutic relationship between providers and patients, a key component of effective care (Kinnear et al., 2016). Additionally, the underlying nuances involved in the treatment of older patients, particularly those suffering from illnesses like dementia, require an acute care specialist service that will enhance comfort and quality of life. Such recognition highlights the absolute importance of acute care to family practice settings, where it not just cures but also respects patients' integrity at vulnerable moments along their health course (Birch et al., 2008).

7.1. Role of Family Practitioners in Acute Care

Learning Outcome

1. Distinguish between primary care and acute care
2. Describe the training and skills requirements for family practitioners
3. Understand the patient-centered approach

In acute care, family physicians are gatekeepers linking the initial patient interface with the broader health care system. They usually are the initial physicians patients seek out when acute health issues arise, with extensive, timely, as well as critical assessment. By producing high-quality initial assessments, family physicians facilitate appropriate diagnostic studies and the initiation of treatment programs tailored to specific patient needs. Their role is particularly crucial in the treatment of conditions that require urgent attention, for example, infections or asthmatic exacerbations of chronic disease. In this role, they possess the expertise required to stabilize patients and make initial decisions regarding referrals to specialists, ensuring care and preventing complications due to delays in appropriate treatment. Also, family physicians must navigate the complexities of delivering acute care to patients from diverse backgrounds. This involves not only the extent of clinical knowledge but also cultural understanding and people skills to effectively engage patients from diverse backgrounds. For instance, general practitioners tend to consult older patients with complex health conditions, particularly in residential aged care facilities (RACF), where transitional care is challenging due to the frailty of the residents (Flicker, 2021). Their understanding of the social determinants of health also enhances their ability to provide individualized advice and support. By fostering trust-based relationships, family practitioners empower patients to become collaborative participants in their healthcare decision-making process, which is crucial in the acute care setting, where timely interventions are indispensable for the best possible outcome. Family practitioners' contribution towards acute care also extends beyond multidisciplinary cooperation with other healthcare professionals. They tend to consult with nurses, specialists, and allied health professionals to develop comprehensive care plans that address both acute and chronic medical concerns. In emergency departments, efficient coordination among emergency rooms and family physicians can strongly influence patients' recovery, as seen in cross-coverage between hospitals (Michael, 2014). This collaboration enables family practitioners to ensure their patients receive timely interventions and appropriate follow-up care—factors integral to improving overall healthcare quality. As coordinators of care, family practitioners assume a leading role in preventing risks associated with acute health conditions and ultimately in improving patient satisfaction and healthcare effectiveness (Figure 7.3).

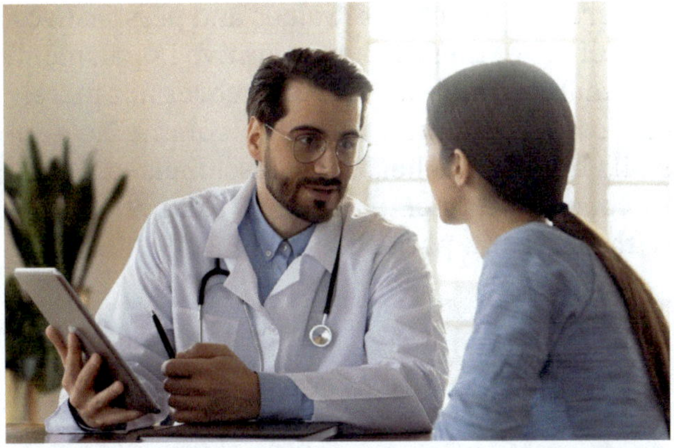

Figure 7.3. The essential roles of a family medicine doctor.

Source: https://wp02-media.cdn.ihealthspot.com/wp-content/uploads/sites/456/2021/0
iStock-1224215467.jpeg.

7.1.1. Primary Care vs. Acute Care

The divergence between primary and acu
care exists at the core of understanding tl
organization and functioning of the health ca
systems. Primary care typically encompass
long-term health and preventive care, serving
the first point of contact for the patient. In thi
family physicians are responsible for treatir
chronic illnesses, providing regular check-up
and maintaining ongoing patient relationship
with an emphasis on holistic health.

This prevention approach is vital in minimizing the risk of sudden health crises, ultimately resulting in better health outcomes. Acute care, on the other hand, addresses immediate and serious health issues requiring urgent solutions, often in hospitals where expert teams handle critical situations. The contrast between the two models of care establishes the worth of an integrated model, with a powerful message that effective primary care can significantly reduce the workload for acute care facilities. When acute care components are integrated into family practice, there is room to enhance patient outcomes, particularly during crisis cases. Acute care practices entail quick assessment, diagnosis, and treatment to stabilize patients presenting with pressing medical conditions. For instance, acute care-capable family practitioners can manage most of the emergencies effectively, like an asthma flare-up or minor trauma, in their own offices. With this capacity, not only is the patient's recovery faster, but practitioners are also empowered to ensure the continuation of care. In addition, studies have indicated that the inclusion of primary palliative care strategies in the acute setting can greatly improve the quality of life for patients with serious illness, thereby providing an empathetic health care experience (Lynn et al., 2024).

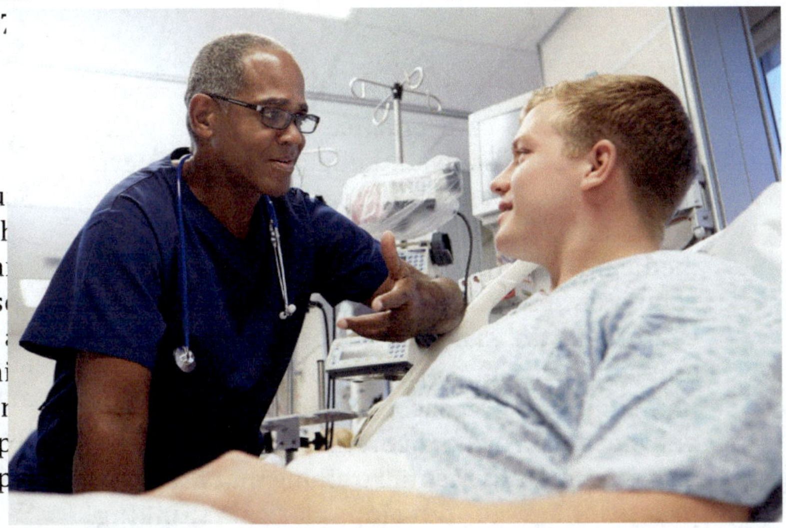

Figure 7.4. Primary care vs. acute care.

Source: https://online.utulsa.edu/images/bee68497-dffa-4de1-9f08-737dcf674d26.jpg.

The integration of primary and acute care yields a holistic model of health care that recognizes the multifaceted needs of patients across the continuum of care. Understanding of the barriers inherent in the primary and acute care distinction is crucial to health care professionals. Socioeconomic status, cultural beliefs, and organizational differences could have a great bearing on patient access to care (Dewez et al., 2023). These could affect the accommodation of patients between primary and acute care systems, predisposing them towards delays in care or suboptimal control of conditions. As health systems strive for more integrated services, training family practitioners in acute care procedures is becoming increasingly prominent, yet again bridging the gap between acute care and these two areas of care. Improved communication between primary care doctors and acute care specialists also leads to more effective patient care methodologies and reduced healthcare spending. Understanding and addressing these complexities is key to creating a more integrated model of health care that emphasizes patient well-being across all levels of care (Figure 7.4).

7.1.2. Training and Skills Required

Effective acute care practice demands a well-rounded set of skills and education to achieve maximum outcomes for patients. Providers must have core knowledge in emergency medicine that encompasses a range of clinical competencies, including the assessment of acute conditions, the management of life-threatening emergencies, and the implementation of immediate care protocols. Training courses not only need to provide theoretical information but also physical, experiential training that prepares practitioners to develop critical thinking and rapid decision-making abilities. This is particularly important in time-constrained situations, where initial evaluation and intervention significantly influence the patient's prognosis. Besides, there is a constant need for education to accommodate new medical practices, technologies, and treatment policies that become available to improve the quality of care delivered in acute environments. Beyond primary medical training, optimizing patient care for special-needs patients, for instance, individuals with dementia, requires specialized information and an understanding of their care requirements. Dementia training courses have stressed the importance of taking on a person-centered approach with values and perspectives, first of all, of those facing cognitive impairment. Optimal staff training needs to cover not merely clinical information but also communication skills to enhance health professionals' capacity to communicate empathetically and effectively with dementia patients.

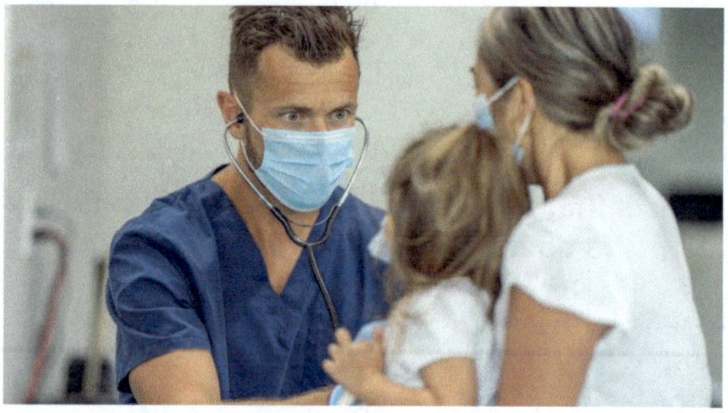

Figure 7.5. Acute and urgent care skills required by family nurse practitioners.

Source: https://onestepnola.org/wp-content/uploads/2023/09/image001-805x452.jpg.

The conclusions of qualitative studies emphasize improving staff training in acute settings to address barriers such as resource limitations and ineffective care pathways, ensuring that healthcare professionals are better positioned to deliver high-quality, patient-centered care to vulnerable groups (Brooker et al., 2016). Moreover, the deployment of formal education systems, such as the Emergency Neurological Life Support (ENLS), significantly enhances acute care doctors' capabilities. Research indicates that these programs significantly enhance cognition and decision-making ability to the advantage not just of the providers but also to better patient care outcomes in settings with limited resources. Crisis management and decision-making training courses ensure that medical professionals are current in managing neurological emergencies so that there is proficiency in their areas. The provision of evidence of retaining skills over the long term underscores the value of ongoing professional development and continuing education in acute care settings, and thus it becomes essential for family practice professionals to engage in lifelong learning to address new health challenges (Acharya et al., 2018) (Figure 7.5).

7.1.3. Patient-Centered Approach

In family practice, patient-centered care is a cornerstone of effective healthcare delivery, particularly in acute care. This approach promotes the tailoring of medical decisions and interventions to patients' personal preferences and values. By involving patients directly in treatment plans, clinicians enhance not only patients' feelings of agency but also treatment compliance. There is evidence that patient feelings of being heard and understood increase the likelihood of favorable health outcomes significantly. The patient-centered model, hence, serves as an essential framework for understanding the complexity of individual health experiences, particularly among populations with diverse backgrounds whose cultural susceptibilities and personal circumstances can greatly shape health behavior and decision-making. One of the main elements of this approach is the integrated coordination of care, required to ensure that patients receive suitable interventions in the right time. Approaches that support the medical home model demonstrate the concept by providing holistic, coordinated care within health care systems. Implementing such programs in the acute care setting would boost quality considerably while, paradoxically, reducing expenditure, offering a double benefit in the delivery of health services. As an illustration, states that have advanced the medical home model have recorded higher levels of patient satisfaction and outcomes, which attest to the efficacy of a coordinated care approach in family practice aimed at the holistic consideration of patients' needs (Takach et al., 2009). This form of integration not only speaks to the philosophy of patient-centered care but also underscores the necessity for continuity in the treatment of acute conditions. In addition, the focus on care after discharge further underscores the importance of transition planning to prevent avoidable hospital readmissions. Patient-centered care recognizes that the stage of discharge is critical in the patient's healthcare life cycle. Engagement in effective intervention activities—ranging from patient and caregiver education, clear communication, and follow-up care—has been shown to significantly reduce readmission rates. Following a definitive four-step methodology throughout hospitalization and discharge helps make the transition less complex for patients, thereby improving the overall care experience and outcome. With patient education and multidisciplinary care coordination, healthcare professionals can focus attention on potential complications, thereby enhancing the patient-oriented role in acute care within family practice offices.

Test Your Knowledge

1. What is the difference between acute and primary care?
2. What is the patient-centered approach?

7.2. Common Acute Conditions Treated in Family Practice

Learning Outcome

1. Describe the respiratory infections
2. Describe the musculoskeletal injuries
3. Understand the gastrointestinal issues

In family practice, acute conditions make up a significant portion of patient presentations ranging from a long list of conditions that must be treated right away. Common conditions treated on a regular basis are infections such as influenza, urinary tract infection, and respiratory infection, where early intervention is necessary to lessen symptoms and prevent further complications. The family practice setting is also best suited to respond to such acute events, given its emphasis on global care and continuity. In the patient demographics, there was a consistent pattern in the most frequent presenting complaints, as likewise indicated by research findings highlighting the importance of attending to patients' needs and expectations within the primary care setting. Such knowledge is not only vital for effective treatment but also for achieving optimal patient satisfaction and outcomes in acute care contexts, such as in the need for accurate data on symptom frequency across various settings (Muscat et al., 1989). Another significant field in family practice is the management of acute musculoskeletal symptoms, which can present as a sprain, strain, or fracture. Patients also commonly present with these acute conditions following trauma or physical activity, necessitating prompt evaluation to rule out other more serious injuries. Family participation in initial treatment may significantly influence recovery time and patient outcome. Family physicians are also well prepared to provide treatments such as immobilization, analgesia, and referral for radiologic imaging where necessary. As seen in various studies, awareness of geographical variability in acute presentation can enhance family practice capacity to respond appropriately. The evidence highlights the need for extensive knowledge of common conditions in local populations, re-emphasizing the need for ongoing education and training of healthcare professionals (Muscat et al., 1989). Lastly, management of acute gastrointestinal illnesses, such as gastroenteritis and food poisoning, is another frequent problem in family practice. These conditions are reported immediately by the patients because their onset is sudden, with vomiting and diarrhea being frequent. Family doctors must be able to differentiate between self-limiting illnesses and those requiring additional treatment or hospitalization. Effective management in such instances relies heavily on prompt diagnosis and appropriate symptomatic therapy, which may include hydration and nutritional counseling. In addition, improved care management strategies can greatly benefit older or chronically ill patients with such acute illnesses, as can innovative interventions that facilitate transitions among providers and sites. By addressing these widespread acute conditions, family practice not only provides required medical attention but also encourages an active response to the overall well-being of a population (Figure 7.6).

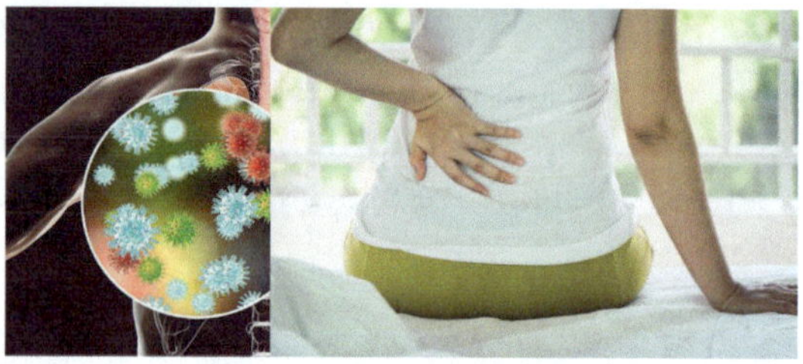

Figure 7.6. Acute conditions.

Source: https://medicalofficeofkaty.com/wp-content/uploads/2023/08/Acute-Condition-Banner.jpg.

7.2.1. Respiratory Infections

Respiratory infections are a high priority in family practice, with a non-specific presentation making diagnosis and treatment difficult. Among them, acute respiratory infections (ARIs) are most prevalent, encompassing a variety of conditions, including viral and bacterial infections of the upper and lower respiratory tract. Practitioners face the challenge of distinguishing between viral and bacterial pathogens to ensure appropriate treatment. Misdiagnosis leads to inappropriately prescribed antibiotics, which not only do not help patients but also contribute to the growing public health issue of antibiotic resistance. Patients' expectations about treatment also guide prescribing practices, with patients expecting antibiotics to be the best treatment for respiratory infections regardless of the cause (Mar et al., 2015). These interactions emphasize the need for an effective method of treating respiratory infections in family medicine. Arguably, the most crucial theme in managing respiratory infections is patient education and shared decision-making. Families tend to present first with existing convictions about the necessity of antibiotics, either as a result of earlier healthcare presentations or general beliefs about best treatment. The trend has the potential to disconnect patient expectations from clinical guidelines, making it harder for clinicians to educate patients with facts and offer treatment plans. Through participation in shared decision-making activities, healthcare professionals reduce the unnecessary prescription of antibiotics to a great degree without adversely affecting patient satisfaction or increasing re-consultation rates (Beller et al., 2015). Thus, it becomes essential to make open discussion of the nature of the illness, the basis on which certain treatments are administered, and the harms associated with unnecessary antibiotic use critical in ensuring evidence-based practice compliance. Preventive measures are also important when treating respiratory infections. Vaccination is a critical intervention in reducing the occurrence and severity of infections such as influenza and pneumococcal illness, which are culprits of substantial morbidity and healthcare costs. Family immunization education on the benefits and schedules of immunization in family practice can reduce the morbidity burden of ARIs in the population. Furthermore, promoting lifestyle interventions—such as smoking cessation, handwashing, and diet—can enhance respiratory health overall and reduce infections. The coupling of prevention with effective communication strategies enhances a balanced approach to acute care that prioritizes long-term health outcomes over short-term symptom relief, ultimately benefiting individual patients and the overall public health environment (Figure 7.7).

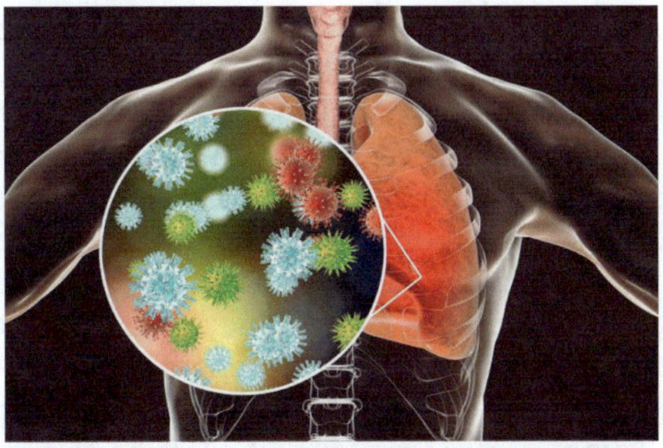

Figure 7.7. Respiratory tract infections.

Source: https://www.omdiagnosticlabs.com/wp-content/uploads/2022/10/Respiratory-Tract-Infections2.jpg.

7.2.2. Musculoskeletal Injuries

In acute care in family practice, musculoskeletal injury is a major challenge for several reasons. It has varied etiologies and long-term implications for the patient's function. In most instances, the injury is caused by multiple sources, such as sports, workplace injuries, and falls among older adults. The acute management of musculoskeletal injuries requires a proper assessment to determine the severity of the injury and its impact on the patient's daily activities. Proper control of pain is necessary, as pain is a disabling complaint that is often associated with these kinds of injuries. The American College of Physicians advocates for robust performance measures of pain management in acute care settings, noting that acute pain interventions should not only relieve discomfort but also enhance patient function and overall quality of life (Qaseem et al., 2024). In treating musculoskeletal injuries, family doctors face a number of challenges that necessitate a multidisciplinary response. The increasing incidence of fragility fractures among elderly patients emphasizes the need for comprehensive care plans addressing not only short-term but also long-term consequences of the injury. Fragility fractures not only compromise the musculoskeletal system but can also initiate a cascade of functional deterioration and increased dependence. As emphasized in the recent controversy surrounding geriatric fracture care, optimal management of this injury includes not just orthopedic treatment but also supportive care and rehabilitation for optimal recovery (Jae-Lim, 2019). The nature of such cases requires general practitioners to engage in ongoing collaboration with specialists to develop coordinated care systems that promote effective treatment of musculoskeletal injury across all patient groups. Besides, the evolving healthcare environment demands that family physicians be competent in the ideal best-practice management of musculoskeletal trauma to achieve the best patient outcomes. Prevention education is also essential, particularly in elderly patients who have a higher risk of falling and subsequent fractures. Implementation of standardized treatment based on evidence-based guideline recommendations can substantially enhance patient care for musculoskeletal injuries. This involves assuming performance measures to improve the assessment and management of pain and the recovery of function. The global call for action by organizations for the treatment of fragility fractures highlights the imperative for systemic reform towards rationalizing the pathways of treatment for such patients, advocating for a cohesive approach integrating acute care with active rehabilitation. Hence, increasing awareness and responsiveness in family practice can significantly improve the health outcomes of patients with musculoskeletal injury (Jae-Lim, 2019; Qaseem et al., 2024) (Figure 7.8).

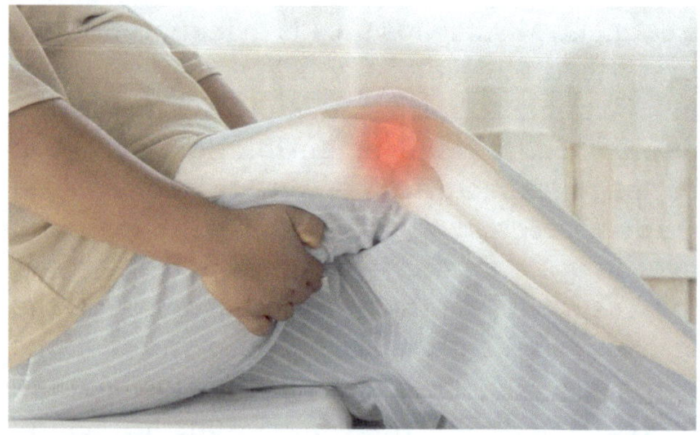

Figure 7.8. Musculoskeletal injuries.

Source: https://modernprimaryhealthcare.com/wp-content/uploads/2024/03/Musculoskeletal-injuries.webp.

7.2.3. Gastrointestinal Issues

Gastrointestinal issues pose a significant challenge in acute care, particularly in family practice, where overall patient management is key. Diseases like gastroesophageal reflux disease (GERD), irritable bowel syndrome (IBS), and inflammatory bowel disease (IBD) present a spectrum of symptoms ranging from mild discomfort to extensive distress. In family practice, clinicians must be able to identify the emotional problems early and appropriately so that proper interventions can be instituted. Education on the wide range of gastrointestinal symptoms and their potential impacts on patients' quality of life must be delivered with a multidisciplinary approach that incorporates diagnostic and therapeutic interventions. The value of patient communication regarding their gastrointestinal health can enhance patient participation and adherence to treatment protocols, thereby improving overall outcomes in family practice. A key aspect to managing conditions of the gastrointestinal tract is the incorporation of evidence-based guidelines into practice. Practitioners must stay current with the latest research on gastrointestinal disorders and their management to enable better care for patients. This entails being aware of when and where referring to specialists is justified, and adhering to guidelines for conditions such as diverticulitis or celiac disease. Besides that, patient and family education regarding dietary modification, management of symptoms, and drug compliance is essential in achieving better health results. As highlighted in the literature, multidisciplinary care, such as consultant-staff interactions among primary care physicians, specialists, and nutritionists, can be effective in establishing good control of acute gastrointestinal disease, hence enhancing the potential for successful patient outcomes (Bultas et al., 2016). Further, an understanding of the psychosocial issues associated with gastrointestinal illness is important in acute care practice. Depression and anxiety caused by chronic gastrointestinal disorders are prevalent among patients, and these aggravate their symptoms and complicate their management. It becomes part of their holistic care plan to respond to patients' psychological well-being. Family practitioners are in the best position to provide integrated care that addresses both physiological and psychological challenges. This approach aligns with recent recommendations to enhance family self-management skills, improve patient-provider relationships, and improve overall health and well-being (Pisani et al., 2010). Emphasis on these elements can greatly improve care management for gastrointestinal disease, leading to enhanced patient satisfaction and improved clinical outcomes (Figure 7.9).

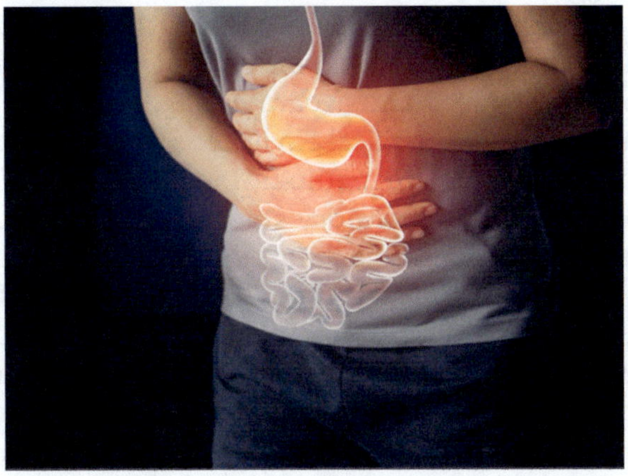

Figure 7.9. Gastrointestinal issues.

Source: https://gastroenterology.smileshospitals.com/wp-content/uploads/2021/07/shutterstock_1135057226.png.

Test Your Knowledge

1. What are respiratory infections?
2. What are the gastrointestinal issues?

7.3. Diagnostic Tools and Techniques

Learning Outcome

1. Understand the physical examination
2. Describe the laboratory tests
3. Understand the imaging studies

Diagnostic tools and methods are of utmost significance in acute care within the practice family environment, enhancing clinicians' ability to deliver rapid and accurate diagnoses. Given the pace of this medical environment, employing various diagnostic methods, including imaging examinations, laboratory studies, and point-of-care testing, is crucial. State-of-the-art imaging with ultrasound and computed tomography (CT) allows for immediate examination of internal anatomy, yielding valuable information about conditions such as appendicitis or fracture. The integration of laboratory studies, from the complete blood count to the metabolic panel, provides a comprehensive picture of the patient's status to support sound clinical decision-making. Thus, the use of a variety of diagnostic tests not only streamlines the assessment process but also underscores the importance of accurate diagnosis to ensure optimal outcomes for patients in family practice (Gordon et al., 1952). Besides, point-of-care testing has revolutionized the diagnostic process in acute family care settings. These are all procedures conducted at or near the site of patient care and enable rapid clinical assessment that is essential for acute illness. Rapid glucose testing, strep testing, and even cardiac biomarkers can all be obtained within minutes, allowing the clinician to initiate treatment without delay. This significantly facilitates the management of acute disease, reducing waiting time for laboratory reports. Furthermore, the portability and ease of use of the majority of point-of-care devices ensure that family doctors can use these diagnostic devices in a variety of settings, ranging from office practices to community health programs, thereby enhancing access to high-quality acute care (Kitsiou et al., 2013). In addition to physical diagnostic equipment, the implementation of digital health technology, such as telemedicine and electronic health records (EHRs), is of high significance in modern acute care diagnostics. Telemedicine enables remote consultations, making it easier for physicians to evaluate patients and determine whether additional diagnostics are required, with fewer patient visits and waiting times. EHRs enhance diagnostic accuracy by integrating patient data, histories, and prior test reports into a single, accessible repository. The large-scale management of data allows clinicians to consider a patient's complete medical history while diagnosing. Combined, such technologies can make diagnostic processes in acute care more effective and efficient while encouraging patient-oriented work in family practice – ensuring time relevance and care tailored to personal needs (Gordon et al., 1952) (Figure 7.10).

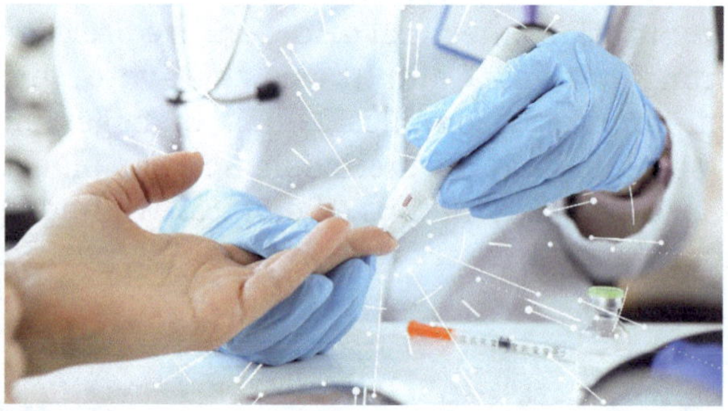

Figure 7.10. Addressing point-of-care diagnostic device.

Source: https://flex.com/wp-content/uploads/2024/02/Point-of-care.jpg.

7.3.1. Physical Examination

The physical exam is a core element of family practice acute care, significantly impacting decision-making in clinical practice. By considering the physical condition of a patient systematically, healthcare practitioners are in a position to note vital signs for underlying conditions that might not be immediately obvious. The comprehensive examination includes assessing cardiovascular, respiratory, and neurological status. The ability to perform an accurate and complete physical assessment not only facilitates the diagnosis of acute illnesses but also enables timely interventions, thereby improving health outcomes. Trained practitioners and nurses play a significant role by supporting the multi-professional care process, ensuring that patients' health across all spheres is tracked and treated. During family practice, the role of the physical examination extends beyond mere symptom detection to include ongoing monitoring of patients' health and well-being. Periodic physical assessment can facilitate monitoring of chronic conditions and changes over time, and allow the healthcare practitioner to modify treatment plans accordingly. This aggressive position is particularly applicable in the wake of numerous common health problems that occur among specific groups, such as students, who have unique challenges, including drug abuse and mental disorders. As Gottlieb et al. (1979) argue, the involvement of nurse practitioners in university health centers maximizes the potential of family practice, particularly in addressing such complex health care needs by means of comprehensive tests and tailored interventions. Further, the physical exam is most often the gateway to teaching patients self-management and preventive care. As practitioners examine patients' health, they are not only capable of identifying areas for improvement but also of empowering patients to take charge of their own health through lifestyle modification. This aspect of education is particularly important in managing behavioral health issues, such as issues with disorders such as autism spectrum disorder. As observed by Bultas et al. (2016), empowering families to perform their daily functions and behaviors enhances their overall health outcomes. Physical examination, in this case, is not merely a diagnostic tool but also a catalyst for patient empowerment and taking responsibility for health care in the family practice environment (Figure 7.11).

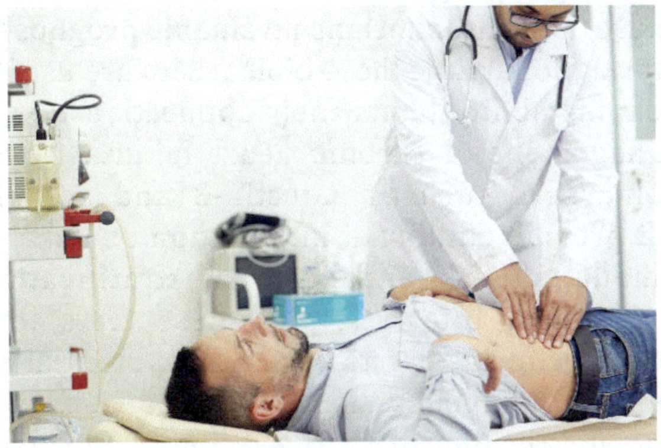

Figure 7.11. Physical examination.

Source: https://www.kellummedical.com/wp-content/uploads/2019/07/AdobeStock_174938098.jpeg.

7.3.2. Laboratory Tests

In acute care settings, laboratory testing is an important element in the early diagnosis and treatment of various medical conditions. Laboratory tests provide vital information that informs clinical decisions, particularly in distinguishing between severe infections and non-severe diseases. Point-of-care testing, such as C-reactive protein testing, is essential in enhancing diagnostic accuracy. One recent study demonstrated that the use of these tests as part of the assessment protocol significantly enhances sensitivity and negative predictive value for serious infection in acutely ill children. It is a particularly valuable approach because it enables earlier detection of patients who must be referred urgently and minimizes the risks that accrue with delayed therapy. Thus, the use of diagnostic technology in family practice can lead to improved patient outcomes and reduced hospitalization among non-critical patients (Aertgeerts et al., 2014). Laboratory tests are also utilized outside the scope of infectious disease diagnosis to other forms of acute medical ailments, for example, heart failure. B-type natriuretic peptide (BNP) and NT-proBNP biomarkers have emerged as an indispensable diagnostic tool in acute decompensated heart failure, offering clinicians invaluable prognostic information. While these biomarkers are useful, their instability limits their application to the management of chronic heart failure. Novel biomarkers such as galectin-3 and soluble ST2 provide additional information on cardiac remodeling and enhance risk stratification in patients. Integration of these tests into routine clinical practice has the potential to improve therapeutic choices to be more specific, ultimately leading to improved clinical outcomes in patients at risk for adverse cardiac outcomes, including death and myocardial infarction (Wu et al., 2012).

This underscores the importance of modifying laboratory practices in family medicine to address patients' complex needs. As family physicians practice acute care situations, the strategic use of laboratory testing becomes more critical. The capacity to read laboratory results correctly directly affects patient management decisions and treatment outcomes. Practitioners need to take into account the specificity and sensitivity of numerous biomarkers and tests to customize their approach to each patient's distinct clinical presentation. For instance, combining past test results with the newer biomarkers may provide a general impression of the patient's condition and inform appropriate interventions. Moreover, ongoing research and development in biomarker science will enable family physicians to adopt new diagnostic algorithms, ultimately enhancing their ability to deliver quality care. Such programs not only benefit individual patients but also contribute to the general objective of optimizing healthcare efficiency and reducing rates of adverse events for acute conditions (Wu et al., 2012; Aertgeerts et al., 2014) (Figure 7.12).

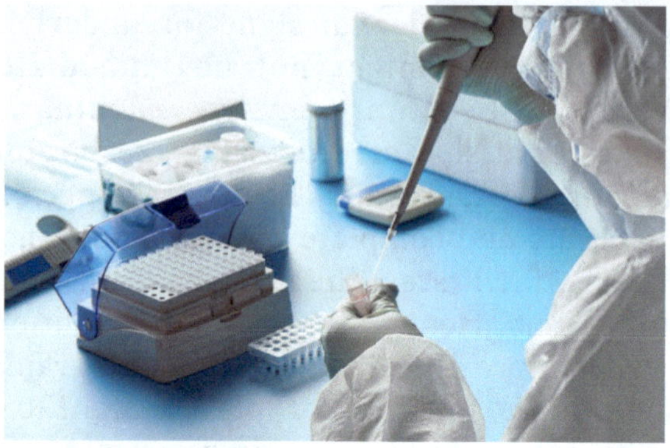

Figure 7.12. Laboratory tests.

Source: https://wp02-media.cdn.ihealthspot.com/wp-content/uploads/sites/522/2020/09/iStock-1209968955.jpg.

7.3.3. Imaging Studies

The integration of imaging examinations into acute care in family practice is increasingly important, especially for the treatment of emergent conditions. Imaging examinations such as X-rays, CT scans, and MRIs provide critical diagnostic information that informs treatment. For example, with acute lower back pain, imaging aids clinicians in deciding on whether to have serious underlying pathology such as fractures, tumors, or infections. However, overuse of imaging tests is associated with the risk of escalating costs, radiation exposure, and the possibility of incidental findings that can lead to inappropriate interventions. The prudent use of imaging must therefore be applied to balance the need for accurate diagnosis and the dangers of excessive exposure to imaging modalities. It is thereby the significance of adherence to clinical guidelines that promote evidence-based family medicine. Despite the importance of imaging tests, a significant gap remains in implementing evidence-based guidelines for their use. Recent studies reveal that clinical practice guidelines, particularly for acute condition management, are not automatically adopted in primary care. For instance, in the acute low back pain management, there was a trial to assess the effect of a theory-informed intervention upon guideline adherence, with imaging referrals being the matter of focus. The intervention was set to reduce unwarranted referrals for plain X-rays while enhancing patient outcomes, such as disability. The findings of such research can provide valuable information on optimal imaging practices, enabling improved care by reducing the risk of avoidable imaging without undermining diagnosis and treatment (Donner et al., 2008). Implementation of imaging studies in acute care necessitates ongoing education and awareness of family practice clinicians to implement best practices. The increasing availability of evidence-based clinical practice guidelines is a significant step towards better-quality care in family practice clinics. By attending training sessions and workshops that elaborate on such guidelines, practitioners can better understand when imaging is necessary and which modalities to apply for particular conditions. This interaction not only enhances diagnostic accuracy but also aligns with the overall context of patient-centered care, which is focused on information-based decision-making and minimizes unnecessary interventions. Last but not least, a culture of adherence to evidence-based imaging guidelines is needed to optimize patient outcomes in family medicine (Kitsiou et al., 2013) (Figure 7.13).

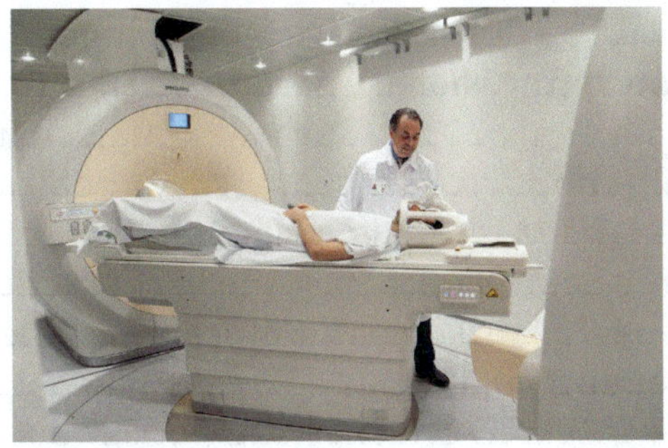

Figure 7.13. MRI scan.

Source: https://www.medifee.com/blog/wp-content/uploads/2017/11/MRI-Scan.jpg.

Test Your Knowledge

1. What is the physical examination of a patient?
2. What are imaging studies?

7.4. Treatment Protocols in Acute Care

Learning Outcome

1. Understand the medication management
2. Know the process of referral to specialists
3. Describe the follow-up care

In acute care, treatment protocols are a pillar of timely and effective intervention for patients. Protocols are designed to standardize care, reduce variability, and maximize patient outcomes by providing clear guidelines for clinicians to follow. In family practice, when one is exposed to a broad spectrum of health conditions, entrenched treatment protocols can guide healthcare practitioners in diagnosing and treating acute illness. These protocols consist of evidence-based guidelines for specific conditions, such as infectious illnesses, acute trauma, or chronic disease flare-ups. Under such protocols, family practitioners can ensure they are meeting patients' clinical needs while maximizing resource utilization and minimizing the risk of injury. Furthermore, integrating multidisciplinary teams into the acute care setting optimizes treatment protocol efficiency. Team approaches involve various healthcare professionals, including physicians, nurses, and allied health professionals, who collaborate to create and implement care plans. The collaboration is particularly valuable in complex cases with multiple acute problems. Treatment options, informed by the collective expertise of the team, can not only address the presenting medical issue but also the psychosocial issues that can affect patient recovery. As has become clear in studies examining healthcare team dynamics, such synergy leads to more holistic patient care, with an emphasis on communication and interprofessional shared decision-making (Braham et al., 2019). Such a multidisciplinary model supports contemporary healthcare trends aimed at delivering holistic, patient-centered acute care. Lastly, the best practice for implementing treatment protocols in acute care is to conduct continuous assessment and update as new research evidence and patient outcome data emerge. Continuous quality improvement processes within the family practice setting can identify gaps in current protocols and respond accordingly, aligned with best practices. Furthermore, educational opportunities for healthcare workers to continue updates in the best clinical guidelines must be sustained so as to ensure a highly skilled workforce. As the face of healthcare evolves and introduces new technology and modes of treatment, family practitioners are forced to remain up-to-date in their approach to acute care management. It is within this repetitive cycle that programs are guaranteed to be not just up-to-date, but responsive to the unique and dynamic needs of the patient populations treated within family practice (Gottlieb et al., 1979).

7.4.1. Medication Management

Effective drug management is an integral component of acute care within family practice, being that middle stage between clinical intervention and patient adherence to therapeutic regimens. Not only an administrative function, but management of the drugs also involves an in-depth understanding of pharmacology, patient education, and ongoing monitoring of therapeutic effects. Family practice clinicians must evaluate patients' reactions to drug interactions and side effects, as well as each patient's unique history, to tailor treatment regimens to each individual's health profile. This multifaceted process not only enhances patient safety but also engages individuals as active participants in their care, possibly lowering readmission and overall enhancing health outcomes. Due to the complexity of medication therapy regimens commonly required in the acute care environment, a successful medication management plan must be in place to ensure optimal patient care. Administration of medication management within the acute care system should be a multidisciplinary process between healthcare providers. Communication is key; family physicians must work closely with pharmacists, nurses, and specialists to ensure a comprehensive review of all aspects of a patient's medication regimen. According to the outcomes of a recent study, effective communication between patients and healthcare workers significantly enhances drug therapy adherence, with fewer adverse effects and treatment failures. The nurse has a great impact in this interaction. Not only do clinical skills make it easy to manage drugs, but they also address adherence as an issue by educating and counseling patients and their caregivers (Hemingway et al., 2014). By establishing a strong chain of communication and trust development, health care teams can optimize the effectiveness of medication management, ultimately resulting in better patient outcomes in the acute care environment. Medication management is also not a one-time event process, but a continuous process that demands ongoing monitoring and revision based on patient response and emergent clinical circumstances. As outlined in various healthcare programs, e.g., those of Princeton HealthCare System and Sutter Health, effective medication management programs typically consist of extensive patient assessment and streamlined care strategies. They support regular follow-up visits and incorporate patient input to further individualize treatment plans. These preventive steps are crucial for identifying and preventing medication-related complications inin identifying and preventing potential complications from medication withinfor identifying and preventing medication-related complications in the acute care environment. By offering an environment in which patient safety and patient education take center stage, family practices not only facilitate adherence but contribute to the quality of care as a whole, an invaluable step forward for the management of acute illness (Figure 7.14).

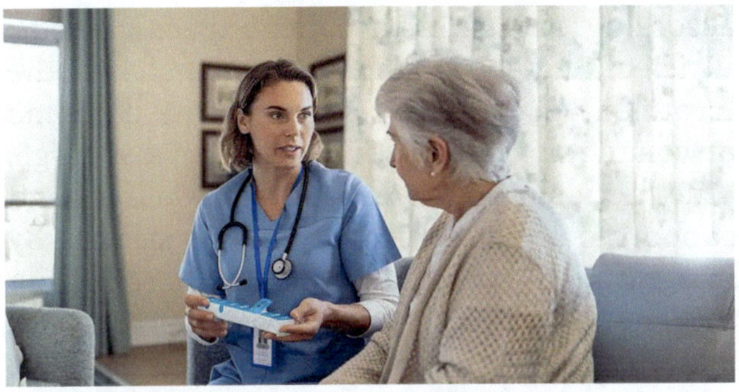

Figure 7.14. Medication management.

Source: https://www.myneva.eu/hs-fs/hubfs/image-png-May-14-2024-09-34-36-4198-AM%20(1).webp?width=1320&height=692&name=image-png-May-14-2024-09-34-36-4198-AM%20(1).webp.

7.4.2. Referral to Specialists

The referral system to specialists is a family practice determinant of acute care, particularly in cases that transcend the main scope. The common dilemma for family practitioners is determining when a patient's needs exceed their capacity and require specialist treatment. For instance, musculoskeletal symptoms, and especially low back pain, frequently lead to referral, but evidence suggests that the majority of them may be handled in a primary care setting. A study collected data on orthopedic outpatient clinic referrals and found that few low back pain patients required specialist treatments such as MRI, demonstrating a pressing need for standardized guidelines to rationalize referral procedures. The findings indicate that the majority of patients can potentially be well treated without specialist care, and hence, effective triage in family practice to provide timely and appropriate treatment is essential (Borg et al., 2014). Moreover, the characteristics of interdisciplinary collaboration are more relevant when specialist referrals are being addressed. Primary care clinicians, specialists, and community services need to be coordinated to provide patients with uninterrupted and comprehensive care. Effective referral processes not only enhance patient outcomes but also prevent unnecessary healthcare utilization. The complexity of operating within healthcare systems is typically an issue for both patients and practitioners, so good communication and collaboration are essential. When there are good relationships between primary care doctors and specialists, patient referral processes can be streamlined and appropriate care pathways established. By drawing lessons from successful care coordination strategies, such problems get resolved, enhancing health outcomes in most areas of medicine (Malley et al., 2009). Finally, a properly planned referral system is important not just for patient care but also for the effectiveness of the whole healthcare system. With an increasing patient population and limited resources, it is essential that referrals are processed with caution and accuracy. Using evidence-based standard protocols and best practices can significantly improve decision-making about referrals. By addressing a wide range of treatments offered through primary care before specialist referral, family doctors can minimize waiting times for outpatient consultations and thereby improve patient satisfaction. Literature shows that it is feasible to establish local guidelines for the management of acute illness, such as low back pain, which will enable family physicians to make well-informed referrals and thereby improve the efficient delivery of health care and patient outcomes in the community (Borg et al., 2014).

7.4.3. Follow-Up Care

There is a requirement for efficient follow-up care in acute care in family practice since it serves as an intermediate between inpatient treatment and sustained management of patients. After the acute care phase, medical professionals use follow-up to assess patients' recovery, manage persistent conditions, and prevent subsequent complications. This continuity of care is particularly important for older adults and patients with multi-morbidities, where transitions between different healthcare settings can lead to fragmented care and increased hospital readmissions. Organizations with established follow-up protocols are better positioned to significantly enhance patient outcomes through ensuring proper communication among healthcare providers and patients, too, addressing issues that tend to arise during the recovery process, and providing the necessary resources for self-management, which can eventually lead to better overall health outcomes (Sochalski et al., 2010). A better integrated care plan in follow-up further involves various interventions that serve to decrease the risk of preventable hospital readmissions. Such interventions typically start at the point of hospitalization and follow up to the discharge process, to ensure that patients receive the necessary education regarding their condition and treatment plan. For instance, multidisciplinary care coordination, in which various healthcare practitioners collaborate, has been found to improve overall quality of follow-up care. With patient and caregiver education, clinicians can help patients understand their own health needs and recognize signs that require immediate follow-up. This approach not only enhances patient satisfaction but also reduces healthcare expenditure related to readmissions, underscoring the usefulness of guideline-based follow-up procedures in family practice. While delivering successful follow-up care, family doctors must also consider the social determinants of health that affect patients' outcomes. Socioeconomic status, access to healthcare, and support networks are determinants that can significantly influence a patient's ability to comply with follow-up care. Identification of these determinants allows health professionals to tailor follow-up interventions according to individual patient-specific needs, which ultimately enhances compliance with the treatment plan. By visiting patients at home or conducting telehealth visits after discharge, practitioners can deliver tailored resources and support to promote recovery. In this manner, by integrating these considerations into follow-up care, not only are practitioners contributing to a more holistic approach to patient health, but also ensuring interventions are equitable and effective across the board in diverse populations, thereby supporting family practice's function of delivering integrated acute care (Figure 7.15).

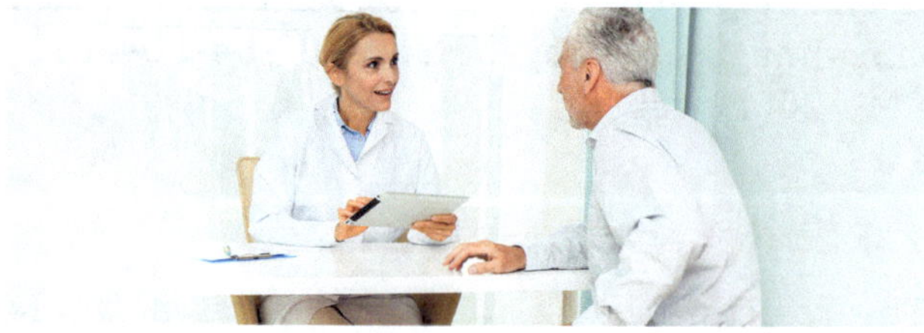

Figure 7.15. Follow-up care.

Source: https://adit.com/storage/files/the-importance-of-follow-up-care-in-patient-retention.jpg.

Test Your Knowledge

1. What is the medication management?
2. What is the process of referral to specialists?

7.5. Challenges in Providing Acute Care

Learning Outcome

1. Describe the time constraints and resource limitations in providing acute care
2. Understand the patient compliance issues

The provision of acute care presents several crucial challenges, foremost among them the accessibility of the service to diverse patient populations. Families with limited resources or those residing in rural settings typically experience barriers preventing them from accessing timely care for acute conditions. Moreover, accessibility is not just a physical proximity to healthcare but also involves financial, cultural, and social factors that prevent an individual from receiving necessary assistance. The integration of culturally relevant practices is required to overcome such barriers, ensuring that every group is appropriately represented and treated in emergent situations. The gap between equity in health policies and the realities faced by patients underscores the need for system changes that favor access and inclusion in the provision of acute care. Coordination of various multidisciplinary teams is another issue in the provision of acute care. Family practice healthcare providers work collaboratively with physicians, nurses, social workers, and specialists. All members have a defined role in patient care; however, inter-member communication can be difficult. For instance, when handling diseases such as eating disorders, non-specialist physicians face difficulties in understanding the complexity of the disease, and this affects their treatment choice. Research suggests that an integrated approach, where input from all members of the medical team is taken into consideration, increases patient outcomes by recognizing the value of teamwork and coordinated care (Braham et al., 2019). Implementation of guidelines for frequent communication and information exchange between team members can help overcome these challenges and provide the impetus towards more effective and coordinated acute care interventions. Ongoing education and training also pose serious challenges in acute care. The professionals are required to be cognizant of evolving best practices, treatment techniques, and emerging public health concerns. However, the rapid pace of medical progress leaves clinicians constantly playing catch-up, with gaps between what they know and what they don't, which affects patient care. Furthermore, specially targeted training is urgently needed in specific conditions that are acute care sensitive, e.g., care of complex disorders like eating disorders. Physicians require support structures that enhance not merely their clinical proficiency but also instill confidence in their ability to make good treatment choices. Enforcing a lifelong culture of learning in family practice settings is imperative to ensure that acute care is appropriately utilized. In summary, the above problems describe the complexity of providing acute care and the various variables that must be managed to improve patient outcomes in family practice (Figure 7.16).

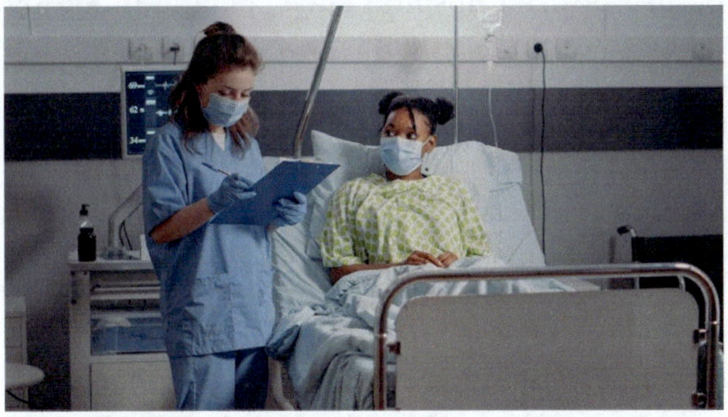

Figure 7.16. Challenges faced by acute care nurses while they save lives.

Source: https://ihm.edu.au/wp-content/uploads/2023/08/medical-assistant-doing-consultation-with-ill-patient-wearing-face-masks-hospital-ward-nurse-discuss.jpg.

7.5.1. Time Constraints

In family practice acute care, time management is the greatest challenge for health practitioners. Large numbers of cases and patient needs place significant pressure on time management, making effective service delivery methods necessary. Such a race leads healthcare providers to make quick decisions at the expense of thorough patient assessment and individualized care. This situation is further compounded by the diversity of skills required across various sub-sectors of health and social care. For instance, the overriding need to deploy higher-level skills in fields such as physiotherapy and radiography requires effective systems for time management to facilitate smooth procedures and alleviate the pressures that come with time constraints (Brown et al., 2000). The consequences of time pressures extend to the health promotion interventions for vulnerable groups, such as obese children. Acute care nurses generally experience the time pressures that deter them from providing complete health advice. Research exploring attitudes among children's nurses about offering health promotion indicates how time pressures can seem to constitute an obstacle to successful communication with families and patients. The demanding nature of brief hospital stays, compounded by inadequate institutional support and training, can discourage health workers' contributions to required health dialogue. Such gaps serve to underscore the need for an organizational framework actively promoting health within acute care environments, facilitating extensive health-oriented discussions capable of producing lasting effects on patient healthcare outcomes (Greenwood et al., 2015). Moreover, time management in the acute care environment involves a holistic approach to the complexity of patient demand. Allocation of funds to training programs with the objective of enhancing staff competence can improve efficiency in patient handling and care provision. By fostering a culture that balances time management and whole-person patient care, healthcare facilities can disentangle the interface between acute medical needs and health promotion interventions. Such an equilibrium is especially relevant to the increasing need for services, one that puts emphasis on care models that also see the value of medical interventions as mattering as much as maintaining long-term health and well-being. Ultimately, facilitating a setting that addresses time pressures can enhance the quality of care provided in family practices for the benefit of patients and healthcare professionals alike.

7.5.2. Resource Limitations

In acute care family practice, resource limitations are a significant constraint that can affect the effectiveness and accessibility of healthcare services. Care delivery highly depends on material, human, and financial resources. For instance, optimal patient outcomes often hinge on timely interventions and coordinated management strategies, which are severely hindered by insufficient staffing or limited access to basic medical facilities. The impacts of these limitations are even more pervasive in community settings, where family doctors must navigate the complex dynamics of care provision. Additionally, according to various projects commissioned by NHS Highland, such resource issues necessitate a concerted approach to building the capacity and competence of community nurses, bringing into sharp focus the need for support systems capable of maximizing resource use and improving patient care outcomes (Gray et al., 2010). The impact of resource constraints is not merely operational but also intrinsically related to the quality of care provided in the case of acute conditions. When healthcare professionals are denied necessary resources, their decision-making is compromised, which can lead to suboptimal patient management. For example, educational programs like the Emergency Neurological Life Support (ENLS) program demonstrate the potential for enhancing certain training in settings with resource constraints. In a Nepalese study, significant gains in knowledge and decision-making competence were observed post-course, even in a setting with limited medical resources. This suggests that while the availability of resources is important, enhancing medical education and decision-making frameworks can also mitigate some of the effects of these constraints, ultimately improving preparedness and patient outcomes in acute care settings (Acharya et al., 2018). Moreover, ongoing assessment of resource limitations must involve a clear understanding of local healthcare environments. Different areas have varying degrees of access to resources, and this affects the extent to which acute care can be controlled. Family doctors are often confronted with ethical dilemmas when deciding on care amid scarce resources, particularly in emergency situations. New models of care, informed by systematic reviews of the evidence and community nursing models, can assist with these complexities. among health workers and incorporating community-based interventions can help the health system better address such resource constraints. This approach not only enhances the quality of care but also builds a responsive model for sustainable practice in family medicine, ensuring effective acute care even in the face of heavy barriers (Gray et al., 2010).

7.5.3. Patient Compliance Issues

Compliance issues among patients are also a significant problem in family practice and acute care, both influencing treatment outcome and patient outcomes generally. Noncompliance with medication or follow-up exercise prescribing regimens can exacerbate disease and drive up healthcare costs. Experiments have identified poor adherence to treatment protocols as endemic, with a tendency to have negative outcomes for patients and professionals alike. Non-adherence is noted as being complicated by its multi-dimensional nature, requiring multiple methods to address the root causes. Without interventions that account for psychological, social, and physical impediments to compliance, it can be challenging for healthcare professionals to effectively address these compliance issues (Airaksinen et al., 2010). In response to combating patient non-adherence, there is a need to initiate far-reaching adherence plans that extend beyond the simple reminder or directive. Motivational cognitive-behavioral interventions have been found to improve attendance at exercise clinics and, therefore, promote better health outcomes. Evidence indicates that interventions aimed at maximizing proximal adherence may achieve some success but lose steam in sustaining long-term compliance.

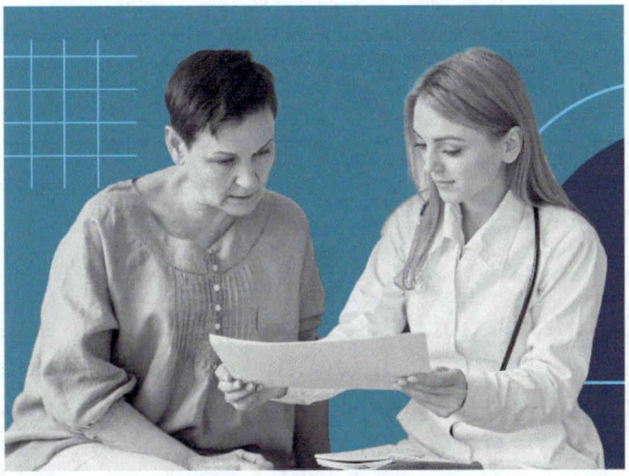

Figure 7.17. Patient compliance issues.

Source: https://creyos.com/hubfs/Patient%20Compliance-1.png.

Hence, a multifaceted intervention design can be helpful, incorporating multiple strategies to improve long-term adherence to both home exercise and clinic visits. An integrated understanding of barriers to adherence is pivotal for designing these interventions so that healthcare providers can apply the strategy accordingly (Airaksinen et al., 2010). Quality improvement activities in family practice are also essential for guiding patient compliance issues. Engaging healthcare providers and staff in redesign processes based on adherence measurement can streamline care for the patient. Through performance data analysis and feedback loops, practices can adjust their strategy based on what is most effective in terms of patient compliance. This process of constant revision is necessary because it establishes a culture of continuous improvement where staff are incentivized to raise compliance to a higher level. The incorporation of best-practice literature into everyday practice can also empower practitioners, equipping them with the tools they need to overcome patient compliance challenges (Figure 7.17).

Test Your Knowledge

1. What are the challenges of acute care nursing?
2. What are patient compliance issues?

7.6. The Impact of Technology on Acute Care

Learning Outcome

1. Know the telemedicine applications
2. Describe the electronic health records
3. Describe the mobile health technologies

The integration of technology into the acute care setting significantly enhances family practice physicians' ability to deliver timely, efficient care. Advanced diagnostic tools, such as telemedicine and mobile imaging, enable medical staff to rapidly access critical patient data in emergencies. This access allows the clinician to act rapidly on facts, optimizing patient outcomes during peak moments. Second, the use of electronic health records (EHR) enables better communication among healthcare teams and seamless care coordination across settings. Not only do EHRs enable real-time reporting of patient conditions, but they also reduce medical errors, thereby enhancing patient safety. With an aging population and a high incidence of chronic illnesses, the contribution of technology to simplifying acute care processes is more crucial now than ever in family practice settings. Secondly, technological innovations lead to improvements in how patient care is managed in family practices. For instance, mobile health apps allow patients to exercise control through self-management of health conditions and remote monitoring resources. The control enhances patient engagement and supports adherence to treatment regimens, which is most crucial during acute care events. As explored in literature, emerging technologies have proven to improve patient empowerment and care coordination—drivers to successful acute care management. Adoption of these applications embodies a shift toward a more integrated model of care, promoting proactive management and intervention strategies for avoiding acute exacerbations of chronic disease. With these technologies, family practices can better position themselves to address the complexities of acute care within their patient base. Healthcare delivery system fragmentation is also something that technology can help reduce, identified as an issue in recent policy proposals. The use of care models, coupled with technological advancements, has the potential to address gaps in service provision while maximizing patient satisfaction. For instance, effective communication and interoperability among healthcare providers can facilitate holistic care plans tailored to address the needs of individual patients. According to reports, policy reforms towards payment models and care coordination mechanisms are also capable of enhancing the role of technology in the efficacy of acute care. With regard to healthcare systems with the correct infrastructure to facilitate collaborative care, family practices can alleviate pressure on acute services. Thus, the intersection of health policy and technology offers a way to enhance the field's response to acute care matters, culminating in improved patient health outcomes in family practice settings.

7.6.1. Telemedicine Applications

The integration of telemedicine into acute care family practice has transformed how healthcare professionals interact with patients. Telemedicine technology enables clinicians to deliver instant care with various technologies, beyond geographical locations, and to widen access to essential services. For instance, remote consultations enable professionals to assess patients' conditions in real time, allowing for timely intervention that can forestall complications. This is particularly beneficial in rural or underserved communities where specialists are less available. By combining technologies such as video conferencing and mobile health applications, family physicians can enhance patient engagement and adherence to treatment regimens, thereby improving overall patient outcomes. Moreover, the utilization of these technologies aligns with the shift towards patient-centered care, facilitating teamwork that is stronger and a more supportive physician-patient relationship. Telemedicine also plays a critical role in the management of chronic diseases and acute episodes, enhancing continuity of care within family medicine facilities. In cases where patients abruptly evolve medical complications, ready access to telehealth centers can trigger needed assessment and management processes, with a significant increase in rates of recovery. Particularly in palliative care, telehealth platforms enable continuous health monitoring and early intervention as patient needs evolve. As highlighted in recent reports, technologically enabled care has the potential to relieve pressure on the healthcare system by reducing hospitalizations and emergency department visits for non-life-threatening conditions. While telemedicine is very promising, it also requires ongoing evaluation of the success of these applications to ensure they meet patients' diverse needs and adhere to clinical guidelines, thereby providing practitioners and patients with a reliable means of care delivery.

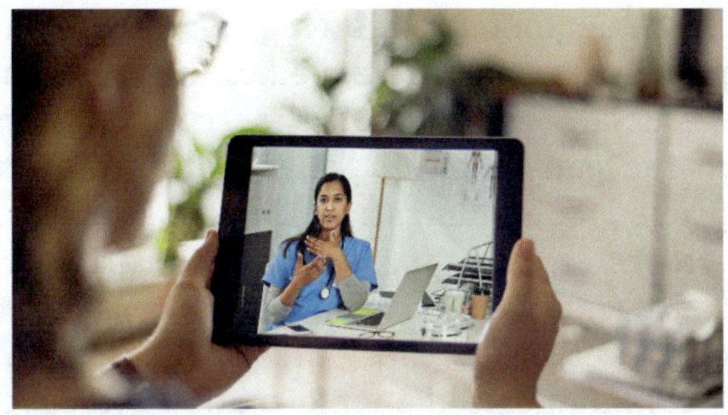

Figure 7.18. Telemedicine applications.

Source: https://images.ctfassets.net/4f3rgqwzdznj/1VkeTZCjmyf6wwYZARI2WL/74af2d10193848bb57059ade7331caaf/woman_online_doctors_appointment_1062130130.jpg.

The role of effective doctor-patient communication cannot be overstated in telemedicine. The more technology encompasses family practice workflows, the more crucial it is to keep lines of communication open. The virtual setting can facilitate more open information sharing, allowing patients to express their concerns more easily than in traditional face-to-face sessions. Furthermore, quality communication during remote visits can lead to better-informed patients who are more engaged in their health care decisions. Studies show that when technology is complemented by effective communication practices, patient involvement and satisfaction increase considerably, ultimately leading to better health outcomes. Here, their family physicians must take precautions to modify their communication style to the unique demands of telemedicine, considering that efficient use of these technologies relies on the existence of good interpersonal relationships with patients to build trust and shared understanding (Downey et al., 2008; Johnston et al., 2014) (Figure 7.18).

7.6.2. Electronic Health Records

Implementation of Electronic Health Records (EHRs) is a landmark advancement in acute care in family practice. EHRs accelerate patient data management, allowing for immediate access to comprehensive medical histories that are crucial during emergency consultations. Such reorganization of patient data facilitates improved communication among healthcare providers, allowing for coordinated care plans. Because various social and family influences affect health outcomes, the ability to share and communicate that information effectively is essential. Numerous states that recognize this have implemented strategies to enhance the medical home model, which focuses on well-coordinated, integrated care. These models not only enhance the quality of care but also aim to contain mounting healthcare spending, thereby demonstrating the dual benefit of employing EHRs in acute care (Takach et al., 2009). Within family practice, where illness typically demands swift attention with consideration, the effectiveness of EHRs is further bolstered by their ability to reduce care fragmentation. With EHR systems, providers can monitor treatment plans, medication histories, and diagnostic findings in real time, helping reduce the risk of redundant treatments or miscommunication. This is particularly relevant for acute care situations where decisions need to be made promptly. To successfully transition to this integrated system, healthcare organizations would do well to examine policy reforms that encourage EHR adoption across different provider settings. By surmounting regulatory barriers and aligning payment systems with coordinated care goals, the stakeholders can optimize the efficiency of electronic systems in family practice. As highlighted in recent research, such adjustments are essential in creating mechanisms to facilitate global care (Gauthier et al., 2008). Despite positive developments attributed to EHRs, implementation and usage are also problematic. Difficulty with data privacy concerns, incomplete integration across platforms, and end-user resistance may hold back the full potential of EHRs in acute care. Family practices need to address these difficulties tactfully to create a culture that supports technological advancements without violating patient confidentiality and consent. Education and ongoing support for the medical staff are critical components of such a transition to ensure EHRs are successfully deployed in acute settings. In addition, the success of EHRs in enhancing patient outcomes will largely depend on the collaborative efforts of providers in leveraging technology in a manner that is supportive of holistic patient care and system interoperability. Emphasizing these factors can significantly improve the quality of acute care provided by family practice (Figure 7.19).

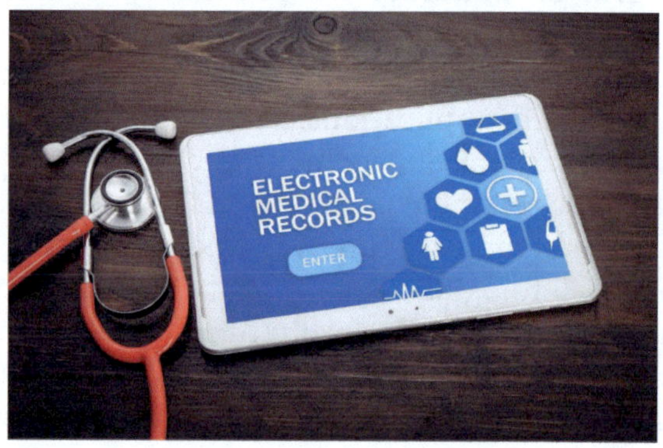

Figure 7.19. Electronic health records.

Source: https://www.softclinicsoftware.com/wp-content/uploads/2024/11/emr-implementation-in-hospitals-1.jpg.

7.6.3. Mobile Health Technologies

The advent of mobile health technologies has revolutionized the acute care setting in family practice, enhancing communication between healthcare providers and patients. As technology is introduced to enable real-time health tracking, such innovations may assist in monitoring vital signs and chronic conditions from the comfort of a patient's home. Mobile health applications can store and compare patient data in order to facilitate more informed treatment recommendations by healthcare professionals. handheld capability and interoperability are essential in fulfilling the diverse requirements of patients as well as the ease of integration into existing healthcare systems. As clinicians increasingly utilize mobile health technologies, patient activation is heightened, promoting proactive health management and the quality of care delivered in family practice settings. Moreover, the integration of mobile health technologies is significant in palliative and home care, particularly given the growing number of older adults. Telehealth platforms allow caregivers to monitor patients remotely and provide timely interventions that alleviate symptoms and maximize quality of life. For instance, research shows that home technologies can help improve communication among family, patients, and healthcare providers during transitions of care. Such a flexible model is critical for patients requiring palliative care, where timely decisions about care can significantly affect treatment outcomes. Although there are barriers, such as patient technology literacy and the effectiveness of these technologies, numerous examples of successful implementation prove the advantage of mobile health technologies to assist patients in their homes (Johnston et al., 2014). Implementing mobile health technologies in family practice not only enhances the direct care patients receive but also encourages a healthier approach to managing health. The ability to consolidate data across multiple health metrics enables providers to design interventions tailored to individual patients' histories and needs. This patient-centric consideration mirrors today's healthcare expectations, moving away from being reactive to being proactive. Further down the line, as mobile health technologies advance, collaboration among healthcare providers, technologists, and patients will also be critical to maximizing their use. Assessing the potential of mobile health technology to enhance the delivery of care processes, clinicians remain advocates for its adoption in routine practice, citing the necessity of ongoing education and training to facilitate effective use in acute family practice settings (Figure 7.20).

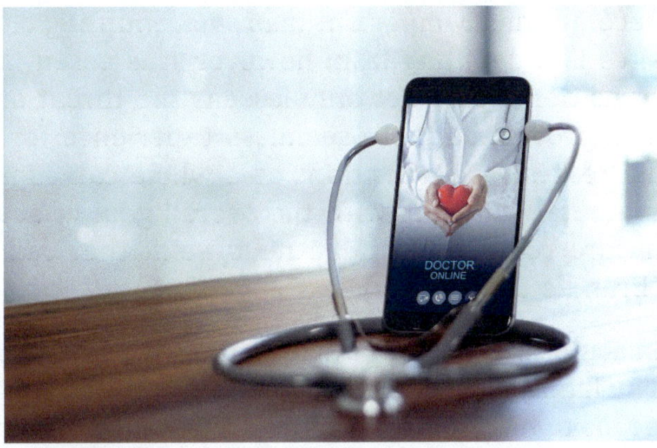

Figure 7.20. Mobile health technologies.

Source: https://images.squarespace-cdn.com/content/v1/5aa96c579772aea9adaa2ef7/1613657281972-BZ9ULI2G6OZOGU5OYCWU/MobileTechnologyinHealthcare_0221.jpg.

Test Your Knowledge

1. What is a telemedicine application?
2. What is the electronic health record?

SUMMARY

In summary, the incorporation of acute care services in family practice is necessary to address the complex conditions of patients, particularly those with complex health conditions. The incorporation intends to improve patient outcomes, particularly for vulnerable groups such as the elderly. As medical practitioners struggle to navigate the complexities of acute care, ranging from managing chronic disease and cognitive impairments to ensuring critical care capability in every unit, it becomes clear that a customized approach is imperative. Ongoing embracement of evidence-based practice guidelines, although strong on paper, often faces practical implementation barriers. Thus, regular training and support of healthcare professionals are critical for these guidelines to not only be understood but also applied effectively in clinical practice (Brandis et al., 2019). Moreover, the findings that relate to the challenges of caring for falls in older adults with cognitive impairment highlight the need for a less conspicuous application of care protocols. The recognition that awareness of falls prevention policy is not sufficient underscores the need to understand patient-specific requirements. Involvement of family, as suggested in the literature, is imperative while planning a comprehensive care plan, proactive with respect to fall risk and fall prevention. By forging interprofessional relationships between healthcare teams and families, practitioners are able to create a care delivery environment that supports quality care (Sochalski et al., 2010). Lastly, with the evolution of healthcare, the emphasis on innovative care management interventions becomes more important than ever. Shuffling older, frail, chronically ill patients through various care sites is a daunting task; however, it is essential in ensuring continuity and quality care. Effective transitional care not only lessens the threat of adverse events, such as hospital readmission, but also provides a more seamless experience for patients. Taking a multidisciplinary approach that addresses care transitions as a whole can significantly enhance the quality of life for the elderly, ultimately aligning with the overall goal of acute care in family practice. The complexity in their nature requires an adaptive system that can address the complexities surrounding their care (Brandis et al., 2019).

In acute care in family practice, though, addressing the complexity of patients' needs remains topmost. The family practitioner is usually the initial responding practitioner to acute health issues and thus needs to have a thorough understanding of the common health issues. A good example would be the rising incidence of asthma, for which evidence-based practice and ongoing professional education are necessary. Studies have shown that although detailed guidelines are available, practitioners do not implement them in practice and get good patient outcomes. Therefore, knowledge translation should be enhanced and practical tools utilized, as seen in the initiatives of the Canadian Thoracic Society, to improve the quality of acute care (Rawlinson et al., 2014). Moreover, the integration of palliative care into family practice is increasingly recognized as an essential component of care for patients with life-threatening illnesses. The expansion of palliative care services in Africa, as exemplified, demonstrates an imperative shift towards integrated patient-centered care. This shift not only improves patients' quality of life but also demands holistic methods to symptom control and alleviation of suffering. Organizational structures like the African Palliative Care Association are a sign of collective efforts towards integrating these essential services, yet they also mark the ever-enduring challenges of access and allocation within healthcare systems. With coordination between healthcare practitioners and the provision of requisite training, family doctors can enhance the integration of palliative care concepts into their practice, thereby empowering them to efficiently manage acute conditions (Rawlinson et al., 2014). Finally, the evolving health climate requires an intense focus on continuing education for family practitioners. This means leveraging technological advances to deliver relevant, accessible educational content. As has been demonstrated through creative programs for enhancing palliative care training in Africa, interactive and informative modules can improve practitioners' competence and confidence in the provision of care. This kind of program demonstrates the need for education materials that are pertinent to the local situation and provide focused solutions for community health problems. Furthermore, continuous evaluation of educational gains is necessary, as it helps maintain high quality and ensures the information remains pertinent to family practice and patient needs. By ensuring ongoing education and the application of guidelines in practice, family physicians can positively impact the care and welfare of patients during acute episodes (McIvor et al., 2008).

KEY TERMS FROM THIS CHAPTER

- Acute care
- Chronic illnesses
- Evidence-based practices
- Hypertension
- Influenza
- Patient satisfaction
- Primary care
- Acute pulmonary edema
- Computed tomography
- Health service delivery
- Infections
- Musculoskeletal injuries
- Patient-centered approach
- Respiratory infections

CRITICAL THINKING QUESTIONS

1. **Which of the following is a common acute condition managed in family practice?**
   a. Type 2 Diabetes Mellitus
   b. Acute Upper Respiratory Tract Infections (URTI)
   c. Chronic Hypertension
   d. Osteoarthritis
2. **What is the first step in managing a patient presenting with acute chest pain in a family practice setting?**
   a. Start high-dose aspirin immediately
   b. Obtain a detailed family history
   c. Perform an ECG and assess vital signs
   d. Refer to a cardiologist
3. **Which of the following is a red flag in acute abdominal pain requiring urgent referral?**
   a. Diffuse mild discomfort
   b. Localized pain relieved by rest
   c. Persistent vomiting and signs of shock
   d. Temporary diarrhea without blood
4. **A 25-year-old patient presents with a fever, sore throat, and swollen cervical lymph nodes. What is the most likely diagnosis?**
   a. Acute pharyngitis
   b. Viral gastroenteritis
   c. Bronchitis
   d. Otitis media
5. **Which of the following is the best initial treatment for an acute asthma exacerbation?**
   a. Inhaled corticosteroids
   b. Short-acting beta-agonists (SABA)
   c. Oral leukotriene receptor antagonists
   d. Long-acting beta-agonists (LABA)

Short Answer Questions

1. What is acute care?
2. Why is acute care important?
3. Describe the role of family practitioners in acute care.
4. What are treatment protocols in acute care?
5. What is the impact of technology on acute care?

Answer to Critical Thinking Questions

1. (b); 2. (c); 3. (c); 4. (a); 5. (b).

REFERENCES

1. McCredie, V. A., Shrestha, G. S., Acharya, S., Bellini, A., Singh, J. M., Hemphill, J. C., & Goffi, A. (2018). Evaluating the effectiveness of the Emergency Neurological Life Support educational framework in low-income countries. *International Health, 10*(2), 116–124. https://doi.org/10.1093/inthealth/ihy003Aertgeerts, B., Bullens, D. M. A., Buntinx, F., de Burghgraeve, T., et al. (2014). Diagnosing serious infections in acutely ill children in ambulatory care (ERNIE 2 study protocol, part A): Diagnostic accuracy of a clinical decision tree and added value of a point-of-care C-reactive protein test and oxygen saturation. https://core.ac.uk/download/55807501.pdf (accessed on 14th July 2025).
2. Agius Muscat, H., & Carabott, P. (1989). *The Content of General Practice in Malta: A Pilot Study Comparing Health Centre and Private Practice in Malta With Each Other And with General Practice (As Reported for Other Countries)*. https://core.ac.uk/download/46601977.pdf (accessed on 14th July 2025).
3. Airaksinen, T., Altman, R. D., Basler, H. D., Beswick, A. D., Campbell, R., Littlewood, C., Damen, L., et al. (2010). Interventions for enhancing adherence with physiotherapy: A systematic review. https://core.ac.uk/download/100492.pdf (accessed on 14th July 2025).
4. Aydın, V., Akıcı, A., Sakarya, S., Akman, M., Fak, A. S., Shabbir, S., Pouliquen, I., et al. (2020). Selected abstracts from Pharmacology 2019. *British Journal of Clinical Pharmacology*. https://www.semanticscholar.org/paper/79c102d9df520004af2b67c23a1a1e72fa391a3d (accessed on 14th July 2025).
5. Beller, E. M., Coxeter, P., Del Mar, C. B., Hoffmann, T. C., et al. (2015). Interventions to facilitate shared decision making to address antibiotic use for acute respiratory infections in primary care. https://core.ac.uk/download/196601007.pdf (accessed on 14th July 2025).
6. Birch, D., & Draper, J. (2008). A critical literature review exploring the challenges of delivering effective palliative care to older people with dementia in the acute hospital setting. https://core.ac.uk/download/82906952.pdf (accessed on 14th July 2025).
7. Borg, J., Cuschieri, S., & Grech, S. (2014). Outcome of low back pain patients referred to orthopaedic outpatient clinic. https://core.ac.uk/download/46602498.pdf (accessed on 14th July 2025).
8. Braham, S., Dasey, L., Davidson, A. R., Reidlinger, C., et al. (2019). Physicians' perspectives on the treatment of patients with eating disorders in the acute setting. https://core.ac.uk/download/222450509.pdf (accessed on 14th July 2025).
9. Brandis, S., Chaboyer, W., Cooke, M., Darch, J., et al. (2019). Caring for the older person with cognitive impairment in hospital: Qualitative analysis of nursing personnel reflections on fall events. https://core.ac.uk/download/196606817.pdf (accessed on 14th July 2025).
10. Brooker, D., Casey, D., Houghton, C., Murphy, K., et al. (2016). Healthcare staffs' experiences and perceptions of caring for people with dementia in the acute setting: Qualitative evidence synthesis. https://core.ac.uk/download/76977844.pdf (accessed on 14th July 2025).
11. Brown, A., Green, A., Pitcher, J., Simm, J., et al. (2000). *Employers' Skill Survey: Case Study: Health and Social Care*. https://core.ac.uk/download/4154238.pdf (accessed on 14th July 2025).

12. Bultas, M. W., Burkett, K., Johnson, N. L., et al. (2016). Translating research to practice for children with autism spectrum disorder: Part 2: Behavior management in home and health care settings. https://core.ac.uk/download/213081290.pdf (accessed on 14th July 2025).

13. Del Mar, C., Hansen, M. P., Hoffmann, T. C., Howlett, M., et al. (2015). Parents' beliefs and knowledge about the management of acute otitis media: A qualitative study. https://core.ac.uk/download/196601013.pdf (accessed on 14th July 2025).

14. Dewez, J. E., Nijman, R., Fitchett, E. J. A., Lynch, R., de Groot, R., van der Flier, M., Philipsen, R., et al. (2023). Adoption of C-reactive protein point-of-care tests for the management of acute childhood infections in primary care in the Netherlands and England: A comparative health systems analysis. *BMC Health Services Research, 23*. https://www.semanticscholar.org/paper/bb43048d43b197894c54f0695c1871da713867ad (accessed on 14th July 2025).

15. Donner, A., Bellg, A. J., Engers, A. J., Australian Acute Musculoskeletal Pain Guidelines Group (AAMPGG), McGuirk, B., Walker, B. F., Walker, B. F., et al. (2008). *IMPLEMENTing a Clinical Practice Guideline for Acute Low Back Pain Evidence-Based Management in General Practice (IMPLEMENT): Cluster Randomized Controlled Trial Study Protocol*. https://core.ac.uk/download/177076.pdf (accessed on 14th July 2025).

16. Downey, K., Eckler, P., & Worsowicz, G. (2008). Improving physician–patient communication. https://core.ac.uk/download/16429557.pdf (accessed on 14th July 2025).

17. Flicker, L. (2021). Why is it so hard to organize healthcare for older people in residential aged care facilities in Australia? *Internal Medicine Journal, 51*. https://www.semanticscholar.org/paper/44d922cd2dfae6bf03987851fa8e151c2a18d1fe (accessed on 14th July 2025).

18. Gauthier, A. K., Shih, A., McCarthy, D., Davis, K., Nuzum, R., & Schoenbaum, S. C. (2008). *Organizing the U.S. Health Care Delivery System for High Performance*. https://core.ac.uk/download/71353608.pdf (accessed on 14th July 2025).

19. Gordon, N., & Laikin, S. (1952). The casework techniques used by the social worker in a medical setting: A study of the casework techniques in fifty closed cases of the social service department of the Massachusetts General Hospital. https://open.bu.edu/bitstream/2144/11515/1/Gordon_Nancy_1952_web.pdf (accessed on 14th July 2025).

20. Gottlieb, M. L., & Moore, C. B. (1979). *Activities of Nurse Practitioners as Identified by Medical Directors of University Student Health Services*. https://core.ac.uk/download/215482198.pdf (accessed on 14th July 2025).

21. Gray, C. M., James, B., Lauder, W., McCulloch, J., et al. (2010). Developing community nursing practice: Promoting case management and skill enhancement to support shifting the balance of care. https://core.ac.uk/download/110605.pdf (accessed on 14th July 2025).

22. Greenwood, N., & Lewis, K. (2015). Opportunistic health promotion among overweight children. https://core.ac.uk/download/30731293.pdf (accessed on 14th July 2025).

23. Hemingway, S. (2014). Medication management in mental health: Nurses' perceptions of their work with service users and carers. https://core.ac.uk/download/30731079.pdf (accessed on 14th July 2025).

24. Johnston, B. (2014). Palliative home-based technology from a practitioner's perspective: Benefits and disadvantages. https://core.ac.uk/download/46559049.pdf (accessed on 14th July 2025).

25. Kinnear, D., Victor, C., & Williams, V. (2016). 'It's the little things that count': Healthcare professionals' views on delivering dignified care: A qualitative study. https://core.ac.uk/download/42370653.pdf (accessed on 14th July 2025).

26. Kitsiou, A., Caforio, A. L. P., Porta-Sanchez, A., Vahanian, A., Iung, B., Carrera, C., Szymanski, C., et al. (2013). *ESC Core Curriculum for The General Cardiologist (2013)*. https://core.ac.uk/download/55756305.pdf (accessed on 14th July 2025).

27. Lashbrook, A., & Silow-Carroll, S. (2009). *St. Charles Hospital: Improving Surgical Care Through Best-Practice Literature and Order Sets*. https://core.ac.uk/download/71355297.pdf (accessed on 14th July 2025).

28. Lim, J. Y. (2019). Fragility fracture care: An urgent need to implement the integrated model of geriatric care. *Annals of Geriatric Medicine and Research, 23*, 1–2. https://www.semanticscholar.org/paper/719cb29ac8b08c5c50e6c39af01d7b8c66aeb773 (accessed on 14th July 2025).

29. Lynn, A., Miller, S. M., Brackett, A., & Kodadek, L. M. (2024). Opportunities for incorporation of primary palliative care in acute care surgery: A narrative review. *The American Journal of Hospice & Palliative Care*. https://www.semanticscholar.org/paper/51a735b57886dff31f22ff712dff24bda21522ae (accessed on 14th July 2025).

30. McIvor, A., & Hodder, R. (2008). Canadian Adult Asthma Update 2008 key messages: A focus on translating knowledge into action in primary care. *Canadian Respiratory Journal, 15*(3), 121, 122. https://www.semanticscholar.org/paper/3ba650fc5771177aa1d9e22e1fc71e992598e92d (accessed on 14th July 2025).

31. Micheal, J. C. (2014). No lost opportunities in the emergency department. *British Journal of Nursing, 23*(15), 830. https://www.semanticscholar.org/paper/a9d6db7a67e299c260ae9d4b997fc1f985031a9e (accessed on 14th July 2025).

32. Morton, S., & Dunn, W. (2015). Addressing the health needs of an aging America: New opportunities for evidence-based policy solutions. https://core.ac.uk/download/75783019.pdf (accessed on 14th July 2025).

33. O'Malley, A. S., Tynan, A., Cohen, G. R., Davis, M. M., & Kemper, N. M. (2009). *Coordination of Care by Primary Care Practices: Strategies, Lessons and Implications*. https://core.ac.uk/download/71350438.pdf (accessed on 14th July 2025).

34. Pilgrim, A. (2023). Acute pulmonary edema and NSTEMI. *Journal of Education & Teaching in Emergency Medicine, 8*, O1–O32. https://www.semanticscholar.org/paper/5c724fdbd5a43f2f52509d5049c4b8d16424ba75 (accessed on 14th July 2025).

35. Pisani, S. (2010). *The Nurse of the Mediterranean*. https://core.ac.uk/download/46602269.pdf (accessed on 14th July 2025).

36. Qaseem, A., Campos, K., MacDonald, S., Mount, C. A., Tierney, S., Fitterman, N., Basch, P., et al. (2024). Quality indicators for pain in adults: A review of performance measures by the American College of Physicians. *Annals of Internal Medicine, 177*, 1539–1546. https://www.semanticscholar.org/paper/7790d4f17a58ec11a5dbc2ea46037013547d53f8 (accessed on 14th July 2025).

37. Rawlinson, F., & Luyirika, E. (2014). Collaboration across continents to produce e-learning for palliative care education in Sub Saharan Africa. *ecancermedicalscience, 8*. https://www.semanticscholar.org/paper/e4c706de6d5ce1e193c4d23158fe728c44b1fb8e (accessed on 14th July 2025).

38. Sochalski, J. A., & Naylor, M. D. (2010). Scaling up: Bringing the Transitional Care Model into the mainstream. https://core.ac.uk/download/71354715.pdf (accessed on 14th July 2025).

39. Takach, M., & Kaye, N. (2009). *Building Medical Homes in State Medicaid and CHIP programs.* https://core.ac.uk/download/71349689.pdf (accessed on 14th July 2025).

40. Wu, A. H. B. (2012). Biomarkers beyond the natriuretic peptides for chronic heart failure: Galectin-3 and soluble ST2. https://core.ac.uk/download/323074780.pdf (accessed on 14th July 2025).

TRAUMA AND INJURY CARE

8

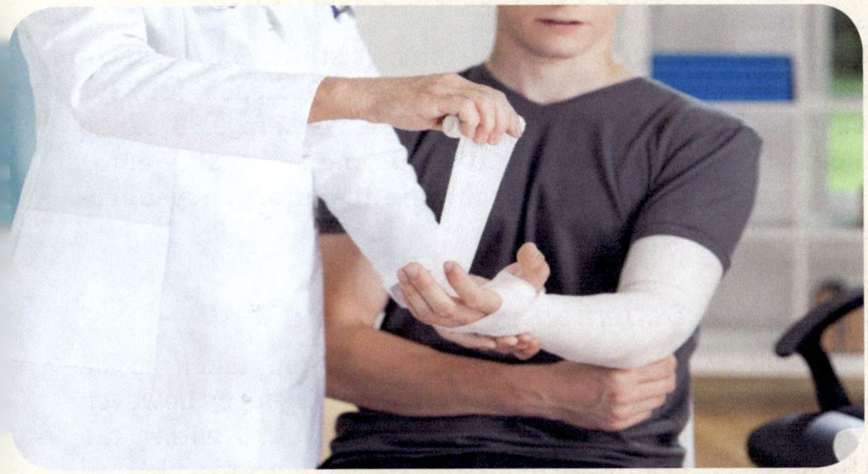

LEARNING OBJECTIVES

After studying this chapter, you will be able to:

1. Describe the types of trauma
2. Understand the mechanisms of injury
3. Describe the initial assessment and triage process in trauma and injury care
4. Know the treatment protocols of trauma and injury
5. Describe the psychological impact of trauma
6. Understand the prevention strategies in trauma and injury

Introduction

From the perspective of trauma and injury management, awareness of the basic concepts and structures is most essential for a proper response to traumatic situations. Trauma care encompasses several dimensions, from immediate injury management to ongoing management and rehabilitation. Multidimensionality that typifies trauma cases can necessitate an intervention with a multidisciplinary approach through several health practitioners collaborating. Such collaboration is particularly important with respect to matters such as the psychological impact of trauma on patients and the need for proper and urgent physical attention. Education and ongoing training are also integral components, wherein specialists must remain up-to-date with new methods, technology, and innovations to achieve maximum patient outcomes. Notably, the evolution of trauma care solutions reflects the dynamic balance between scientific advances and the realities of the situation, highlighting the need for consistent education in a rapidly evolving medical context. The decisive role of institutions dedicated to improving trauma care, such as that of the Association of Osteosynthesis (AO), must not be belittled. Started enhancing fracture treatment over six decades ago, AO has spread its influence through science, education, patient care, and MedTech. Examining the impact it has had on publications it sponsored, it can be seen that there has been a drastic increase in frequency of citations of such publications, with certain top publications receiving up to 2000 citations annually. Moreover, the broad distribution of AO courses, covering more than 645,000 students, underscores the organization's objective of educating professionals in trauma care. Such an interdependent effort not only strengthens professional education but eventually leads to improved patient care, as seen in cost savings and improvements in health through enhanced treatment strategies.

The interdependence between education and field practice strategies mirrors the shifting dynamics of trauma management within well-established institutions. New technologies have revolutionized trauma diagnosis, particularly that of intra-abdominal injuries. Diagnostic peritoneal lavage (DPL), although old and historical, has been surpassed by non-invasive imaging technologies such as ultrasonography. Although a reliable one, DPL is fraught with complications and high false-positive rates, which can lead to unnecessary surgeries at risk to patient health.

On the other hand, ultrasound has proven more specific and sensitive, with quick, comprehensive diagnostics and absolutely no risk associated with invasive maneuvers. This trend towards non-invasive diagnostics is part of a broader effort in trauma treatment to reduce patient injury while maximizing the efficiency of care. Hospitals with 24-hour ultrasonographic capabilities are therefore in a better position to manage blunt abdominal trauma effectively, boosting patient outcomes and satisfaction in the trauma continuum of care (Figure 8.1).

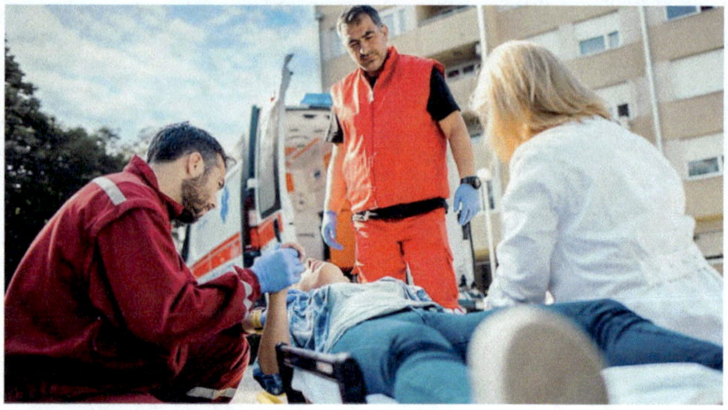

Figure 8.1. Trauma and injury care.

Source: https://static.wixstatic.com/media/491b63_57519d1bb7534c609efaeabe7f28736c~mv2.jpg/v1/fill/w_724,h_406,fp_0.38_0.27,q_80,usm_0.66_1.00_0.01,enc_avif,quality_auto/UPDATED_-Trauma-and-Emergency-Care-1536x864.jpg.

Definition of Trauma and Injury

Trauma and injury are often taken to be synonymous in everyday language; however, they have different connotations within the healthcare industry. Trauma refers to a physical wound or damage that is induced by an external agent, which may present as blunt trauma or penetrating trauma to induce a varying degree of physical harm. Injury is generally taken to be the long-term consequences of the trauma, for example, psychological trauma and long-term rehabilitation. In understanding trauma, its multi-dimensionality should be acknowledged so that patients may either present with immediate life-threatening conditions or have extended periods of recovery. The available evidence indicates that the majority of trauma patients also have serious complications even after the acute critical phase, and thus, multidisciplinary care of trauma extending beyond acute care to long-term prognosis of the patient is required. This is particularly important in intensive care settings, where the ability to recognize complications early largely dictates recovery trajectories (Eriksson et al., 2022). Farther down the hierarchy of trauma classification, recognition must be given for the various types that can exist, including but not limited to physical, psychological, and emotional trauma. Physical trauma is primarily injuries sustained by accidents, falls, and violence, and may range from minor injuries to severe conditions requiring surgery. Psychological trauma, however, is caused by subtle exposures such as abuse, neglect, or witnessing violent acts, which have adverse impacts on mental well-being and health. Emotional trauma is observed in children and adults, rendering trauma care more difficult and demanding an interdisciplinary intervention involving psychological support.

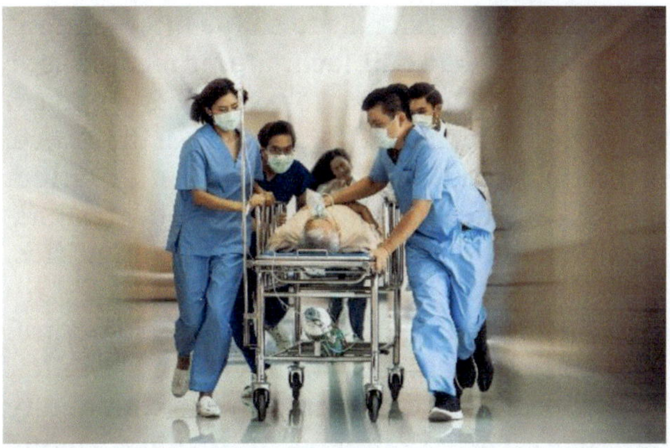

Figure 8.2. Traumatic injury.

Source: https://mitrauma.org/wp-content/uploads/2022/07/what-is-traumatic-injury.jpg.

Information regarding these layers is important for professionals who deal with trauma care, as treatment through different modes might be required to cater to the specific requirements of various types of trauma, resulting in a holistic process of healing and recovery for affected individuals (Babl et al., 2019). In short, injury and trauma each present unique challenges in the healthcare profession, and there needs to be a thorough understanding of what each entails. Trauma treatment and assessment must be multidisciplinary to allow for immediate physical care as well as attention to psychological and social factors that affect rehabilitation. As trauma treatment evolves as a science, constant updating of definitions and treatment protocols is necessary. This ongoing growth will help in the development of better patient outcomes for those who go through the trauma and injury realities. Therefore, the integration of research, clinical evidence, and patient-oriented care models is key to strengthening the resilience of individuals facing the aftereffects of trauma and to eventually create a superior trauma care system (Babl et al., 2019) (Figure 8.2).

Importance of Timely Care

Early treatment in trauma and injury management is crucial to optimizing patient outcomes. The relationship between the timeliness of medical intervention and healing rates has been well established, with delays tending to produce complications or increased mortality. Studies have shown that patients gain significant improvement in their state of health when treated with early definitive therapy, especially when there is a traumatic injury. For instance, streamlined trauma care has been shown to reduce the time from emergency department presentation significantly to needing imaging studies, and then affect the care of pediatric blunt trauma injuries. Through minimizing critical imaging acquisition times, such as computed tomography (CT) scans and focused assessment with sonography for trauma (FAST), healthcare providers can accurately diagnose injuries earlier, and treatment can be initiated earlier, ultimately enhancing the potential for a positive outcome in these vulnerable patients (Cross et al., 2019). Even the psychological dimension of trauma care is similarly significant, pointing to the necessity of prompt interventions. Too frequently, the psychological effects after acute traumatic injuries deeply affect the recovery of patients. In a recent pilot study, the importance of employing screening instruments like the Primary Care-Posttraumatic Stress Disorder (PC-PTSD) was emphasized by bedside nurses. It facilitates early identification of high-risk patients for traumatic stress and enables timely intervention in psychology. Although its use did not have a major impact on the number of consultations during the period compared to past periods, it enabled access to a large number of patients in need of appropriate psychological care. This brings about the importance of early psychological intervention in the overall treatment of trauma patients and ultimately towards better overall health outcomes (Alexander et al., 2017). Also, enhancing treatment timeliness is more than just providing prompt physical treatment; it involves establishing effective protocols and training for medical personnel. Since it has been realized that trauma treatment productivity can be greatly improved by structured systems and regular training, medical centers are increasingly adopting formal trauma protocols. These procedures not only maximize the trauma care logistics but also establish an environment where healthcare professionals are able to work at their best capacity. Evidence from experiments in research confirms that implementing such measures results in drastic reductions in critical reaction times, which is essential for both physical and mental assessments. The proactive approach that healthcare systems use in delivering timely treatment is crucial to ensuring that all aspects of trauma care, ranging from imaging and surgery to psychological evaluation, are adequately addressed without delay (Alexander et al., 2017; Cross et al., 2019).

8.1. Types of Trauma

Learning Outcome

1. Recognize the physical trauma
2. Describe the psychological trauma
3. Understand the distinctions between acute and chronic trauma

Trauma occurs in varying forms, each with causal factors and treatment implications. Physical trauma, for example, usually occurs due to accidents, violence, or catastrophes. This type has immediate medical concerns such as fractures, wounds, or internal injuries, and therefore, intervention is rapid. Emotional and psychological trauma, on the other hand, comes from experiences that are traumatic in nature but may not present physically, but rather affect one's psyche with ease. Abuse, neglect, and traumatic loss can lead to such conditions as Post-Traumatic Stress Disorder (PTSD), which requires empathetic understanding and multi-faceted treatment strategies that consider psychological and emotional healing. The identification of such differences will enable healthcare professionals to shape interventions in a manner that will facilitate proper, holistic recovery mechanisms for subjects exposed to various forms of trauma. Furthermore, interconnected factors significantly affect the experience and occurrence of trauma, particularly for marginalized communities. Boys and young men of color (BYMOC) are often at heightened risk due to structural disparities, including implicit and explicit racism, economic disadvantage, and community violence. The treatment of trauma among this population involves taking into account the ways social determinants of health can heighten vulnerabilities and restrict treatment access. The work of healthcare workers and policymakers is then crucial in an effort to make sure that services are not only equitable but also culturally competent. By acknowledging the adverse effects of societal institutions on trauma experience, the health system is able to better address high-risk populations and facilitate resilience and recovery. Hence, the convergence of social determinants and trauma places focus on an interdisciplinary approach in any model of trauma-informed care, particularly among vulnerable populations, as advanced by Rich (2016). The role of service providers in delivering trauma care goes beyond direct medical intervention to encompass holistic approaches that meet the diverse needs of the patients. The conclusion drawn from stakeholders within the health sector shows the complexity of delivering effective trauma care since gaps highlighted are typically based on limited capacity, resources, or knowledge of special challenges faced by trauma survivors. These findings identify the added value in integrating psychosocial support within mechanisms for trauma response to enable improved patient need understanding and improving models of service delivery. Providers are best positioned to advocate for change in the system so that trauma care not only heals physical trauma but also the associated emotional and psychological effects. Finally, enhancing trauma and injury care will mean working together among various stakeholders to create an integrated system in which healing and care become the central focus for everyone, as postulated by Aiken et al. (2014) (Figure 8.3).

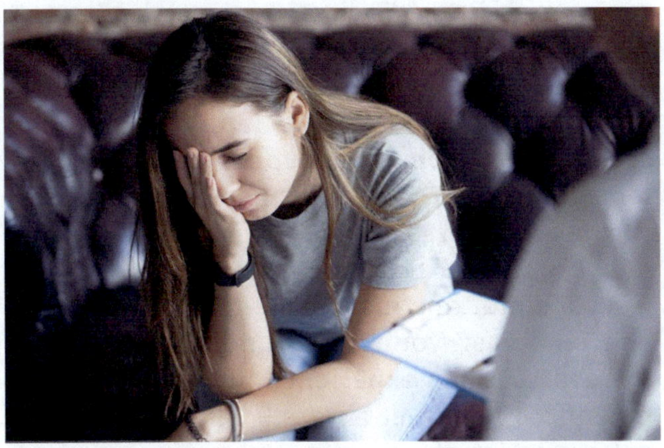

Figure 8.3. Common types of trauma.

Source: https://www.midwestrecoverycenter.com/wp-content/uploads/2020/07/types-of-trauma.jpg.

8.1.1. Physical Trauma

Physical trauma, as used in trauma and injury care, is recognized as a significant area of concern with a wide variety of injuries that can be brought about by environmental and situational factors. Physical trauma conceptually refers to the damage inflicted upon body tissues, organs, and systems, which can happen in numerous circumstances, from car crashes to sports and violence between individuals. Such trauma needs to have a structured approach, as early intervention produces a significant effect on outcomes of recovery. In addition, the effects of physical trauma extend past the initial medical response to reach psychological well-being and mechanisms of rehabilitation. Understanding the nuances of such a double effect is crucial for healthcare professionals who have to manage the complexities of trauma healing, with emphasis on adopting holistic care strategies that treat physical injuries as well as resultant psychological repercussions. Damage control (DC) surgery has emerged as a revolutionary concept in managing complex traumatic cases, echoing the shift in surgical paradigms with patient outcomes in mind. Where once therapeutic liver packing was used, a method abandoned due to negative outcomes, DC has gravitated toward more conservative surgical techniques, including truncated laparotomy. This is evidence of a respect for the multifaceted physiology of trauma patients and the necessity of a controllable approach tailored to the severity and nature of injuries sustained. Based on DC research, this type of surgical innovation is continually assessed for effectiveness and appropriateness across contexts, such as abdominal compartment syndrome. Therefore, the growing body of literature on DC surgery demonstrates the importance of adapting medical practice to meet modern trauma care and highlights the necessity of continuous assessment and adaptation of surgical techniques (Ball et al., 2017). In addition to the sudden physical trauma sustained during traumatic episodes, there are profound implications in the way of psychological response, particularly in traumatic birth. The conditions during the birth can create immense distress in addition to disturbing the physical well-being of the mother and child, as well as their psychological state. Despite the established relationship between physical trauma and traumatic birth experience, the term traumatic birth reveals the complexity, which generally goes beyond the boundaries of physical injury. Added to the trauma experience are the psychological and emotional consequences that can far outlast the event. Understanding such experiences lies at the core of trauma and injury care as it requires an integrated approach to treatment that treats both physical traumas and their lasting emotional effects, ultimately enabling better outcomes for mothers and their families (Glover et al., 2016) (Figure 8.4).

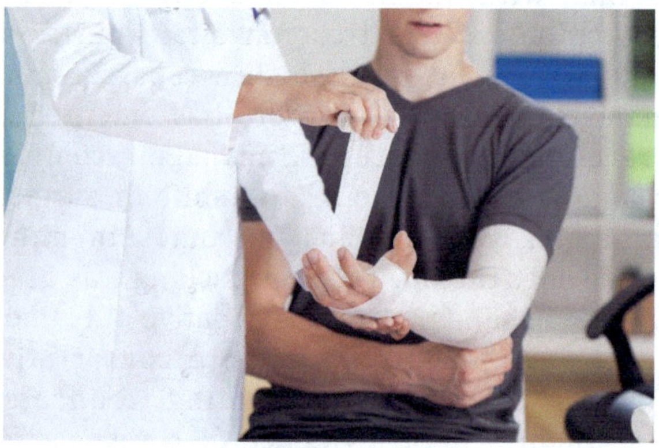

Figure 8.4. Physical trauma.

Source: https://carolinauc.com/wp-content/uploads/2023/08/Physical-Trauma-Image.jpg.

8.1.2. Psychological Trauma

Psychological trauma encompasses a wide variety of experiences that might profoundly affect one's mental health as well as general well-being. It most often results from events overwhelming one's ability to cope, such as physical violence, emotional mistreatment, or structural domination. The events can lead to long-lasting psychological effects, including anxiety, depression, as well as post-traumatic stress disorder (PTSD). The consequences of trauma do not remain limited to individual incidents alone but may rather create a cycle of adversity that extends beyond the direct victim to impact families and societies as well. As trauma-informed care is making it to the headlines in sectors in general, it becomes more crucial to learn about such difficult experiences and the consequent impact they have on treatment practice. The treatment of psychological trauma in marginalized groups requires an integrated response that addresses the social determinants of health that are accountable for mental health inequalities. The need to treat psychological trauma is particularly relevant among boys and men of color, who are faced with unique challenges of exposure to violence, discrimination, and social stigmatization.

Many of these individuals carry a disproportionate burden of trauma owing to socio-economic determinants as well as systemic inequalities. There has been evidence to show that the accumulation of these experiences has adverse impacts on health, hence a proper comprehension of traumas social context becomes crucial. Trauma-informed practices can be implemented in healthcare organizations, community environments, and educational settings to strengthen support mechanisms for such groups. This shift not only improves the health status of the individual but also has broad social reform. Addressing these issues simultaneously can instill resilience and empower young men and boys of color to reverse their experience and realize their potential (Wilson et al., 2009). In addition, the determination of the effect of trauma emphasizes the imperative for policy programs that aim to create healthier environments for traumatized subjects. The role of community care systems, mental health care, and social welfare cannot be overstated at this juncture. Initiatives that combine trauma awareness with violence prevention, health care, and juvenile justice can significantly improve the mental health of boys and young men of color. Such policies will also have to engage the implicit and explicit racism they suffer, which compounds their trauma. By establishing environments that prioritize healing and resilience, society can seek to dismantle the cycles of trauma. Lastly, an obligation to understanding and mitigating the effects of psychological trauma is central in building a healthier, more equitable future for all youth (Rich, 2016) (Figure 8.5).

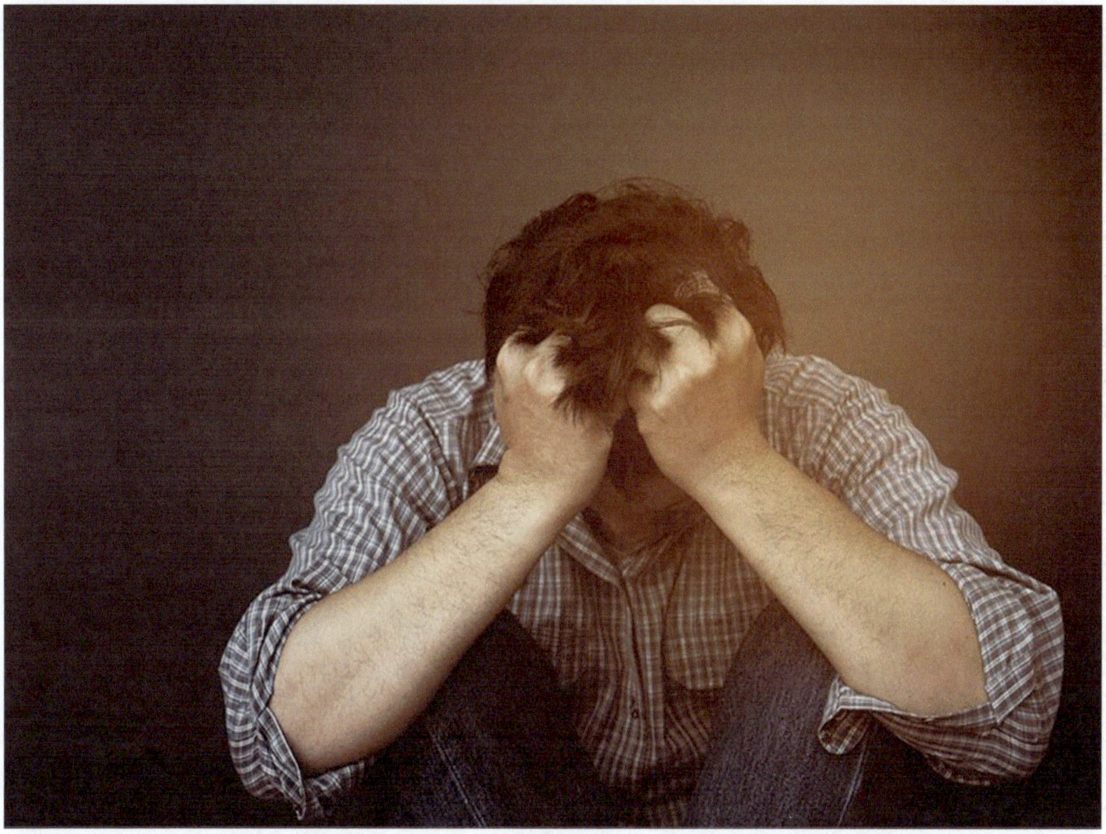

Figure 8.5. Psychological trauma.

Source: https://www.dbe.com.tr/upload/trauma-in-adults-16035139565665-b.jpg.

8.1.3. Acute vs. Chronic Trauma

It is necessary to understand how acute and chronic trauma differ in order to offer appropriate trauma and injury care. Acute trauma refers to injuries that occur suddenly and typically as a result of a direct causative factor, such as a car accident or a fall. Acute injuries typically require immediate medical intervention and may be fractures, cuts, or concussions. The physiologic response to acute trauma involves a predictable pattern of inflammatory processes designed to trigger healing. For instance, patients who require resections of the lung as a result of traumatic lung injury have demonstrated varied outcomes depending on the type of surgical intervention, with the high significance of evaluation in acute states (Doben et al., 2020). The major issue in acute trauma is the stabilization of the patient, pain control, and avoidance of complications that have a direct impact on the long-term course of recovery. Chronic trauma, on the other hand, entails persistent or repeated aversive exposure with resulting long-term physical and psychological outcomes. Chronic trauma develops over time, typically as a sequela to stressors, such as chronic domestic violence or abuse history. This type of trauma may result in conditions like post-traumatic stress disorder (PTSD), anxiety, or pain syndromes that permanently impair the quality of life for the patient. As opposed to acute trauma, in which symptoms and effects are more visible, chronic trauma progresses slowly and may only be noticed through the cumulative effect over time. Chronic disease is a more complex and multifaceted approach to treatment, in that it can include interdisciplinary approaches like psychological counseling and long-term physical rehabilitation. The impact of the various forms of trauma transfers over into systemic response within the organism. For instance, in a study on extremity injuries, researchers documented that severe extremity injury initiates a cascade of inflammatory events, resulting in prolonged hospital stays and additional pathology (Abboud et al., 2019). This brings to light the need to take both immediate and long-term care into consideration for trauma patients, as those with chronic traumatic conditions can't be helped with the same acute care methods that work for acute injuries. Treatment of both acute and chronic trauma is crucial in order to achieve better health outcomes and to create successful healthcare methods that provide for the distinctive challenges with each form of trauma. A thorough appreciation of the differences enables healthcare professionals to provide individualized interventions that enhance recovery and prevent long-term complications (Figure 8.6).

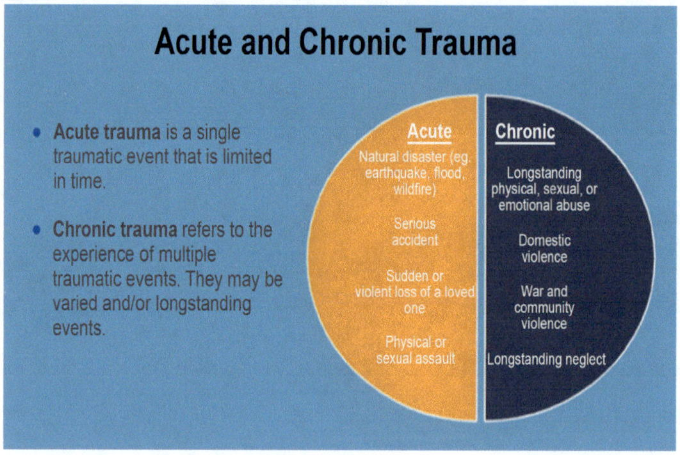

Figure 8.6. Acute and chronic trauma.

Source: https://img.oercommons.org/oercommons/media/editor/None/Screen_Shot_2021-06-21_at_2.53.18_PM_LTIGF6r.png.

Test Your Knowledge

1. What is the physical trauma?
2. What is the psychological trauma?

8.2. Mechanisms of Injury

Learning Outcome

1. Describe the blunt force trauma
2. Describe the penetrating trauma
3. Know the environmental factors in injury

Understanding mechanisms of injury is a central part of trauma and injury care, particularly in the context of the most frequent causes of injuries globally. Various mechanisms yield distinct patterns of injury, based on external factors to the person, including environment and activity level. As an illustration, traumatic spinal injuries (TSIs) resulting from road traffic accidents (RTAs) differ from those resulting from non-traffic-related accidents. Researchers in one study conducted at Tanzania's Muhimbili Orthopedic Institute concluded that RTAs accounted for a considerable proportion of TSIs, with notable demographic trends influencing injury severity. This indicates the necessity to face certain mechanisms of injury in order to develop specific interventions that can be utilized to limit the risk of such trauma, ultimately improving patient outcomes across different populations (Cheserem et al., 2024). The second key factor in injury-mechanism analysis is the injury environment, particularly for part-time soldiers in combat situations, where involvement entails exclusive exposures. Reserve Army data in Australia report knee injuries as the most prevalent category of injury documented, with a significant proportion involving soft tissue injury under combat and physical training maneuvers. Combat training, which is more risky because tasks are so strenuous, has been identified as a common environment in which these injuries are sustained. This suggests that there must be prevention programs, specific to this group, that address the mechanisms of injury in this population. Finally, appreciation of the unique mechanisms involved enables the formulation of injury prevention programs that account for the subtleties of activities that influence the frequency and severity of injury (Dey et al., 2012).

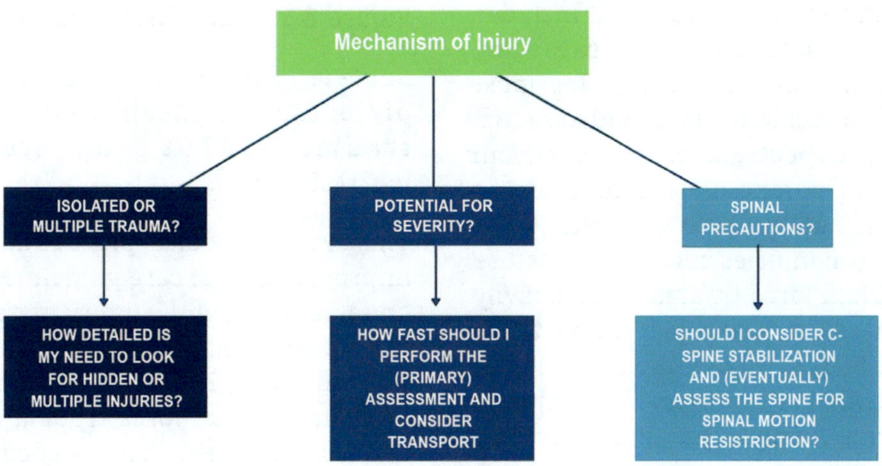

Figure 8.7. Mechanism of injury.

Source: https://limmereducation.com/storage/media/trauma-assessment_mechanism-of-inury_flowchart.jpg.

When one considers the mechanisms of injury, it is clear that multiple factors, such as demographics, context, and activity, intersect to shape outcomes. Installation of integrative systems for trauma care requires an integrated response that includes effective pre-hospital management, specialized care, and robust prevention systems. Viewing injury mechanisms from various perspectives serves to appreciate the sophisticated dynamics of trauma. Implications of recent studies advocate for equitable allocation of resources within trauma care programs, particularly in low- and middle-income countries where some types of injury, such as cervical spinal injuries, are more likely to result in fatalities. With the ongoing evolution of the field of trauma care, an appreciation of the multifaceted mechanisms of injury remains central to shaping policy and practice within the discipline, where interventions are both efficacious and equitable (Cheserem et al., 2024) (Figure 8.7).

8.2.1. Blunt Force Trauma

Blunt force trauma is a prominent focus of practice in trauma and injury care and includes a broad spectrum of injuries that are caused by non-penetrating trauma. These injuries most likely occur due to accidents, falls, and assaults, occurring along a spectrum of severity from mild contusion to potentially life-threatening organ injury. It is important to understand the mechanisms of such injuries because the nature of the effect of blunt force trauma relies heavily on factors such as the severity of impact, the character of the body part, and the condition of the patient's health. For example, blunt injuries can cause internal hemorrhage and laceration of organs, especially of life-supporting organs such as the spleen and the liver. This intricacy demands an advanced approach to trauma care, prioritizing early diagnosis and appropriate management methods specific to the nature of each case. Recent studies indicate a trend towards nonoperative management of certain types of blunt trauma, namely in hemodynamically stable patients. The evolution away from emergency surgery in the initial management of such accidents as blunt liver injury is indicative of the importance of incorporating new advances in imaging techniques and critical care interventions. Research shows that nonoperative strategies yield good results with no surgical side effects, especially if the injury does not require urgent treatment. The modalities used include careful observation, percutaneous drainage, and embolization for hemorrhage control.

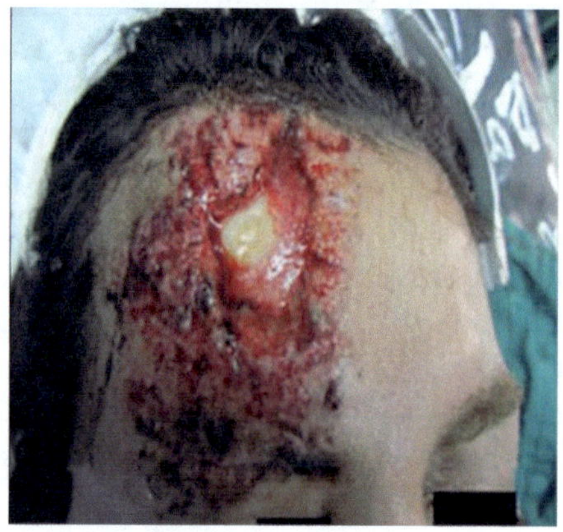

Figure 8.9. Blunt force trauma.

Source: https://img.medscapestatic.com/pi/features/slideshow-slide/blunt-force-trauma-6007991/updated2022/fig2.jpg?resize=580:*.

This evolving medical practice has been fueled by improved critical care guidelines and increased understanding of the injury patterns that dictate the optimal management of trauma patients (Ferrada et al., 2017). The financial implications of treating blunt force trauma are substantial, underscoring the necessity of cost-effective care in the health system. A thorough examination of patients who were hospitalized due to blunt trauma found that the costs of care are greatly dependent upon elements of injury severity, hospital stay, and surgical needs. Approximately 69% of the patients afflicted needed a minimum of one surgical operation, with dramatic cost variations depending upon the Glasgow Coma Score and the nature of trauma. By strengthening public health measures to reduce both the incidence and severity of blunt trauma, medical systems can save significant amounts of money and improve patient outcomes overall. Some measures that could be effective include prevention, safety protocol training, and the utilization of best-trauma care resources to avoid hospitalization and its associated costs (Christensen et al., 2008) (Figure 8.9).

8.2.2. Penetrating Trauma

Penetrating trauma is a significant problem in trauma and injury management, which refers to injuries that pass through the skin and inner tissues. They result from various mechanisms, with gunshots, stabbings, and impalements being some of the most common. The injuries are likely to result in complex clinical presentations, and therefore their rapid assessment and management are crucial to avoid complications. In the majority of cases, penetrating trauma can damage vital organs, blood vessels, and nerves and lead to serious morbidity and mortality. Trauma care practitioners should know the mechanisms of injury, the character of the forces, and the probable courses of associated complications to provide time-sensitive and effective treatment. With the prevalence of such trauma on the rise globally, particularly in urban areas, it brings into focus the need for increased preventive strategies as well as enhanced emergency intervention strategies in trauma care services. Penetrating trauma treatment is generally a multi-disciplinary approach with the integration of surgical management, intensive care, and rehabilitation services. The initial evaluation generally follows the Advanced Trauma Life Support (ATLS) algorithm, with stabilization of airway, breathing, and circulation being the priority. At the center of this is the use of imaging technology, such as computed tomography (CT) scans, which can better delineate the extent of internal injuries. Current research shows that associated injuries, especially chest or abdominal injuries, significantly affect patient outcomes and length of hospital stay (Kalliopi et al., 2011). Furthermore, the emergency operation would be laparotomies or thoracotomies based on the extent of the damage, with the focus being on the preservation of life as much as the restoration of function.

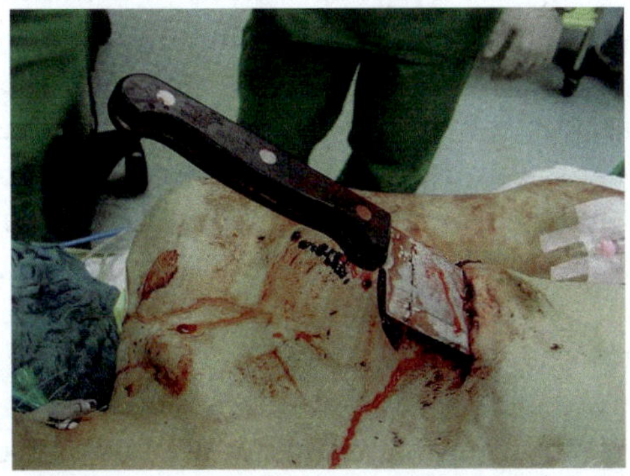

Figure 8.10. Penetrating trauma.

Source: https://media-us.amboss.com/media/thumbs/big_5081d9411945f.jpg.

Because patients are heterogeneous, each patient will require individualized regimens to optimize recovery and prevent late sequelae. Penetrating trauma will often manifest immediate dangers, but secondary complications of infection, in addition to a long-term hospital stay, also need to be managed. The occurrence of concomitant infections, such as HIV, among trauma patients, is an occupational hazard to healthcare workers and hinders the determination of the overall treatment strategy (Chalya et al., 2010). Such complications can result in extended durations of hospitalization and higher rates of morbidity, which necessitate the implementation of standardized infection control within trauma care facilities. Trauma infections can also delay healing and influence the overall prognosis of a patient. Delineation of both direct and indirect effects of penetrating trauma can result in enhanced management planning, ensure a better recovery process, and ultimately improve patient outcomes in injury and trauma management (Figure 8.10).

8.2.3. Environmental Factors in Injury

Environmental factors play a significant role in influencing the prevalence and type of injuries among populations, thereby influencing the responsiveness of trauma and injury care. Urban populations tend to have more cases of trauma due to partly increased population density and the resultant risks for accidents on the road, violence, and other accidental trauma. A Scott County, IA study has demonstrated that demographic data, coupled with spatial analysis, can illuminate distinctive environmental circumstances that lead to higher trauma incidence. Mapping hot spots of trauma occurrence through geographic information systems (GIS) can assist stakeholders in understanding which mechanisms of injury are most prevalent and how spatial factors, such as emergency access to services or geography, might affect outcomes. This strategy focuses on the need to transform trauma care resources to be provisioned based on the unique environmental characteristics and challenges of diverse populations (Koch et al., 2018). The combination of environmental factors and individual patient features further complicates the injury profile. Military and civilian populations, for instance, are likely to encounter unique threats surrounding traumatic injuries based on their environment. Of particular interest are invasive fungal infections caused by serious injuries sustained in environments such as war or disaster relief zones. The post-trauma IFI's peculiar epidemiological context demonstrates how health outcomes are shaped by environmental factors, e.g., exposure to specific pathogens and the presence of health infrastructure. Understanding these dynamics is essential to the creation of specialized prevention measures. By identifying common risk factors, including injury patterns and comorbidities, health practitioners can maximize the practice of trauma care by targeting underlying environmental etiologies that promote injury risk and complicate recovery (Bochicchio et al., 2017). To address environmental factors in injury prevention, there must be a multi-component plan involving community education, policymaking, and resource allocation. Safety awareness programs in urban areas or special schemes in rural areas can significantly minimize the occurrence of injuries. Local government, healthcare facilities, and community organizations need to collectively formulate measures that are appropriate to the environment. For instance, the provision of pedestrian walkways for safety in urban areas, the stiffening of traffic regulations, or the decongestion of emergency services in rural areas are all essential factors. As shown by Scott County's combined data, the intelligent deployment of trauma assets based on environmental analysis not only speeds up response times but also has the potential to reduce injury severity. An effective trauma and injury care model would focus on acknowledging and redefining injury-related environmental factors to create a better environment for all community stakeholders (Koch et al., 2018).

Test Your Knowledge

1. What is the blunt force trauma?
2. What is a penetrating trauma?

8.3. Initial Assessment and Triage

Learning Outcome

1. Know the primary survey techniques
2. Describe the secondary survey procedures
3. Understand the importance of triage in emergency settings

Initial triage and evaluation in trauma and injury management are of utmost significance for effective patient care in emergency settings. This systematic approach enables healthcare professionals to provide care according to the severity of injuries and the immediate needs of each patient. With rapid evaluation of vital signs, mechanism of injury, and clinical presentation, medical personnel can allocate patients to particular triage categories. The importance of such an approach is typically highlighted by the accuracy of triage classification systems that can utilize complex computer algorithms to process patient data. The use of these models in pre-hospital settings facilitates effective and quick decision-making, which, in turn, improves patient outcomes by enabling caregivers to distribute resources optimally, with important cases receiving early intervention (Holcomb et al., 2019). Triage procedures not only enhance patient care but also significantly influence mortality and morbidity rates following traumatic incidents. In the majority of emergency rooms, the procedures are applied on a daily basis to assess myriad presentations, including those with chest pain that may be drug-induced, such as cocaine. The significance of such an evaluation is that it enables medical personnel to easily diagnose underlying conditions and prepare for possible complications due to dual diagnoses. Patients may also have concomitant symptoms, making evaluation difficult, which underscores the need for a structured triage program. Identifying such patients not only facilitates rapid treatment but also ensures consideration of longer-term rehabilitation plans as part of total trauma care (Bandeeri et al., 2004). This process of triage and assessment thus becomes an essential component in optimizing the outcomes for trauma patients. Effective initial evaluation and triage should also be complemented by interdisciplinary collaboration between healthcare professionals. Such collective practice recognizes the fact that trauma care often involves contributions from a number of specialists, including trauma surgeons, emergency physicians, and nursing staff, all of whom bring essential roles to the outcome of the patient. By facilitating communication and shared decision-making, teams can more effectively manage the complexity of traumatic injuries. Patient prioritization through triage not only identifies which patients are treated immediately, but it also impacts the emergency department workflow overall. Furthermore, as technology continues to improve, the use of digital tools and data analysis can optimize triage processes to ensure that best practices are applied and tailored to each individual patient. This emerging environment underscores the ongoing necessity for training and acclimatization in first assessment and triage processes in trauma and injury treatment (Figure 8.11).

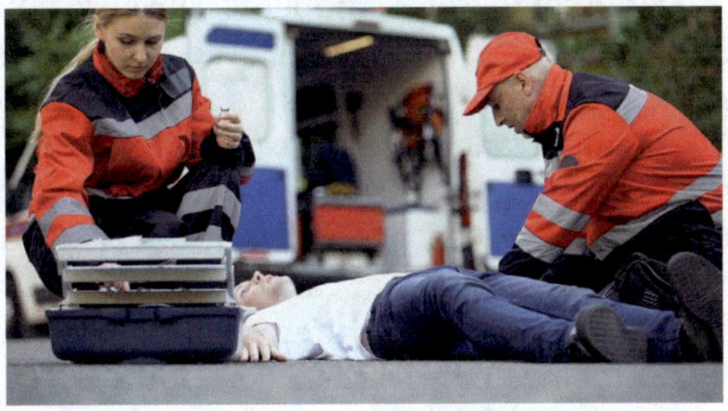

Figure 8.11. Learning the steps of great trauma care: initial patient assessment.

Source: https://projectheartbeat.com/wp-content/smush-webp/2019/10/trauma-care.jpeg.webp.

8.3.1. Primary Survey Techniques

Primary survey techniques form part of the initial patient assessment and management in the context of injury and trauma. The primary survey is an organized method of promptly identifying life-threatening conditions, enabling interventions that significantly affect outcomes. Following the ABCDE principle—Airway, Breathing, Circulation, Disability, and Exposure—caregivers can address key issues effectively. This structured method not only helps to set priorities for treatment but also enhances the safety of both responder and patient. Taking a careful primary survey, if done correctly, means that life-threatening issues are identified and addressed, and the risk of complications from incorrect or delayed intervention is reduced. Effective training in primary survey skills is essential, particularly for healthcare staff with varying levels of experience. Evidence indicates that deficits in basic assessment skills, confidence, and competency can lead to suboptimal practices of care, particularly in acute settings. As an illustration, improper splinting is a common finding among musculoskeletal-untrained clinicians and can trigger complications such as skin breakdown and fracture instability. By providing targeted educational workshops, as the outcomes of orthopedic surgery clinic results illustrate, healthcare practitioners can significantly enhance their skills and confidence in these important maneuvers (Dart et al., 2020). Such educational interventions underscore the power of continued professional development in maximizing trauma care outcomes. With traditional evaluation methods, integrating newer technologies such as point-of-care ultrasound (POCUS) is crucial to enhance the quality of the primary survey in trauma patients. The imaging modality offers the clinician a mechanism to rapidly diagnose traumatic and also uncommon but serious conditions, such as retrobulbar hemorrhage. Evidence indicates that even clinical professionals at various stages of training can successfully apply POCUS to identify such complications and improve diagnostic precision and clinical decision-making (Bajaj et al., 2020). Incorporating these technologies also improves medical professionals' abilities and results in improved patient safety and quality of care. Lastly, constant innovation in primary survey techniques, complemented by targeted training and technology, is required to optimize results in the management of trauma and injury (Figure 8.12).

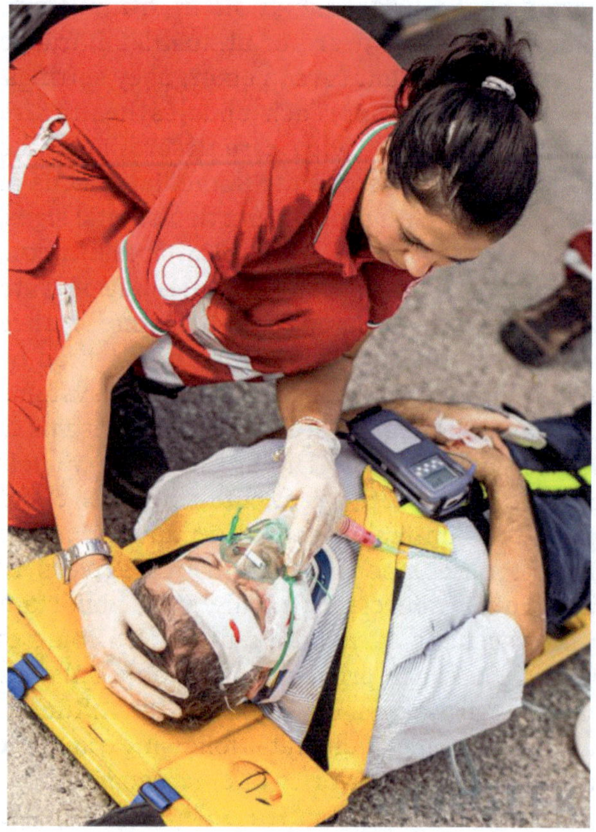

Figure 8.12. Primary survey techniques.

Source: https://upload.medbullets.com/topic/120633/images/primarysurvey.jpg.

8.3.2. Secondary Survey Procedures

Secondary survey protocols are the foundation of trauma care, providing a careful examination of patients once the initial impression is obtained. The methodical approach enables health care professionals to identify any injuries not yet apparent from the primary survey. Unlike the primary survey that treats life-threatening injuries, the secondary survey involves a general inspection of the patient's medical history, physical checkup, and pertinent diagnostic examinations. This multi-faceted evaluation is of paramount importance for verifying that no injuries are overlooked, especially in complex mechanisms of injury or altered level of consciousness presentations in patients. Clinical practice guidelines have a tendency to emphasize the need for early imaging investigations since they not only aid in the initial evaluation but can also significantly enhance outcomes through the enablement of timely interventions (Cross et al., 2019). One of the most critical components of the secondary survey is integrating imaging and laboratory tests, which provide crucial information about internal trauma and necessitate surgery. Timing has a critical place in trauma situations; any delay in performing imaging tests can increasingly complicate the conditions of the patient. Research indicates that the use of an effective trauma response team can significantly decrease the time required for critical imaging tests such as CT scans and FAST exams. For instance, the research found a reduction in CT acquisition time from an average of 37 minutes to 28 minutes after the adoption of standardized trauma protocols, demonstrating the actual dividends of optimized processes (Cross et al., 2019). Not only does this hasten diagnosis, but definitive care can be initiated as soon as possible, which is important with trauma. Additionally, the secondary survey involves repeated monitoring for complications that occur during treatment. Clinicians must be supplied with adequate screening tools, especially in conditions like TBIs, which manifest in a subtle fashion but can have devastating consequences if not diagnosed. Research indicates that the majority of primary care providers are not confident in their ability to identify TBIs, a condition largely attributed to inadequate experience and improper use of existing screening devices. Therefore, improvement in training and education on such evaluation protocols is needed, with the providers being able to identify and successfully treat secondary injuries that can occur later on. Both trauma care policies and powerful screening tools need to work together in an effort to optimize patient outcomes within trauma care settings (Figure 8.13).

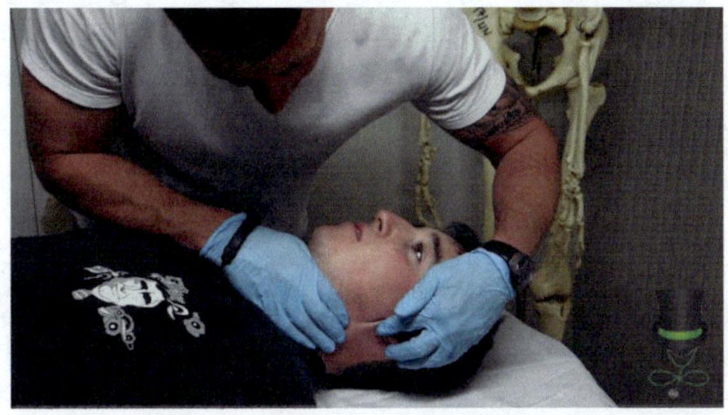

Figure 8.13. The secondary survey trauma.

Source: https://i.ytimg.com/vi/48GH_qQO96s/maxresdefault.jpg.

8.3.3. Importance of Triage in Emergency Settings

In emergency conditions, triage cannot be overstressed, as it is the cornerstone of effective trauma and injury care. Triage processes inherently relate to the organization of patient treatment based on the severity of injuries and the urgency of medical need. Through effective allocation of medical resources, triage ensures that those who require immediate treatment receive it in a timely manner. For instance, the implementation of improved care teams (ECT) in the pre-hospital environment has significantly improved scene times and adherence to triage and hence reduced mortality among penetrating trauma victims. Such structured approaches demonstrate the overriding importance of prompt assessment and that prompt, informed decision-making during triage can have a significant bearing on patient outcomes, not only in acute episodes but across all emergency care (Aldred et al., 2019). Further, in the case of mass casualty incidents (MCI), the necessity for triage is even greater. With more patients, there is more complexity in medical care. Appropriate triage intervention is very important in managing patient flow, determining treatment priorities, and ensuring a systematic response from healthcare practitioners. Recent simulations of MCI indicate that organization among medical personnel regarding triage procedures improves interactions and treatment based on injury severity, as demonstrated by the use of wearable proximity sensors in these drills. With the application of technology, real-time monitoring of patient care dynamics becomes possible, thus illuminating how triage priority aligns with the adequacy of healthcare delivery in disordered environments (Carenzo et al., 2018). These observations further support the argument that good triage systems are essential components of emergency medical response, thereby improving preparedness and ultimately saving lives. The scope of effective triage extends beyond the direct outcome of patients to encompass overall organizational effectiveness of emergency medical services. Incorporating full triage procedures can significantly reduce scene time, particularly in severe cases. Studies have shown that the presence of ECT not only reduces on-scene time but also enhances overall compliance with established medical protocols during critical incidents. Emergency services can create an environment that streamlines patient management, reduces delays, and addresses the needs of all patients, regardless of the magnitude of the incident, by implementing standardized triage protocols. Thus, investment in training and resources for triage systems is a proactive action in trauma and injury care that is critical to meet the urgent demands of today's emergency healthcare settings (Aldred et al., 2019). The initiative not only enhances the patient's survival rate but also provides a long-term model of care for emergency services (Figure 8.14).

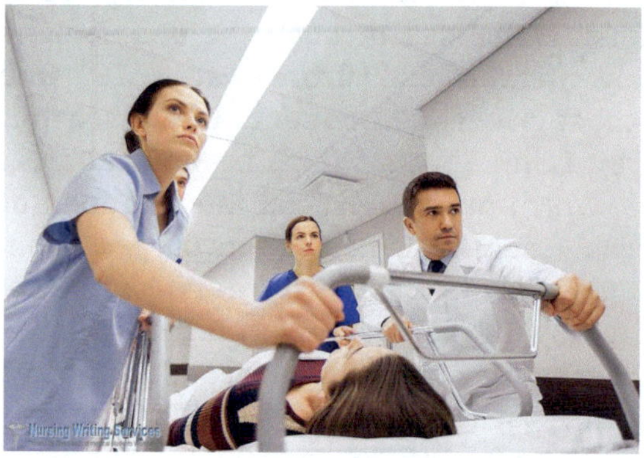

Figure 8.14. Importance of triage: prioritizing patient care in emergency situations.

Source: https://www.nursingwritingservices.com/images/blog/emergency-care-hospital.jpg.

Test Your Knowledge

1. What are the primary survey techniques?
2. What is the importance of triage in emergency settings?

8.4. Treatment Protocols

Learning Outcome

1. Describe the immediate care interventions
2. Know the surgical options for severe injuries
3. Describe the rehabilitation and recovery processes

Effective treatment protocols play a crucial role in trauma and injury management because they dictate clinical care and the management of the injured patient. Protocols are generally characterized by the nature of the injury, patient factors, and the setting of care. For chest injuries, for instance, which represent a significant proportion of trauma cases, the treatment can vary based on the type of injury, whether penetrating or blunt. A study has revealed that the most common cause of chest trauma is road traffic accidents, which highlights the need for the implementation of some protocols to deal with such a prevalent cause. Most patients are treated non-operatively, but a subgroup may require more severe methods, i.e., thoracotomy, especially when the presenting complications are life-threatening, e.g., hemopericardium. These differences in treatment modalities bring into sharp focus the necessity for evidence-based practices to advance patient outcomes in trauma care with an emphasis on evidence-based care (Kalliopi et al., 2011). Additionally, pediatric patients' treatment protocols must be adjusted to meet their unique anatomical and physiological requirements. The Pediatric Emergency Care Applied Research Network (PECARN) spearheads the creation and standardization of these protocols, emphasizing evidence-based practice among children. PECARN's overall strategy includes the development of research capacity, the training of investigators, and the dissemination of results so that best practices are optimally translated into practice. This strategic growth not only promotes innovation in pediatric emergency treatment but also enhances the overall quality of treatment provided to young patients suffering from trauma. The role of dedicated networks like PECARN in streamlining treatment protocols is thus vital to enhancing treatment for sensitive populations, thereby underscoring the significance of protocol development in the management of injury and trauma (Kim et al., 2014). In summary, developing treatment protocols for trauma care is necessary not only to optimize clinical performance but also to standardize care across various healthcare settings.

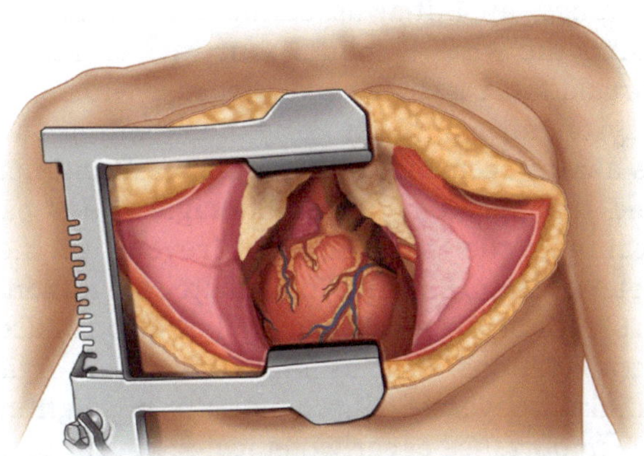

Figure 8.15. Clamshell thoracotomy.

Source: https://i0.wp.com/basicmedicalkey.com/wp-content/uploads/2020/10/467973_1_En_2_Fig6_HTML.png?w=960.

The protocols enable medical practitioners to make informed decisions for trauma cases such that they are treated appropriately and quickly. Parameters such as the nature of the injury, patient demographics, and comorbidities must continuously inform the crafting and adjustment of treatment strategies. The dynamic nature of trauma and injury management necessitates ongoing research and education to enhance these protocols. As demonstrated by the heterogeneity in treatment needs across populations, healthcare systems must be adaptive to address emerging challenges as and when they arise. By applying data collected from research networks and studies, health practitioners can make treatment models meaningful and effective in the quest for better trauma care (Kalliopi et al., 2011; Kim et al., 2014) (Figure 8.15).

8.4.1. Immediate Care Interventions

Such urgent care interventions are central to trauma and injury treatment because they directly impact patient outcomes. The pathophysiology of trauma often results in complex physiological responses that require immediate assessment and management. For instance, an initial assessment is performed using the ABCDE model—Airway, Breathing, Circulation, Disability, and Exposure—to enable a systematic approach. Early interventions such as airway securing, intravascular resuscitation, and management of hemorrhagic shock can stabilize the patient and prevent further deterioration. Effective immediate care not only provides a basis for recovery but also reduces complications such as brain injury or organ failure in severely injured patients, highlighting the importance of early medical intervention in trauma again. Damage control surgery (DCS) is a paradigm of immediate intervention in critically injured patients. DCS is a sequence of staged injuries to manage traumatic injury, allowing for rapid hemorrhage and contamination control with deferral of definitive repair. The evolution of DCS, which originally emerged from post-World War II operations, has been further supplemented by greater insight into the physiology of the trauma patient. According to the literature, the development of DCS has been extensively documented, underscoring its central role in managing complex abdominal injuries and its broader use across a wider range of trauma cases (Ball et al., 2017). Application of quick conservative surgical techniques can decrease complications, streamline the process of surgery, and ultimately boost patient survival rates; hence, it is an essential part of the initial management of trauma victims. In the case of traumatic brain injury (TBI), initial interventions are absolutely essential in adherence to established clinical practices. Effective TBI management is based on repeated assessment of intracranial pressure (ICP) and cerebral perfusion pressure (CPP), thereby enabling timely modification of therapeutic measures to avoid secondary brain damage. Research has shown that systematic surveillance of TBI guideline compliance can optimize clinical outcomes through validation that interventions align with best-practice guidelines (Moss et al., 2018). Integration of real-time ICU data into process models enables strong tests of treatment adherence. Hence, personalized interventions become essential in the moment according to individual physiology, underlining the need for ongoing assessment, adaptive flexibility of intervention methods, and commitment to adherence to prescribed protocols for optimizing recovery in trauma and injury care.

8.4.2. Surgical Options for Severe Injuries

In the treatment of trauma and injury, surgical procedures for severe injuries tend to rely on the nature and degree of injury sustained. With advanced surgical methods at hand, physicians have various options for repairing and restoring functional activity with healing. Of these methods, liver trauma management exemplifies the use of a tailor-made approach tailored to specific injuries. Based on the grade that has been supplied by the American Association for the Surgery of Trauma (AAST), treatments can vary from conservative treatment to operative repair, based on the patient's hemodynamic status and severity of the injury itself. The physiological and anatomical considerations of managing liver injuries emphasize that surgery is not an off-the-shelf maneuver but requires a tailor-made approach to ensure optimal patient outcomes and prevent complications during healing (Abu-Zidan et al., 2016). Surgical management of open fractures emphasizes careful planning and execution. In an open fracture with severe injury, the initial management's first steps are immediate debridement and irrigation to prevent infection and maintain limb function. The policy recommends definitive fixation in all cases except where severity warrants a staged method of management. Reconstruction of solid bone defect is achieved through a number of approaches, including induced membrane methods, which permit staged bone grafting, as well as distraction osteogenesis.

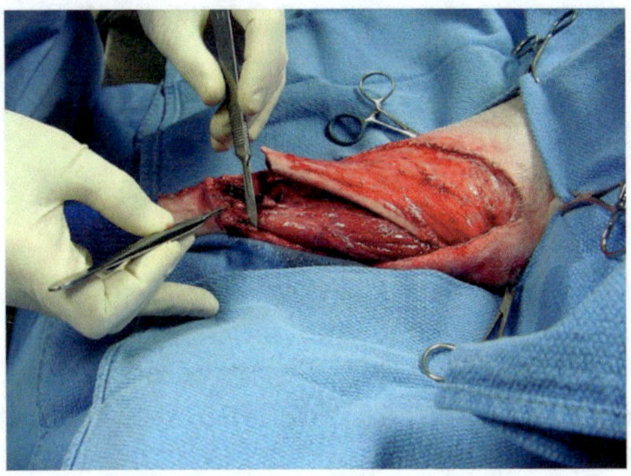

Figure 8.16. Surgical repair of open fractures.

Source: https://images.ctfassets.net/4dmg3l1sxd6g/0eYcrmAhNEdRbuKB9kpx5/02a0cdf774232070337f956e0a07243d/surgical-repair-of-open-fractures-figure-3-23436-gallery.jpg_-_en.

These methods offer adequate healing, but the challenge lies in preserving soft tissues, an element that is vital in cases of extensive injury. Negative pressure wound therapy is a worthwhile addition to surgical treatment, promoting healing and reducing complications in these severe injuries (Abell et al., 2017). Lastly, the evolving face of surgery in trauma care reflects heightened sensitivity to injury patterns and patient demand. Emerging developments in surgical practice, complemented by established protocols, demonstrate that timely and appropriate surgical intervention is life-saving. The integration of evidence-based interventions within surgical trauma care not only maximizes recovery but also personalizes treatment to account for the subtleties of the case. Moreover, ongoing developments and research in operating room technologies continue to influence best practices in trauma care, underscoring that a holistic approach, tailored to the specific conditions of a given injury, is required to achieve optimal clinical outcomes in severe injury management. Exploration of these surgical avenues is part of an overall campaign towards patient-centered care, a hallmark of effective trauma care programs (Figure 8.16).

8.4.3. Rehabilitation and Recovery Processes

Rehabilitation and recovery procedures are a critical component of injury and trauma management, attending to both the physical and mental aspects of rehabilitation. The multifaceted role of rehabilitation not only includes restoring physical function but also facilitating emotional and cognitive rehabilitation. For those who have experienced traumatic brain injury (TBI), this double focus is critical to the preservation of long-term health. One longitudinal study of survivors of TBI found that, despite injury severity, many reported long-term positive shifts in their outlook in the years following the accident, reflecting the ability of rehabilitation to promote psychological adaptation and resilience (Hawley et al., 2008). This reflects the need to incorporate holistic rehabilitation approaches that include psychological as well as physical therapy, ultimately enabling them to take back their lives and respond adequately to their environment. Augmenting traditional rehabilitative strategies, novel modalities such as adapted sport and adventurous training have emerged as effective interventions in fostering recovery. Participants are provided with the opportunity to engage in meaningful physical activity that can enhance their psychological well-being. Studies on military personnel with physical and/or emotional disability found that involvement in such programs gave the members an ability to reestablish a sense of self, create new social relationships, and regain a sense of purpose. The findings emphasized how these experiences led to present- and future-oriented outcomes, as proof that recovery is more than physical recuperation but also the reintegration of personal identity and social incorporation (Anthony et al., 2013). Secondly, the recovery process may vary extremely from one person to another, requiring individualized rehabilitation strategies. These interventions need to be sensitive to the unique needs and circumstances of every patient, adjusting both for the severity of the injury and the psychological state. Professionals involved should engage an ecological recovery process, aware that positive psychological adaptation can take place at various stages following injury, as justified by the TBI survivors' narratives. This integrated approach to rehabilitation and recovery guarantees that both physical capabilities and mental health are touched upon at the same time, ultimately resulting in a better quality of life for those healing from injury and trauma. An integrated approach to trauma and injury treatment promotes the idea that healing is a process, one that is extremely personal and largely determined by the social and emotional context in which it occurs (Figure 8.17).

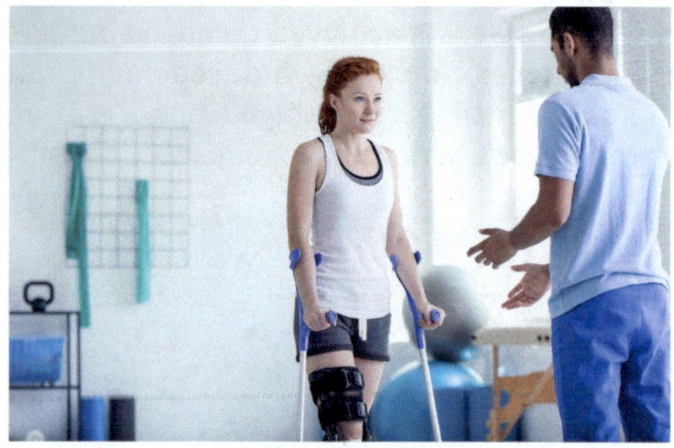

Figure 8.17. Rehabilitation after injury.

Source: https://www.majortraumagroup.co.uk/wp-content/uploads/2020/06/rehabilitation-1000-667-768x512.jpg.

Test Your Knowledge

1. What are immediate care interventions?
2. What are the surgical options for severe injuries?

8.5. Psychological Impact of Trauma

Learning Outcome

1. Describe the common psychological responses
2. Know the long-term effects of trauma
3. Understand the importance of mental health support

The psychological impact of trauma is profound, typically extending way beyond the acute physical trauma experienced. After trauma, victims typically present with an array of psychological symptoms, including depression, anxiety, and post-traumatic stress disorder (PTSD). These symptoms can be seriously impairing to everyday living, impacting a person's ability to engage in social interactions, employment, and family functioning. Current studies indicate a close correlation between impairments in the physical, psychological distress, and general role performance. Specifically, pain, mobility issues, and psychological distress have been identified to predict later impairment in functioning, which emphasizes the need for an integrated recovery plan addressing physical as well as psychological recovery concurrently (Bakker et al., 2024). It is also significant to comprehend the psychological impact of trauma and how patients perceive recovery. If what patients and families perceive as needed for recovery is not taken into account during trauma treatment, then the overall treatment plan can be unsuccessful. A study with trauma patients, their families, and professionals found that indicators of successful recovery included resumption of work, emotional stability, and resumption of everyday roles (Anke et al., 2016). Patients reported an evident change in their recovery priorities, with greater understanding of the interconnectedness between physical and emotional recovery.

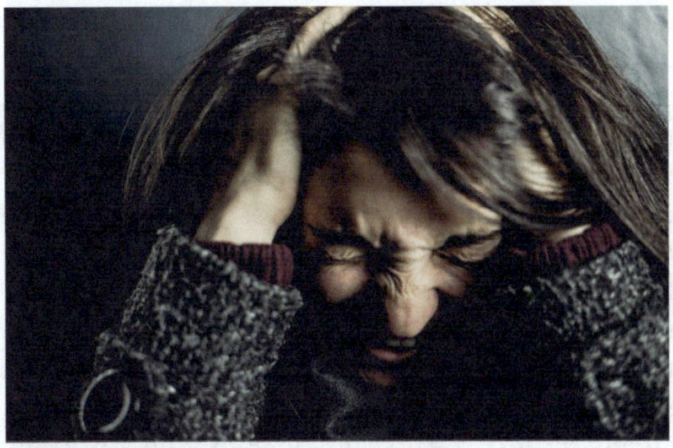

Figure 8.18. Understanding the psychological impact of trauma.

Source: https://psychology-spot.com/wp-content/uploads/2025/01/psychological-impact-of-trauma-pexels-scaled.webp.

They better recognized the reality that psychological recovery was not one process but was interlocked with physical rehabilitation and readmission to everyday living. This emphasizes the importance of health professionals involving patients in establishing personalized recovery goals, so that trauma care aligns with patients' overall needs. Added to the psychological impact of trauma is the potential for long-term effects. Long-term conditions due to persistent psychological states are not only harmful to the mental condition of the patient but also to their health. Furthermore, social and family outcomes are significant, as patients will find it hard with altered relationships and an altered sense of self. The fact that these problems have to be addressed renders them paramount in the treatment of trauma. Evidence dictates initial assessment of physical trauma and psychological symptoms alike in a bid to provide individualized aftercare that provides excellent long-term results (Bakker et al., 2024). The establishment of a therapeutic setting that allows for psychological healing can enhance resiliency, improve the quality of life, and facilitate a simple return to society and ultimately result in an integrated practice that defines modern trauma and injury care (Figure 8.18).

8.5.1. Common Psychological Responses

The experience of trauma can elicit a range of psychological responses, which it is vital for healthcare caregivers to recognize in the treatment of injuries. Normal responses are acute stress reactions, where patients exhibit higher anxiety, avoidance, or intrusive memories of the trauma. Not only are such responses normal, but they can also be adaptive, allowing individuals to give meaning to what has happened to them. But when these reactions last more than a month, they may become post-traumatic stress disorder (PTSD), a more severe condition of long-term anxiety and emotional anguish. Identification of such mental conditions is a vital part of the job of healthcare professionals, as interventions at early stages can eliminate the long-term impacts of trauma on mental well-being, which explains why more training in psychological assessment is needed in trauma care settings. To successfully treat psychological trauma effects, screening tools such as the Primary Care-Posttraumatic Stress Disorder (PC-PTSD) have an important role to play. Their deployment by bedside nurses can assist in increasing identification of traumatic stress-at-risk patients, hence promoting early intervention. There is proof that while psychiatric consultations within overall health psychology will not always produce a mass increase, screening can yield referrals that are indicated for many patients, revealing a vital unmet mental health requirement within the trauma centers (Alexander et al., 2017).

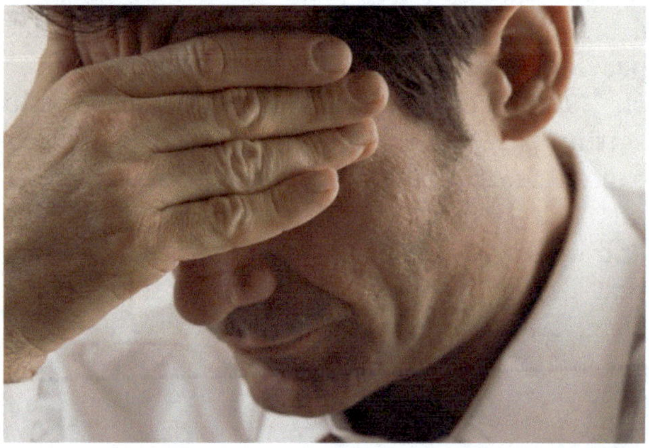

Figure 8.19. Common psychological responses.

Source: https://www.neurocaregroup.com/hubfs/Imported_Blog_Media/stress-feat-3-1-1-2.png.

Active intervention of this sort is aligned with the values of full care of trauma, which cultivates the welfare of body and mind, both of which are necessary to improve patient lives. In addition, the interaction between trauma exposure and PTSD symptom occurrence needs serious monitoring by healthcare providers. Evidence indicates that victims of accidents, such as motor vehicle crash survivors, are at a higher risk of developing physical and mental health issues, suggesting an interaction between injury severity and mental health (Kennedy-Moffat et al., 1997). These are pre-existing psychological illnesses, the severity of the incident, and the degree of body injuries. All are linked with greater PTSD symptoms. These results support the necessity of an integrated model of trauma treatment involving assessment of mental health and counseling, so that patients receive physical as well as psychological care under one umbrella. By integrating these variables into trauma care practices, medical practitioners can develop a more conducive recovery environment (Figure 8.19).

8.5.2. Long-Term Effects of Trauma

The chronic effects of trauma extend far into physical harm, profoundly impacting psychological well-being and social adaptation. Individuals who have been exposed to severe trauma, like traumatic brain injury (TBI), may experience persistent cognitive and emotional challenges that disrupt everyday function. This is particularly so in diffuse axonal injury, where recovery complexity extends to chronic symptoms that span decades. Research has shown that the caregivers of TBI survivors also carry heavy psychological burdens, often mirroring the trauma experienced by the victims. The shared exposure to trauma among family members complicates recovery, with each going through the emotional landscape left behind by the trauma. Awareness of these shared long-term effects further underscores the necessity of establishing comprehensive support systems that address the needs of both the survivor and the caregiver. Evolving opinions regarding TBI also illuminated the long-term consequences of trauma, and today, researchers consider it a chronic disease rather than an acute injury that requires instant intervention. This evolving thought foretells a demand for ongoing interventions to cater to the long-term rehabilitation of individuals who have suffered from TBI. Specifically, studies have proven that non-neurological complications, such as hospital-acquired complications, play an important role in the influence of recovery patterns and overall disability following the injury. Through the scrutiny of the intersection between acute medical care and long-term health consequences, we can establish preventive interventions and therapeutic interventions that minimize harmful effects. The coming together of both the biological model and the psychological model in establishing the spectrum of TBI recovery can enhance trauma and injury care practice through increased awareness of the chronic effects of trauma. Finally, the impact on family and community relationships cannot be overstated, as the continuity of harm tends to reverberate through social relationships. Trauma survivors tend to leave behind prolonged stress on families with the emotional and financial burden of care and rehabilitation. In other cases, this strain can contribute to increased conflict or even the breakdown of family relationships, highlighting the need for integrative care approaches that include the entire family system. The positive impact of caregiver involvement can foster resilience and attachment; however, these benefits are often overwhelmed by the omnipresent stressors inherent in caregiving. Therefore, long-term interventions should address not only the injured individuals but also their families to ensure that the trauma related to recovery and injury is tackled in a holistic manner. Based on a broader understanding of trauma and its effects, we can highlight how to design improved environments to care for the injured, as seen in studies on TBI and caregiving relationships (Raman et al., 2013; Kumar et al., 2018) (Figure 8.20).

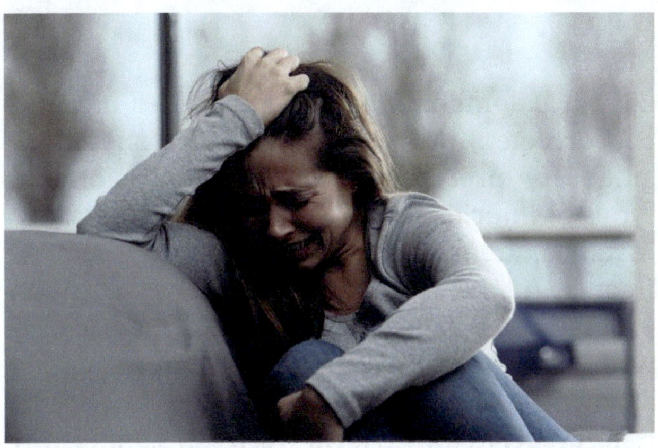

Figure 8.20. Long-term effects of trauma.

Source: https://www.northpointrecovery.com/wp-content/uploads/2017/02/The-Long-Term-Effects-of-Trauma-and-How-to-Deal-with-It.jpeg.

8.5.3. Importance of Mental Health Support

Mental health is not overemphasized, particularly when it comes to treating trauma and injury. Trauma has serious psychological consequences, normally more so than physical injuries. People who experience trauma, whether caused by an accident or disease, tend to develop stress disorders, anxiety, and depression. This stress psychologically makes recovery a challenging task, leading to poor outcomes if not treated appropriately. Mental health treatment, in the form of therapy and counseling, is vital in helping people deal with their experiences, overcome emotional suffering, and learn to adapt. Recognizing the intersection of mental and physical health enables medical providers to create comprehensive treatment plans that significantly enhance overall recovery and wellness. Informal care is also important in mental illness, as informal caregivers would typically face undue physical and emotional exertion in caring for the long-term disabled or severely traumatized. The caregivers would most likely face stressors that may lead to burnout and poor mental health. Psychological needs of the caregivers need to be attended to so that the caregiver-patient relationship can be established and thus affect the quality of care rendered. Research has indicated that the optimization of carer resilience has short-term dividends for both caregiver and their cared-for individuals. Intervention was seen to be highly promising in fostering resilience and suggesting that investment in caregivers' mental health proportionally transfers to dividends across the broader system of care (Piccenna et al., 2025). Moreover, the applicability of mental health services extends to occupational fields that have been traumatized, such as police departments. Policemen tend to encounter traumatic incidents and are subjected to extreme psychological duress, with resulting high levels of burnout and suicide. An urgent demand currently exists for mental health interventions that have been tailored to this population. Existing resources must adjust in a bid to effectively destigmatize mental health conditions and provide certain interventions for officers with difficulties in emotional coping with their exposures. Including learning programs that focus on psychological well-being from the initial stages of training can foster better coping methods and resilience in the long term (Dombroski et al., 2017). In general terms, putting mental health care first through various levels of trauma and injury treatment is key to enhancing individual and community wellness (Figure 8.21).

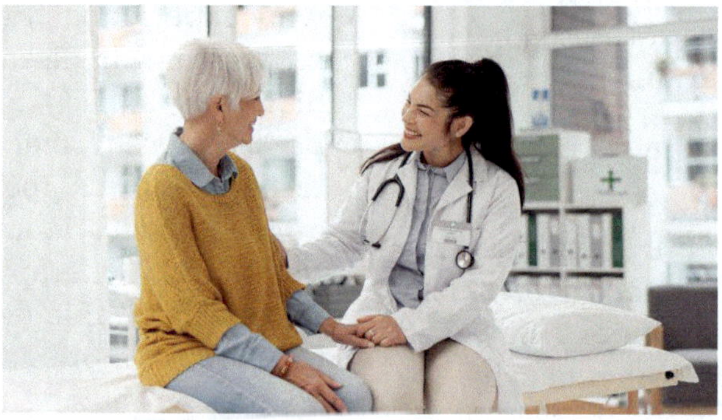

Figure 8.21. The importance of mental health support for aging adults.

Source: https://www.chenmed.com/sites/default/files/styles/blog_post_teaser/public/2024-11/The%20Importance%20of%20Mental%20Health%20Support%20for%20Aging%20Adults.jpg?itok=w8bZ5cor.

Test Your Knowledge

1. What are the common psychological responses?
2. What is the importance of mental health support?

8.6. Prevention Strategies

Learning Outcome

1. Describe the education and awareness programs
2. Know the safety regulations and policies
3. Understand the role of community involvement in trauma and injury prevention

Effective prevention measures are crucial in reducing the incidence of injury and trauma, particularly in high-risk environments such as farming. Farming has been recognized by Deasy et al. (2018) as being one of Ireland's most dangerous occupations, with rising numbers of farm accidents mainly affecting older men. To be corrected, prevention programs should be guided by precise data on the population and types of injuries that occur among farmers. For instance, identifying common injuries, such as fractures of the tibia/fibula, can inform education programs to enhance safe practices when dealing with farm animals. In addition, implementing awareness campaigns that describe the specific risks associated with farm work can significantly enhance workers' awareness and help them adopt appropriate precautionary measures. By putting the spotlight on tailored strategies, the focus can shift from retrospective medical care to future prevention of trauma, resulting in improved safety in farms. In addition to demographic-specific interventions, establishing a culture of continuous education and upgrading competence in trauma nursing is also crucial. The required trauma care competencies are diverse and must cover a broad spectrum of prevention strategies. A scoping review cited in 최모나 (2019) emphasizes that trauma nursing competencies encompass care-giving across various contexts, such as prehospital care, hospital care, and rehabilitation. It also foregrounded the existence of an overwhelming gap in the incorporation of the aforementioned competencies, along with the prevention of injury. Participating in this disconnect is essential; by not including injury prevention in the curriculum for trauma nurses, a probable means of minimizing trauma through proactive action is left untapped. Incorporating training on identifying risk and preventing injury into nurse education can therefore produce a workforce concerned with health promotion and protection in trauma care. Last but not least, stakeholders such as healthcare providers, safety regulatory agencies, and community groups must work together to formulate effective prevention strategies. The intricate relationship between trauma calls for an integrative response by matching medical knowledge with knowledge from the community to build effective preventive measures. For example, joint work between local farmers, teachers, and health workers can lead to community-based safety programs tailored to specific populations, thereby making them more effective. Furthermore, by promoting free information exchange between the groups, it is possible to share best practices and new prevention techniques, thereby reducing risks. In adopting a common prevention strategy, the overall strategy transcends the management of injury to establish sustainable practices that substantially reduce the incidence of trauma in the population. The combined effect created through these collaborations will progress a culture of safety and prevention of injury in trauma and injury care significantly.

8.6.1. Education and Awareness Programs

Education and awareness schemes are highly significant to preventing and managing trauma and injury care, particularly among susceptible groups. They provide individuals with education on the risks involved in certain activities and situations to enable them to make decisions that will limit injury. For instance, programs like the P.A.R.T.Y. (Prevent Alcohol and Risk-related Trauma in Youth) program have worked to effectively target youth, particularly those who are involved within the juvenile justice system. By taking real-life trauma scenarios, such programs confront the realities of risk-taking behavior. Research on this program demonstrates a significant reduction in violence and traffic offenses among participants in the future, presenting an economic approach to trauma prevention that not only instructs but also engages high-risk youth in an immersive learning experience (Burrell et al., 2012). Education and awareness programs have not only individual but also societal impacts. Informal caregivers often play a key role in trauma care, particularly for patients with severe and chronic disability, by providing essential support for medical and daily needs. Through educating these caregivers in educational content and psychosocial treatments, programs can enhance their resilience and effectiveness as caregivers. Studies show that psycho-educational and educational interventions have proved effective in supporting the capacity of informal carers to meet the challenges of their roles, thus limiting the formal healthcare system's workload. Not only does this multi-component intervention support the enhancement of quality care, but it also promotes a more sustainable care culture for people with long-term disabilities (Piccenna et al., 2025). Moreover, the success of education and awareness programs depends on periodic screening and updating to align them with community needs. Even though some interventions have been shown to be effective, the context for trauma and injury care is constantly evolving, due to new research discoveries as well as social change. Programs must adapt in an attempt to integrate evidence-based practices that take into consideration the special threats and challenges of specific demographic groups. Diversity requires a holistic approach with emphasis on continuous stakeholder involvement, feedback mechanisms, and integration of new findings. With awareness and education, communities can build resilience to harm and trauma, leading to healthier outcomes and improved care approaches for all concerned (Burrell et al., 2012; Piccenna et al., 2025) (Figure 8.22).

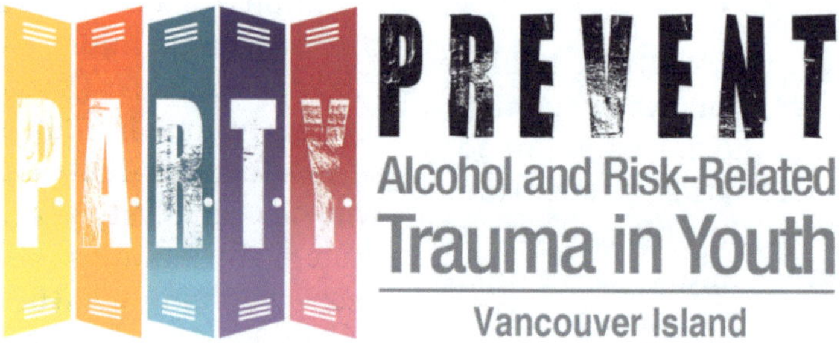

Figure 8.22. Prevent alcohol and risk-related trauma in youth (P.A.R.T.Y.).

Source: https://www.islandhealth.ca/sites/default/files/styles/banner_image/public/children-youth-family/PARTY/party-program-banner.png?itok=6NgOx5v6.

8.6.2. Safety Regulations and Policies

Good safety practices and policies are essential in trauma and injury care because they protect both patients and health workers from harm. They are designed to ensure that all medical personnel adhere to standard procedures to lower the risk of errors or unwanted effects during treatment. For instance, the establishment of procedures for data gathering and validation in clinical trials enhances the validity of findings, particularly in such complex cases as brain injuries. The coordination facilitated by IT-based solutions, including the efforts exemplified by efforts such as BrainIT, illustrates how systematic information management can enhance safety in trauma care by providing institutions with vital information securely across institutions. Without such regulatory frameworks, clinical procedures would no longer be cohesive enough to ensure the safety of patient well-being, potentially jeopardizing recovery processes in those who suffer debilitating injuries (Piper et al., 2009). In college athletics, safety legislation plays a fundamental role in protecting student-athletes from the effects of injury sustained through athletic competition. The National Collegiate Athletic Association (NCAA) has set up regulations governing the participation of athletes, but there are significant loopholes in responsibility that expose student-athletes to the long-term effects of illness. The existing system, at times providing an appearance of informed consent, fails to adequately disclose the risks associated with high-level sporting activity. As indicated by current criticism, coercive relationships between NCAA and student-athletes result in the absence of transparency with regard to potential injuries (Jacinto et al., 2020). This is a reason why the mandate of the NCAAs should be reinterpreted to ensure athletes receive full disclosure of potential risks involved, thereby creating a safer environment within college sports. Moreover, the effectiveness of safety regulations also relies on continuous evaluation and reshaping based on newly emerging evidence as well as from practitioners' experiences on the ground. Reviewing current policies can reveal gaps, such as insufficient training for athletes and medical staff in injury prevention and response measures. The adoption of collaborative research activities, such as those undertaken by COSBID and similar groups, is critical for generating data to guide future safety programs (Piper et al., 2009).

By leveraging technological progress and developing improved regulatory models, stakeholders can foster a safe environment that prioritizes the welfare of patients and athletes alike. With the evolving environment of injury and trauma treatment, embracing a proactive approach to safety standards will minimize risks and enhance the quality of care delivered in hospitals and other healthcare facilities.

8.6.3. Community Involvement in Prevention

The role of community engagement in preventing injury and trauma lies at the heart of brokering the intricate aspect of violence and adversity that individuals, particularly young men and boys of color, endure. Community engagement provides a healthy space where individuals are able to engage together in brokering the causes of trauma, such as poverty and discrimination. By accessing local resources, organizations can make programs possible that educate families about trauma-informed care, thereby improving the resilience of the populations. Further, as community members become actively involved in developing prevention measures themselves, more culturally congruent interventions are likely to be created that meet the community's specific needs. This not only enables effective education but also fosters a sense of ownership among community members, which is critical to ensuring lasting success in managing trauma and injury (Wilson et al., 2009). Effective community-based programs have the potential to transform the violence prevention paradigm by collaborating with stakeholders such as the police, schools, and healthcare professionals. By building coalitions, these organizations can share resources, knowledge, and best practices to guide trauma-informed solutions tailored to communities.

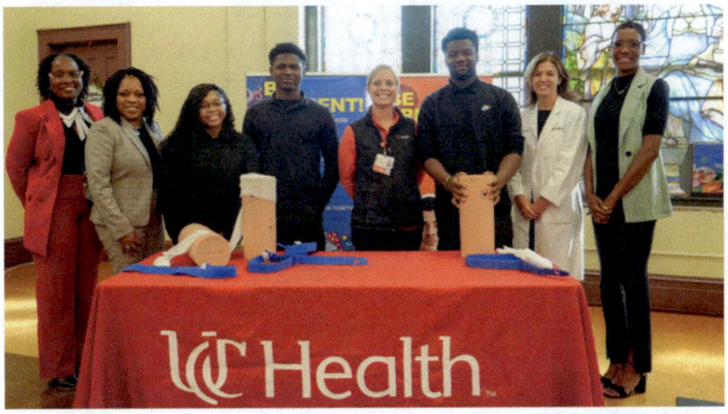

Figure 8.23. Role of community engagement in preventing injury and trauma.

Source: https://www.uchealth.com/content/dam/uchealth/images/media-room/articles/stop-the-bleed1.png.

When programs also involve parents, youth, and community leaders, they can enhance the protective factors that reverse the effects of trauma. Community involvement also raises awareness of the physical and emotional impacts of violence, allowing local advocates to influence policy change.

These programs can also address systemic problems that cause a cycle of trauma. For these programs to be as effective as possible, stakeholders within the community must be well-informed and responsive to their constituents' evolving needs (Rich, 2016). The integration of voices from the community into a framework of trauma prevention also entails understanding the implicit and explicit racism that men and boys of color endure, further complicating their pathways with trauma. It is critical to grasp this in creating interventions that are not only trauma-informed but also culturally responsive. Community discussion of their experiences can outline unique challenges while promoting healing and resilience. By addressing both systemic and personal problems through community participation, programs can increase the social networks needed for healing. Through this, ultimately is a preventative model that not only deals with present issues but also establishes paths of long-term healing and empowerment so that young men and boys are helped to be their best selves (Wilson et al., 2009; Rich, 2016) (Figure 8.23).

Test Your Knowledge

1. What are the safety regulations?
2. What is the role of community involvement in trauma and injury prevention?

SUMMARY

The concluding chapter summary on trauma and injury care consolidates the most important findings and implications raised throughout the book. Prehospital care and patient outcome remain in focus, with the question of how on-scene times and provided care influence mortality rates being a highlighted concern. Surprisingly, findings demonstrate a strong correlation between longer on-scene times and a higher risk of mortality, highlighting the importance of effective emergency medical services. As Frankema et al. (2007) imply, variation in on-scene duration of care might affect assessments of trauma severity, which in turn influences treatment processes. The optimization of response times and EMS is therefore important for improving patient survival rates and overall performance in trauma care. In addition to this, the psychological impact of trauma cannot be overlooked in the overall framework of injury care. Survivors of the traumatic event experience long-term impairment of emotional and professional functioning that requires integrated intervention from healthcare professionals. The work conducted on survivors of fire shows that trauma's impact is more multidimensional than physical harm, with a significant decline in mental health and quality of life. As put by Fregni et al. (2012), emotional trauma tends to overpower physical injuries, implying the need for integrated support systems that incorporate both psychological and physical healing. This identification calls for trauma care systems that provide priority to mental health treatment alongside traditional injury care, with emphasis on a balanced care approach. Generally, trauma and injury care must involve an integrated approach with both short-term medical attention and long-term mental health care. The interplay between physical and mental health increases the complexity of recovery in trauma patients, which elucidates the need for paradigms of integrated care. Optimal systems, where prehospital response strategies are maximized and mental health facilities are allocated, can lead to improved patient outcomes. Overall, the study presents an urgent imperative for policymakers and healthcare professionals to enhance trauma systems of care that consider the biological and psychosocial principles of recovery. Embracing this all-encompassing methodology will ultimately result in a more effective system of addressing trauma and its inevitable effects on populations and individuals.

With a focus on trauma and injury treatment, it is important to emphasize the growing importance of joint clinical research, especially in multi-center trials. Effective treatment and care for injuries due to trauma, such as those brought about by brain injury, need extensive data collection among institutions. The severity of cases with multi-trauma, particularly those related to brain injury care, demands more advanced technical infrastructures that provide safe access and sharing of information among hospitals. As highlighted by collaborative efforts such as the BrainIT and COSBID initiatives, overcoming obstacles to data accessibility can go a long way in improving the quality of clinical research and trials, which ultimately translates into improved patient outcomes. It is thus important to invest in IT-based solutions for data collection and validation, with collaborative research a pillar in driving trauma and injury care practices forward (Piper et al., 2009). Another crucial aspect of trauma care is timing in surgery, particularly in spinal cord injury (SCI). There is some evidence now that indicates early decompression is very helpful to patients with SCI, as timely surgery is linked with improved outcomes. Early surgery adoption is heterogeneous, with controversy regarding the optimal window of intervention; adopted thresholds are typically between ultra-early (8–12 hours) and late (>48–72 hours). Current reviews have determined that optimal outcomes are associated with more rapid surgical timelines. Prehospital and hospital logistical barriers still stand to delay access to prompt surgical intervention for most patients. Additional studies should be conducted to establish fine-tuned surgical criteria and to surmount these logistical hurdles to treat patients in a timely and efficient manner (Badhiwala et al., 2020). Lastly, care for trauma and injury requires an integrated model with collaborative research and immediate clinical interventions. Integration of cutting-edge data-sharing infrastructures and implementation of evidence-based surgical practices hold promise for improved outcomes in trauma cases. Through cooperation of medical institutions and focus on innovations in data gathering and surgery, the specialty can enhance the quality of care provided for the traumatized. Serious efforts in overcoming present obstacles—both access to data and logistics of interventions in a timely fashion—will play a crucial role in shaping the future of trauma and injury care and eventually benefit patients in need of specialized treatment and rehabilitation. This integrated approach to trauma management ensures ongoing improvement and resilience within the health system, facilitating optimal recovery trajectories in victims of injury (Badhiwala et al., 2020; Piper et al., 2009).

KEY TERMS FROM THIS CHAPTER

- Acute trauma
- Chronic pain
- Emotional trauma
- Injury care
- Physical trauma
- Psychological trauma
- Spatial analysis
- Blunt force trauma
- Chronic trauma
- Geographic information systems
- Penetrating trauma
- Post-traumatic stress disorder
- Sonography
- Trauma care

CRITICAL THINKING QUESTIONS

1. **What is the primary assessment step in trauma care?**
   a. Administering oxygen
   b. Securing intravenous access
   c. Airway, Breathing, Circulation (ABC) evaluation
   d. Performing diagnostic imaging
2. **In the case of suspected spinal injury, what is the most important initial step?**
   a. Move the patient to a sitting position
   b. Immobilize the spine and maintain cervical alignment
   c. Provide pain relief with oral medications
   d. Administer intravenous fluids immediately
3. **What is the primary imaging modality for assessing trauma patients in the emergency department?**
   a. MRI
   b. Ultrasound
   c. CT Scan
   d. X-ray
4. **Which of the following is a red flag for internal bleeding in trauma patients?**
   a. Normal blood pressure
   b. Tachycardia with hypotension
   c. Warm, dry skin
   d. Regular pulse and respiratory rate
5. **Which of the following is the most common cause of blunt abdominal trauma?**
   a. Stabbing
   b. Motor vehicle accidents
   c. Gunshot wounds
   d. Falls from height

Short Answer Questions

1. What is trauma?
2. Why is timely care important?
3. List the types of trauma.
4. What are the mechanisms of injury?
5. What is the psychological impact of trauma?

Answer to Critical Thinking Questions

1. (c); 2. (b); 3. (d); 4. (b); 5. (b).

REFERENCES

1. Almahmoud, K., Abboud, A., Namas, R. A., Zamora, R., Sperry, J., Peitzman, A. B., Truitt, M. S., Gaski, G. E., McKinley, T. O., Billiar, T. R., & Vodovotz, Y. (2019b). Computational evidence for an early, amplified systemic inflammation program in polytrauma patients with severe extremity injuries. *PLoS ONE, 14*(6), e0217577. https://doi.org/10.1371/journal.pone.0217577Abdul Raman, R., Jamaludin, H., Khaw, W. F., Mohd Riji, S., et al. (2013). Mental trauma experienced by caregivers of patients with diffuse axonal injury or severe traumatic brain injury. https://core.ac.uk/download/153811106.pdf (accessed on 14th July 2025).
2. Abell, A., Apostle, B., Benson, D., Blum, M., Bosse, M., Breccia, A., Brewster, R., et al. (2017). Critical-sized bone defects: Sequence and planning. https://core.ac.uk/download/287623796.pdf (accessed on 14th July 2025).
3. Abu-Zidan, F. M., Ansaloni, L., Biffl, W., Catena, F., et al. (2016). WSES classification and guidelines for liver trauma. https://core.ac.uk/download/84403004.pdf (accessed on 14th July 2025).
4. Aiken, L. H., Bate, P., Beckett, A., Black, N., Braun, D., Centre for Workforce Intelligence, Edwards, M., et al. (2014). Providing effective trauma care: The potential for service provider views to enhance the quality of care (qualitative study nested within a multicenter longitudinal quantitative study). https://core.ac.uk/download/30627896.pdf (accessed on 14th July 2025).
5. Aldred, D., Cowley, A., Crabb, R., Crouch, R., et al. (2019). Presence of a pre-hospital enhanced care team reduces on-scene time and improves triage compliance for stab trauma. https://core.ac.uk/download/287582487.pdf (accessed on 14th July 2025).
6. Alexander, D. A., Bell, J., Bertelson, P., Bryant, R., Freedy, J., Hanley, C., Harvey, M., et al. (2017). Addressing traumatic stress in the acute traumatically injured patient. https://core.ac.uk/download/213086871.pdf (accessed on 14th July 2025).
7. Anke, A. G., Ardolino, A., Ashford, R. L., Bayley, M., Bergner, H., Bertisch, H., Berwick, D. M., et al. (2016). Indicators of injury recovery identified by patients, family members and clinicians. https://core.ac.uk/download/76982230.pdf (accessed on 14th July 2025).
8. Anthony, W., Cooke, C., Crossley, M., Carless, D., Guttman, L., McKenna, J., Lieblich, A., et al. (2013). Psychosocial outcomes of an inclusive adapted sport and adventurous training course for military personnel. https://core.ac.uk/download/29018278.pdf (accessed on 14th July 2025).
9. Babl, F. E., Borland, M., Bressan, S., Cheek, J. A., et al. (2019). Traumatic brain injury in young children with isolated scalp hematoma. https://core.ac.uk/download/327951027.pdf (accessed on 14th July 2025).
10. Badhiwala, J., Fehlings, M. G., Harrop, J., Kwon, B. K., et al. (2020). Early surgery for traumatic spinal cord injury: Where are we now? https://core.ac.uk/download/288122076.pdf (accessed on 14th July 2025).
11. Bajaj, T., Carlin, E., Nelson, M., Palmieri, J., et al. (2020). Ultrasound identification of retrobulbar hematomas by emergency physicians in a cadaveric model. https://core.ac.uk/download/305124074.pdf (accessed on 14th July 2025).
12. Bakker, M., de Jongh, M. A. C., Enting, M., Geuze, E., et al. (2024). The cross-sectional and longitudinal interconnectedness of physical, psychological and role functioning following

physical trauma: A network analysis. https://core.ac.uk/download/620820046.pdf (accessed on 14th July 2025).

13. Ball, C. G., Fabian, T. C., Feliciano, D. V., Ivatury, R., et al. (2017). History of the innovation of damage control for management of trauma patients: 1902–2016. https://core.ac.uk/download/84402892.pdf (accessed on 14th July 2025).
14. Bandeeri, N., Henry, J. A., Meredith, C., Treacy, P. J., et al. (2004). The prevalence of cocaine-associated chest pain in a London hospital. https://core.ac.uk/download/5230488.pdf (accessed on 14th July 2025).
15. Bizon, L. J., Jr. (2017). *Traumatic Brain Injury Screening Tools in Primary Care.* https://core.ac.uk/download/79664900.pdf (accessed on 14th July 2025).
16. Bochicchio, G., Bochicchio, K., Kronen, R., Liang, S. Y., et al. (2017). Invasive fungal infections secondary to traumatic injury. https://core.ac.uk/download/129069519.pdf (accessed on 14th July 2025).
17. Brügger, U., Denk, E., Eichler, K., Gutzwiller, F., et al. (2019). The impact of the AO Foundation on fracture care: An evaluation of 60 years AO Foundation. https://core.ac.uk/download/289121729.pdf (accessed on 14th July 2025).
18. Burrell, M., Geelhoed, E., Gope, M., Ho, K., et al. (2012). An injury awareness education program on outcomes of juvenile justice offenders in Western Australia: An economic analysis. https://core.ac.uk/download/77142602.pdf (accessed on 14th July 2025).
19. Carenzo, L., Cattuto, C., Colombo, D., Della Corte, F., et al. (2018). Wearable proximity sensors for monitoring a mass casualty incident exercise: A feasibility study. https://core.ac.uk/download/653699673.pdf (accessed on 14th July 2025).
20. Cassar, K. (2006). Diagnostic peritoneal lavage: An obituary? https://core.ac.uk/download/46602096.pdf (accessed on 14th July 2025).
21. Chalya, P. L., Dass, R. M., Kalluvya, S. E., Mayala, B. K., et al. (2010). Prevalence of HIV infection among trauma patients admitted to Bugando Medical Centre, Mwanza, Tanzania and its influence on outcome. https://core.ac.uk/download/pdf/18410768.pdf (accessed on 14th July 2025).
22. Cheserem, B., Härtl, R., Ikwuegbuenyi, C., Lazaro, R., et al. (2024). Is mechanism of injury associated with outcome in spinal trauma? An observational cohort study from Tanzania. https://core.ac.uk/download/615460267.pdf (accessed on 14th July 2025).
23. Christensen, M. C., Lecky, F. E., Morris, S., Munro, P., et al. (2008). Outcomes and costs of blunt trauma in England and Wales. https://core.ac.uk/download/335446.pdf (accessed on 14th July 2025).
24. Cross, K., Fallat, M. E., Laniewicz, M., Nti, M., et al. (2019). A novel streamlined trauma response team training improves imaging efficiency for pediatric blunt abdominal trauma patients. https://core.ac.uk/download/187423820.pdf (accessed on 14th July 2025).
25. Dart, B., Davis, N., Patel, O., Vopat, L., et al. (2020). Enhancing splinting confidence through inter-residency education: An educational workshop. https://core.ac.uk/download/289166202.pdf (accessed on 14th July 2025).
26. Deasy, C., & Sheehan, M. (2018). A descriptive study of the burden of animal-related trauma at Cork University Hospital. https://core.ac.uk/download/149224823.pdf (accessed on 14th July 2025).

27. Dey, P., Mukhopadhyaya, B., Roy, S., Vempati, R., et al. (2012). A profile of knee injuries suffered by Australian Army Reserve soldiers. https://core.ac.uk/download/196606976.pdf (accessed on 14th July 2025).

28. Doben, A. R., Dolich, M., Grigorian, A., Gross, J., et al. (2020). Outcomes after pneumonectomy versus limited lung resection in adults with traumatic lung injury. https://core.ac.uk/download/323308579.pdf (accessed on 14th July 2025).

29. Dombroski, M. (2017). Changing police culture: Raising awareness of the importance of mental health. https://core.ac.uk/download/162579322.pdf (accessed on 14th July 2025).

30. Eriksson, J. (2022). Aspects of risk factors, pathophysiology and outcomes in trauma. https://core.ac.uk/download/516463999.pdf (accessed on 14th July 2025).

31. Ferrada, P., & Peysha, J. (2017). Operative and nonoperative management of blunt liver injuries. https://core.ac.uk/download/84404215.pdf (accessed on 14th July 2025).

32. Frankema, S. P. G., Patka, P., Ringburg, A. N., Schipper, I. B., et al. (2007). Helicopter emergency medical services (HEMS): Impact on on-scene times. https://core.ac.uk/download/19192458.pdf (accessed on 14th July 2025).

33. Fregni, F., Ryan, C. M., Salles, S. S., Schneider, J. C., et al. (2012). The long-term impact of physical and emotional trauma: The Station Nightclub Fire. https://core.ac.uk/download/28942158.pdf (accessed on 14th July 2025).

34. Glover, L., Greenfield, M., & Jomeen, J. (2016). What is traumatic birth? A concept analysis and literature review. https://core.ac.uk/download/151161006.pdf (accessed on 14th July 2025).

35. Hawley, C., & Joseph, S. (2008). Predictors of positive growth after traumatic brain injury: A longitudinal study. https://core.ac.uk/download/49380.pdf (accessed on 14th July 2025).

36. Holcomb, J. B., Radhakrishnan, H., Scerbo, M., Wade, C. E., et al. (2019). System and method for determining triage categories. https://core.ac.uk/download/211343488.pdf (accessed on 14th July 2025).

37. Jacinto, A. (2020). Should the NCAA have to pay? Long-term injuries in college athletics, improper assumptions of risk, and coverage of medical expenses after college. https://core.ac.uk/download/322983775.pdf (accessed on 14th July 2025).

38. Kalliopi, A., Kuzuku, A., Adem, A. A., Cooper, C., Raul, C., Aylwin, C. J., Wisner, D., et al. (2011). Pattern and outcome of chest injuries at Bugando Medical Centre in Northwestern Tanzania. https://core.ac.uk/download/pdf/16666644.pdf (accessed on 14th July 2025).

39. Kennedy-Moffat, J. (1997). *The Psychological Impact of Motor Vehicle Accidents: A New Zealand Study: A Thesis Presented in Partial Fulfilment of The Requirements for The Degree of Master of Science in Psychology at Massey University*. https://core.ac.uk/download/159449347.pdf (accessed on 14th July 2025).

40. Kim, E., Kuppermann, N., & Tzimenatos, L. (2014). The Pediatric Emergency Care Applied Research Network: A history of multicenter collaboration in the United States. https://core.ac.uk/download/323069086.pdf (accessed on 14th July 2025).

41. Koch, M. (2018). Spatial epidemiology of summer trauma in Scott County, IA: Use of GIS to identify trauma incidence in urban and rural areas. https://core.ac.uk/download/234816903.pdf (accessed on 14th July 2025).

42. Kumar, R. (2018). Acute inflammation and infection: The effects on recovery following moderate-to-severe traumatic brain injury. https://core.ac.uk/download/163106577.pdf (accessed on 14th July 2025).

43. Moss, L., Piper, I., & Stell, A. (2018). Automated measurement of adherence to traumatic brain injury (TBI) guidelines using neurological ICU data. https://core.ac.uk/download/151169979.pdf (accessed on 14th July 2025).

44. Piccenna, L., Pattuwage, L., Bragge, P., & Gruen, R. (2025). Optimizing support for informal carers of the long-term disabled to enhance resilience and sustainability. https://core.ac.uk/download/pdf/30672597.pdf (accessed on 14th July 2025).

45. Piper, I., & Sinnott, R. O. (2009). E-infrastructures fostering multi-center collaborative research into the intensive care management of patients with brain injury. https://core.ac.uk/download/1396979.pdf (accessed on 14th July 2025).

46. Rich, J. (2016). *Moving Toward Healing: Trauma and Violence and Boys and Young Men of Color.* https://core.ac.uk/download/71338671.pdf (accessed on 14th July 2025).

47. Wilson, A., Rich, J., Rich, L., Bloom, S., Evans, S., & Corbin, T. (2009). *Healing the Hurt: Trauma-Informed Approaches to The Health of Boys and Young Men of Color.* https://core.ac.uk/download/71360851.pdf (accessed on 14th July 2025).

ALLERGY AND IMMUNOLOGY

9

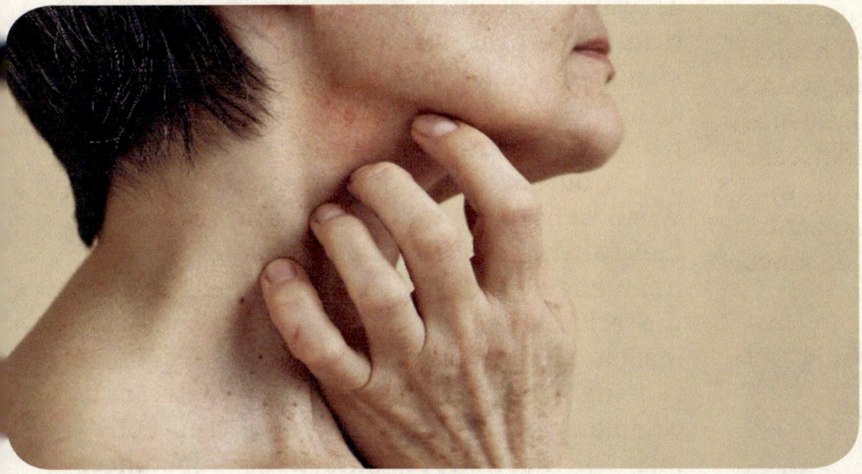

LEARNING OBJECTIVES

After studying this chapter, you will be able to:

1. Give an overview of the immune system
2. Understand the mechanisms of allergic reactions
3. Describe the common allergies in humans
4. Discuss the diagnosis of allergies
5. Understand the treatment and management of allergies
6. Describe the role of genetics in allergies

Introduction

Allergy and immunology research in humans gives an insight into the complex interaction between the immune system and the surroundings. Allergic reactions result from aberrant immune responses to previously harmless substances called allergens. Hypersensitivity is increasingly frequent, particularly in industrialized nations, due to lifestyle and environmental causes that contribute significantly to its prevalence. Allergy pathophysiology is intricate and often IgE-mediated, as in canine atopic dermatitis (CAD). CAD and human atopic dermatitis have similar pathophysiologic characteristics, and thus, researchers undertook to explore the cause of their increasing incidence, particularly in urban areas where environmental burdens vary uniquely (Nødtvedt et al., 2007). One of the hallmarks of the discipline of allergy is to identify the pathway through which parasitic infection, such as helminths, modulates the immune system. Intestinal helminths coexist in most developing countries in association with humans and shape immune tolerance, and can act to prevent autoimmune disease and allergy. The reverse relationship between the elimination of helminths in industrialized nations and the rising trend of allergic conditions is a fundamental focus of immunology research. The current theories propose that the absence of such parasites, which humankind has co-evolved with for centuries, can lead to an overactive immune response against harmless allergens, consequently developing diseases such as allergic rhinitis and asthma (Else et al., 2014). The link points towards the evolutionary aspects of immunological defenses and the fine balance needed to maintain health. Furthermore, this evolving notion of allergy and immunology has again emphasized the influence of environmental and genetic factors in disease expression. Current evidence indicates that food changes, air pollution, and urbanization may influence immune function and enhance susceptibility to allergy.

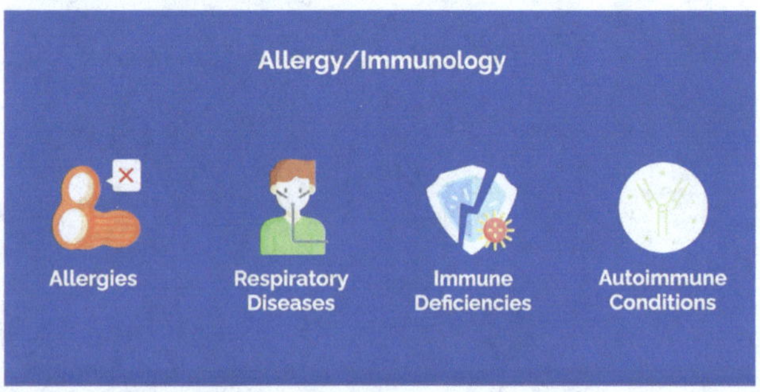

Figure 9.1. Allergy and immunology.

Source: https://medschoolinsiders.com/wp-content/uploads/2023/09/allergy-immunology-examples-graphic-1024x498.png.

Some segments of the population, particularly children, are at particular risk because their emerging immune system reacts to a wide variety of progressively complex allergens. Investigation of dietary interventions and preventive measures is gaining momentum, particularly regarding the potential merits of certain feeding patterns during very critical early periods of life (Nødtvedt et al., 2007). By integrating data from diverse disciplines such as epidemiology, genetics, and environmental science, researchers are striving to develop comprehensive methods to control and even prevent allergic disorders, with a view toward enhancing public health outcomes across diverse populations (Figure 9.1).

Definition of Allergies

An examination of immune response mechanisms underlying the development of allergies is necessary to understand allergies. Allergies result when the immune system confusingly identifies harmless particles, known as allergens, as harmful and mounts an overactive immune response. A few common allergens include pollen, dust mites, pet dander, and certain foods. When sensitized individuals are exposed to these allergens, their immune systems produce Immunoglobulin E (IgE) antibodies, causing the release of histamine and inflammatory mediators. It results in a spectrum of symptoms ranging from mild respiratory distress to complete anaphylactic responses. The body's misidentification of innocuous substances contributes to the complexity of immune system function and the need to balance reactivity and immune tolerance. Allergic conditions such as asthma, eczema, and allergic rhinitis are characterized by a heterogeneous clinical presentation that engages numerous organ systems. Each allergic reaction, while based on a common IgE pathway, can be radically different in severity and symptomatology between individuals. Some research suggests that allergic reactions may be linked to other immunological conditions, such as granulomatous-lymphocytic interstitial lung disease (GLILD), particularly in patients with associated immunodeficiency. The definition of GLILD, for instance, as a distinctive clinic-radio-pathological interstitial lung disease that is associated with a typical immune profile reflects the complexity of diagnosing allergic diseases in immunocompromised individuals. Such interdependencies in immunology reveal the broadest possible prevalence of allergies and emphasize the necessity of nuanced diagnosis and treatment protocols in practice (Avery et al., 2017). Furthermore, epidemiological research has suggested intriguing correlations between various infections and allergic sensitization, with particular interest in the role of helminth infections. Experiments have shown a negative correlation between helminth prevalence and allergic diseases, which suggests that immune responses elicited by the parasites might be protective against allergies. Helminth products induce regulatory immune responses that can suppress allergic sensitization, underscoring the intricate interplay among immune pathways. The observations have far-reaching consequences, as they raise questions about evolutionary adaptations and immunological balance in immune regulation. The illumination of the modes by which helminth infections and allergens engage the immune system expands our understanding of allergy mechanisms and intensifies debate about possible therapeutic interventions and prophylactic measures in allergy and immunology (Mutapi et al., 2012) (Figure 9.2).

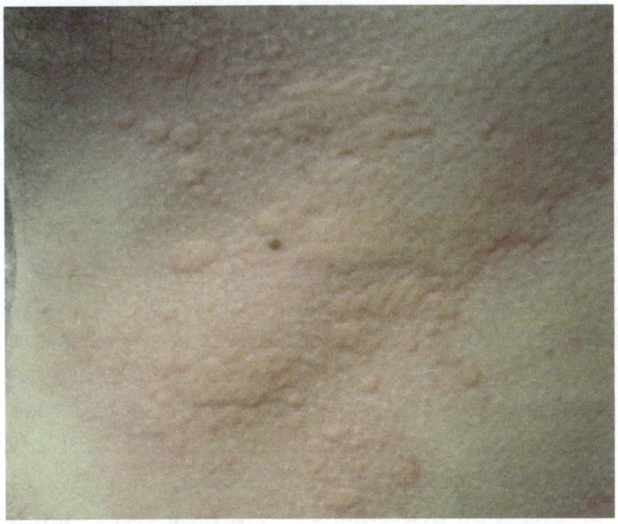

Figure 9.2. Allergies.

Source: https://upload.wikimedia.org/wikipedia/commons/6/6f/Hives2010.JPG.

Importance of Studying Allergies and Immunology

The rising prevalence of allergies and allergic diseases in some populations underscores the relevance of allergy and immunology research. The topic is significant for understanding the mechanisms of allergy, which often involve complex interplay between environmental factors and the immune system. For instance, the frequency of canine atopic dermatitis (CAD) provides hints about shared pathophysiologic mechanisms in humans and animals, thereby underscoring comparative studies as a means of understanding allergenic processes. CAD is linked with IgE-mediated responses to environmental allergens and has been found to be comparable in nature to atopic dermatitis, particularly in industrial environments where altered lifestyles would have caused them to rise (Nødtvedt et al., 2007). With our increasing knowledge of these interactions, it is more important than ever that researchers work to develop specific treatments and prevention strategies aimed at the root causes of allergic disease. Additionally, the role of environmental influences, including climate change and pollution, on the increasing prevalence of allergy is an important area of research in immunology. Studies show that pollen exposure, one of the main provoking factors for respiratory allergies, is worsened by both global change and increased air pollution levels. Pollen from plants such as Kentucky bluegrass and white birch has been found to damage respiratory epithelial cells, making one more vulnerable to infections (Gevaert et al., 2019). This exchange between allergens and the immune system highlights the necessity of comprehensive research into how outside agents influence the onset and increase of allergies. By understanding these dynamics, researchers can create public health policy aimed at reducing exposure to allergens, ultimately benefiting patient outcomes and reducing the financial toll of allergic diseases. Finally, the study of allergies and immunology also facilitates the development of personalized medicine and treatment strategies tailored to the patient. A better understanding of the environmental and genetic factors that induce allergic responses enables clinicians to design individualized interventions tailored to each patient's background. For example, through the epidemiology of diseases such as CAD, the knowledge gained would help identify promising preventive treatments, i.e., dietary changes at crucial stages of development in allergy-prone individuals (Nødtvedt et al., 2007). Furthermore, as a result of advances in immunotherapy and biologic therapies, future research will enable doctors to identify which patients are most likely to benefit from specific therapies. The formulation of treatment modalities based on solid immunological research ultimately promises to enhance the quality of life for those suffering from allergies, thereby making the case that the topic of allergy and immunology is not merely an abstract academic concern but a pressing public health concern.

9.1. The Immune System: An Overview

Learning Outcome

1. Describe the components of the immune system
2. Describe the types of immunity
3. Understand the role of white blood cells in immune response

The immune system defends the human body from pathogens, such as viruses and bacteria, and attains a balance so that it does not respond unnecessarily to harmless substances. The immune system is made up of a subtle interaction of cells, tissues, and organs and operates through innate and adaptive mechanisms. The innate immune response provides immediate defense through barriers such as skin and mucous membranes, and it employs phagocytic cells that identify and destroy invading microbes. The adaptive immune response, involving particular lymphocytes and immunologic memory, takes time to develop and provides particular defense against previously encountered pathogens. This double use is an example of the sophisticated architecture of the immune system, allowing adequate responses while keeping the risk of allergic reactions to a minimum, where the immune response could mistakenly identify innocuous substances as dangerous. The sophistication of the immune system has particularly significant implications for immunological disorders such as Primary Immune Regulatory Disorders (PIRD). They arise from genetic defects in immune regulatory mechanisms and result in inappropriate immune responses. PIRD patients, for instance, may have hypo- and hyperimmune responses that cause immunodeficiency as well as autoimmunity of multiple organ systems. PIRD is challenging to treat; standard immunosuppressive therapy tends to be ineffective. Most importantly, hematopoietic cell transplant (HCT) has been a therapeutic option, with resolution of disease in over half of patients who have received it. The 5-year survival rate following such interventions is promising at 67%, drawing attention to further studies aimed at standardizing treatment protocols for the management of PIRD (Allenspach et al., 2020). As the field of allergy and immunology continues to develop, the assessment of immunological responses, particularly food allergies, becomes increasingly sophisticated. Using an Adverse Outcome Pathway (AOP) framework, there is a systematic investigation into the mechanistic basis of IgE-mediated food allergies. The framework provides a biological context to the existing *in vitro* tools for assessing the sensitizing capacity of various food proteins. By gaining a clear vision of molecular initiating events and key stages of the allergic sensitization process, researchers can more critically evaluate which tests are optimal. Significantly, the use of novel *ex vivo* culture methods may enhance current testing protocols and, potentially, avoid the need for animal models. Such a convergent comprehension of food allergen sensitivities is significant for ensuring the safety of new food sources, bridging opportunities for new food allergen risk evaluations (Benedé et al., 2019) (Figure 9.3).

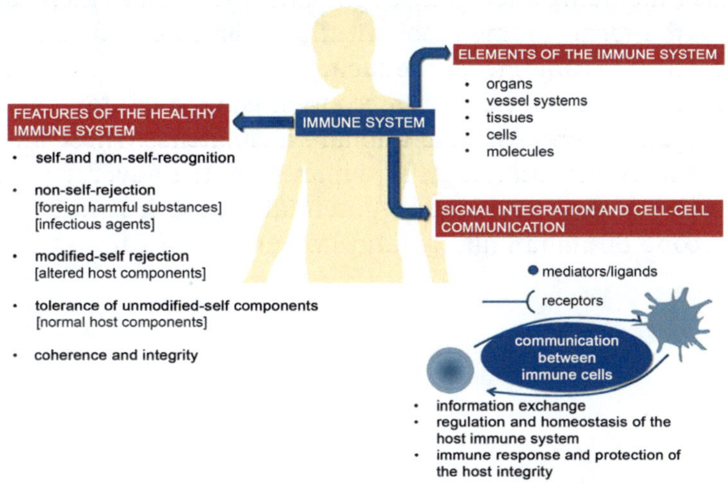

Figure 9.3. Overview of the immune system.

Source: https://cdnintech.com/media/chapter/54266/1512345123/media/F1.png.

9.1.1. Components of the Immune System

The immune system is an intricately organized collection of cells, tissues, and organs that work together to safeguard the body against infection-causing agents. At the core of this system are the white blood cells, or leukocytes, which detect and destroy harmful pathogens such as bacteria, viruses, and allergens. Among all leukocytes, lymphocytes, such as T cells and B cells, are particularly significant. T cells, which are produced in the thymus, are responsible for cell-mediated immunity, killing infected cells and coordinating the immune response. B cells, on the other hand, primarily function on humoral immunity, producing antibodies that specifically attack antigens. The intricate interaction between these cell types is guided by a set of molecules called cytokines, which not only regulate the immune response but also influence allergic reactions and autoimmunity; hence, it is more important to comprehend immune factors in the context of allergy and immunology in humans. With the exception of leukocytes, the inborn system is the body's first line of defense against foreign pathogens, providing physical barriers and numerous immune cell types. Epithelial cells that form layers on surfaces such as the skin and mucous membranes, for example, are physical barriers, while phagocytes such as macrophages and neutrophils actively engulf and destroy pathogens. Complement proteins also play a role, increasing inflammation and enhancing the capacity of antibodies and phagocytes to eliminate microbes. Another significant characteristic of the innate immune response is its more rapid activation than that of the adaptive immune system, which has a longer time for antigen recognition and response development. This two-way mechanism of defense mechanisms is a reflection of the immune response's sophistication, particularly in light of how allergens can exploit these mechanisms to cause hypersensitivity reactions, and is a primary theme in research on allergies and the immunological principles that govern them. Recent studies also indicate the significant role of the microbiome in maintaining the immune system's operation. The human microbiome is a community of trillions of microbes within and on the body that contributes to immune homeostasis and susceptibility to allergic disease. This association suggests that a diminished microbiome could be responsible for the rise in non-infectious diseases, including allergy, through pathways such as increased immune tolerance dysfunction. To this end, the term "biome reconstitution" has emerged as a promising therapeutic approach for rebalancing the microbiome and reducing allergic and autoimmune reactions. Through the reintroduction of specific missing helpful microorganisms in contemporary lifestyles, one can correct the immune dysregulation-relevant evolutionary mismatches. These methods track in parallel with innovative methods within immunology, as depicted by the adverse outcome pathway (AOP) method of evaluating food protein sensitization potential, where it is noted that extensive testing is required within the scope of human allergy and immunology (Adler et al., 2013; Benedé et al., 2019) (Figure 9.4).

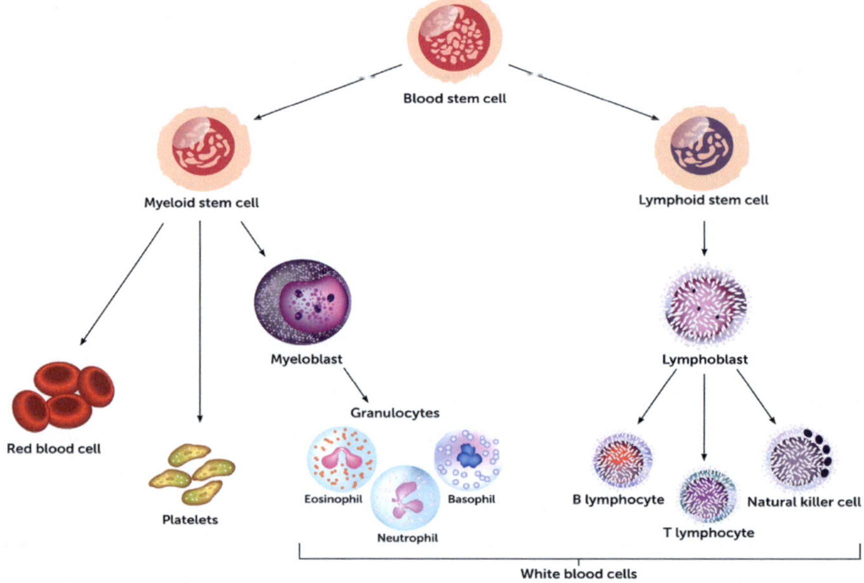

Figure 9.4. Blood cells.

Source: https://m2.healio.com/~/media/images/education-lab/learning-sites/learn-immuno-oncology/the-immune-system/learnimmunoblood.jpg.

9.1.2. Types of Immunity: Innate vs. Adaptive

The human immune system comprises two very important components: innate and adaptive immunity, both of which are essential to the body's defense against disease-causing organisms. The body's first line of defense is innate immunity, which contains non-specific mechanisms that respond rapidly against a wide range of pathogens. The response by the innate system includes physical barriers such as the skin and mucous membranes, and biochemical mechanisms, including phagocytosis by neutrophils and macrophages. One of the major characteristics of innate immunity is its ability to produce inflammatory responses that favor the recruitment of additional immune cells to the site of infection. Although rapid, the innate immune response lacks memory, a characteristic of adaptive immunity that guarantees a more precise and effective response during repeated infections by the same pathogen. Unlike innate immunity, adaptive immunity takes time to develop and is a very specific response to some antigens.

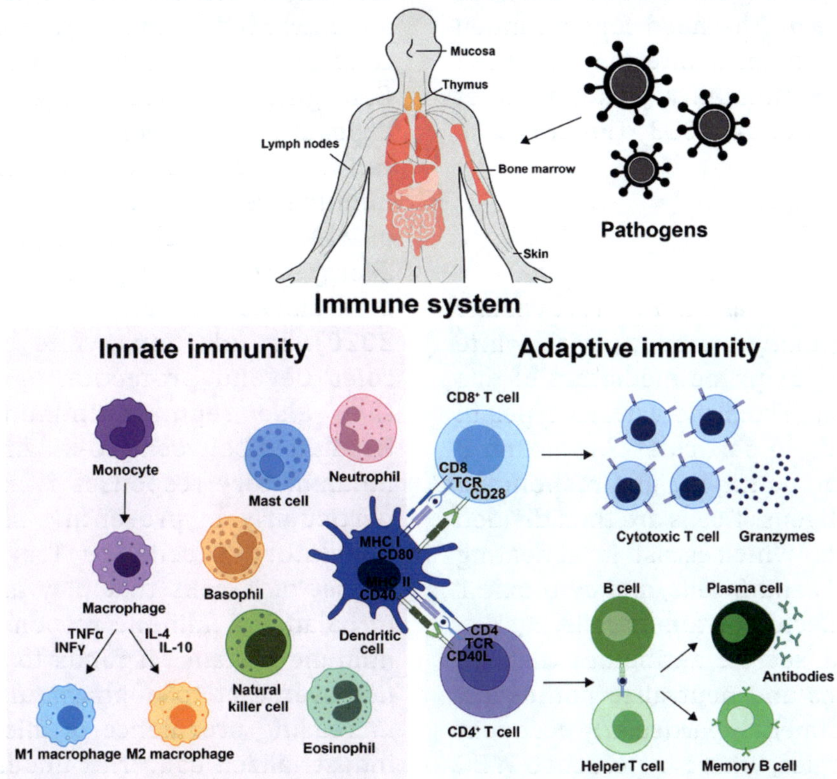

Figure 9.5. Types of the immune system.

Source: https://www.biointron.com/static/upload/image/20241128/1732726698157923.jpg.

This component of the immune system is primarily mediated by lymphocytes, including B cells and T cells. B cells secrete antibodies that neutralize pathogens, while T cells can kill infected host cells directly or help coordinate other immune responses. The adaptive immune system is perhaps most often invoked for its capacity to remember past infections, enabling it to react faster and more vigorously on subsequent exposure to the same pathogen. It is that memory aspect that is of such value in vaccination, where the goal is to trigger the adaptive immune system to detect and eliminate infectious agents without causing disease. These mechanisms emphasize the roles of innate and adaptive immunity in maintaining host health. The coordination between innate and adaptive immunity is essential for an effective immune response, particularly in allergic disorders, where the immune system responds abnormally to harmless substances. Allergies can be simply explained as a nonadaptive response in which sensitization against specific allergens leads to the production of immunoglobulin E (IgE) antibodies. Such hyper-sensitive reactions have been found to depend upon previous exposure to an allergen, revealing a loss of regulatory mechanisms typically present in normal immune responses. New findings have highlighted the role of innate immune cells in modulating the adaptive response, as seen in experiments documenting immune dysfunction across a variety of infections, including the SARS-CoV-2 pandemic. An improved understanding of these mechanisms will help to fill knowledge gaps and could lead to new therapy approaches for the management of allergic as well as infectious diseases, emphasizing the need for continued research into the complex interplay between innate and adaptive immunity (Sokolowska et al., 2020; Sandstedt et al., 2023) (Figure 9.5).

9.1.3. Role of White Blood Cells in Immune Response

The immune response is an interactive, dynamic process involving many elements, with white blood cells (WBCs) as prime mediators of this defense mechanism. From the various types of WBCs, lymphocytes, in particular T cells and B cells, are pivotal in identifying and responding against foreign antigens. T cells are then divided into helper T cells, which assist in activating other immune cells and B cells, and cytotoxic T cells, which kill infected or tumor cells. B cells, on the other hand, secrete antibodies that are specific to antigens and neutralize pathogens. This immune adjustment is particularly pertinent in the case of allergies, where hyperactive WBC responses to harmless stimuli can trigger a range of allergic reactions, highlighting the fine line the immune system must walk in its regulatory process. The white blood cell response to allergens is an ideal case of the tribulations faced in the immune response. Under allergic reactions, B-cell synthesis of Immunoglobulin E (IgE) is at the basis of the reaction, facilitating immediate hypersensitivity upon re-exposure to the allergen. This is typically followed by the release of histamine and other mediators from activated mast cells and basophils, thereby exacerbating allergy symptoms such as inflammation, itching, and difficulty breathing. Understanding these mechanisms is especially relevant in studies of allergic diseases, where an unwanted immune response can lead to conditions like asthma and atopic dermatitis. Emerging theories suggest that early-life exposure to a diverse microbial community can influence the development and activity of immune cells, underscoring the significance of white blood cells in shaping an individual's allergy susceptibility profile over time, as argued by available research evidence (Apostol et al., 2020). In addition, white blood cells have roles beyond protection against pathogens; they also regulate immune homeostasis. Regulation between pro-inflammatory and anti-inflammatory responses is extremely crucial, particularly in preventing allergic reactions. Regulatory T cells, or Tregs, are a unique subset of T cells that play an important role in balancing immune responses, ensuring the immune system responds to threats but does not overreact to nonharmful substances. The increasing prevalence of allergic illnesses in industrialized countries underscores the need to examine the role of lifestyle in the activity of these immune cells. For instance, restricted microbial exposures, as proposed by the hygiene hypothesis, might predispose immune reactions and skew them toward allergic manifestations (Nødtvedt et al., 2007). Thus, the study of the intricate activities of white blood cells in this context not only enhances our understanding of immune response but also sheds light on therapeutic strategies for allergy control.

Test Your Knowledge

1. What are the components of the immune system?
2. What are the 2 types of immunity?

9.2. Mechanisms of Allergic Reactions

Learning Outcome

1. Describe the types of allergens
2. Understand the process of sensitization
3. Describe the immediate and delayed allergic responses

The allergic pathological processes are multifactorial and involve subtle host environment interactions of the immune system and allergens. The allergic response usually begins with sensitization, in which an individual initially encounters an allergen and activates T-helper (Th) cells. The Th cells activate B cells to produce immunoglobulin E (IgE) antibodies against the allergen. Upon repeated exposures, the binding of the allergen to these IgE antibodies on the surfaces of mast cells and basophils leads to degranulation, such as histamine and other inflammatory mediators. This series of events leads to the classic symptoms of allergy, such as itching, swelling, and bronchoconstriction. Effective therapy of allergic reactions not only relies on understanding of such initial immune events but also on understanding how environmental factors can influence these reactions across various populations. Unsurprisingly, the presence of parasitic helminths sheds light on the control of allergic reactions. There is evidence of an inverse relationship between helminth infection and the prevalence of allergic sensitization or atopy, and it is suggested that helminths can induce regulatory immune responses capable of suppressing allergic reactivity (Mutapi et al., 2012). In many rural communities, helminths are paired with other immune challenges, possibly leading to adaptive immune responses that suppress inappropriate reactions to non-parasitic allergens. The dialogue between the immune system and helminth products appears to elicit a form of immunomodulation that suppresses allergen-related mechanisms while simultaneously favoring responses to helminthic infection. These findings pose intriguing evolutionary questions about host defense and the development of allergic diseases across varying environmental contexts. Moreover, chronic encroachment of westernized health behaviors that eliminate helminth infection has been associated with rising rates of autoimmune disease and allergy in developed nations (Else et al., 2014).

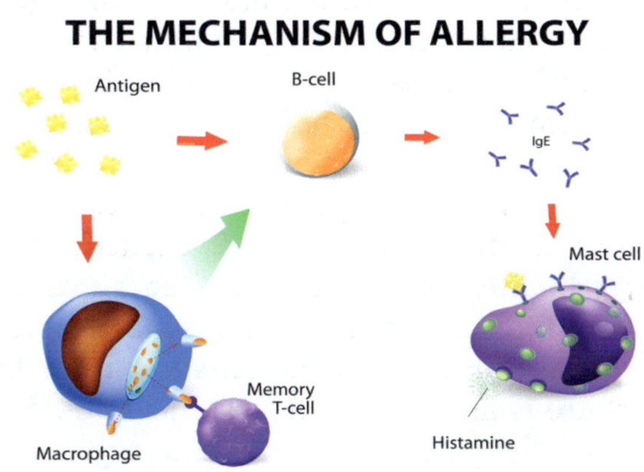

Figure 9.6. Mechanisms of allergy.

Source: https://allergie-geneve.com/wp-content/uploads/2023/08/Meca-1-1536x1238.webp.

This paradox explains the importance of understanding the role that helminths play in immunity homeostasis. In occupying a niche within the immunity landscape, helminths have the ability to regulate the host's immune responses, draining energy from hyper-reactive allergenic pathways. Therefore, investigation into the sophisticated interactions between the host and the helminth at the mucosal surface can reveal the therapeutic potential, i.e., novel vaccination strategies that exploit such immune modulatory activities. They are significant because they can inform public health interventions towards the control of the endemic wave of allergic disorders globally, with a reevaluation of our infectious disease eradication policy in preparation for the maintenance of healthy immune status (Figure 9.6).

9.2.1. Types of Allergens

Allergens, typically proteins that can elicit immune reactions, can be further classified into several types, viz., environmental, food, and arthropod allergens. Environmental allergens encompass a broad range of substances, including pollen, dust mites, fungal spores, and animal dander. Environmental allergens typically cause respiratory conditions, such as allergic rhinitis or asthma. For instance, pollen emitted at a specific season can cause severe allergic reactions in some individuals, underscoring the significance of temporal factors in allergen exposure. Identification and grouping of such environmental stimuli are required to effectively enforce management programs for allergic patients, as reducing exposure is most often the first line of defense against allergic reactions. Food allergens are of particular interest due to their potential to trigger potentially lethal reactions such as anaphylaxis. Common food allergens include proteins from milk, eggs, peanuts, tree nuts, fish, shellfish, soy, and wheat. The proteins have the potential to cause sensitization, whereby the immune system reacts unfavorably upon exposure. Research has advanced the molecular foundations of food allergies, yielding models such as the adverse outcome pathway (AOP) for categorizing allergens by their capacity to stimulate immune responses. This focused classification enables researchers and practitioners to identify sensitizing potential more easily, thereby helping people with food allergies receive precise dietary guidance to avoid accidental consumption of these poisonous proteins (Benedé et al., 2019). Insect allergens constitute yet another large group, primarily those from stinging insects such as bees and wasps. Their symptoms range widely, from local swelling to severe anaphylactic shock. Urban residents may experience more exposure to such allergens in terms of increased human-insect contact or increased population density, as has been researched in atopic diseases (Nødtvedt et al., 2007). The intricacy of insect allergy also makes its management more challenging and requires both avoidance of the allergen and possible immunotherapy to ensure lasting relief. Awareness of the type of allergens involved and the corresponding immunological response is important in the formulation of comprehensive strategies encompassing prevention and treatment, and therefore the quality of life in the affected subjects (Figure 9.7).

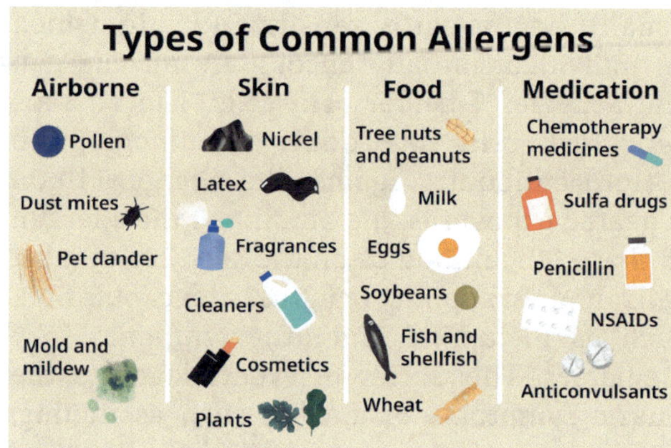

Figure 9.7. Types of common allergens.

Source: https://www.verywellhealth.com/thmb/VY-XGkcVbs8Q1uNM1JW7L8lORWc=/1500x0/filters:no_upscale():max_bytes(150000):strip_icc()/VWH-MichelaButtignol-AllergensTypes-4000x2700-736b224d42bf4961b60059a0c24ae8cc.png.

9.2.2. The Process of Sensitization

Sensitization is an important process in the pathogenesis of allergic diseases, in which the immune system comes to perceive a harmless material as harmful. Initially, when an individual who is sensitized comes into contact with an allergen, T cells are presented with allergen fragments by specialized immune cells, e.g., dendritic cells. This interaction converts naïve T cells to Th2 cells, which produce cytokines that further activate B cells to produce immunoglobulin E (IgE), an allergen-specific antibody. Over time, repeated exposure to the same allergen results in IgE binding to mast cells and basophils, leading to histamine release and other allergy-related mediators, such as itching, swelling, or anaphylaxis. Such an immunological response not only unravels the mechanisms underlying allergic reactions but also highlights the importance of understanding the sensitization pathways as the future in finding preventative strategies. Research has also clarified the role of risk assessments in sensitization processes, especially regarding dietary sources. Regulatory precepts prior to introducing new food proteins to the market require stringent assessments aimed at establishing potential food allergenicity (Benedé et al., 2019). By applying the adverse outcome pathway (AOP) framework, researchers can organize current knowledge of molecular and cellular processes in IgE-mediated food allergy into a systematic framework. This is crucial for developing efficient *in vitro* test methods. The merits and demerits of various current methods provide a foundation for understanding what drives food sensitization, offering insights into the typically complex interactions between food allergens and innate immunity. These observations are relevant to the identification and management of dietary allergens in risk groups, including children and pregnant women, who are at higher risk of developing allergy. Further, new research identifies that food allergies are on the rise, mainly in children and adults, and thus there is a need to look further into the cause of sensitization. For instance, recent studies indicate that while food allergies have been proven to be the second most common allergic illness in children, there has been insufficient focus on the adult experience (Seita et al., 2013). This research gap highlights the necessity of extensive studies that examine the relationship between mothers' allergies and their health conditions, as well as those of their infants. Such research is important for both determining food allergy prevalence and assessing its possible impact on perinatal health. Therefore, a multimodal approach, combining AOP frameworks and epidemiological research, is essential for addressing the challenges posed by rising sensitization rates and their broader public health implications (Figure 9.8).

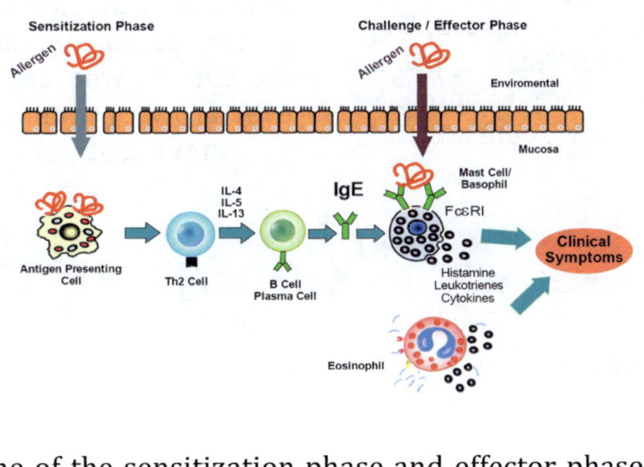

Figure 9.8. General scheme of the sensitization phase and effector phase in the immune response to food allergens.

Source: https://www.creative-diagnostics.com/blog/wp-content/uploads/2021/12/General-scheme-of-the-sensitization-phase-and-effector-phase-in-the-immune-response-to-food-allergens.png.

9.2.3. Immediate vs. Delayed Allergic Responses

The immune response to allergens can be classified into two types: immediate and delayed. Immediate allergic responses, also known as Type I hypersensitivity, occur within minutes of allergen exposure. They are mediated by IgE antibodies, which bind to allergens and trigger the release of histamine and other inflammatory mediators from mast cells and basophils. Common presentations for acute allergic responses are allergic rhinitis, urticaria, and anaphylaxis. The acute onset may lead to extremely severe symptoms, with a need for rapid medical assistance, particularly when anaphylaxis occurs. Understanding the underlying mechanisms of acute responses is essential because environmental factors and individual vulnerabilities still influence their incidence, particularly in an aging population, where allergic disease is spreading (Bonini et al., 2017). On the other hand, delayed allergic reactions, or Type IV hypersensitivity reactions, typically manifest hours to days following exposure to an allergen. They are T lymphocyte-mediated, specifically CD4+ T helper 1 cells, and do not involve antibody. Instead, the immune response is predicated on macrophage activation and cytotoxic T cells. This is typically seen in contact dermatitis, where irritants like poison ivy induce a reaction after sensitization. Delayed reactions are more often associated with chronic inflammation, which in turn can trigger more long-term conditions like asthma and eczema. The physiologic characteristics of the aged immune system can complicate such reactions, as aging changes may increase susceptibility to prompt and delayed allergic reactions (Bonini et al., 2017). The impact of immediate and delayed allergic reactions extends beyond individual health, influencing public health policy and research agenda for allergy and immunology. Therapeutic strategies are increasingly focused on interpreting and manipulating the immune response, most importantly with regard to regulatory T cells (Tregs), which play a key role in inducing tolerance and preventing unacceptable immune responses. The promise of Treg expansion as a therapeutic option offers a fascinating avenue for the treatment of allergic disease and the prevention of adverse reactions. An integrated approach that targets both acute and latent responses can lead to improved management techniques and outcomes for patients with allergies. How the two responses interact and influence one another through a detailed examination will enable the discipline to develop efficient strategies that address increasingly diverse patient populations, especially among the elderly, who are at risk of developing an ever-growing number of allergic disorders (Bonini et al., 2017).

Test Your Knowledge

1. What are the types of allergens?
2. What is the process of sensitization?

9.3. Common Allergies in Humans

Learning Outcome

1. Know the impact of environmental allergens
2. Understand the food allergies
3. Describe the phenomenon of drug allergies

Allergies are more prevalent conditions that afflict a considerable majority of the human population in the form of immune responses against otherwise harmless substances. The most prevalent allergens are pollen, dust mites, dog and cat dander, foods, and insect stings. In sensitive individuals, exposure to these allergens triggers an inappropriate immune response, which is usually the formation of Immunoglobulin E (IgE) antibodies. This immune reaction can lead to as mild as sneezing and itching or as severe as anaphylaxis. The increasing incidence of allergic disorders, particularly among urban dwellers, suggests a complex interplay between environmental factors and genetic predisposition. Notably, these reactions can significantly affect quality of life, rendering it crucial to take appropriate measures to curtail the allergenic load on individuals' health. Food allergy is a common allergy, affecting millions of people worldwide and causing different harmful reactions when particular allergens such as peanuts, tree nuts, fish, and shellfish are ingested. Recent advances in clarifying the immunological processes that orchestrate these allergic responses have underscored the need for extensive research into food safety assessments. According to emerging evidence, gut absorption and digestion of dietary proteins are crucial factors to consider before introducing new dietary proteins into the food supply. Evidence covers the molecular and cellular processes involved in IgE-mediated food allergies, as reported in validated frameworks like the adverse outcome pathway (AOP) (Benedé et al., 2019). It aids not only in the detection of susceptible individuals but also in the production of safe foodstuffs for human use, thereby eliminating the risk of extremely severe allergic reactions. The interaction between the immune system and human microbiota is significant for the frequency and severity of allergy. Environmental changes, such as urbanization and dietary modifications, have led to a drastic decrease in microbial diversity, thereby affecting the immune system's ability to distinguish between harmful and harmless agents. This aspect, also known as the biodiversity hypothesis, suggests that reduced exposure to natural environmental microbes may contribute to increased allergy and other inflammatory disorders (Lehtimäki et al., 2017). When the microbiota is changed, the complex balance of the immune reaction is disturbed, and individuals are susceptible to allergy. Encouraging multidiverse exposure to microbes through lifestyle choices—such as dwelling outdoors or maintaining traditional farming—can thus be fundamental to optimizing immune regulation and preventing the prevalence of allergic disease in modern populations (Figure 9.9).

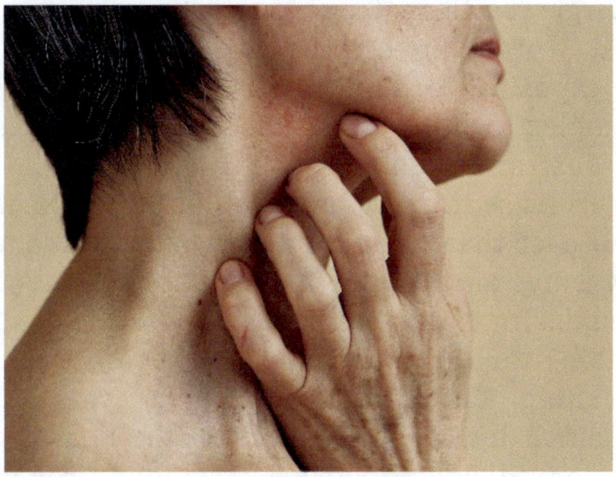

Figure 8.9. Common allergy.

Source: https://www.health.com/thmb/_-ZjWrLdiFlD_8FKQqFh77y9Aeo=/6720x0/filters:no_upscale():max_bytes(150000):strip_icc()/Health-GettyImages-1765432668-00434bbc48ed43f691b4bd9cc5a9aca5.jpg.

9.3.1. Environmental Allergens (Pollen, Dust Mites)

The impact of environmental allergens, including pollen and dust mites, on human health is significant and multifaceted. Pollen from grasses, trees, and weeds is a main trigger for seasonal allergic rhinitis, also known as hay fever. The inhalation of pollen grains induces a hypersensitivity response, leading to symptoms such as sneezing, a runny nose, and watery eyes. This is due to sensitization of the immune system, which, in error, identifies otherwise harmless particles as dangerous. The increase in allergic diseases such as asthma and dermatitis worldwide can be partly accounted for by environmental and lifestyle factors that increase exposure to such allergens, making it ever more critical to conduct broad studies on their frequency and management in urban centers, where such phenomena are most pronounced. Dust mites, small animals that inhabit warm and moist environments, are another major environmental allergen. Dust mites feed on organic material, much of which is human skin shed, and their fecal pellets harbor very potent allergens that can cause severe allergic reactions. Chronic coughing, wheezing, and worsening eczema are manifestations of exposure to dust mites, which are highly complex for individuals affected. Management of dust mite numbers in homes, particularly in urban settings, requires an interdisciplinary approach that includes education on avoidance measures and housing modifications. Evidence demonstrates that reducing exposure to dust mites, through actions such as intensive cleaning, can decrease allergic symptoms significantly, thereby improving the quality of life for individuals with sensitizations. Growing evidence suggests intriguing interactions between environmental allergens and the immune system. For instance, studies have indicated that patients infected with helminths have lower rates of allergic diseases, potentially due to the immunomodulatory activity of these parasites that inhibits mechanisms of allergic sensitization. The link is counterintuitive in both the evolutionary mechanisms of immune response and the environmental influences on allergen exposure. These findings illustrate the complexity of the immune system, as it must function in a world that contains both allergens such as pollen and dust mites and potentially beneficial agents such as helminths. Further investigation into how these systems interact may provide insights into new therapeutic management strategies for allergies, enabling better understanding and intervention within the broader context of allergy and immunology in human populations (Nødtvedt et al., 2007; Mutapi et al., 2012) (Figure 9.10).

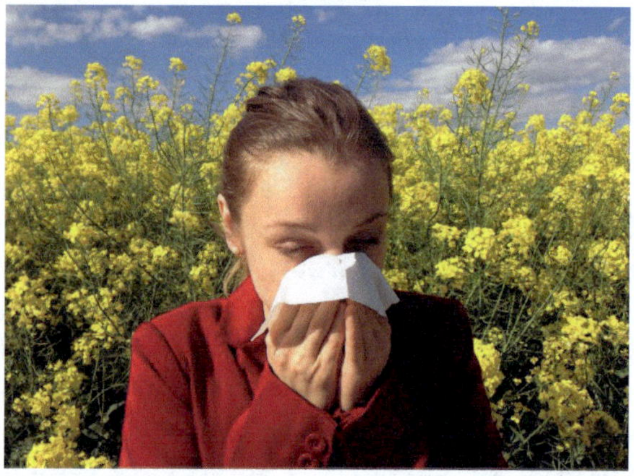

Figure 9.10. Environmental allergies.

Source: https://nationaleczema.org/wp-content/uploads/2017/05/allergy-1738191_1920-e1495510204937.jpg.

9.3.2. Food Allergies (Nuts, Shellfish)

Food allergies, particularly to nuts and shellfish, are a serious public health problem, affecting millions of individuals all over the globe. Allergies result from an overactive immune response, in which proteins from nuts and shellfish are mistakenly identified as harmful by the body. When exposed repeatedly, the immune system unleashes histamines and other chemicals, which lead to potentially life-threatening allergic reactions. The increasing prevalence of food allergies in developed countries has been explained by various factors, from genetic predisposition to environmental reasons. With the increasingly sterilized life of city residents, there is a possibility of decreased exposure to diverse microbiomes, which can lead to inadequate immunological development. This result is consistent with the Hygiene Hypothesis, which posits that reduced exposure to childhood microbials may be responsible for increased allergic responses, and therefore a better understanding of allergy mechanisms and public health measures for prevention and treatment is warranted (Ell et al., 2024). Food allergies can severely lower the quality of life of afflicted individuals, particularly among youth. Social dining opportunities, such as eating together and socializing, can be sources of worry for individuals with allergies due to the potential for exposure. Avoidance is perpetuated out of fear of unwilled ingestion, with a negative impact on mental health and social adaptation. Isolation continues to escalate during adolescence, a crucial period in social bonding. Also, inadequate food allergen labeling policies exacerbate this stress because consumers are exposed to misleading or missing information about allergens on pre-packed and unpacked foods. By addressing these labeling issues and fostering allergen awareness among food providers, significant improvements can be made in reducing the pressure and social limitations experienced by people with food allergies, thereby improving their quality of life (Ell et al., 2024). Current research emphasizes the complex interplay between novel foods, including insect-based foods, and food allergies. As alternative foods gain wider use owing to global resource limitations, their allergenic potential needs to be thoroughly investigated. For instance, tropomyosin, an allergen-related protein, has been identified in various invertebrate species, including insects and mollusks. The most commonly used insect employed in natural dyeing, Dactylis's coccus, has been implicated to cause allergic reactions, which indicates the necessity for comprehensive allergenic assessment of new foods. Awareness of cross-reactivity among homologous proteins is also important because shellfish-allergic patients could potentially react with proteins from insects, too. This altered food source environment and its potential allergenic impact require new approaches to regulation and allergen education, particularly as diets shift towards sustainability (Figure 9.11).

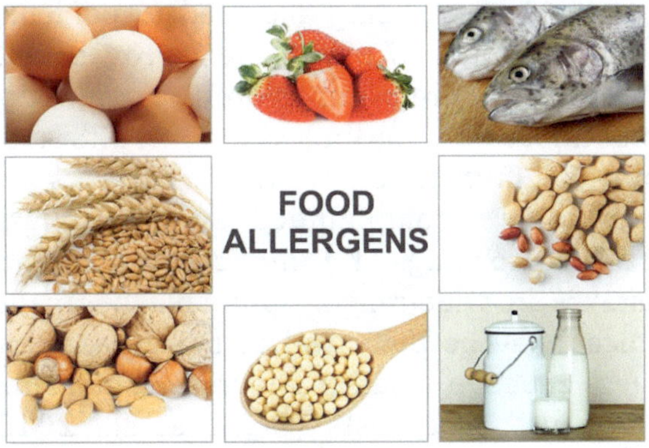

Figure 9.11. Food allergies.

Source: https://foodallergiesatlanta.com/wp-content/uploads/2019/07/What-are-the-8-Most-Common-Food-Allergies.jpg.

9.3.3. Drug Allergies (Penicillin, Sulfa Drugs)

The phenomenon of drug allergy, particularly with regard to penicillin and sulfa drugs, is a significant interaction between immunological reactions and pharmacologic agents. Penicillin and sulfa drugs are commonly used antibiotics; nevertheless, they are two of the most commonly reported allergens in clinical practice. The immune reaction to penicillin and sulfa drugs usually involves the production of hapten-like metabolites, which become bound to proteins, leading to an allergic response mediated by immunoglobulin E (IgE). In their more sophisticated versions, this can lead to life-threatening anaphylactic reactions that demand instant medical intervention. The sophistication of such responses thus justifies understanding drug-specific IgE mechanisms, e.g., for therapeutic control and prevention strategy planning, utilizing IgE-allergen interaction disruptors (Bilgicer et al., 2019). In a recent research on the credibility of self-reported drug allergy, one of the notable points was that the majority of the patients misname their reaction, and this creates a chain reaction, such as avoiding useful therapies. For instance, despite 39.2% of drug allergies being allocated to penicillin, as many as just 67.8% of them proved to be actual drug allergies on rigorous examination. This misunderstanding often results from poor communication between patients and practitioners, compounded by poor allergy history recording. The implications of these mistakes are wide-ranging; probable therapeutic choices may be perceived as more hazardous or less effective, leading to increased morbidity and health care costs (Grant et al., 2015). Management of drug allergy not only involves accurate recording but also patient education, particularly in hospital drug administration settings, where dosing is more intensive. Pharmacists also play a key role in assessing the validity of reported drug allergy and preventing inappropriate medication of patients. This entails not only clearing up misinterpretations of allergist histories but also establishing a culture of transparency where patients will disclose their problems. The use of detailed allergy assessment can reduce the likelihood of prescribing contraindicated medications, thereby improving patient outcomes (Grant et al., 2015). The complexities of drug allergies, namely to penicillin and sulfa medications, need to be appreciated to advance allergy and immunology practice in humans (Figure 9.12).

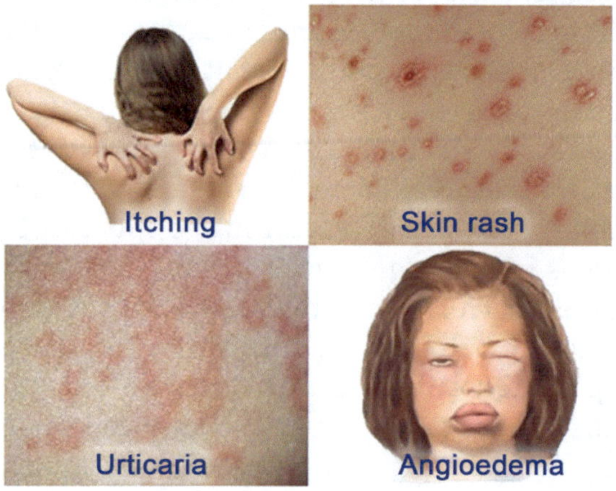

Figure 9.12. Drug allergy.

Source: https://asthmaallergyclinic.in/wp-content/uploads/2023/03/Drug_Allergy_2.png.

Test Your Knowledge

1. What are the environmental allergens?
2. What are the most common drug allergies?

9.4. Diagnosis of Allergies

Learning Outcome

1. Describe the skin prick tests
2. Understand the role of blood tests in the diagnosis of allergies
3. Understand the role of elimination diets in allergy and immunology

The allergy diagnosis requires an integrated approach that combines the patient's medical history, physical examination, and laboratory investigations. Medical history is crucial, as it provides evidence of potential allergens and the severity of the allergic response, which may range from mild to life-threatening. Physicians will usually use questionnaires to assess symptom patterns and potential environmental irritants. A physical exam following a quality history assists in ascertaining the nature and degree of allergic reactions encountered. Such findings are essential for assessing the impact of allergens on patients' quality of life and for guiding future testing and management strategies. Diagnostic allergy tests typically involve skin prick tests, blood work, and, in certain cases, oral food challenges.

Skin prick tests involve a small amount of potential allergens being put on the skin to monitor for an immediate response, which reflects IgE-mediated reactions. Serum specific IgE tests, however, quantify antibody titers against some allergens in the blood. These tests are highly useful for establishing diagnoses and personalized management regimens. Additionally, knowledge of the differential diagnosis is crucial, as related symptoms can be caused by diseases such as asthma or eczema, underscoring the importance of thorough evaluation and individualized patient management. Current research highlights the importance of environmental and genetic influences in the increasing incidence of allergic disease in industrialized nations. The theory of biome depletion, which captures the loss of diverse microorganisms essential to human well-being, suggests that such depletion could lead to several immune disorders, including allergies. Research has shown that city dwelling and sanitation have been associated with higher rates of allergy, supporting the hygiene hypothesis. Addressing these factors with therapies such as biome reconstitution may provide new avenues for the prevention of allergic disease and general enhancement of immune function, thus offering hope for preventive as well as therapeutic interventions in the treatment of allergies (Nødtvedt et al., 2007; Adler et al., 2013) (Figure 9.13).

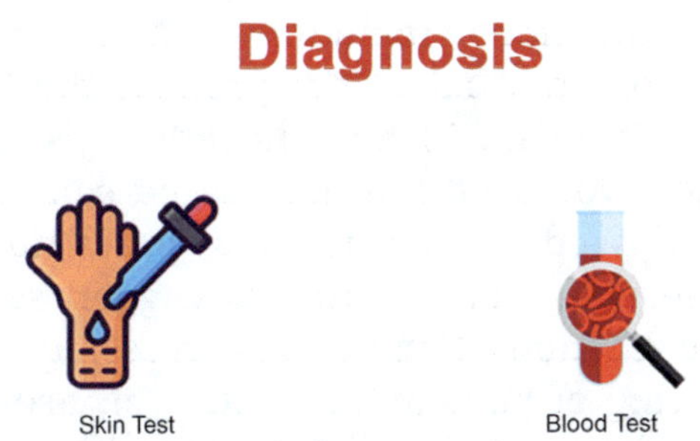

Figure 9.13. Diagnosis of allergies.

Source: https://www.lalpathlabs.com/blog/wp-content/uploads/2023/02/skin-allergy-diagnosis.png.

9.4.1. Skin Prick Tests

Skin prick tests are an important diagnostic tool in immunology and allergy because they allow medical professionals to assess individuals' sensitivities to various allergens. The procedure involves injecting a small amount of allergen into the skin's epidermis, typically using a pricking device, and observing the region for a local reaction, such as redness or swelling. This immediate hypersensitivity response is achieved by activating IgE antibodies bound to skin mast cells, revealing each patient's allergen sensitivities. In addition to providing rapid results, this test helps physicians create patient-specific management plans, potentially preventing life-threatening allergic conditions such as anaphylaxis triggered by exposure to specific allergens. Therefore, skin prick tests are a vital component of comprehensive allergy testing, allowing determination of a patient's immune response in real-world situations. Reliability and validity of skin prick tests are enhanced by adherence to standardized practices that delineate allergen selection and the test method. Several factors, including time of year, geography, and even diet, can influence allergen sensitivity and must be taken into consideration when interpreting results. The tests are very safe, but, like all tests, it is important to know contraindications, including skin issues or medications that might compromise the test's validity or result in false negatives. Notably, the tests would indeed have to be conducted and followed up by trained practitioners because they can, at times, trigger severe allergic reactions. Hence, valid assessment and monitoring of patients are critical in order to preserve both the validity of test results and the safety of concerned individuals, validating the requirement for trained allergy professionals during interpretation. Furthermore, the uses of skin prick testing extend beyond immediate clinical practice; they also teach us about immunological reactions more broadly. Age has been shown to have a demonstrable influence on atopy prevalence, with findings indicating that sensitization diminishes with age (Auguglaro et al., 2011). This raises significant questions about immunosenescence and its relationship to allergic illness in older populations. In addition, the need to develop age-related allergy tests is evident, as the geriatric patient could potentially have a presentation different from that of his younger counterpart. The complexity of interpreting skin prick tests across various population groups underscores their value not only in diagnosing allergy but also in directing research efforts to understand age-related immune changes and their clinical significance in allergy treatment, including the development of customized therapeutic plans (Figure 9.14).

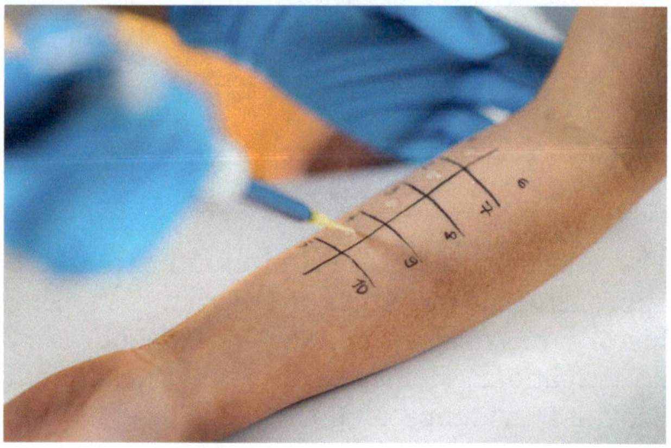

Figure 9.14. Skin prick allergy testing.

Source: https://www.imc-healthcare.com/wp-content/uploads/2022/12/imc-skin-prick-allergy-testing.jpg.

9.4.2. Blood Tests (IgE Testing)

Blood testing, such as Immunoglobulin E (IgE) tests, is pivotal for diagnosing and managing allergies. With exposure to an allergen, the immune system produces IgE antibodies, which bind to mast cells and basophils and trigger the release of histamines and inflammatory mediators during subsequent exposures. The IgE process is crucial for physicians to diagnose specific allergies and institute appropriate treatment. Diagnostic procedures such as the enzyme-linked immunosorbent assay (ELISA) can quantify individual IgE in blood, thereby enabling healthcare practitioners to correlate clinical symptoms with identifiable allergens. This technique is critical for distinguishing allergic from non-allergic disease, ultimately guiding treatment paradigms tailored to unique patient needs. The incidence of allergies and associated conditions has increased exponentially in the past few decades, necessitating investigation into the immunological basis of these diseases. Research has established that both genetic disposition and external influences are implicated in increased IgE secretion. Comprehending the intricacies of IgE-dependent allergies is imperative, especially as concerns grow about the increasing prevalence of food allergies in humans and domesticated animals, including canine atopic dermatitis (CAD) research. New research projects are examining the epidemiological patterns and risk factors of such allergies and finding that urban living and seasonal influences might worsen such ailments. The correlations observed between human and dog immune responses reveal a broader pattern among environmental shifts and allergy cases, suggesting that data from one species might inform treatment strategies in another with regard to IgE testing (Nødtvedt et al., 2007). Treatment strategies themselves are evolving alongside these diagnostic advancements, particularly in food allergies, where traditional therapy remains limited.

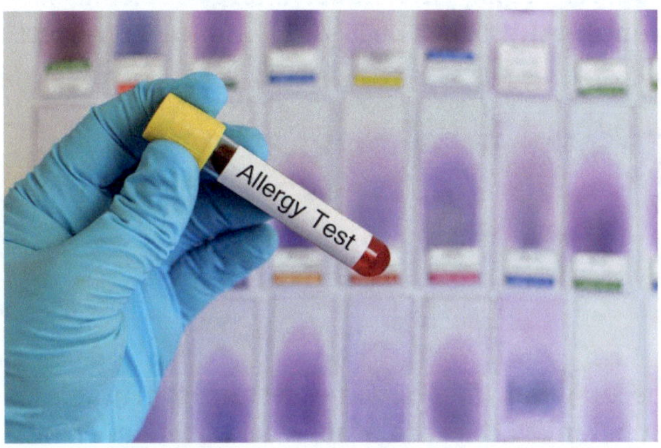

Figure 9.15. Allergy blood test.

Source: https://www.houstonent.com/hubfs/blog%20images/allergy%20blood%20test%201.jpg.

Sublingual immunotherapy (SLIT) has shown promise in human research so far and is now being explored in veterinary medicine, particularly for diseases involving IgE sensitization. The ability of SLIT to control IgE responses without triggering side effects represents a significant milestone in the management of allergic diseases in both animals and humans, as shown by initial safety trials with dogs. Such trials not only confirm an increase in food allergen-specific IgG following treatment but also demonstrate a failure to sensitize in clinical trials, thereby providing a foundation for further research (Cox et al., 2017). The integration of diagnostic testing with innovative therapeutic modalities underscores the critical importance of IgE testing in the ongoing effort to understand and effectively manage allergies in the practices of allergy and immunology (Figure 9.15).

9.4.3. Elimination Diets

Elimination diets, in which foods suspected to be causing allergic or intolerance reactions are removed in a systematic manner, are a valuable tool in the specialty of allergy and immunology. Diets are most beneficial in patients with symptoms of food allergy, such as urticaria, an all too frequent allergic condition characterized by swelling and hives. By eliminating foods suspected of being allergenic, patients can identify culprits, while physicians can order appropriate diagnostic testing and treatment. The new urticaria guidelines emphasize the importance of identifying the above stimuli and managing symptoms appropriately, as chronic spontaneous urticaria may negatively affect quality of life and everyday functioning in affected individuals (Zuberbier et al., 2021). Elimination diets are based on a simple, evidence-based approach for both people with food allergies and practitioners aiming to improve their patients' health outcomes. The proper application of an elimination diet is a systematic process because inappropriate application can lead to nutritional deficiencies or unintentional exposure to allergens. An elimination diet is typically initiated by removing common allergens—such as dairy, eggs, nuts, gluten, and soy—for a predetermined time, typically four to six weeks. An individual monitors symptoms throughout this interval because the reintroduction of removed foods can be employed to determine precise causes. Additionally, keeping a full food diary can simplify the process by documenting reactions to reintroduced foods. New research on the human microbiome also reveals the relevance of an evenly balanced diet to sustaining immune function. Dysbiosis, or distorted microbial equilibrium in the gut, can amplify allergic responses, hence modulating the effectiveness of elimination diets (Pessemier et al., 2021). Understanding these interactions can help develop dietary regimens to optimize immune function. Aside from revealing food allergies, elimination diets might contribute to the general benefit of health. Diets have been shown to control immune function, quite possibly decreasing symptoms of most skin diseases and other allergic disorders. By inducing a healthier gut microbiome through dietary variety, elimination diets are expected to improve overall immune function, which in turn may mitigate allergic reactions and skin disease (Pessemier et al., 2021). It is important that individuals following these diets do so under professional supervision to ensure nutritional adequacy and effective symptom control. This approach not only teaches people to take control of their health but also heightens awareness of the interrelated nature of eating, immunity, and the clinical presentation of allergies (Figure 9.16).

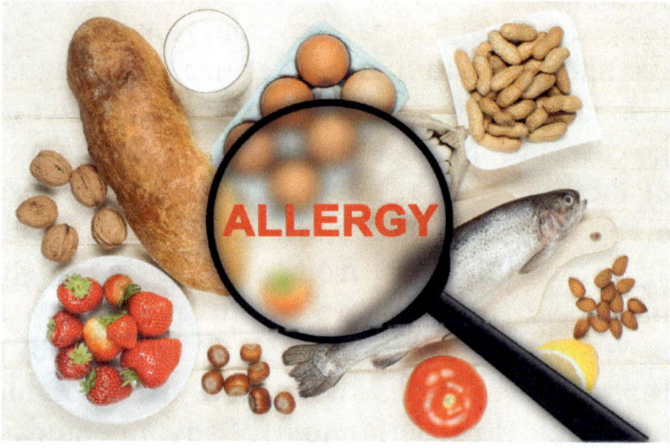

Figure 9.16. Elimination diets.

Source: https://deliciouslyallergyfree.com/wp-content/uploads/2017/11/Elimination-Diets.jpg.

Test Your Knowledge

1. What disease does skin prick test for?
2. What blood tests are done for allergies?

9.5. Treatment and Management of Allergies

Learning Outcome

1. Know the avoidance strategies in managing allergies
2. Describe the pharmacological treatments for allergies
3. Describe the immunotherapy

Therapy and treatment of allergies require a thorough understanding of the processes that control such immune responses. Allergies occur when the immune system overreacts to substances that are otherwise harmless. These reactions manifest as specific symptoms, which can range from mild to lethal. Treatment options present today are all about allergen avoidance, drug management, and immunotherapy. Avoidance forms the first line of therapy; patients must identify and shun the triggers. Pharmacotherapy involves antihistamines, corticosteroids, and bronchodilators, which calm symptoms by slowing allergic response or suppressing inflammation. Immunotherapy may be prescribed by allergists for more long-standing cases, in which patients are slowly desensitized to allergens over time, thereby building longer-term tolerance. This multi-level approach is necessary, as it not only treats proximal symptoms but also seeks to address durable immunological changes that can result in meaningful improvements in patients' quality of life. Furthermore, severe allergic reactions like anaphylaxis need to be managed by a proactive and educated response from patients and caregivers. Anaphylaxis is an acute condition necessitating urgent medical intervention through the administration of epinephrine. Education of the patient cannot be overstressed; at-risk individuals must be given self-management education and skills, as well as identification of early signs. Unfortunately, there are well-known barriers to compliance with prescribed auto-injectors that are critical for the treatment of anaphylaxis. Research has identified inconsistencies in health professional advice, perceived stigma of possessing weapon-type objects, and insufficient training as fundamental barriers.

Their resolution through increased training and public awareness campaigns is key to enhancing self-care practice and reducing the potential risk of anaphylactic episodes (Barnett et al., 2013). Finally, the development of targeted therapies and novel therapeutic modalities promises improved control of allergies. New advances in genetics and immunotherapy paradigms are paving the way for individualized treatment regimens tailored to different patient profiles. For instance, biologic drugs that target specific immune processes involved in inducing allergic conditions are becoming more prevalent in clinical practice. Moreover, guidelines developed through consensus emphasize the importance of evidence-based diagnosis and management practices for complex cases such as Hereditary Angioedema (HAE) (Aygören-Pürsün et al., 2012). Guidelines are helpful resources for healthcare practitioners that promote uniform care and access to effective treatments globally. Ultimately, an integrative approach that utilizes patient self-management, robust educational interventions, and cutting-edge therapeutics will be indispensable to enhancing the overall environment of allergy treatment and management.

9.5.1. Avoidance Strategies

Avoidance strategies are the centerpiece of the approach in the management of allergies and immune responses. The centerpiece of these strategies is the deliberate avoidance of known allergens, thereby reducing the likelihood of allergic responses. This preventive action is particularly crucial in the management of food allergies, where the goal is to avoid specific allergens, such as peanuts or shellfish, that trigger adverse immune responses. Education plays a vital role in the successful implementation of avoidance methods because both the subjects and caregivers must be aware of the causes of allergens in their environments. Proper labeling of food ingredients and awareness also play a significant role in everyday life, particularly when dining out or buying processed food products. Through reinforcement of these behaviors, high-risk groups can significantly reduce the risk of allergic responses and improve the quality of their lives. In addition to food allergies, avoidance strategies are also included for environmental causes such as pollen, dust mites, and pet dander. Environmental allergy victims can manage their symptoms by making pragmatic modifications at their workplaces and homes. For example, they use HEPA filters, clean often to minimize dust accumulation, and create allergen-free zones to drastically reduce exposure. Besides this, outdoor activities may require specific timing to avoid peak pollen months or protective gear when necessary. All these actions not only help eliminate allergens from daily environments but also allow individuals to reclaim control of their health and well-being, demonstrating the importance of an inclusive approach to allergy control. Such practices are consistent with the general recommendations of allergy and immunology experts, underscoring the importance of customized avoidance strategies. The effectiveness of avoidance steps in allergy control is also underscored by recent studies examining their impact on allergic symptoms and sensitization. For instance, studies have highlighted the significance of long-term avoidance as a mechanism to prevent violent allergic reactions and anaphylaxis. Particularly, rigid adherence to avoidance measures is crucial in situations of high-risk exposure where contact could lead to life-threatening consequences. For patients who have life-threatening allergic responses, e.g., anaphylaxis, administration of epinephrine auto-injectors becomes part of their avoidance protocol. Patient and provider partnership in developing individualized avoidance protocols not only protects against exposure but also facilitates patient education regarding potential risk factors and emergency management. Such initial steps are required to efficiently control allergies, as various clinical guidelines and studies in allergy and immunology emphasize the foremost importance of avoidance in managing patients (Alvarez-Twose et al., 2014; Cox et al., 2017) (Figure 9.17).

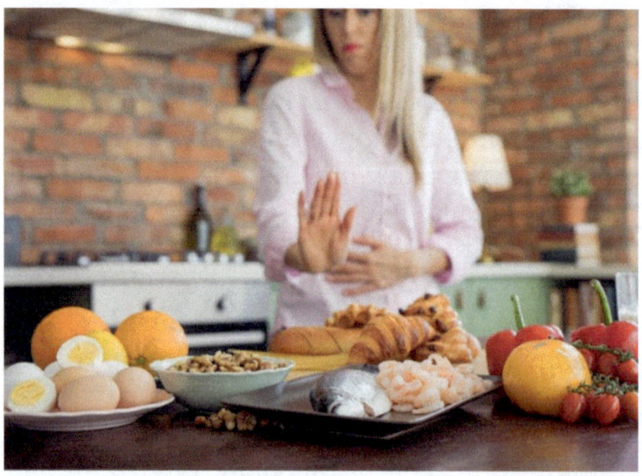

Figure 9.17. Avoiding food allergy reactions.

Source: https://www.emjreviews.com/wp-content/uploads/2025/05/9am-Allergy-4.jpg.

9.5.2. Pharmacological Treatments (Antihistamines, Corticosteroids)

Pharmacotherapy for allergies, in particular antihistamines and corticosteroids, plays a central role in managing symptoms associated with allergic reactions. Antihistamines, by inhibiting histamine, a pivotal mediator of allergic inflammation, represent an initial measure against conditions such as allergic rhinitis and urticaria. The drugs have the ability to effectively reduce symptoms such as itching, sneezing, and nasal stuffiness. Additionally, newer antihistamines are less sedating than older types and thus more suitable for use on a daily basis.

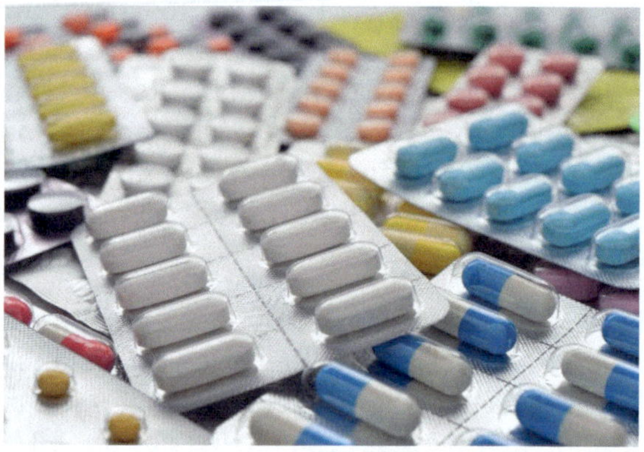

Figure 9.18. Drug allergy treatment.

Source: https://www.jaxallergy.com/wp-content/uploads/bb-plugin/cache/jacksonville-drug-and-medication-allergy-treatments-landscape-4018303a393a9c71c7c4d6e07ef4ea84-c1lbh8vxjg47.jpg.

Their clinical efficacy in the management of acute allergic attacks is presented in different clinical situations, such as that of a three-year-old boy who presented with chronic nasal blockage and rhinorrhea, and in whom significant benefit was gained from utilizing such therapeutic measures (drkvassallo@yahoo.co.uk et al., 2007). Corticosteroids constitute another group of drugs that are vital in the management of allergy, particularly in more serious or chronic cases. Corticosteroids act by inhibiting inflammation and immune function and thereby reducing the whole allergic response. Intranasal corticosteroids are indicated for moderately to severely affected patients with allergic rhinitis and have been shown to substantially improve quality of life. Studies indicate that corticosteroids can also treat long-term allergy-related complications, such as sinusitis, by reducing nasal obstruction and improving drainage. The use of corticosteroids in treatment strategies underscores the importance of multimodal therapy for allergies, particularly for individuals with complex backgrounds and symptoms (Bosnic-Anticevich et al., 2017). The combination of antihistamines and corticosteroids generally results in synergistic action, providing widespread relief for allergy patients. This personalized treatment plan allows medical practitioners to not only alleviate the causative symptoms of the allergic reaction but also the resulting inflammation, thereby reducing the risk of chronic diseases. In addition, the development of several formulations, i.e., oral, intranasal, and topical corticosteroids, ensures that the patient has options based on individual symptoms and personal preference. With a greater understanding of the mechanisms of allergic reactions, strategic use of these pharmacologic treatments now encompasses personalized medicine, where the treatment is more specifically directed to individual patient profiles, thus enhancing outcomes in allergy and immunology (drkvassallo@yahoo.co.uk et al., 2007) (Figure 9.18).

9.5.3. Immunotherapy (Allergy Shots)

Immunotherapy, or, as it is usually referred to, allergy shots, is a standard treatment for allergic disease in humans. By injecting escalating doses of allergens into the patient's body, the treatment will ultimately desensitize the patient to the specific allergen, thereby reducing their allergic reactions. Subcutaneous injections are the route of administration used to stimulate the immune system with allergens in a controlled manner. A number of recent studies have suggested the efficacy of immunotherapy in the treatment of a variety of allergies, particularly environmental and food allergies, with long-term relief even after therapy is withdrawn. The therapeutic approach is particularly pertinent given the growing incidence of allergies in populations, warranting new approaches to their treatment that can enhance patients' quality of life and potentially reduce healthcare costs for life-threatening allergic reactions. Peanut allergy research illustrates the urgent need for effective immunotherapy treatment, as peanut allergies have a tendency to induce life-threatening reactions and have increased over the years. The nature of peanut allergy is complex, so creating an effective treatment that can treat a large number of patients is crucial. Immunotherapy research has not only focused on subcutaneous administration but also on other methods, such as oral and sublingual administration. These approaches aim to alter the immune response to minimize undesirable effects while optimizing desensitization outcomes. There are promising research results indicating that immunotherapy can reduce the severity of allergic reactions and improve quality of life for patients with peanut and other food allergies, underscoring the need for further research in this critical area of allergy treatment (Rauscher et al., 2015). Future directions for immunotherapy aim to improve both the efficacy and safety of treatment protocols. Therapeutic advances in subcutaneous immunotherapy (SCIT) for respiratory allergy, such as allergic rhinosinusitis and bronchial asthma, demonstrate the potential of this modality in treating complex allergic disease. It has been reported that traditional SCIT regimens, due to their higher compliance and safer patient profiles, remain significant in the clinic (Lukan et al., 2017). Moreover, the identification of new administration pathways, such as intradermal or intratympanic, holds the prospect of quicker and more effective desensitization. However, as science advances, there is an emerging need for targeted biomarkers to evaluate successful therapeutic results. By pairing biological specimens with measures of quality of life, clinicians can establish more effective monitoring regimens, which, in turn, will guide clinical decisions and maximize patient care in the new landscape of allergy and immunology (Figure 9.19).

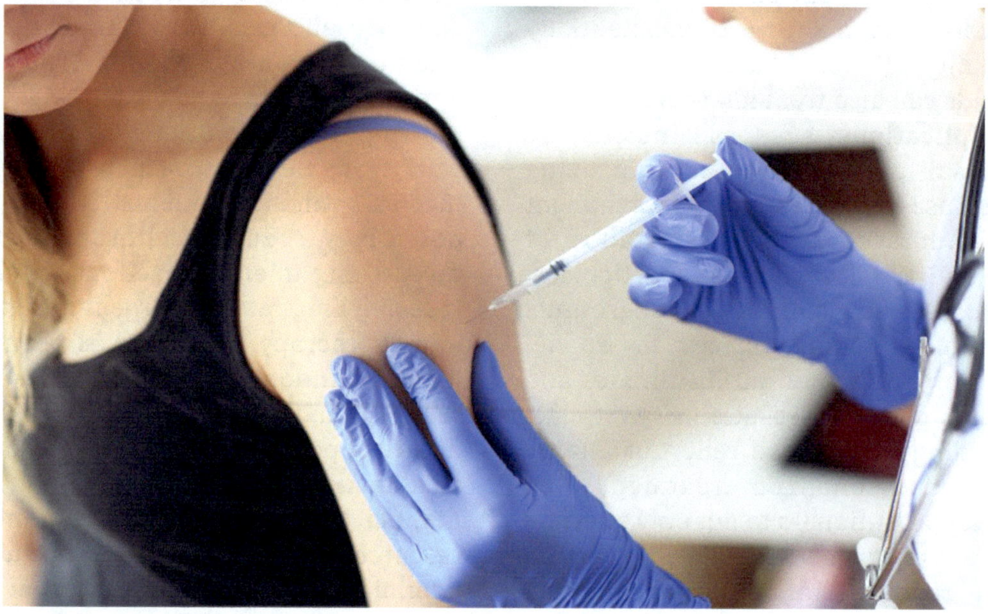

Figure 9.19. Allergy shots (immunotherapy).

Source: https://cdn-prod.medicalnewstoday.com/content/images/articles/320/320402/allergy-shot-injection-being-given-to-young-woman.jpg.

Test Your Knowledge

1. What are the avoidance strategies in managing allergies?
2. What is the best medication for allergies?

9.6. The Role of Genetics in Allergies

Learning Outcome

1. Describe the influence of family history and genetic predisposition on the development of allergic conditions
2. Understand the environmental factors influencing genetic expression
3. Explore ongoing research in allergy genetics

The intricate relationship between allergies and genetics has garnered a lot of attention in recent times, with emphasis on the role hereditary factors play in making individuals vulnerable to allergic diseases.

Genetic contributions can take numerous forms, including the expression of specific genes that regulate immune responses. An area of important research focuses on polymorphisms in immunoglobulin E (IgE) receptor genes and related pathways involved in heightened allergic responses. As persons with a family history of allergy have higher levels of IgE, it is essential to understand these genetic components better for the diagnosis and management of allergic disorders. In addition, the study of genetic syndromes that predispose patients to various allergic disorders underscores the complexity of allergic pathophysiology and calls for targeted therapeutic interventions. The study of animal models has also significantly advanced the current understanding of the genetic basis of allergies. Studies in domestic animals, particularly dogs, have demonstrated similarities between the human and canine genetic determinants of atopic disorders. For instance, canine atopic dermatitis has been proposed as an analogue of human allergic responses, and both share similar immune mechanisms. Canine genetic variants regulating allergy-related genes, such as those involved in IgE production and allergic inflammation, provide insight into the evolutionary conservation of these processes. Research into the role of certain genetic markers in breed-specific allergic susceptibility highlights crossover potential for using these findings in both pet and human populations, with a case made for shared genetic etiology across species (Nødtvedt et al., 2007). Moreover, research now focuses on the extent to which environmental factors interact with genetic susceptibilities to influence allergic reactions. Current research indicates that lifestyle, dietary intake, and allergen exposure can influence the expression of genes that cause allergy susceptibility. Additionally, environments like those in the urban environment have been shown to exacerbate allergic disorders due to heightened exposure to possible allergens and pollutants. For example, service animal breeding has similarly sought to decrease allergenic potential linked with specific genetic traits, suggesting that genetic control of expression would suppress allergic reactions. All these discoveries not only increase our understanding of the interaction between genetics and the environment but also open opportunities to design individualized preventive and therapeutic interventions for managing allergies (Belanger et al., 2016) (Figure 9.20).

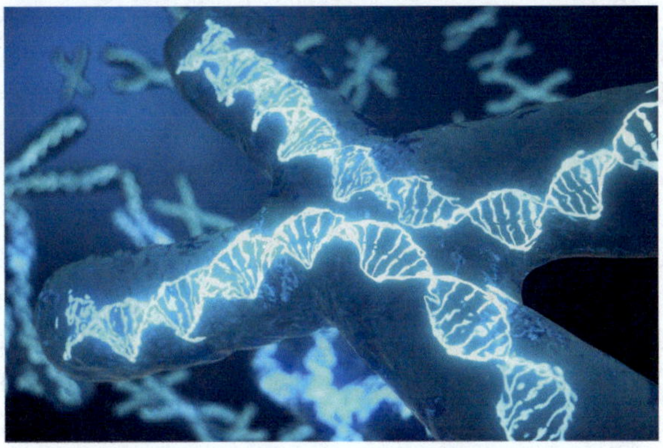

Figure 9.20. The role of genetics in allergies.

Source: https://premiumallergy.com/wp-content/uploads/2024/09/bigstock-d-Illustration-X-chromosomes-262273369.jpg.

9.6.1. Family History and Genetic Predisposition

The contribution of family history and heredity to the causation of allergic disease cannot be overstated. A significant amount of evidence indicates that individuals with a history of allergies, asthma, or atopic diseases in their families are at higher risk of having these conditions themselves. This hereditary factor means that there are specific alleles that predispose certain individuals to hypersensitivity reactions, which are underlying biological processes to most allergic diseases. For instance, the inheritance of immune system-regulating characteristics has been linked to susceptibility to environmental allergens, indicative of a higher genetic inclination towards such immunological responses. In addition, the combination of genetic predispositions with environmental cues can further exacerbate the development of allergies and lead to an increased rate of conditions such as hay fever or allergic rhinitis in individuals with genetic predispositions in today's environments. The genetic predisposition theory is not so much about family trends; it also accounts for environmental factors that affect an individual's immune profile. For example, (Nødtvedt et al., 2007) draws attention to the increasing prevalence of allergic disorders in parallel with lifestyle, particularly in developed countries. Here, the existence of genes that mirror immune function intersects with environmental factors such as urban living, dietary patterns, and microbial exposure. The multilateral character of this relationship demonstrates that genetic predisposition cannot act on its own; instead, it is regulated by a wide range of lifestyle and environmental factors. Such evidence also confirms the importance of a multifactorial approach in allergy research, as it underscores how environment and heredity cooperate to shape individual immune responses. On top of that, recent research has identified new methods for fighting allergies based on genetic predispositions. Emerging theories, such as the hygiene hypothesis, suggest that modern lifestyles may disrupt the normal microflora that support the development of robust immune responses. As Adler et al. (2013) outline, biodepletion syndrome, which refers to the removal of diverse microbial populations from our environment, accounts for the emergence of immune-related pathologies, including allergic diseases. This growing understanding of the microbiome's function offers the potential for the use of interventions, such as biome reconstitution, to restore balance and suppress allergic response. With an emphasis on the interaction between genetic predisposition and environmental context, future studies have the potential to yield personalized strategies for allergy prevention and treatment that target not just symptoms but also root causes that bridge the genetic to the ecological.

9.6.2. Environmental Factors Influencing Genetic Expression

Environmental factors play an important role in the manifestation of genetic factors, particularly in gene expression related to allergies and immunology. Various external factors, such as air pollutants, dietary factors, and allergens, can directly modulate gene function and influence the human immune system. For instance, outdoor ozone exposure has been shown to exacerbate allergic diseases and influence immune regulatory gene expression. These changes can affect the synthesis of key proteins involved in immune protection and inflammation, suggesting environmental effects on genetic susceptibility to allergy development. Ozone exposure, for example, will inhibit the expression of surfactant protein-D (SP-D), an essential protein in maintaining lung integrity and controlling inflammatory reactions, hence indicating the intricate connection between environmental stressors and gene expression in allergic disease (Belanger et al., 2016). The dog allergen example further illuminates environmental control of gene expression. Experiments have shown that the amount of the dominant dog allergen, Can f 1, varies widely across dog breeds and that selective breeding for specific traits might inadvertently modify allergenic potential through genetic variation in the Lipocalin 1 (LCN1) gene. Such diversity highlights the contribution of genetic susceptibility and environmental context in allergen expression. For service animals, often bred with specific characteristics in mind, prioritization towards reducing allergenicity can substantially contribute to compatibility with individuals who are allergic. Understanding how genetic expression intersects with the environment is thus key to both breeding and allergy management in humans (Belanger et al., 2016). Moreover, glucocorticoid modulation by environmental stimuli such as ozone provides evidence of the complexity of gene regulation in allergic disease. Glucocorticoids are largely used to treat asthma and other allergies due to their anti-inflammatory properties. However, research has shown that environmental factors such as ozone compromise the efficacy of glucocorticoids, impairing the drug's capacity to regulate gene expression in the immune system. This impairment could complicate therapeutic strategies, particularly in asthmatics with high pollutant exposure. Grasping how environmental factors influence the effectiveness of genetic responses to therapy is essential for developing individualized strategies for the management and treatment of allergy (Flayer et al., 2019). In this light, the study of environmental influences on genetic expression provides valuable data for health professionals and researchers investigating allergy and immunology (Figure 9.21).

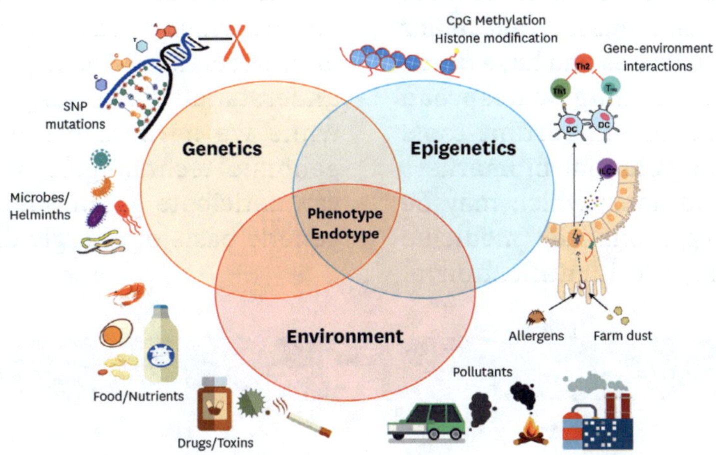

Figure 9.21. The complex interactions between genetic, epigenetic, and environmental factors in the development of allergic disorders.

Source: https://www.researchgate.net/publication/357530364/figure/fig1/AS:1108266100760576@1641242637001/The-complex-interactions-between-genetic-epigenetic-and-environmental-factors-in-the.png.

9.6.3. Ongoing Research in Allergy Genetics

The genetics of allergy has advanced significantly in recent years, as researchers seek to unravel the array of genetic factors that contribute to the development of allergic disease. The genetics of allergy is a multifaceted interaction involving multiple genes and environmental factors, and thus a highly difficult field of study. Recent studies indicate that some genotypes may be associated with increased susceptibility to diseases such as atopic dermatitis and allergic rhinitis. Despite a growing literature on the role of cytokines in allergy pathogenesis, the genetic basis of the process remains poorly defined. (Martyna, 2013) highlights the genotype-phenotype correlation in the progression of atopic dermatitis and the need for further work to explain these in simple terms so that interventions may be effective. Beyond individual genetic factors, studies are now also attempting to explain the impact of gene-environment interactions in the development of allergic responses. This is a two-way approach, since genetic predisposition is typically a function of environmental exposure to substances such as allergens, toxins, and lifestyle. Genome-wide association studies (GWAS) have identified numerous loci that confer susceptibility to allergic diseases and have paved the way toward understanding widespread genetic variation. GWAS are important tools for the identification of potential biomarkers for allergen-related conditions, which may be employed to facilitate personalized medicine strategies. Furthermore, the identification of the role of epigenetic modifications in altering gene expression in response to an allergen is a novel and interesting field to explore, which may lead to novel therapeutic targets and interventions. The intricacy of these interactions is central to advancing our knowledge of allergy pathogenesis. Despite the progress that has been made in the field of allergy genetics, there still exist monumental hurdles to be cleared. One of the biggest stumbling blocks is the lack of large, heterogeneous datasets upon which to base conclusions about genetic risk factors in various populations. Additionally, the field faces methodological challenges in distinguishing real genetic correlations from those driven by confounding factors. Researchers continue to stress the importance of joint approaches in allergies as multi-disciplinary research can provide more conclusive results. (Kinney et al., 2007) also notes the value of employing robust metrics like the h-index for evaluating research output, which can also assist in the stratification of projects that have major contributions to our understanding of allergy genetics. Ultimately, while we harness the potential of advanced genomic technologies and data analysis, we can anticipate gaining further insight into the genetic basis of allergic diseases.

Test Your Knowledge

1. What is the genetic predisposition for allergies?
2. What are the environmental factors influencing genetic expression?

SUMMARY

With the integration of vast amounts of information on allergy and immunology, the complex interaction between human health and the environment becomes the focal point. Allergens, often underrated, are significant to a myriad of health conditions, as is evident from diseases related to the air. The information not only underscores the ubiquity of these agents but also underscores the necessity for a structured method for understanding their impact on human health. Addressing the multifaceted effects of allergens requires awareness of the scientific credibility of claims about them and of their implications for public health initiatives more broadly. In a society confronted with an increased incidence of allergic reactions, particularly in urbanized societies where exposure rates are higher, there is a need to anchor debates in empirical facts to avoid the fallacy of ungrounded fear and disinformation (Borchers et al., 2006). The pattern in related fields, where conditions such as canine atopic dermatitis (CAD) have escalated, mirrors the parallel between human and animal health in allergies. As in humans, the incidence of CAD has been linked to environmental factors, mirroring a shared vulnerability across species. Above all, factors such as urban residence and dietary intake during critical developmental periods demonstrate that interventions can mitigate risk factors for allergic diseases. Such findings place greater importance on prevention strategies that can be adjusted on both sides of veterinary and human medicine. Recognition of these associations not only refines understanding of immune processes but also points to the utility of integrated approaches to treatment of allergic conditions and thus to the development of an integrated perspective to allergy and immunology (Nødtvedt et al., 2007). Last, a general appreciation of allergy and immunology in humans needs an integrated paradigm that encompasses environmental, genetic, and life factors. With advancing research, interdisciplinary collaboration becomes more evident. Incorporating findings from various fields—such as epidemiology, immunology, and environmental science—we can develop more effective prevention and intervention strategies. Moreover, public health communication should aim to make people aware of the facts about allergens and the scientific evidence supporting them, so that informed lifestyle decisions are made. As we reach the end of this venture, it is clear that vigilance against the subtleties of allergies is essential for navigating the future of human health, as the relationship between the environment and immunity continues to evolve (Borchers et al., 2006; Nødtvedt et al., 2007).

The field of allergy and immunology has seen significant advances, particularly in the treatment and diagnosis of allergic conditions. The efficacy of sublingual allergen immunotherapy (SLIT) has recently emerged, and it has now taken a prominent position as an alternative treatment. A pivotal phase III trial in adult patients with birch pollen allergy demonstrated a clinically significant reduction in symptom scores compared with placebo. This benchmark study not only determined the safety profile of SLIT but also demonstrated improved quality of life among patients, underscoring the therapy's promise in reducing symptoms of allergic rhinitis. These results represent an important step toward optimized allergy control protocols, further reiterating the pivotal role of immune modulation in effectively managing allergic reactions. The implications of this study portend a shift towards personalized therapeutic regimes in immunotherapy. Increased research in allergy and immunology has highlighted the importance of understanding the various factors that influence drug safety and effectiveness. Research has progressed from individual treatments to cover areas such as antigen presentation, which is a key to the puzzle in the development of immunotherapies. The Global HIV Vaccine Enterprise, for instance, convened a working group on the rational design of vaccine ingredients with active debate among key scientific leaders. Such debates have extensive implications for the design of targeted therapies and for the explanation of T and B cell interactions in allergic diseases. Ongoing cooperation among members of the scientific community, including allergists and immunologists, ensures a multidimensional response to complex immune-related diseases, ultimately facilitating innovation in treatment and prevention. As research continues to uncover more information, cumulative findings further confirm a multifaceted picture of allergies and their immunological substrates. For instance, the pioneering work on SLIT supports the growing recognition of the advantages of immunotherapies, ultimately contributing to better patient outcomes. Furthermore, the cross-disciplinary discourse in debates such as those of the Global HIV Vaccine Enterprise illustrates the value of collaborative science. Through the convergence of various perspectives and knowledge, the study of allergy and immunology is poised to explore new approaches and treatment potential specific to the evolving landscape of the immune response. This spirit of cooperation not only enhances the understanding of allergies but also underscores the commitment to advancing public health by innovative and judicious immunological practice.

KEY TERMS FROM THIS CHAPTER

- Allergens
- Anaphylaxis
- Diet
- Environmental science
- Genetics
- Parasitic infections
- Pollen
- Allergy research
- Canine atopic dermatitis
- Dust mites
- Epidemiology
- Immunology
- Pet dander
- Pollution

CRITICAL THINKING QUESTIONS

1. **What type of hypersensitivity reaction is involved in anaphylaxis?**
   a. Type I
   b. Type II
   c. Type III
   d. Type IV
2. **Which antibody is primarily responsible for mediating allergic reactions?**
   a. IgG
   b. IgA
   c. IgE
   d. IgM
3. **What is the gold standard for diagnosing food allergies?**
   a. Serum IgE testing
   b. Skin prick testing
   c. Oral food challenge
   d. Elimination diet
4. **Which of the following is a primary treatment for anaphylaxis?**
   a. Antihistamines
   b. Corticosteroids
   c. Epinephrine
   d. Beta-blockers
5. **A patient with recurrent sinusitis and nasal polyps should be evaluated for which condition?**
   a. Allergic rhinitis
   b. Cystic fibrosis
   c. Aspirin-exacerbated respiratory disease (AERD)
   d. Systemic lupus erythematosus

Short Answer Questions

1. What are allergies?
2. What is the immune system?
3. What are the mechanisms of allergic reactions?
4. Name the three types of allergies.
5. What are the tests for allergy diagnosis?

Answer to Critical Thinking Questions

1. (a); 2. (c); 3. (c); 4. (c); 5. (c).

REFERENCES

1. Adcock, I. M., Garssen, J., Kazempour Dizagie, M., Mirsaeidi, M., et al. (2017). What immunological defects predispose to non-tuberculosis mycobacterial infections? https://core.ac.uk/download/157859147.pdf (accessed on 14th July 2025).
2. Parker, W., & Ollerton, J. (2013). Evolutionary biology and anthropology suggest biome reconstitution as a necessary approach toward dealing with immune disorders. *Evolution Medicine and Public Health, 2013*(1), 89–103. https://doi.org/10.1093/emph/eot008Allenspach, E. J., Andolina, J. R., Aquino, V. M., Bacchetta, R., et al. (2020). Hematopoietic cell transplantation in patients with primary immune regulatory disorders (PIRD): A Primary Immune Deficiency Treatment Consortium (PIDTC) survey. https://core.ac.uk/download/288432976.pdf (accessed on 14th July 2025).
3. Alvarez-Twose, S., Muraro, A., Arga, M., Armstrong, M., Arroabarren, M., Sheikh, A., Barnett, D., et al. (2014). International consensus on (ICON) anaphylaxis. https://core.ac.uk/download/28978204.pdf (accessed on 14th July 2025).
4. Apostol, A. C., Beaudin, A. E., & Jensen, K. D. C. (2020). Training the fetal immune system through maternal inflammation: A layered hygiene hypothesis. https://core.ac.uk/download/288432714.pdf (accessed on 14th July 2025).
5. Augugliaro, G., Bellia, V., Callari, A., Marchese, R., et al. (2011). The impact of age on prevalence of positive skin prick tests and specific IgE tests. https://core.ac.uk/download/53271530.pdf (accessed on 14th July 2025).
6. Avery, G. R., Babar, J. L., Baxendale, H. E., Buckland, M. S., et al. (2017). British Lung Foundation/United Kingdom Primary Immunodeficiency Network consensus statement on the definition, diagnosis, and management of granulomatous-lymphocytic interstitial lung disease in common variable immunodeficiency disorders. https://core.ac.uk/download/151162017.pdf (accessed on 14th July 2025).
7. Aygören-Pürsün, E., Bork, K., Bowen, T., Boysen, H., et al. (2012). WAO guideline for the management of hereditary angioedema. https://core.ac.uk/download/17179867.pdf (accessed on 14th July 2025).
8. Bachert, C., Boot, J. D., de Kam, P. J., Džupinová, S., et al. (2019). Sublingual allergen immunotherapy with a liquid birch pollen product in patients with seasonal allergic rhinoconjunctivitis with or without asthma. https://core.ac.uk/download/237011131.pdf (accessed on 14th July 2025).
9. Barnett, J., Kuljis, J., Lucas, J., Money, D., et al. (2013). Patient perceptions of epinephrine auto-injectors: Exploring barriers to use. https://core.ac.uk/download/29140206.pdf (accessed on 14th July 2025).
10. Belanger, J. M., Breitenbuecher, C., Famula, T. R., Fates, M., et al. (2016). Protein expression and genetic variability of canine Can f 1 in golden and Labrador retriever service dogs. https://core.ac.uk/download/323071242.pdf (accessed on 14th July 2025).
11. Benedé, S., Bouchaud, G., Costa, A., Denery-Papini, S., et al. (2019). Applying the adverse outcome pathway (AOP) for food sensitization to support *in vitro* testing strategies. https://core.ac.uk/download/232112908.pdf (accessed on 14th July 2025).

12. Bilgicer, B., Deak, P. E., Kaplan, M. H., Kim, D., et al. (2019). Covalent heterobivalent inhibitor design for inhibition of IgE-dependent penicillin allergy in a murine model. https://core.ac.uk/download/395674816.pdf (accessed on 14th July 2025).

13. Bluestone, J. A., Bonyhadi, M. L., Earle, K. E., Liu, W., et al. (2005). *In vitro* expanded human CD4+CD25+ regulatory T cells suppress effector T cell proliferation. https://core.ac.uk/download/323073865.pdf (accessed on 14th July 2025).

14. Bonini, M., Canonica, G. W., Del Giacco, S., Gangemi, S., Lombardi, C., Minciullo, P. L., et al. (2017). Allergic diseases in the elderly: Biological characteristics and main immunological and non-immunological mechanisms. https://core.ac.uk/download/80193935.pdf (accessed on 14th July 2025).

15. Borchers, A. T., Chang, C., Gershwin, M. E., Keen, C. L., et al. (2006). Airborne environmental injuries and human health. https://core.ac.uk/download/323069620.pdf (accessed on 14th July 2025).

16. Bosnic-Anticevich, S. Z., Carney, A. S., Carter, V., Christian, L., et al. (2017). Seasonal patterns of oral antihistamine and intranasal corticosteroid purchases from Australian community pharmacies: A retrospective observational study. https://core.ac.uk/download/131024570.pdf (accessed on 14th July 2025).

17. Cox, E., Hesta, M., Maina, E., Pelst, S., et al. (2017). Food-specific sublingual immunotherapy is well tolerated and safe in healthy dogs: A blind, randomized, placebo-controlled study. https://core.ac.uk/download/84042228.pdf (accessed on 14th July 2025).

18. De Pessemier, B., Grine, L., Debaere, M., Maes, A., Paetzold, B., & Callewaert, C. (2021). Gut–skin axis: Current knowledge of the interrelationship between microbial dysbiosis and skin conditions. *Microorganisms, 9*, 353–353. https://doi.org/10.3390/microorganisms9020353 (accessed on 14th July 2025).

19. Ell, A. (2024). The increase of allergies in developed countries: A comparison of the quality of life and psychosocial burden of individuals with food allergies in Switzerland and the United States of America. https://core.ac.uk/download/619721873.pdf (accessed on 14th July 2025).

20. Else, K. J., Garcia, F. T., McSharry, C., Nakajima, H., Oku, Y., Pawlowski, Z., Petit-Frere, C., et al. (2014). Mucosal immune responses following intestinal nematode infection. https://core.ac.uk/download/29469509.pdf (accessed on 14th July 2025).

21. Flayer, C. H., Ge, M. Q., Haczku, A., Hwang, J. Y., et al. (2019). Ozone inhalation attenuated the effects of budesonide on *Aspergillus fumigatus*-induced airway inflammation and hyperreactivity in mice. https://core.ac.uk/download/323070060.pdf (accessed on 14th July 2025).

22. Gevaert, K., Impens, F., Laval, K., Nauwynck, H., et al. (2019). Pollens destroy respiratory epithelial cell anchors and drive alphaherpesvirus infection. https://core.ac.uk/download/222452376.pdf (accessed on 14th July 2025).

23. Grant, E. (2015). Validity and accuracy of self-reported drug allergies. https://core.ac.uk/download/145038969.pdf (accessed on 14th July 2025).

24. Kinney, A. L. (2007). National scientific facilities and their science impact on non-biomedical research. http://arxiv.org/abs/0705.1797 (accessed on 14th July 2025).

25. Lehtimäki, J. (2017). *The Biodiversity Hypothesis of Allergy: The Interrelations Between the Skin Microbiota, Allergic Diseases and Exposure to Microbes in Residential Environments.* https://core.ac.uk/download/132491171.pdf (accessed on 14th July 2025).

26. Lukan, N. (2017). Present and future of subcutaneous aero-allergen immunotherapy. https://core.ac.uk/download/322428948.pdf (accessed on 14th July 2025).

27. Mascola, J., Steinman, R., King, R. C., & the Working Group convened by the Global HIV Vaccine Enterprise. (2010). Immunogens and antigen processing: Report from a Global HIV Vaccine Enterprise Working Group. https://core.ac.uk/download/pdf/289325.pdf (accessed on 14th July 2025).

28. Mutapi, F., Rujeni, N., & Taylor, D. W. (2012). Human schistosome infection and allergic sensitization. https://core.ac.uk/download/28974396.pdf (accessed on 14th July 2025).

29. Nødtvedt, A. (2007). Epidemiology of canine atopic dermatitis. https://core.ac.uk/download/11695161.pdf (accessed on 14th July 2025).

30. Palmer, L. (2016). Edible insects as a source of food allergens. https://core.ac.uk/download/77945692.pdf (accessed on 14th July 2025).

31. Rauscher, B. (2015). Use of immunotherapy in the treatment of peanut allergies in the pediatric population. https://core.ac.uk/download/58826198.pdf (accessed on 14th July 2025).

32. Sandstedt, M., Vukusic, K., Johansson, M., Jonsson, M., Magnusson, R., Hultén, L. M., Dellgren, G., et al. (2023). Regional transcriptomic profiling reveals immune system enrichment in nonfailing atria as well as all chambers of the failing human heart. *American Journal of Physiology. Heart and Circulatory Physiology*. https://www.semanticscholar.org/paper/b4f30277285e6477aed4fe9435348e2154fcf0c2 (accessed on 14th July 2025).

33. Seita, H. M. (2013). Food allergies in pregnant women: A study of prevalence in expecting mothers and association with neonatal outcomes. https://open.bu.edu/bitstream/2144/12219/6/Seita_Helene_2013.pdf (accessed on 14th July 2025).

34. Sokolowska, M., Lukasik, Z., Agache, I., Akdis, C., Akdis, D., Akdis, M., Barcik, W., et al. (2020). Immunology of COVID-19: Mechanisms, clinical outcome, diagnostics, and perspectives—A report of the European Academy of Allergy and Clinical Immunology (EAACI). *Allergy, 75*, 2445–2476. https://www.semanticscholar.org/paper/1576d54368c68c1d335068c654a10a95408c88c5 (accessed on 14th July 2025).

35. Vassallo, K. (2007). Rhinitis in general practice. https://core.ac.uk/download/46602128.pdf (accessed on 14th July 2025).

36. Wesserling, M. (2013). Role of genetic aspect in pathogenesis of atopic dermatitis. https://core.ac.uk/download/71976799.pdf (accessed on 14th July 2025).

37. Zuberbier, T., Abdul Latiff, A. H., Abuzakouk, M., Aquilina, S., Asero, R., Baker, D. R., Ballmer-Weber, B., et al. (2021). The international EAACI/GA^{2}LEN/EuroGuiDerm/APAAACI guideline for the definition, classification, diagnosis, and management of urticaria. *Allergy, 77*, 734–766. https://doi.org/10.1111/all.15090 (accessed on 14th July 2025).

INFECTIOUS DISEASES

10

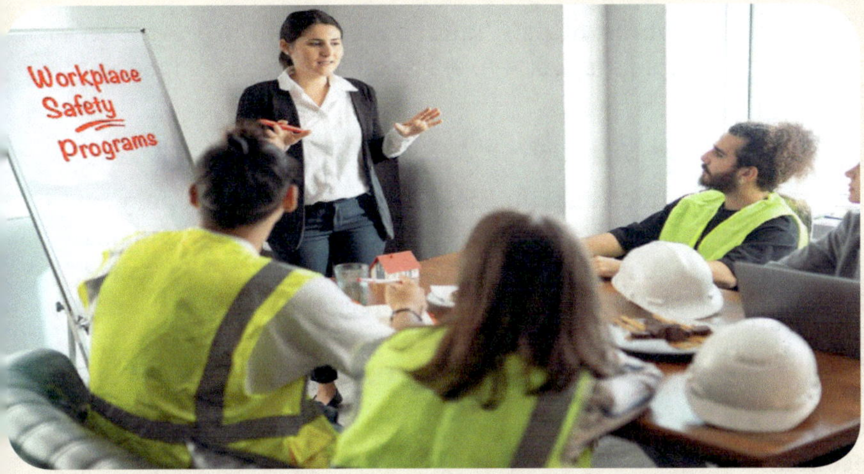

LEARNING OBJECTIVES

After studying this chapter, you will be able to:

1. Describe the types of infectious diseases
2. Describe the transmission of infectious diseases
3 Understand the symptoms and diagnosis of infectious diseases
4. Know the treatment options for infectious diseases
5. Understand the prevention strategies for infectious diseases
6. Know the impact of infectious diseases on society

Introduction

Infectious diseases are a major public health problem globally, impacting millions of people every year. This is due to the intricate dynamics involving the pathogens—e.g., bacteria, viruses, fungi, and parasites—and their hosts, including humans. The study of infectious diseases requires that one deal with a detailed analysis of the factors that enable the transmission and emergence of the diseases. With globalization and urbanization on the rise, the potential for outbreaks increases, underscoring a serious need for effective surveillance and prevention practices. Furthermore, societal behaviors and environmental factors have significant impacts on the spread of disease. Given the multiplicity of infectious diseases, there is a need for interdisciplinary approaches, including epidemiology, public health, and environmental science. This chapter seeks to describe the mechanisms of infectious disease in human populations, emphasizing their public health significance as well as potential lines of intervention (Devos et al., 2017). Of particular interest here is the link between environmental change, agriculture, and the emergence of infectious diseases. A systematic review recognizes that agricultural intensification and environmental change are most directly linked to zoonotic disease—disease spread from animals to humans. As human numbers grow, they exert pressure on natural habitats and alter ecosystems, thus raising contact between wild and domesticated animals. It is this contact that is a major driver of new disease emergence, as indicated by research showing that most zoonoses are driven by the evolving agricultural landscape and changing human practices. Unless there is an appropriate conception of this agriculture-environment interface, attempts to anticipate and prevent disease outbreaks could be unfruitful.

Therefore, the interconnectivity among biological, environmental, and socio-economic determinants must be recognized to craft effective public health interventions to combat infectious diseases in humans (Artois et al., 2013). The impacts of infectious diseases extend far beyond human well-being, affecting economic stability, social arrangements, and global politics. As the globe continues to grapple with the ongoing pandemic risk of infectious diseases, the call for a strong public health infrastructure has never been more urgent. Public health investment in prevention, education, and rapid-response capacity is important for minimizing the effects of outbreaks. Moreover, support for international cooperation and information exchange among states is necessary to effectively respond to pandemics and enhance surveillance mechanisms. Infectious diseases need to be tackled through a combination of responses that take their complexities and interconnectedness into account. As we move through the various facets of infectious diseases in this chapter, it is clear that an engaged, informed response is required to defend public health and enable the well-being of future generations (Figure 10.1).

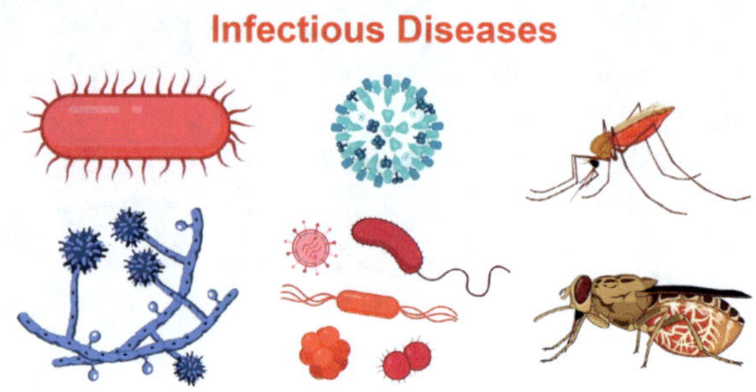

Figure 10.1. Infectious diseases.

Source: https://microbenotes.com/wp-content/uploads/2024/04/Infectious-Diseases.jpeg.

Definition of Infectious Diseases

Infectious diseases are a broad category of diseases caused by pathogenic microorganisms, such as bacteria, viruses, fungi, and parasites. Microorganisms can infect the host body and multiply, causing a range of clinical signs that may vary in severity. Infectious diseases are transmitted in various ways, e.g., through direct contact with infected individuals, via contaminated surfaces, or via vectors such as mosquitoes. The resulting diseases affect not only individual patients but also have far-reaching implications for public health, particularly in overcrowded areas or where healthcare infrastructure is poor. As the nature of multihost parasites has been visualized, the transmission ecology and ecological relationships of such pathogens need to be understood to develop efficient disease control strategies in humans and animals (Adamo et al., 2015). Zoonotic infections are a significant category of infectious diseases, originating in animals before they leap to humans. The World Health Organization has emphasized addressing such infections through a One Health approach that is centered on the connection between human, animal, and environmental health (Buttigieg et al., 2015). This framework recognizes that most emerging infectious diseases are zoonotic, necessitating collaboration among veterinary and medical scientists to develop effective prevention and control strategies. Because such diseases tend to thrive in ecosystems with close human-animal coexistence, an integrated understanding of both the ecological dynamics and the evolutionary responses of pathogens to anthropogenic changes is essential. Such an approach not only aims to eliminate infections but also to reduce the risk of future outbreaks by addressing the drivers of disease emergence. Furthermore, the continuous adaptation of infectious pathogens poses a challenge for controlling these diseases. Pathogens adapt to environmental pressures, including antimicrobial use and host behavioral changes.

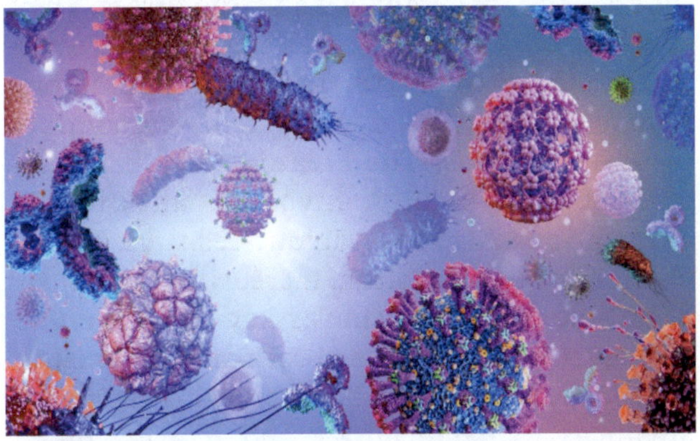

Figure 10.2. Definition of infectious diseases.

Source: https://www.yourgenome.org/wp-content/uploads/2023/11/1600-shutterstock_2112088307.jpg.

This shift can lead to increased virulence, antibiotic resistance, and spillover from animal reservoirs to human populations. In the context of these dynamics, researchers recommend a more integrative approach to infectious disease prevention that involves cautionary exploration of disease ecology and host-pathogen interactions. Methods for conducting empirical research and theory modeling can inform the most influential drivers of disease spread and provide a solid basis for evidence to inform public health programs (Adamo et al., 2015; Buttigieg et al., 2015). By working on prevention and control, the public health community can make efforts to significantly reduce the infectious disease burden in humans (Figure 10.2).

Importance of Studying Infectious Diseases

The study of infectious diseases remains relevant in the field of international health, especially given the increasing number of severe zoonotic infections. Management of such diseases requires a strong background understanding of epidemiology, patterns of transmission, and associated risk factors. To address these challenges in an interdisciplinary way, multidisciplinary research is required, as emphasized by the roadmap to Combat Zoonoses in India initiative, which prioritizes research options for zoonosis control by converging different expertise. Identification of pre-eminent knowledge gaps and evidence-based research agendas, such as in health policy and systems, also underscores the necessity of acknowledging the complexities of infectious disease management. This self-initiated measure not only promotes disease prevention and control but also forms inter-sectoral coordination, ultimately leading to healthier communities and individuals (Kakkar et al., 2011). Furthermore, environmental factors play an essential role in the transmission and epidemiology of infectious diseases, particularly those caused by microparasites. Key environmental parameters such as temperature and rainfall have been shown to affect disease transmission dynamics in complex ways, but the relationship remains poorly understood. The extent of knowledge gaps regarding environmental determinants from existing models underscores the need to incorporate such determinants into disease control strategies. Transmission of schistosomiasis is a suitable model to investigate how environmental changes affect the viability and infectivity of disease stages, for instance. Including time-varying environmental processes in mathematical models of disease allows scientists to improve predictive capacity and plan more effective intervention measures. Thus, the study of infectious diseases is unavoidably connected with the knowledge of environmental settings that affect their evolution, which is crucial for the implementation of evidence-based health policy (Remais et al., 2010). Moreover, infectious disease research is not only necessary for immediate public health reaction but also for preparedness to avert pandemics.

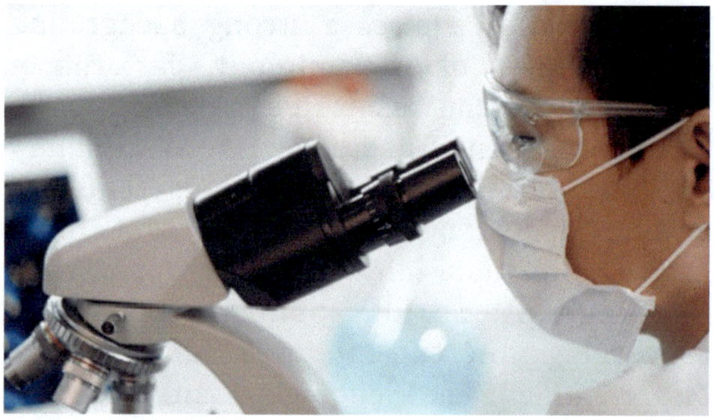

Figure 10.3. Importance of studying infectious diseases.

Source: https://nanocellect.com/wp-content/uploads/2020/06/12.png.

Experience has shown that emerging infectious diseases can destabilize societies, economies, and health systems. The COVID-19 pandemic is a case in point, highlighting the benefits of continuous surveillance, research, and investment in health systems to mitigate the impact of infectious outbreaks. Information on the determinants of the occurrence and spread of infectious diseases enables effective readiness operations when emergencies occur. By fostering a research culture and public health education, communities can develop immunity to both known and emerging pathogens. This cutting-edge model for research into infectious diseases not only aims to promote personal health but also international security through the safeguarding of communities against the multifaceted threats of infectious agents (Figure 10.3).

10.1. Types of Infectious Diseases

Learning Outcome

1. Understand the bacterial infections
2. Understand the viral infections
3. Describe the fungal infections

Infectious diseases are divided into a variety of types, primarily based on the causative agents. Bacterial infections are among the most common and include diseases such as tuberculosis, pneumonia, and strep throat. They are caused by pathogenic bacterial growth in the host, which can trigger inflammatory responses that range from mild discomfort to severe illness. The treatment of bacterial infections typically involves antibiotics, although advances in antibiotic-resistant strains complicate this situation. Increasing awareness of antibiotic stewardship is key to controlling the development of these resistant organisms, as recent studies underscore the need for advances in bacteriology and pharmacology (Barton et al., 2012). The other predominant category of infectious diseases is viral infections, caused by viruses such as influenza, HIV, and SARS-CoV-2. Viral infections vary widely in pathogenicity, modes of transmission, and public health significance. Viruses cannot replicate on their own and require host cells to propagate. This unique characteristic has led to numerous prevention and treatment strategies, such as vaccines and antiviral medications. The COVID-19 pandemic is a hallmark illustration of the ruinous effects of a viral epidemic on global health systems and underscores the need for rapid research and development of effective vaccines and treatments to manage viral infections. Therefore, viral mutations and vaccine efficacy remain the focus of public health discussion and concern (Burke et al., 2013). Fungal infections are another critical group of infectious diseases, particularly in the immunocompromised host. Opportunistic fungal infections such as candidiasis and aspergillosis can cause tremendous morbidity and mortality in susceptible hosts. These issues are aggravated by the delayed diagnosis and inadequate therapeutic options, highlighting the need for rapid improvement in antifungal research. Recent patent analyses depict a rising pattern of enthusiasm in developing new forms and treatments for the infections, as seen in the stress laid on research of effective antifungal therapies. In addition, the rising incidence of invasive fungal infections globally calls for enhanced monitoring and public health responses to curb their impact, underscoring the importance of vigilance in combating this oft-overlooked spectrum of infectious illnesses (Barton et al., 2012; Burke et al., 2013) (Figure 10.4).

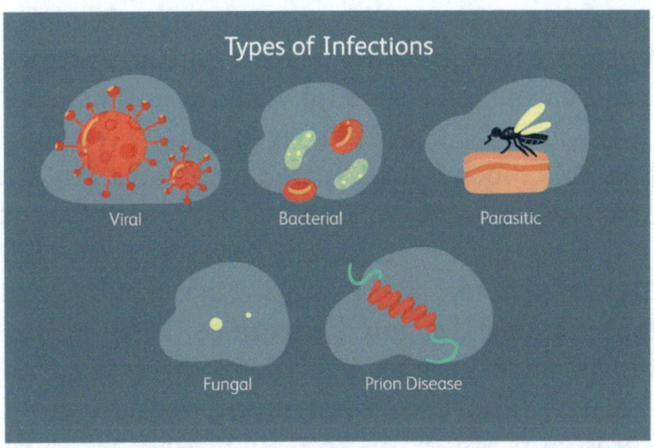

Figure 10.4. Types of infectious diseases.

Source: https://www.verywellhealth.com/thmb/HVLoB-Gfeddv1Zb1Wh67TKHi-Fo=/1500x0/filters:no_upscale():max_bytes(150000):strip_icc()/infection-5096014-Final-eaf7a90b39fd4eb69b3a1776b721d975.gif.

10.1.1. Bacterial Infections

Bacterial infections constitute one of the principal classes of infectious human diseases, characterized by their ability to grow and multiply extensively and to cause complex health complications. Some of the most notorious bacteria are Escherichia coli, Klebsiella pneumoniae, and Staphylococcus aureus, all of which are notorious for their ability to cause severe infections and serious morbidity and mortality. The emergence of multidrug-resistant strains of such pathogens has further compounded treatment challenges, as standard antibiotic therapy is often ineffective. It is a matter of particular concern in low- and middle-income countries, where the healthcare setup is poor, and surveillance systems for antimicrobial resistance are not yet well established. Management of such bacterial infections necessitates an integrated approach that incorporates public health interventions, medical treatment, and local health infrastructure development to address resistance and improve patient outcomes. Antibiotic resistance is more and more moving into the limelight in the management of bacterial infections, fundamentally revolutionizing treatment practice and outcomes. New studies evidence an alarming rise in resistance rates among various types of bacteria, particularly nosocomial pathogens. For instance, the prevalence of methicillin-resistant Staphylococcus aureus (MRSA) and extended-spectrum beta-lactamase (ESBL) producing organisms is on the rise. The reports point towards the fact that without an effective public health response, the effectiveness of available antibiotics will be greatly diminished, thereby leading to extended hospital stays, higher healthcare costs, and higher mortality rates. Efforts to enhance clinical microbiology services and stimulate systematic surveillance in animal and human medicine are essential. These efforts, informed by systematic data gathering, can help establish efficient treatment protocols and national policies to curb antibiotic resistance, thereby improving patient care and public health. The incorporation of systematic frameworks, such as the Infectious Disease Ontology (IDO), can help our understanding and containment of bacterial infections. IDO provides a structured approach to classify and study infectious diseases, such as many bacterial pathogens. Unifying disease data in a single system helps medical professionals and researchers better analyze epidemiological trends and patient outcomes. Ongoing development of specialized extensions, such as those for specific pathogens, enables detailed research and improves data exchange among health care practitioners. The application of IDO facilitates a collaborative approach to infectious disease control, driving research and treatment development. It primarily facilitates reproducibility and consistency in bacterial infection studies, essential in developing effective public health policy and interventions to mitigate the infectious disease burden in human populations (Matee et al., 2013; Babcock et al., 2021) (Figure 10.5).

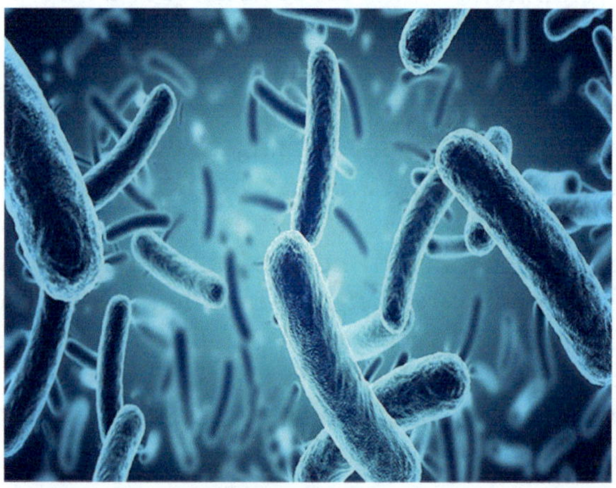

Figure 10.5. Bacterial infections.

Source: https://www.drpriyaskinandhairclinic.com/imageuploads/pages/2019/04/16/bacterial-infection-treatment-in-bangalore.jpg.

10.1.2. Viral Infections

The study of viral infection involves an investigation into its mechanisms and roles in human health. Viruses are characterized by their ability to infect host cells and hijack their machinery for replication, and, in doing so, destroy or kill the cell. In contrast to bacterial infections, which are usually treatable with antibiotics, viral infections pose unique challenges in treatment and prevention. Vaccine development has been a pillar in the management of viral diseases, significantly reducing infection rates for diseases like measles, mumps, and rubella. Nonetheless, as detailed in current research, vaccines are not effective against all viral infections, necessitating other intervention measures for specific populations. This deficiency is increasing the need for continued research in therapeutic development and vaccine development, especially given that some of these patients will not tolerate vaccines (Fang et al., 2004).

In recent years, viral infection control has seen new therapeutic strategies, indicating a paradigm shift in therapy. Traditional immunizations have dominated the field of prevention, yet scenarios under which vaccines are not feasible call for new solutions. A prime example is monoclonal antibodies, a class of agents that represents a quantum leap in the prevention and treatment of specific viral infections, such as respiratory syncytial virus (RSV). Not only does this biochemical option block entry by the virus, but it also terminates viral replication at the cellular level itself, providing credible alternatives for risk groups. Furthermore, the application of targeted therapies, such as RNA interference, is more specific to the replication process. These advancements constitute a significant shift in the fight against viral infections, improving the means available to medical professionals (Eijck et al., 2003). Aside from these advancements, the complexity of viral infection remains a significant challenge. Strain heterogeneity of the virus, host immunity, and dynamic epidemiological patterns are complicating factors for successful prevention and control. faster pace than research can keep up with, hence the outbreaks that bedevil public health systems worldwide. There is also an urgent need to understand the relationship between non-communicable diseases and viral infections, which worsens the victim's condition.

Consequently, multidisciplinary models that incorporate genetics, immunology, and the environment have the potential to introduce a multidimensional awareness to the prevention of viral infection. Public education and awareness about such diseases and prevention of disease are essential in preventing outbreaks and mitigating risk for individuals in different populations, and highlighting the intersection of individual health decision-making and community well-being in the infectious disease model framework (Fang et al., 2004) (Figure 10.6).

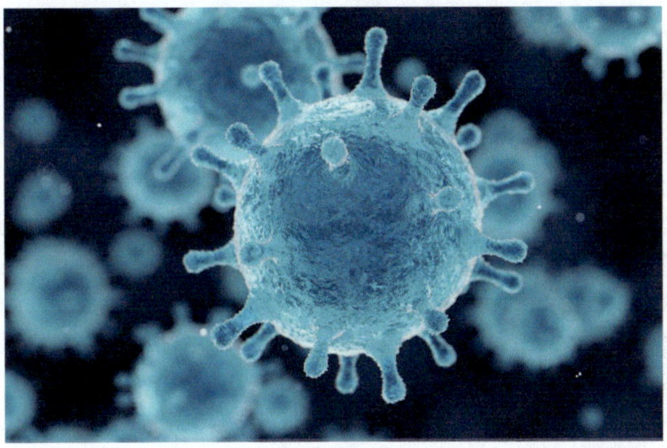

Figure 10.6. Viral infections.

Source: https://www.dzne.de/fileadmin/_processed_/4/7/csm_WEB-AdobeStock_333092093_a2a03c449d.jpg.

10.1.3. Fungal Infections

The growing incidence of fungal infections is a new problem in infectious diseases, particularly amid population changes and medical progress, creating new vulnerabilities. Opportunistic fungi exploit patients' compromised immune systems in diseases such as cancer, diabetes, and post-transplant immunosuppression. The ability of these pathogens to cause infections ranging from mild to deadly is intricately linked to their biology, including their ability to form biofilms. Biofilms are intricate communities of fungal cells that bind to a surface, which allows the organisms to be resistant to antifungal medications and live inside the human body. Hence, understanding the dynamics of fungal infections is crucial for addressing epidemiological trends and designing effective therapeutic regimens to thwart these cunning pathogens. Antifungal resistance has emerged as a key issue over recent years in managing fungal infections, which underscores the need for novel modes of therapeutic intervention. Current antifungals tend to be limited in their activity, and therefore scientists have been interested in identifying substitutes that can improve therapeutic outcomes. Experimental evidence demonstrated that the use of anti-inflammatory agents alongside antifungals could potentially treat pathogens and host inflammatory responses.

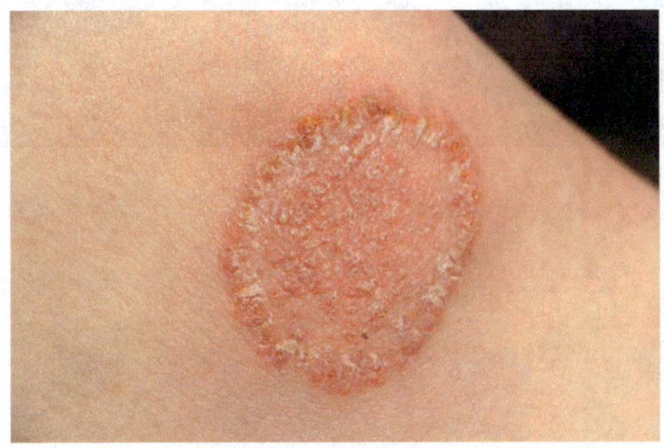

Figure 10.7. Fungal infections.

Source: https://images.squarespace-cdn.com/content/v1/61266e982104fd1fe23f9fba/245213c6-1a39-422e-8d20-d378ecc5572f/Fungal-infections.jpg.

Myriocin, Fulvic Acid, and Acetylcholine are a few substances found to possess potent antifungal and anti-inflammatory effects and are therefore worthy of investigation as dual-action therapeutics. This approach not only treats the fungal infection better but also can reduce the chronic inflammation that is common with fungal infections and therefore enhances patient outcomes as a whole (Eijck et al., 2003). Fungal infection control requires a multi-faceted approach that includes prevention, early diagnosis, and optimal therapeutic modalities.

Surveillance systems to monitor fungal pathogens and resistance patterns are important since they alert clinicians and public health practitioners to emerging threats. Additionally, increased sensitization among patients and health workers to the risk factors causing fungal infections can enable timely interventions. The interplay between human health and determinants in the environment also underscores the importance of examining the ecological reservoirs from which the fungi are sourced. Investigation of the correlation between farming methods, such as organic cattle production, and the incidence of fungal infection can yield data to assist in the development of integrated control strategies to mitigate risks entailed by such pathogens (Eijck et al., 2003) (Figure 10.7).

Test Your Knowledge

1. What is a bacterial infection?
2. What is a viral infection?

10.2. Transmission of Infectious Diseases

Learning Outcome

1. Describe the direct and indirect transmission methods of infectious diseases
2. Understand the vector-borne transmission of infectious diseases

The spread of infectious diseases is a multifaceted process with various factors involved in their causation, including biological, environmental, and socio-economic factors. When man comes into contact with the environment, he creates conditions that naturally facilitate the spread of the causative agents of disease, particularly zoonotic diseases that begin in animals and cross over to man. These interactions can be regulated by land-use change, climate, and urbanization patterns, leading to ecosystem disturbance and altering species interactions. These changes enhance contact between human populations and wildlife, thus amplifying the risk of infectious disease emergence. Therefore, knowledge of these biological and environmental interactions is critical when developing effective public health interventions to control the spread of infectious diseases in humans. Among the core pillars of infectious disease transmission research is the role of genomics in pathogen identification and characterization. Recent advancements in genomic technology, such as high-throughput sequencing and microarray-based detection, have enhanced researchers' ability to analyze the genetic variation of emerging pathogens. By examining the genomic characteristics shared by closely related pathogens infecting different host species, researchers can uncover how zoonotic infections adapt to new human hosts. Comparative studies not only clarify the molecular basis of the host's response to disease but also permit predictions of potential zoonotic transmission outcomes. Such genomic data are invaluable for developing preventive measures and tailoring vaccine design against infectious diseases, thereby boosting global health security. Furthermore, the increasing occurrence of zoonotic diseases calls for an interdisciplinary approach towards comprehending their spread across different disciplines of study, i.e., biological, environmental, and social sciences. The upscaling of zoonotic infections demands an integrative framework dividing research into its corresponding components. An interdisciplinary approach that spans fields such as psychology, economics, and environmental science can provide a comprehensive perspective on the drivers of infectious disease transmission. The integration of human behavior—habitual and motivated—as well as environmental and biological constraints into the analysis allows researchers to better appreciate the complexities of zoonotic transmission. They are embracing this interdisciplinarity not only to assist in clarifying the dynamics of disease transmission but also to enhance public health responses to newly emerging infectious threats, thereby ensuring human health in the face of changing ecological challenges (Andeweg et al., 2009; Barnett et al., 2012) (Figure 10.8).

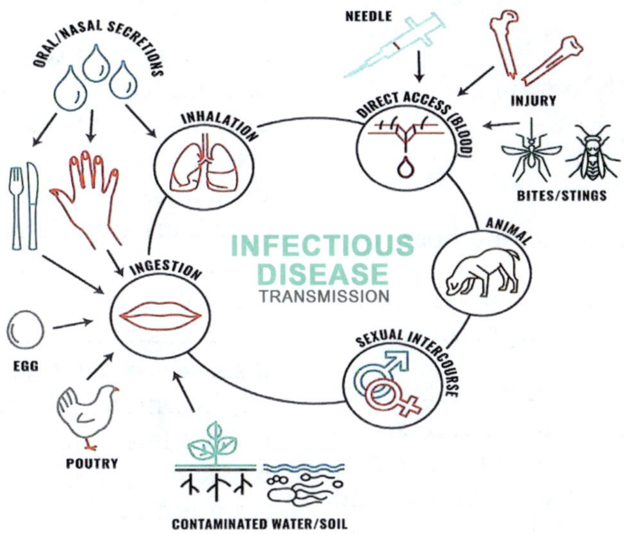

Figure 10.8. Mode of transmission of infectious disease.

Source: https://www.researchgate.net/profile/Oduwe-Ugochukwu/publication/361860777/figure/fig2/AS:1175659565068288@1657310491215/Mode-of-Transmission-of-Infectious-Disease-18.png.

10.2.1. Direct Transmission Methods

Direct modes of transmission in infectious diseases are significant in the comprehension of how diseases pass through the media through which pathogens are transmitted from humans to humans. Direct transmission facilitates the transfer of a pathogen from an infected individual to another individual who is an implied or unknown susceptible, without passing through an intermediary vector. Direct transmission usually occurs through contact, respiratory, and bodily fluids. Distance is significant since most pathogens require intimate contact for their transmission. For instance, the influenza and SARS-CoV-2 viruses spread through respiratory droplets when speaking, coughing, or sneezing, indicating how infections can easily spread in a densely populated environment. Regulation of such direct transmission of infection is integral to public health management, underscoring the requirement for hygiene protocols and social distancing to limit contact-based transmission in communities. One of the most striking aspects of direct transmission is the phenomenon of zoonotic diseases, in which pathogens can move from animals to humans. Farming activities and environmental modification tend to facilitate such transmission, say, for instance. A systematic review established the interface between more intensive agricultural practices and a higher risk of zoonotic diseases, and the interaction between environmental factors and human behavior in disease emergence (Artois et al., 2013).

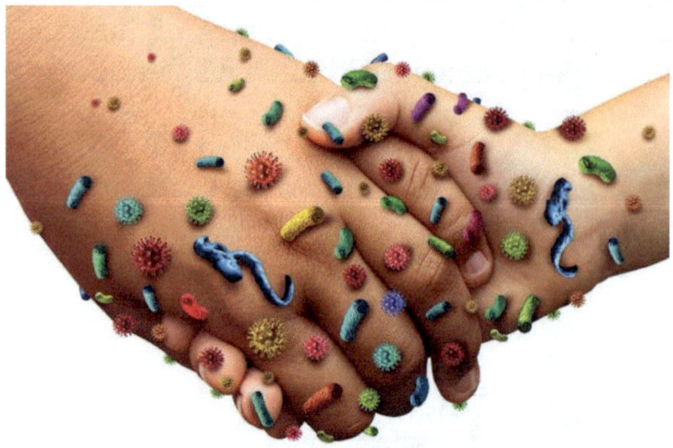

Figure 10.9. Direct transmission methods.

Source: https://api.parashospitals.com/uploads/2019/07/pathogens-airports.jpg.

This phenomenon sheds light on the complexity of direct transmission mechanisms, as these mechanisms mostly involve intricate interactions among wildlife, livestock, and human communities. Emerging pathogenicity in human groups related to animal reservoirs points to the need for interdisciplinarity in approaches to predict and combat such risks as effectively as possible. As human encroachment into wildlife habitats increases, the risk of zoonotic transmission via direct mechanisms heightens, and this must be vigilantly monitored and countered. Besides, although migratory birds may serve as mechanical vectors for many pathogens, direct transmission from birds to humans is uncommon. Research has established that many diseases are associated with wild birds, but few have been confirmed with concrete evidence for direct transmission (Bauchinger et al., 2008). This illustrates the complex mechanisms of pathogen transmission and the rare instances where direct human infection occurs. Understanding these dynamics is essential for formulating targeted interventions for the protection of public health. In the presence of a few confirmed cases of direct bird-to-human transmission, future studies must examine further the ecological determinants of wildlife-to-human pathogen spillover and develop a preventive strategy to reduce the risk of emerging infectious diseases through direct modes (Figure 10.9).

10.2.2. Indirect Transmission Methods

It is important to comprehend the complexity of indirect transmission mechanisms so that one may appreciate how infectious diseases are transmitted in human populations. Indirect transmission occurs when disease-causing agents are transferred by intermediate carriers or reservoirs in the environment rather than directly through host-to-host contact. Some good examples include the transmission of disease via contaminated surfaces, water, or air, in which pathogens survive independently of their initial hosts. The inclusion of wild birds, particularly migratory birds, complicates this situation further. Scientific evidence indicates that, while wild birds are vectors of diseases such as the influenza A virus and arboviruses, direct infection is relatively rare, with only a single case reported (Bauchinger et al., 2008). This provides evidence that information on indirect routes remains important for controlling outbreaks and developing targeted interventions for wildlife-associated diseases. Agricultural management is also important in promoting the indirect transmission of zoonotic diseases. The contact between wild and domestic animals creates niches for cross-species pathogen transmission. Agricultural intensification combined with environmental change has been associated with an increased risk of the emergence of zoonotic diseases, mainly because of the interactions among human, livestock, and wildlife populations. This overlap of agriculture and environment is a broader challenge for public health: how to respond optimally to the multifaceted dynamics of disease transmission. As suggested by evidence from a systematic review, the intricate relationships among these variables tend to limit our ability to forecast and respond to emerging zoonotic threats (Artois et al., 2013).

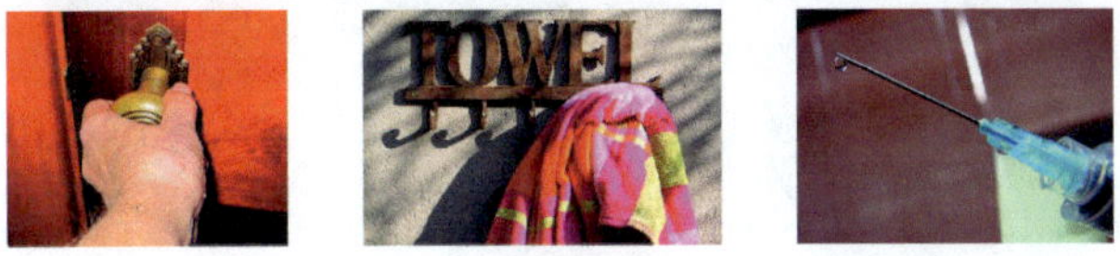

Figure 10.10. Fomites are nonliving objects that facilitate the indirect transmission of pathogens. Contaminated doorknobs, towels, and syringes are all common examples of fomites.

Source: https://s3-us-west-2.amazonaws.com/courses-images/wp-content/uploads/sites/1094/2016/11/03165458/OSC_Microbio_16_03_Indirect.jpg.

The consequences of these indirect transmission routes underscore the need for interdisciplinary methods in public health programs. The solution to infectious diseases will not be achieved merely by understanding the biological processes of pathogens; it also entails exploring the environmental, economic, and social determinants that drive their spread. Strong surveillance systems and active communication across sectors can help identify and control outbreaks early, before they become unmanageable. In this regard, professional education programs for agricultural professionals, as well as the community at large, can sensitize the population to the mechanisms of transmission and preventive measures. By addressing the factors that lead to indirect transmission and leveraging interdisciplinary collaboration, society can strengthen its defenses against the threat of new infectious diseases via the indirect pathway (Figure 10.10).

10.2.3. Vector-Borne Transmission

Vector-borne transmission is a significant route by which infectious diseases affect human populations. Vector-borne transmission occurs when pathogens are carried by vectors, usually arthropods such as mosquitoes, ticks, and fleas, from one host to the next. The relationship between the pathogen and the vector is complex; vectors usually must pass through specific developmental stages that bring them into contact with the microorganisms they carry. Malaria, dengue, and West Nile virus are examples of the major role vector-borne transmission has on the disease burden in the public. They have high potential for morbidity and mortality, particularly where preventive measures are few or where the healthcare system is inadequate. Understanding vector population ecology and how it interacts with pathogens is a cornerstone for reducing disease impact through control measures. Climate change has introduced additional complexities into vector-borne disease control by altering the geographic range of vector species. Temperature increases and changes in rainfall favor vector breeding and enable them to move into new geographical regions that were previously unsuitable. As the ecosystem evolves, human exposure to vector-borne diseases also rises. For instance, factors such as increased temperature or humidity will enhance the vectors' lifespan and reproduction levels, and extend their range. According to research, climate change significantly influences disease transmission patterns for conditions such as the Zika virus and Lyme disease, thereby increasing the complexity of tracking public health responses. Effective modeling and predictive analysis will have to incorporate environmental and climatic data to assess such risks and refine strategies (Nikolaos et al., 2008). Aside from environmental factors, the wildlife reservoir potential for pathogens cannot be excluded in describing vector-borne transmission. Although direct infection of humans by pathogens from wild birds is relatively rare, wild birds serve as vectors and reservoirs of a number of pathogens and contribute to the complexity of disease dynamics. Those pathogens carried by wild birds, such as avian influenza, demonstrate how wildlife indirectly influences the health of humans via intermediate vectors, i.e., mosquitoes or ticks. The dynamics among wildlife, vectors, and human populations explain the need for a One Health system that integrates human, animal, and environmental considerations. Additional research is required to elucidate these dynamics and develop effective responses to mitigate the dangers vector-borne illnesses pose to humans (Bauchinger et al., 2008) (Figure 10.11).

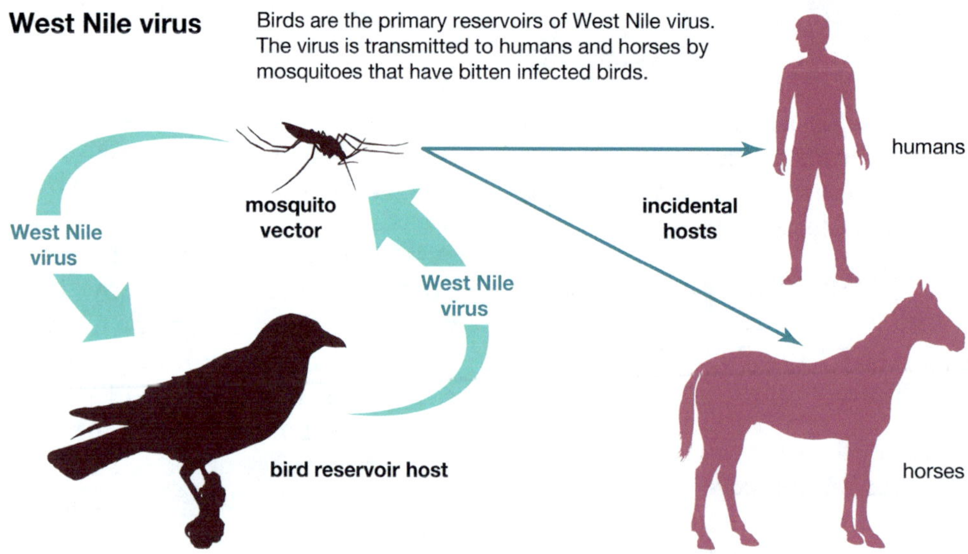

Figure 10.11. Birds are the primary reservoirs of West Nile virus. The virus is transmitted to humans and horses by mosquitoes that have bitten infected birds.

Source: https://cdn.britannica.com/96/78596-050-3FB7591F/virus-Birds-reservoirs-West-Nile-humans-birds.jpg.

Test Your Knowledge

1. What is the direct method of disease transmission?
2. What is a vector borne transmission of an infectious disease?

10.3. Symptoms and Diagnosis

Learning Outcome

1. Know the common symptoms of infectious diseases
2. Describe the diagnostic methods used in infectious diseases
3. Understand the importance of early diagnosis in infectious diseases

The distinction between symptom and sign is essential to the diagnosis of infectious illness, since symptoms are the patient's subjective complaints, while signs are objective phenomena quantifiable by healthcare professionals. For instance, if the patient reports fever, fatigue, and ill feeling, these symptoms guide the clinician's initial assessment. These types of subjective complaints are likely to direct hypotheses towards the infectious cause. However, the objective evidence, such as a raised white blood cell count or specific radiological findings, is used as proof of the suspected diagnosis. The correlation between the history obtained and the sign observed is critical in distinguishing various infectious diseases since a similar presentation can be caused by different organisms. For proper diagnosis, medical systems currently rely virtually entirely on curated ontologies, such as the Infectious Disease Ontology (IDO), that permit systematic consideration of symptoms alongside signs in infectious disease research (Babcock et al., 2021). Diagnosis is further complicated by the manifestation of a wide variety of overlapping symptoms of infectious diseases. For example, conditions such as influenza, COVID-19, and viral infections may present with fever, cough, and body aches, making early diagnosis difficult. Overlapping symptoms emphasize the importance of attentive clinical evaluation and diligent taking of the patient's history. In an era of emerging infectious diseases, where conditions like COVID-19 introduce new pathogens, the identification of unique symptom patterns becomes increasingly important. Diagnostic innovation, such as rapid antigen testing and molecular diagnosis, has significantly enhanced the ability to distinguish between diseases that present with comparable symptomatology. In addition, integrating symptomatology with lab results allows medical practitioners to apply holistic data when making informed decisions about diagnosis, thereby improving patient outcomes and facilitating timely interventions in infectious disease control (Babcock et al., 2021).

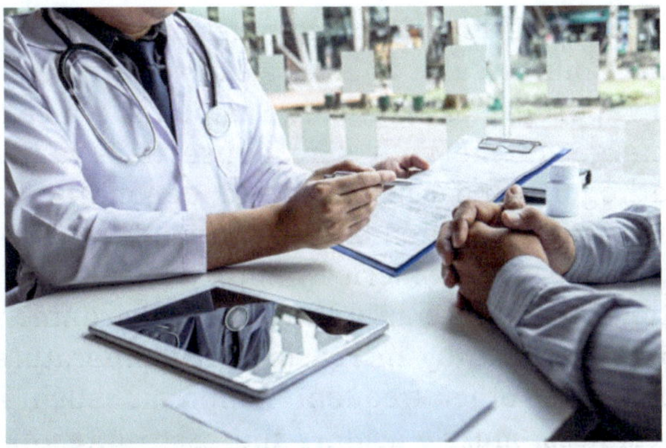

Figure 10.12. Infectious disease diagnosis.

Source: https://dc-whi.org/wp-content/uploads/2021/02/disease-managment-DC-600x400.jpeg.

Some infectious diseases present with unique diagnostic challenges because they exhibit atypical symptom complexes that are not necessarily typical presentations. Take prion diseases, for instance; these neurodegenerative illnesses can have an initial presentation of a wide range of nonspecific symptoms, including cognitive dysfunction and behavioral abnormalities, before progressing to more typical neurological features such as ataxia or myoclonus. Because prion diseases are largely fatal and difficult to diagnose, familiarity with their clinical presentation is important for timely diagnosis. The character of prion diseases is critical in emphasizing the importance of improved diagnostic tests that can differentiate these conditions from other neurological conditions whose presentations are similar. By drawing upon state-of-the-art research in the area of infectious diseases, the medical community can improve diagnostic sensitivity, with the potential to maximize earlier intervention measures to combat neurodegenerative infections more strongly (Figure 10.12).

10.3.1. Common Symptoms of Infectious Diseases

It is essential to understand generic symptoms of infectious diseases to ensure early intervention and appropriate treatment. Symptoms typically emerge as the body's response to invading pathogens and can be varied depending on the type of infection and the patient's immune system. Fever, a generic symptom, is the body's attempt to create an unfavorable environment for pathogens by increasing its temperature. These are other frequent symptoms, such as weakness, muscle aching, and gastrointestinal discomfort, including vomiting and diarrhea. These symptoms are not just uncomfortable but also can produce significant morbidity and, in perilous cases, death if left untreated. As scientists continue to explore the relationships between disease phenotypes and genetic variation, pattern identification of symptoms facilitates the elucidation of infectious disease pathogenesis and their effective treatment (Gkoutos et al., 2014). In addition to fever and generalized malaise, coughing, shortness of breath, and sore throat are typical presentations of infectious respiratory diseases, including influenza and COVID-19. The presentation of these symptoms usually signifies an infectious process of the respiratory system, and there is a risk of community transmission. Zoonoses, or animal-to-human transmissible diseases, further complicate the interpretation of symptoms due to overlapping presentations. For instance, pastoral communities exhibit local syndromic patterns that map animal and human symptoms, with the goal of uncovering the interconnectedness between zoonoses and public health (Catley et al., 2017). Increasingly, this interconnectedness is key as infectious diseases can affect animal populations and human health alike, demonstrating the need for an integrated approach towards combating such diseases. Variation in population perception and knowledge is another essential factor of shared signs of infectious diseases. In some communities, particularly low-resource communities, there may be a lack of awareness or terminology of infectious diseases that can influence access to medical care in a timely manner. For example, among Tanzanian pastoralists, knowledge of zoonotic diseases is often framed in terms of observable signs on animals rather than through a biomedical conceptualization. This environment demonstrates how cultural and social factors shape the nature of perceived diseases and symptoms, impacting healthcare-seeking behavior (Catley et al., 2017). Thus, there is a need for in-depth studies that elaborate on local notions of symptoms and infectious diseases to guide public health interventions and augment response mechanisms across diverse populations (Figure 10.13).

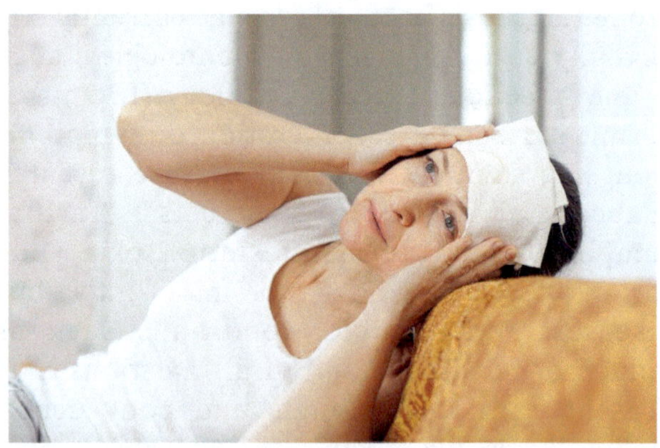

Figure 10.13. Symptoms of infectious diseases.

Source: https://www.shalby.org/wp-content/uploads/2018/04/viralinfection.jpg.

10.3.2. Diagnostic Methods Used

In infectious diseases, speed and accuracy in diagnostic equipment are the most vital aspects for effective treatment and control. Various techniques have been devised to isolate the infecting pathogens, ranging from traditional culture technology to advanced molecular techniques. Culture techniques, although time-consuming, enable the growth and isolation of pathogens in a controlled environment. But recent advances in molecular diagnostics, such as polymerase chain reaction (PCR) and next-generation sequencing, have revolutionized the field. These technologies not only enable rapid detection of pathogens but also identify genetic mutations and resistance markers, thereby informing treatment decisions. The growing reliance on molecular diagnostic tests indicates an intrinsic paradigm shift in the treatment of infectious diseases, with greater emphasis on diagnostic accuracy to yield quantifiable gains in patient outcomes. Among the most valuable diagnostic agents gaining popularity is real-time reverse transcriptase polymerase chain reaction (qRT-PCR), particularly for viruses. This has demonstrated tremendous superiority over traditional fluorescent antigen tests, with significantly higher sensitivity and specificity. As an illustration, a two-step generic lyssavirus qRT-PCR has been shown to be effective for detecting various lyssavirus species, with 100% diagnostic specificity and a record limit of detection. This indicates the ability of the method to detect viral infections effectively, including in low-concentration cases, thus enabling timely medical treatment. Besides, the prospects of qRT-PCR for monitoring the progression of viral infections in models, for instance, rabies virus infection in mice, also increase its use. Hence, diagnostic innovation in such cases pushes the frontier of infectious disease information and improves clinical interventions for new pathogens (Craeye et al., 2014). In addition to molecular techniques, advances in computational methods have become increasingly crucial for diagnosing infectious diseases. Boolean network models are a powerful method of diagnosis and uncovering the disease dynamics, particularly in intricate cases where network interactions play a significant role. The models can aid in determining global states that lead to particular outcomes, thereby enabling pre-processing of control actions in complex infectious disease cases. While the challenge in this case is the inherent complexity of such models, fresh algorithms have since been developed that make the identification of such states easier without further reducing computation and the accompanying processing demand typical of exhaustive search methods. This not only enhances diagnostic accuracy but also sheds light on the forces driving infectious disease dynamics, leading to more effective public health policy initiatives and interventions (Abo-Shehada et al., 2007) (Figure 10.14).

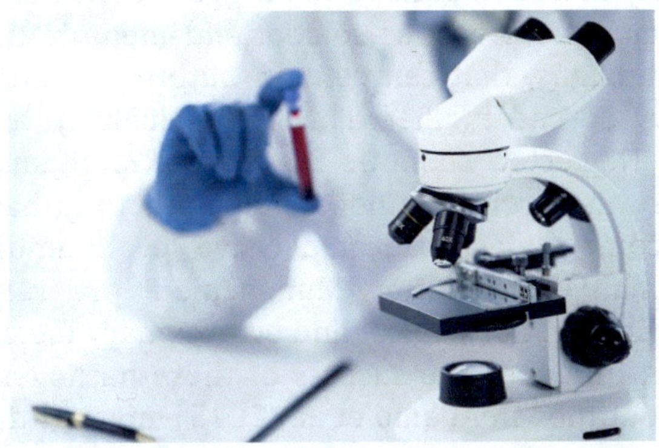

Figure 10.14. Infectious disease diagnostic method.

Source: https://www.news-medical.net/image-handler/ts/20221017072925/ri/950/src/images/news/ImageForNews_728228_16660493650569716.jpg.

10.3.3. Importance of Early Diagnosis

The significance of early diagnosis of infectious diseases cannot be overstated, as it directly affects treatment efficiency and patient outcomes. Early detection of pathogens enables early interventions, which not only enhance the chances of recovery but also minimize complications and long-term health implications. For example, most infectious diseases can progress rapidly if not diagnosed early; early diagnosis allows healthcare professionals to intervene with appropriate therapies tailored to the pathogens in question. Furthermore, early detection of infections can help prevent secondary infections and reduce the overall burden on healthcare systems, particularly in low-resource settings where complex therapies are not readily available. One of the key roles of early diagnosis is in disease spread prevention, most importantly, those that are zoonotic. Recognition of the complex interplay between animal and human reservoirs is vital for reducing transmission rates within populations. Early detection of cases can trigger public health interventions, such as isolation and immunization campaigns, that can contain outbreaks before they spread further. This is particularly true for Neglected Zoonotic Diseases (NZDs), since they may remain undetected until they have become widespread at decisive levels among human communities. Management programs must target ecological and evolutionary factors that influence the success of these pathogens, as outlined in Adamo et al. (2015), highlighting the necessity of early and accurate diagnosis. Beyond its immediate clinical utility, early diagnosis is important for informing broader health programs and research. It allows health authorities to gain critical epidemiological intelligence, which can assist in shaping public health policy and resource allocation. Hence, investment in robust diagnostic capacity serves not only individual patient care but also the overall health infrastructure. Besides, information about the diagnostic difficulty challenges, particularly in certain species such as cats, illustrates the importance of developing comprehensive biomarker methods, as shown by Rodríguez et al. (2019). This can significantly improve early detection rates and, in turn, the quality of life for individuals and communities targeted, underscoring the key role of early diagnosis practices in combating infectious diseases in humans (Figure 10.15).

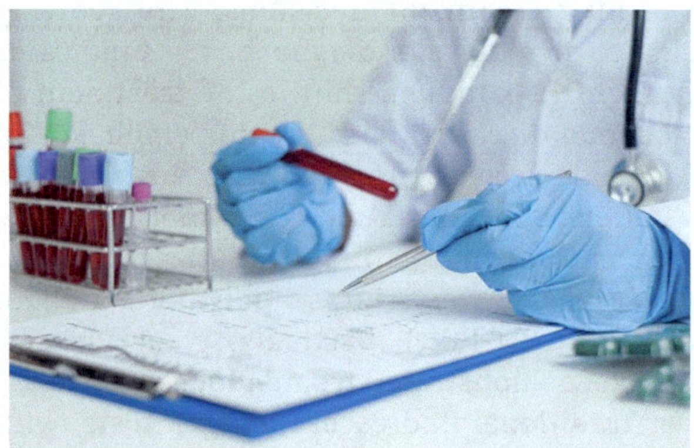

Figure 10.15. Importance of early diagnosis in infectious diseases.

Source: https://www.news-medical.net/images/Article_Images/ImageForArticle_22742_16565105034628224.jpg.

Test Your Knowledge

1. What are the common symptoms of infectious diseases?
2. What is the importance of early diagnosis in infectious diseases?

10.4. Treatment Options

Learning Outcome

1. Describe the antibiotics for bacterial infections
2. Learn about antivirals for viral infections
3. Describe the antifungals for fungal infections

The spread and causation of infectious diseases call for a comprehensive approach to treatment strategies, particularly given the growing concern about antimicrobial resistance (AMR). Treatment strategies must adapt not only to the infections themselves but also to the political and socio-economic determinants of health care systems. Effective policy-making to counter AMR is crucial but far from uniform across the globe. A comprehensive review of infection prevention, surveillance, and judicious use underscores the need to address these issues. Cost-effectiveness analysis in great detail is necessary, especially in middle-income and low-income countries, where resources are limited. Sensitive policy development with sectoral needs integrated, as promoted by the One Health approach, will be important in crafting treatments that are sustainable and equitable. This approach is going to enhance overall public health outcomes by promoting interdisciplinarity among human health, animal health, and environmental health (Aarestrup et al., 2015). When thinking about treatment plans for zoonotic diseases, particularly in low- and middle-income nations, it is significant to note the importance of multidimensional studies to fill current knowledge gaps. The systematic approach developed by initiatives such as the Roadmap to Combat Zoonoses in India (RCZI) is a better model for identifying and ranking research options needed to control zoonoses. A panel of mixed experts formally sorts out the options to produce a strong tool for health policy-makers. Treatment strategies with social, political, and economic implications are found to be an influential factor compared with merely biological interventions. The emphasis on action-oriented research both stimulates intersectoral collaborative action and attends to the multidimensionality of zoonosis problems. This highlights the need for interventions that account for the multidimensionality of human and animal health in treatment (Kakkar et al., 2011). Finally, alternative treatments must consider the contribution of public awareness and education to infectious disease control. As the populations continue to understand the importance of infectious diseases in their lives, the demand for specialized treatment procedures will increase. Awareness campaigns can empower populations to adopt preventive strategies against the disease, thus reducing infection rates and enhancing the effectiveness of existing treatments. Public health campaigns can prove to be the solution to eradicating false perceptions about treatments, particularly vaccination and the use of antibiotics. Involvement of the public in the development of treatment guidelines can ensure that health interventions are acceptable to society and are culturally relevant. While the scientific fraternity is striving towards the development of better treatments, the attainment of the best results will rely to a greater extent upon public participation and cooperation, once again highlighting the need for an integrated approach in the combat against infectious diseases (Kakkar et al., 2011; Aarestrup et al., 2015).

10.4.1. Antibiotics for Bacterial Infections

The invention of antibiotics has revolutionized the treatment of bacterial diseases, reducing mortality and public health burdens significantly. Initially discovered in the early 20th century, antibiotics such as penicillin were the pillars upon which the war against bacterial infections was waged, which had previously been thought to be lethal. Their effectiveness stems from their ability to inhibit bacterial growth or kill bacteria. However, overuse and abuse of antibiotics have driven the evolution of antibiotic-resistant bacteria, which pose a severe threat to modern medicine. Bacteria evolve as they mutate and develop resistance to antibiotics, making some old-fashioned remedies useless. This growing problem demands an overriding policy on the use, stewardship, and research on antibiotics to maintain infectious diseases at bay and prevent a return to the pre-antibiotic era morbidity and mortality. To address the growing issue of antibiotic resistance, scientists have already begun investigating alternative therapies, including bacteriophage therapy. Bacteriophages, or "phages," are viruses that infect and destroy bacteria and are a promising tool for combating resistant strains. In growing skepticism toward the use of conventional antibiotics, phages as medicines have been brought to the center stage. It has emerged that phages can be engineered to target specific bacterial pathogens, providing a specific therapy that is not available in antibiotics. However, the journey toward building phage therapies is long with many obstacles, particularly in patent protection and regulatory approval. Later developments in patent law jurisprudence have challenged the propriety of phage treatments being qualified for robust patent protections necessary to spur investment in their research and development. Grasping such legalities is crucial to unlocking the potential of phage therapies for their delivery in clinical uses. In order to strengthen the antibacterial treatments of the future, something more than one-dimensional must occur, that is, something more than just innovative research coupled with complementary policy structures. New therapies, such as phage therapy, may revolutionize how bacterial infections are treated, particularly given the crisis in antibiotic resistance. But in addition to advancing new treatments, a sincere effort must be made to provide incentives for pharmaceutical companies to invest in such alternatives. This might entail measures such as trade secrecy, regulatory exclusivities, and payment-for-value schemes, which would minimize the cost risks associated with developing new treatments. Furthermore, public awareness about judicious use of antibiotics remains key to avoiding resistance. Ultimately, collaboration among researchers, doctors, and policymakers will be required to achieve a sustainable solution to combat infectious diseases in humans and to ensure that effective treatments remain available to future generations (Figure 10.16).

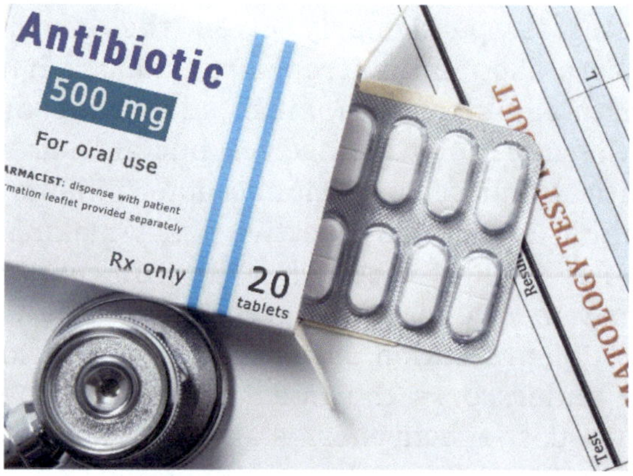

Figure 10.16. Antibiotics for bacterial infections.

Source: https://www.center4research.org/wp-content/uploads/2016/06/shutterstock_504085291-scaled.jpg.

10.4.2. Antivirals for Viral Infections

The quest for effective antivirals has significantly impacted the management of viral diseases, which have a high health burden worldwide. Antivirals work by inhibiting viral replication, interfering with specific stages of the viral life cycle, and thereby reducing the severity and duration of diseases caused by various pathogens. Interestingly, the influenza virus best showcases the importance of developing antiviral strategies. New developments in influenza vaccine technology demonstrate how advances in science, such as recombinant and reverse genetics, have enabled the creation of vaccines that elicit robust immune responses to pandemic strains. Based on the conclusions of the patent landscape analysis, new formulations and production processes for influenza vaccines have increasingly been reported, highlighting a proactive approach to pandemic preparedness and underscoring the critical role that new vaccine technology plays in the battle against infectious disease (Barton et al., 2012). Apart from vaccines, defective interfering (DI) genomes also possess a prospective key to antiviral research. With the aid of faulty viral genomes, scientists are formulating antiviral medications that simultaneously inhibit replication and stimulate the innate immune response. The novel mechanisms employed by DI genomes constitute a multifaceted antiviral treatment that can impart extended protection against an array of viral strains, as shown in preclinical models of influenza A.

This new strategy not only targets the specific virus from which the DI genome is derived but also benefits the host by providing immunity against other respiratory viruses (Dimmock et al., 2015). Such methods emphasize the hope of translating fundamental virology research into the clinic and, eventually, into the creation of the tools needed for the effective control of infectious diseases. The future of antiviral therapy shall likely be marked by the synergy between novel antiviral agents and multimodal therapeutic regimens that employ both medication and vaccine technology. Through the combined strategy, the human immune response can be augmented while viral reproduction is controlled.

As testified by growing patent filings for antiviral breakthroughs, the scientific community is increasingly acknowledging the importance of combating well in the face of evolving viral challenges. Medical professionals and policymakers must remain vigilant in funding virology research and development so society can cope with emerging viral threats. Collaborative efforts among research centers, drug companies, and public health organizations will prove to be the determining factor in extending the boundaries of antiviral medications and reducing the impact of infectious diseases on global health (Figure 10.17).

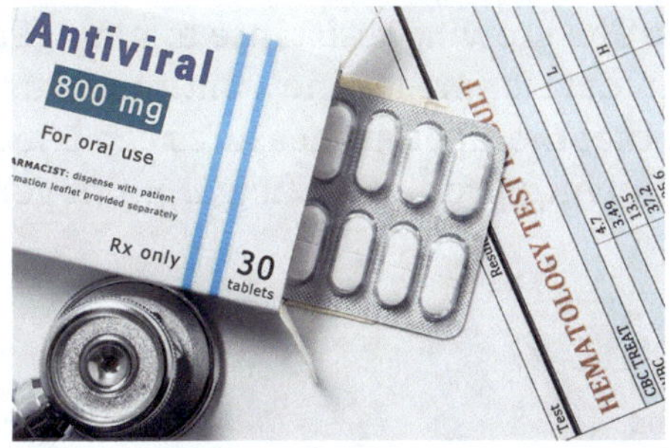

Figure 10.17. Antivirals for viral infections.

Source: https://www.eehealth.org/-/media/images/modules/blog/posts/2021/06/hd-life-covid-antiviral-medication.jpg.

10.4.3. Antifungals for Fungal Infections

Antifungal therapy has emerged as important in combating numerous fungal infections that have become increasingly prevalent, particularly among immunocompromised hosts. Due to the rising incidence of diseases such as cancer and chronic conditions, as well as the greater use of biomedical devices, the interfaces between the host and fungi have become more complex. Opportunistic fungal infections may cause severe complications in health, ranging from mild to lethal. Therefore, it is essential to understand how antifungals work to develop effective treatments. Antifungals such as azoles, echinocandins, and polyenes target various aspects of fungal physiology, yet drug resistance necessitates ongoing research into new antifungal agents and treatment strategies. Antifungal resistance is a new challenge in the antifungal therapy of fungal infections, usually resulting from selective pressure exerted by antifungal therapy itself. Studies have indicated that certain soil-dwelling fungi have developed resistance to common antifungal therapies such as Fluconazole and Nystatin, complicating treatment and highlighting the need for alternative treatment modalities (Kamat et al., 2010). Multidrug-resistant fungal isolates can lead to treatment failures, which are clinically serious. The growing resistance to fungi requires constant development of new antifungal drugs to ensure that therapeutic measures can effectively treat evolving profiles of fungal pathogens.

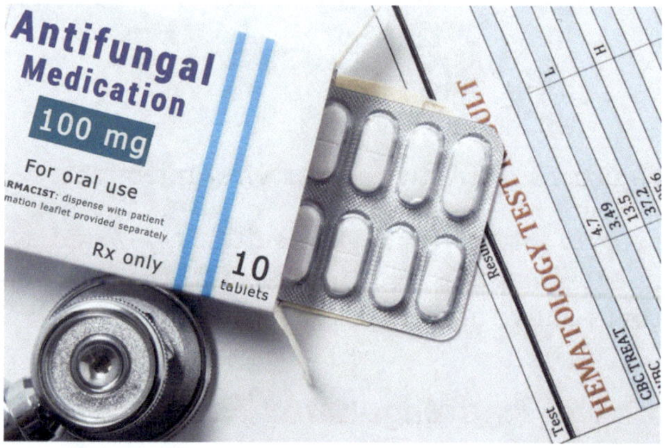

Figure 10.18. Antifungals for fungal infections.

Source: https://images.theconversation.com/files/238436/original/file-20180928-48647-12ud27s.jpg?ixlib=rb-4.1.0&q=45&auto=format&w=926&fit=clip.

In addition, identifying the genetic factors responsible for antifungal resistance can inform measures to prevent such tolerance in the clinic. To combat the menace of antifungal resistance, researchers are seeking dual-purpose drugs that, in addition to curing fungal pathogens, also target the host immune response. Novel drugs like Myriocin, Fulvic Acid, and Acetylcholine have been tested for antifungal activity in addition to showing anti-inflammatory activity, promising a two-way treatment approach (Borghi et al., 2015). By addressing both the fungal disease and the coincident chronic inflammatory responses, such candidates are likely to offer greater advantages over traditional antifungal treatments. The interest in research in this type of dual-functioning compounds underscores the need to unravel the complex interfaces between fungi, host immunity, and therapeutic interventions. While scientific researchers continue to search for innovative antifungal solutions, hope prevails in managing and treating the growing impact of fungal infections in vulnerable populations (Figure 10.18).

Test Your Knowledge

1. Which antibiotic is best for bacterial infection?
2. Which antifungal is best for fungal infection?

10.5. Prevention Strategies

Learning Outcome

1. Describe the vaccination programs
2. Know the hygiene and sanitation practices
3. Understand the public health initiatives

An effective step in avoiding the risk of contagious diseases relies heavily on overall prevention measures, including individual behavior and public health policy. An essential factor in the measures is enhancing public health education to raise awareness about the transmission and risk of various pathogens. Such education should emphasize practices such as vaccination, hygiene, and cleanliness, which are essential for preventing outbreaks. In addition, social mobilization plays a significant role in countering the cultural and behavioral complexities that shape health practices in communities. Through the implementation of behavior-change interventions, it becomes feasible to foster a positive disease-prevention attitude, resulting in an overall healthier population and lower rates of infectious diseases (Djoko et al., 2010). Yet another critical component of prevention measures is managing zoonotic diseases, which are transmitted from animals to humans. New infectious agents emerge constantly at the boundary between animal and human populations, so one needs surveillance programs that monitor their interactions. Effective preventive measures must therefore include monitoring animal health, regulating wildlife trade, and vaccinating domestic animals. Public policy must be developed in accordance with these management practices to help predict and prevent probable outbreaks.

Coordination between the veterinary and human health sectors is necessary in this aspect. Sharing efforts across professions, communities can enhance preparedness for and response to infectious disease threats, resulting in healthier, more resilient health systems that can better address future challenges (Djoko et al., 2010). Prion diseases, though less common than numerous other infectious diseases, present especially difficult prevention regimes due to their atypical modes of transmission and infection, and to the lack of treatment options. Transmission pathways of prion infection can offer insight into potential avenues for prevention. Enhanced surveillance of meat products for BSE and other prion diseases, for example, is essential for public health. Prompt regulation and monitoring of food stocks can also prevent human contact with contaminated materials. Moreover, further research into the molecular dynamics of prion diseases can inform subsequent intervention strategies, either by developing diagnostic techniques or by developing preventive interventions that can presumably reduce risk factors associated with prion transmission. Investment in prion research is therefore necessary, not just to control prion diseases but to enhance strategies generally against neurodegenerative disorders with infectious causes (Figure 10.19).

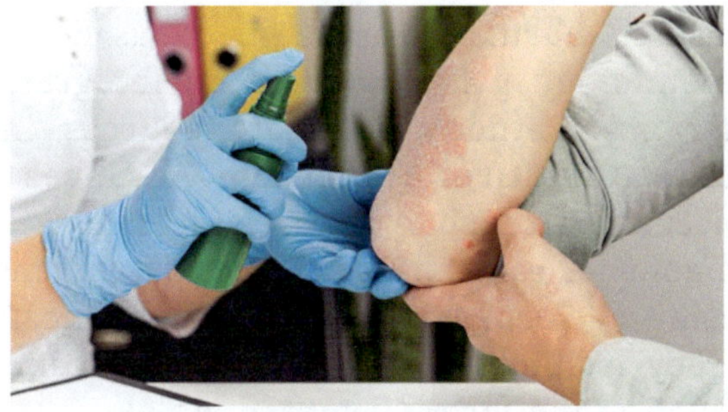

Figure 10.19. Fungal infection prevention.

Source: https://images.onlymyhealth.com/imported/images/2024/October/09_Oct_2024/mn-fungal.jpg.

10.5.1. Vaccination Programs

Vaccination campaigns are a backbone of the global struggle against infectious diseases and have made enormous contributions to public health outcomes. Vaccination campaigns aim to produce immunity against a range of pathogens, thereby reducing the rates of diseases that have traditionally resulted in high morbidity and mortality. The success of vaccination campaigns can be more clearly observed in controlled settings, such as the successful campaign against rabies in Bali. In this, extensive dog vaccination campaigns with high coverage were identified as the key to preventing the spread of rabies, emphasizing the impact of herd immunity on the elimination of zoonoses. This effectiveness demonstrates how strategic vaccination can lead to significant health gains among animals and human populations by reducing zoonotic transmission and preventing outbreaks (Putra et al., 2013). Roll-out of immunization schemes is not without challenges, as logistics, finance, and social acceptance can hinder success. Having adequate coverage is essential; even small exclusions can jeopardize overall vaccination campaigns, as the rabies outbreak in Bali shows, where failing to vaccinate all areas left continued contagion to spread. The need for coordination across regions highlights the importance of planning and coordination in public health measures. Furthermore, as infectious disease epidemiology gains momentum, integrating emerging methods and data sources into vaccine initiatives is needed. Advances in molecular epidemiology and health information technologies can enhance disease surveillance, vaccine performance, and population health, thereby facilitating more effective and timely vaccination efforts (Lewnard et al., 2019). Besides, the universality of vaccine programs challenges their equitable access and provision, and therefore, reacting to health inequalities is vital. Poor and marginalized groups lack access to healthcare, resulting in under-vaccination and vulnerability to outbreaks of infectious diseases. Public health responses should therefore provide equal access to vaccines so that all populations, regardless of socioeconomic factors, can benefit from these preventive measures. Evaluating and adapting immunization programs to meet the distinctive needs of different populations strengthens public health systems. Inclusion not only enhances individual immunity but also ultimately reinforces community immunity, thereby facilitating the broader goal of global infectious disease control while fostering public health trust (Putra et al., 2013) (Figure 10.20).

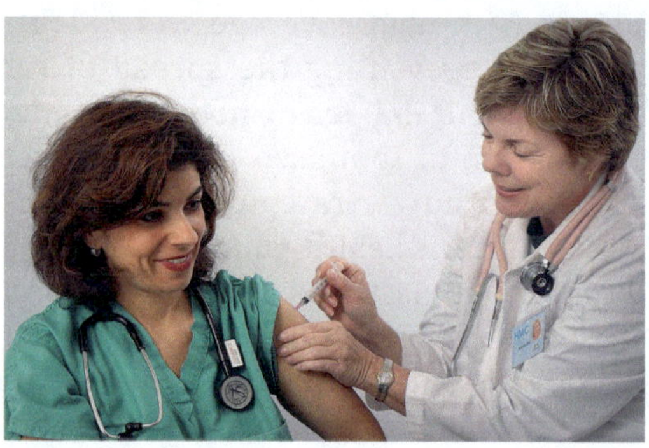

Figure 10.20. Health worker being vaccinated.

Source: https://miro.medium.com/v2/resize:fit:4800/format:webp/0*oeA7BYzHbGk5Welw.jpg.

10.5.2. Hygiene and Sanitation Practices

Good hygiene and sanitation practices are at the heart of interventions to prevent infectious disease transmission, particularly where animal husbandry intersects with human life. It is critical that high levels of hygiene be maintained by populations in contact with livestock, as zoonotic diseases pose enormous health threats. Studies conducted in Laos highlighted the seroprevalence of Trichinella spiralis and hepatitis E virus among human populations, with findings indicating a direct relationship between hygiene and disease exposure. The study found that was associated with the highest risk of contracting pathogens, a reason for the inclusion of effective hygiene practices within livestock management. Enforcing improved sanitation practices within communities can significantly reduce the incidence of zoonoses, safeguarding public health and, as such, calling for interventions targeting specific hygiene practices among pig-farming groups (Ito et al., 2016). Moreover, the multifaceted nature of hygiene practices calls for comprehensive knowledge of microbial interactions in various ecosystems. Effective infection prevention and control needs an integrated approach that recognizes the interplay of animal, human, and environmental health. This is reaffirmed in antimicrobial resistance literature, where appropriate use and stewardship are central to messages across all healthcare sectors. Through advocating for policies supporting rigorous cleaning regimes and prudent uses of antibiotics, it is possible to achieve synergy between veterinary and human healthcare practices. Enhanced surveillance will alert practitioners to new infectious diseases triggered by poor hygiene or unacceptable animal care practices, thereby enabling active public health interventions. Such intersectoral collaboration is crucial for developing effective sanitation and hygiene plans to avert infectious disease risks (Aarestrup et al., 2015). Lastly, the adaptation process towards improved hygiene practices cannot be overstated, particularly in low-income or resource-constrained settings. These barriers, such as inadequate access to clean water, poorly designed waste disposal systems, and inadequate public sensitization, play a major role in limiting the success of effective sanitation programs. Policymakers must prioritize addressing this by critically evaluating existing hygiene policy, identifying weaknesses, and outlining areas for improvement. Frameworks for evaluating the cost-effectiveness and overallizability of sanitation programs can be employed as models for targeted interventions driven by individual community needs. In One Health, addressing such obstacles through sustainable approaches and education will enable communities to improve their hygiene practices, thereby reducing the prevalence of infectious diseases. Incorporating cultural aspects into planning programs will further enhance the likelihood of success in promoting hygienic environments and public health (Aarestrup et al., 2015) (Figure 10.21).

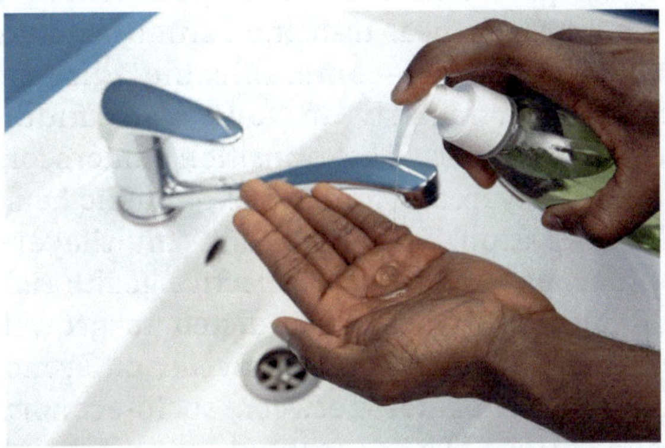

Figure 10.21. The importance of hygiene & sanitation.

Source: https://humanitarianglobal.com/wp-content/uploads/2022/02/A-person-washing-their-hands.jpg.

10.5.3. Public Health Initiatives

Public health programs play an important role in minimizing the impact of infectious diseases on human populations. The programs are typically comprised of vaccination programs, disease surveillance systems, and measures for response to outbreaks aimed at controlling disease spread. Examples include the development and availability of vaccines against diseases such as measles, polio, and influenza, which have previously led to significant reductions in morbidity and mortality. One of the most important strategies is to embrace the One Health philosophy, which emphasizes the interconnectedness of human, animal, and environmental health. This is an increasingly important strategy given the increasing number of zoonotic diseases with their origins in animal reservoirs. In order to address these challenges efficiently, public health workers should be working with veterinary specialists and environmental scientists, with a comprehensive approach to new infectious diseases threatening global health security and ecosystem integrity (Buttigieg et al., 2015). Further, the complexity of contemporary infectious diseases warrants public health action coordinated at local, regional, and international levels. In recent history, such outbreaks of illnesses such as Ebola and Zika have highlighted the necessity of having strong health systems that transcend disciplinary lines. Such efforts, such as the establishment of multidisciplinary teams comprising public health officials, veterinarians, and ecologists, bring together different parties for collaboration, enhancing response readiness for such outbreaks. The recognition of the interdependence among human, animal, and environmental health allows an integrated response, orchestrating resources and expert capabilities to manage disease spread effectively. Public health policy must find it fit to establish systems to facilitate communication and cooperation between sectors so that the international response to infectious disease can be built on (Alagaili et al., 2016). In summary, strategic deployment of public health interventions is key to addressing infectious disease threats. The integration of approaches like One Health not only enhances interdisciplinary collaboration but also maximizes the collective impact of disease prevention and control measures. By understanding the intricate relationships among humans, animals, and the environment, public health workers can uncover innovative solutions that are hazard-free and provide effective protection against future epidemics. As the globe struggles with emerging infectious diseases, commitment to cooperative public health systems will be most critical to safeguard human well-being and the world's ecosystems. Finally, building trust and communication among stakeholders will ensure that public health programs can adapt dynamically to the evolving contexts of infectious diseases (Buttigieg et al., 2015).

Test Your Knowledge

1. What is the role of vaccination in infection control?
2. Describe the hygiene and sanitation practices.

10.6. Impact on Society

Learning Outcome

1. Describe the economic implications of infectious diseases
2. Know the social consequences of infectious diseases
3. Describe the global health challenges related to infectious diseases

The social impact of infectious diseases extends far beyond individual health concerns, transforming social organization, economic security, and public health policy. Historical evidence shows that pandemics can steer the course of society, as the COVID-19 pandemic revealed intricate patterns of collective cooperation among individuals. Controlling infectious diseases typically involves utilizing concerted efforts, with compliance with health guidelines becoming essential. This dynamic highlights the tragedy of the commons; as infection rates decline, social compliance can deteriorate, which in turn creates peaks of transmission. These patterns of action must be clarified to create interventions that sustain cooperation and prevent outbreaks. The impact can be seen in advanced public health policies that incorporate evolutionary dynamics, illustrating how optimal responses can reduce the risks posed by infectious diseases to collective well-being (Glaubitz et al., 2024). Societal problems are also supplemented by the epidemiological transition from infectious diseases to non-communicable diseases (NCDs), particularly in low- and middle-income countries. The transition underscores the multi-layered complexities of public health administration, which require multilayered approaches to address prospective health risks. NCD burden, which is predicted to grow by 17% over the next decade, reveals differences in health outcomes between socio-economic inequalities. The targeted interventions encompass regulatory policies, such as food labeling, and incentives encouraging healthier lifestyle choices, indicating a transition towards preventive care. The interconnectedness of health problems calls for a global response, as the impact of globalization complicates localized solutions. The UN General Assembly's call to reduce premature NCD-related deaths by 25% by 2025 is a reflection of the urgency required of a global response to address such issues (Gostin et al., 2013). Finally, the social burden of infectious diseases necessitates an adaptive response with both individual and collective responsibility. Public health interventions are required to involve communities in assuming their responsibilities to halt transmission and foster health, while fostering an environment that sustains commitment. Reputation systems and collaborative incentives play a pivotal role in spurring public compliance with health regulations, reframing compliance as a requirement rather than a purely obligatory commitment, one shared by society. Additionally, as integrity is integrated into community health, understanding how to hold the delicate balance between facilitating cooperation and confining defectors is essential. The capacity to traverse this ground successfully conditions not only the success of current public health efforts but also society's resilience in the face of forthcoming infectious disease attacks. As challenges evolve, it will be essential to build a culture of shared responsibility and collaboration to safeguard community well-being and enhance societal resilience (Glaubitz et al., 2024).

10.6.1. Economic Implications

The economic impact of infectious diseases extends far beyond the direct cost of medical care, permeating every sector in society. For instance, an epidemic can cause significant disruption to the labor market because infected individuals remain absent from work, leading to reduced productivity and output. The entire economy suffers as businesses face low demand due to fear of infection, leading to lower revenues and potential layoffs. (Barnett et al., 2012) advocates the incorporation of a range of factors—economic drivers included—into knowledge of zoonotic infections. Policymakers might lose vital support systems for successful economic recovery during and following an outbreak by failing to appreciate economic factors. In addition, infectious disease has high indirect costs, particularly through long-term impacts on health and public health infrastructure. If there is an epidemic, it usually forces governments to divert resources to immediate containment at the expense of other valuable services, such as education and public health. The diversion can compromise the ability to respond to future public health challenges, creating vulnerability in populations. The epidemiology modeling of social and economic determinants comes in to explain how health crises can help strengthen existing inequalities between communities. (Anderson et al., 2015) highlights emergent properties such as community resilience and hope as fundamental components that could reverse such cascading economic impacts.

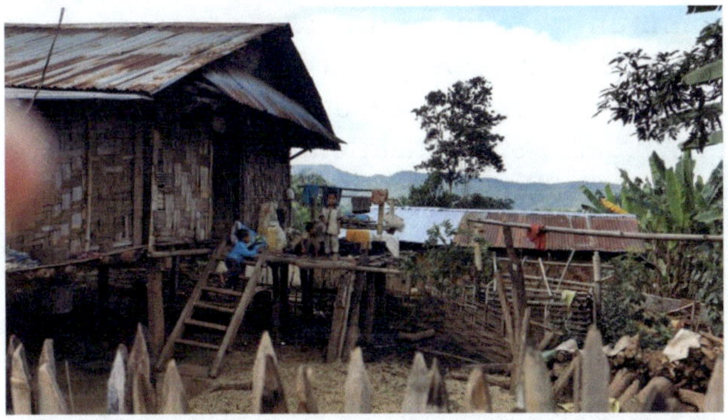

Figure 10.22. Economic impacts of infectious diseases of poverty.

Source: https://media.springernature.com/lw725/springer-cms/rest/v1/content/17667912/data/v2.

Moreover, the ongoing interplay between human behavior and economic drivers can significantly shape the trajectory of infectious disease epidemics. Compliance by the public with public health interventions, such as vaccination and distancing, may rely on economic incentives and perceived gains from investing in preventive assets. Understanding how individuals assess threat in everyday economic conduct, especially during outbreaks, is central to effective intervention strategies. Public education campaigns that emphasize the economic benefits of disease avoidance can improve compliance among populations.

A unified response leveraging knowledge from behavioral economics, biological, and environmental constraints could enhance overall public health responses. Such a unified perspective aligns with the call for a holistic framework encompassing all factors influencing zoonotic infection patterns, as mentioned by Barnett et al. (2012) (Figure 10.22).

10.6.2. Social Consequences

The social influence of infectious diseases extends beyond immediate health consequences, affecting cultural attitudes, societal behavior, and interpersonal relationships within the community. When illnesses spread, fear deepens, forcing people to alter their lifestyles and interactions. Increased anxiety comes with unavoidable stigmatization, where groups are labeled as disease carriers, further expanding the social cleavages. The complexity of this phenomenon is achieved in its realization in spatiality, which opens up the ways in which fear manifests itself in various spaces in society. People may begin associating certain places or groups with greater dangers and thereby socially exclude them. This sets the loop of violence where fear of infection leads to isolation and discrimination, impacting people psychologically and socially. Epidemic space captures social desires to seek protection but simultaneously promotes fragmentation and hostility between groups, mirroring the dualism of disease and social structure (Anderson et al., 2005). Secondly, infectious disease responses are apt to reveal underlying social inequalities, particularly among vulnerable populations. For instance, research on swine flu in Malaysia pointed out that some groups, such as pig farmers, had strong fears about infection risk, which was partly driven by identification with the supposed cause of the epidemic. Those who expressed heightened fear of infection were more likely to narrate the danger of infection within specific societal out-groups, such as homeless people and other stigmatized groups. Though direct discrimination was reported by only a minority, social impacts were present, as nearly half of the interviewees stated that peers had ostracized them due to the epidemic. This case illustrates how contagious diseases can both amplify underlying societal anxieties and perpetuate harmful stereotypes, thereby reinforcing the importance of cultural representation in shaping public responses to health crises (Dhanoa et al., 2011). Besides, the ripple effects of infectious diseases foster social behavior changes that spread to most areas of communal life, including economic and psychological. For instance, the risk of contagion may lead to decreased economic activity, particularly in areas that are human-contact-dependent, e.g., the service sector. This economic downturn also worsens social relations, with job losses heightening fears of resource inadequacy and communal fragmentation. Concurrent with this, the psychological cost of living in a disease-infested environment can manifest in heightened cases of depression and anxiety within afflicted populations, disrupting family and interpersonal relations. As populations grapple with the synonymous double burden of health crises and their impacts, the social glue is destroyed, necessitating holistic interventions to rebuild hope and solidarity following the threat of infectious diseases. Finally, knowing these social impacts is critical for successful public health interventions that meet not only short-term health requirements but also long-term community stability (Anderson et al., 2005).

10.6.3. Global Health Challenges

In the global health context of our time, infectious diseases constitute a significant threat, driven by environmental and socio-economic determinants. Globalization of society facilitates easy spread of pathogens across borders, opening up increased possibilities of overwhelming healthcare systems in outbreaks. Migrant groups, typically displaced under the pressure of conflict, climate change, or economic crisis, pose particular infectious disease vulnerabilities. Their special circumstances create a complex interplay between existing health issues and heightened susceptibility to new infections. As highlighted by current evidence, forced migrant displacement is linked to a triple hazard of non-communicable, infectious, and mental morbidity that calls for a global response to their health care that addresses not only their physical disease but also the social determinants of their health, shaping their well-being and health care access (Jablonka et al., 2018). Increased numbers of outbreaks globally underscore the necessity for efficient health surveillance systems. Infectious diseases possess the ability to evolve and mutate extremely rapidly, leading to public health emergencies that not only pose threats to individual lives but also economic stability and national security. For instance, a recent review of infectious disease outbreaks in February-March 2023 has offered startling trends that can serve as an alarm for policymakers. It emphasizes the need for using integral surveillance systems that can track the timing and location of such outbreaks. That data is crucial to infectious disease epidemiology knowledge and to the creation of effective public health interventions. An inter-country, cooperative approach to monitoring and responding to such threats may facilitate timely action and the deployment of resources required to mitigate disease impacts on human and economic health (Gu et al., 2023). Addressing global infectious disease-related health issues requires multi-sectoral and multi-disciplinary collaborations. All these measures should also consider the vulnerability of the vulnerable populations, including migrants and refugees. Government policies should promote universal coverage of healthcare in accordance with the doctrine in the UN Sustainable Development Goals. It is critical to ensure basic health care, including prevention, treatment, and education, is attained. This becomes a top priority for reducing the overall disease burden and enhancing resilience among vulnerable communities. Such steps also enhance the host population's health security, thereby strengthening the system's ability to withstand the threats posed by infectious diseases in an increasingly globalized world. Such a progressive and compassionate response is not just a matter of health equity but also a global public health and security requirement (Jablonka et al., 2018) (Figure 10.23).

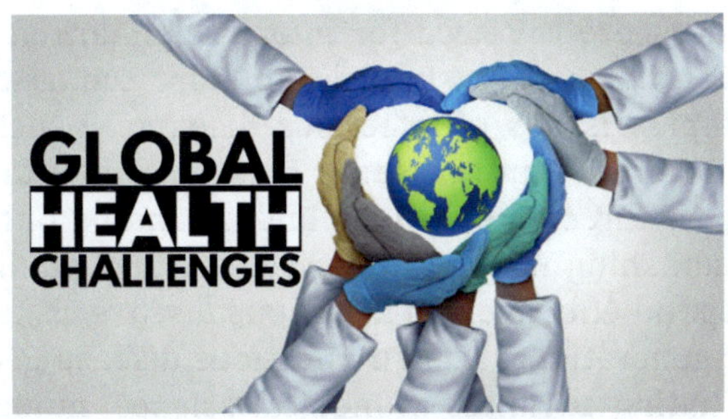

Figure 10.23. Global health challenges.

Source: https://i.ytimg.com/vi/fgcFKes2PMw/maxresdefault.jpg.

Test Your Knowledge

1. What are the economic implications of infectious diseases?
2. What are the social consequences of infectious disease?

SUMMARY

Briefly, the intricate relationship between human activities and the emergence of infectious diseases underscores the crucial need for a comprehensive, forward-looking approach in public health. As extensive research has indicated, the intensity of agricultural development and environmental alteration significantly increases the risk of zoonotic disease transmission from wildlife to human populations. This is particularly alarming in the wake of the expanding human population, which causes tremendous pressure on ecosystems and creates new pathways for pathogens to evolve. Emphasizing the complexity of this relationship can help policymakers and health institutions make decisions that can mitigate the threats posed by these continuously evolving infectious diseases, again reinforcing that public health must be considered in the context of environmental and agricultural dynamics (Artois et al., 2013). Moreover, the overview of this research highlights the dual challenge posed by infectious diseases to both conventional and organic farming practices. Organic farming methods are often hailed for their environmental benefits, but studies also suggest they can be responsible for causing or re-emerging zoonotic diseases, such as Campylobacter and Toxoplasma. This statement raises concerns regarding the safety and health implications of organic food compared to its conventional alternatives. While individuals increasingly turn to organic food due to perceived health benefits, an extensive study of the health issues associated with organic livestock production is necessary. This involves understanding the prevalence of zoonotic infections and evaluating farm management practices to ensure that organic does not inadvertently subvert public health (Eijck et al., 2003). Finally, insights from infectious diseases research in humans underscore the need for interdisciplinary studies that bridge agriculture, environmental science, and epidemiology. Interdisciplinary teams comprising these fields are required to address the complex issues of infectious diseases, which are biological, environmental, and socio-economic in nature. Future research must untangle the intricacies of such interfaces so that interventions can be directed by a deep understanding of how human behavior influences disease dynamics. By establishing integrated agriculture and public health policies, society can better prepare for and respond effectively to infectious disease risks, safeguarding both environmental and human health for generations. Human infectious disease geography is complex and influenced by several factors, including advances in medical science, human activities, and environmental changes. One aspect that is quite significant relates to the enduring burden of arthropod-borne diseases, which continue to be significant health problems despite extensive control initiatives. Researchers have pointed to the need for novel vector control paradigms, and, more specifically, vector behavior modification, as a key strategy for disease control. This has shed light on sub-lethal substances, such as spatial repellents, and on how they can open new avenues for research and implementation under global health initiatives. The problem lies in defining a clear role for such products, since public health communities are often challenged to translate frontier innovations into real practice, limiting the potential impact of advances in vector control (Achee et al., 2012).

Moreover, the relationship between the socio-cultural perceptions and biosecurity controls within infectious diseases highlights significant inconsistencies in risk management approaches. In the case of Chittagong's live bird trading network, key players carry a temporal risk lens with inclinations towards focusing on the present and past states more than foresight. The reduced emphasis on strict biosecurity management, coupled with limited recent outbreak experience, illustrates flawed reasoning in decision-making. With the application of Black Swan theory principles, the normalization of disease threats in such markets complicates prevention and control, as actors justify the past rather than being prepared for high-impact, unforeseen events. This highlights an intrinsic shortcoming in the overlap between sociocultural perspectives and public health readiness models (Appadurai et al., 2018). Finally, an understanding of the sociocultural forces surrounding infectious disease is essential to truly confronting global health challenges. Risk and biosecurity perceptions within society shape paradigms within which disease prevention and control interventions are created and deployed. This necessitates a multidisciplinary effort that transcends traditional epidemiologic paradigms, drawing on anthropological insights to grasp the lived experience of populations. By a socially understandable and pragmatically grounded emphasis, stakeholder engagement is the solution for guaranteeing effective interventions. Referring to everyday risk as normal may undermine biosecurity investments and thus underscore the significance of harmonized approaches that address both the scientific and socio-cultural aspects of disease control. Through encouraging collaboration between health professionals and communities, a more inclusive approach could result in more robust health systems with the ability to respond to emergent infectious diseases effectively.

KEY TERMS FROM THIS CHAPTER

- Antibiotic resistance
- Antifungal research
- Bacteria
- Ecosystems
- Fungi
- Infectious diseases
- Influenza
- Klebsiella pneumoniae
- Parasites
- Pneumonia
- Staphylococcus aureus
- Strep throat
- Tuberculosis
- Viruses

CRITICAL THINKING QUESTIONS

1. **Which of the following is the causative agent of tuberculosis?**
   a. Streptococcus pneumoniae
   b. Mycobacterium tuberculosis
   c. Escherichia coli
   d. Clostridium difficile
2. **What is the primary vector for transmitting dengue fever?**
   a. Anopheles mosquito
   b. Aedes aegypti mosquito
   c. Culex mosquito
   d. Sandfly
3. **Which of the following is NOT a viral infection?**
   a. Polio
   b. Hepatitis C
   c. Typhoid fever
   d. Rabies
4. **Which of the following is a fungal infection?**
   a. Giardiasis
   b. Candidiasis
   c. Hepatitis B
   d. Malaria

5. The BCG vaccine is used for the prevention of:
   a. Diphtheria
   b. Tuberculosis
   c. Measles
   d. Tetanus

Short Answer Questions

1. Define the infectious diseases.
2. Why is it important to study infectious diseases?
3. Name the 3 types of Infectious Diseases.
4. What is the transmission of infectious disease?
5. What is the treatment of infectious diseases?

Answer to Critical Thinking Questions

1. (b); 2. (b); 3. (c); 4. (b); 5. (b).

REFERENCES

1. Dar, O. A., Hasan, R., Schlundt, J., Harbarth, S., Caleo, G., Dar, F. K., Littmann, J., Rweyemamu, M., Buckley, E. J., Shahid, M., Kock, R., Li, H. L., Giha, H., Khan, M., So, A. D., Bindayna, K. M., Kessel, A., Pedersen, H. B., Permanand, G., . . . Heymann, D. L. (2015d). Exploring the evidence base for national and regional policy interventions to combat resistance. *The Lancet, 387*(10015), 285–295. https://doi.org/10.1016/s0140-6736(15)00520-6Abo-Shehada, M. N., Guitian, J., Hegazy, Y. M., Holt, H. R., et al. (2007). Systematic review of brucellosis in the Middle East: Disease frequency in ruminants and humans and risk factors for human infection. https://core.ac.uk/download/pdf/36779249.pdf (accessed on 14th July 2025).
2. Achee, N. L., Bangs, M. J., Farlow, R., Grieco, J. P., et al. (2012). Spatial repellents: From discovery and development to evidence-based validation. https://core.ac.uk/download/9657620.pdf (accessed on 14th July 2025).
3. Adamo, R., Akopyants, N. S., Anderson, J. M., Antia, R., Azevedo, S., Berry, A., Betson, M., et al. (2015). One Health–An ecological and evolutionary framework for tackling neglected zoonotic diseases. https://core.ac.uk/download/36778696.pdf (accessed on 14th July 2025).
4. Alagaili, A. N., Alagaili, A. N., Zumla, A., Arabi, Y., Arabi, Y., Azhar, E., Briese, T., et al. (2016). Taking forward a 'One Health' approach for turning the tide against the Middle East respiratory syndrome coronavirus and other zoonotic pathogens with epidemic potential. https://core.ac.uk/download/45467901.pdf (accessed on 14th July 2025).
5. Anderson, M., Beck, U., Beck, U., Bouter, L., Brewster, D. D., Cann, A. J., Cannon, G., et al. (2005). Epidemic space. https://core.ac.uk/download/30636149.pdf (accessed on 14th July 2025).
6. Anderson, R. M., Aunger, R., Banaji, M., Barnett, T., Denton, D., et al. (2015). Some considerations concerning the challenge of incorporating social variables into epidemiological models of infectious disease transmission. https://core.ac.uk/download/36778292.pdf (accessed on 14th July 2025).
7. Andeweg, A. C., Haagmans, B. L., & Osterhaus, A. D. M. E. (2009). The application of genomics to emerging zoonotic viral diseases. https://core.ac.uk/download/19197722.pdf (accessed on 14th July 2025).
8. Appadurai, A., Bouma, A., Lakoff, A., Martinot, A., Kleinman, A. M., Kousky, C., Lowe, C., et al. (2018). Competing biosecurity and risk rationalities in the Chittagong poultry commodity chain, Bangladesh. https://core.ac.uk/download/161515025.pdf (accessed on 14th July 2025).
9. Artois, M., Jones, B. A., Belotto, A., Boureau, E., Brown, C., Childs, J., Chomel, B., et al. (2013). Zoonosis emergence linked to agricultural intensification and environmental change. https://core.ac.uk/download/36776760.pdf (accessed on 14th July 2025).
10. Babcock, S., Beverley, J., Cowell, L. G., Smith, B., et al. (2021). The Infectious Disease Ontology in the age of COVID-19. https://core.ac.uk/download/305120399.pdf (accessed on 14th July 2025).
11. Barnett, J., Ceddia, G. M., Cook, N., Goodwin, R., et al. (2012). Interdisciplinary approaches to zoonotic disease. https://core.ac.uk/download/29139953.pdf (accessed on 14th July 2025).
12. Barton, J., Cavicchi, J. R., Janovetz, J., Kowalski, S. P., et al. (2012). Patent landscape of influenza A virus prophylactic vaccines and related technologies. https://core.ac.uk/download/72052387.pdf (accessed on 14th July 2025).

13. Bauchinger, U., Falagas, M. E., Kelesidis, I., Kelesidis, T., et al. (2008). Human infections associated with wild birds. https://core.ac.uk/download/323062291.pdf (accessed on 14th July 2025).

14. Borghi, E., Borgo, F., Morace, G., Nile, C. J., et al. (2015). New strategic insights into managing fungal biofilms. https://core.ac.uk/download/42365456.pdf (accessed on 14th July 2025).

15. Burke, R., Cavicchi, J. R., Kowalski, S. P., Michaud-King, P., et al. (2013). Patent landscape of helminth vaccines and related technologies. https://core.ac.uk/download/72052224.pdf (accessed on 14th July 2025).

16. Buttigieg, M. (2015). A review of the One Health concept: Increasing awareness and collaboration between the Maltese medical and veterinary professionals. https://core.ac.uk/download/46603760.pdf (accessed on 14th July 2025).

17. Catley, A., Catley, A., Roug, A., Chengula, A. A., Majule, A. E., Kilale, A. M., Kiwara, A., et al. (2017). Exploring local knowledge and perceptions on zoonoses among pastoralists in northern and eastern Tanzania. https://core.ac.uk/download/76981015.pdf (accessed on 14th July 2025).

18. De Craeye, S., Francart, A., Kalai, M., Lamoral, B., et al. (2014). A two-step lyssavirus real-time polymerase chain reaction using degenerate primers with superior sensitivity to the fluorescent antigen test. https://core.ac.uk/download/55799610.pdf (accessed on 14th July 2025).

19. Devos, I., & Janssens, A. (2017). Introduction. https://core.ac.uk/download/147045679.pdf (accessed on 14th July 2025).

20. Dhanoa, A., Goodwin, R., Haque, S., Hassan, H., et al. (2011). Representations of swine flu: Perspectives from a Malaysian pig farm. https://core.ac.uk/download/20257824.pdf (accessed on 14th July 2025).

21. Dimmock, N. J., & Easton, A. J. (2015). Cloned defective interfering influenza RNA and a possible pan-specific treatment of respiratory virus diseases. https://core.ac.uk/download/42608638.pdf (accessed on 14th July 2025).

22. Djoko, C. F., Fair, J. N., Lebreton, M., Pike, B. L., et al. (2010). The origin and prevention of pandemics. https://core.ac.uk/download/323077529.pdf (accessed on 14th July 2025).

23. Eijck, I., Groot, M., Kasteel, D., Kijlstra, A., et al. (2003). Analysis of black holes in our knowledge concerning animal health in the organic food production chain. https://core.ac.uk/download/10919416.pdf (accessed on 14th July 2025).

24. Fang, F., Le Calvez, H., & Yu, M. (2004). Biochemical prevention and treatment of viral infections – A new paradigm in medicine for infectious diseases. https://core.ac.uk/download/pdf/3550099.pdf (accessed on 14th July 2025).

25. Gkoutos, G. V., Hoehndorf, R., & Schofield, P. N. (2014). Analysis of the human disease reveals phenotype modules across common, genetic, and infectious diseases. https://core.ac.uk/download/185488701.pdf (accessed on 14th July 2025).

26. Glaubitz, A. (2024). *Exploring Group Behavior Through Evolutionary Game Theory: Disease Dynamics, Cooperation, And Reputation.* https://core.ac.uk/download/617915727.pdf (accessed on 14th July 2025).

27. Gostin, L. O., & Thomas, B. P. (2013). Tackling the global NCD crisis: Innovations in law and governance. https://core.ac.uk/download/70375002.pdf (accessed on 14th July 2025).

28. Gu, D., Liu, D., Li, G., Zou, J., He, M., Xiang, Q., Su, Q., et al. (2023). Global infectious diseases in March 2023: Monthly analysis. https://core.ac.uk/download/586281272.pdf (accessed on 14th July 2025).

29. Gutiérrez Rodríguez, A. (2019). Diagnosis of some diseases through biomarkers. https://core.ac.uk/download/288157992.pdf (accessed on 14th July 2025).

30. Herms, J., Kretzschmar, H. A., & Vassallo, N. (2004). The molecular pathology of prion diseases. https://core.ac.uk/download/46601891.pdf (accessed on 14th July 2025).

31. Ito, A., Steyer, A., van den Hurk, A. F., Willingham III, A. L., Phongmany, A., Donnelly, B., Khamlome, B., et al. (2016). Endemicity of zoonotic diseases in pigs and humans in lowland and upland Lao PDR: Identification of socio-cultural risk factors. https://core.ac.uk/download/45467782.pdf (accessed on 14th July 2025).

32. Jablonka, A., Kamarulzaman, A., Tagliabue, A., Trovato, A., Vernon, A., Afkhami, A. A., Gerritsen, A. A. M., et al. (2018). Migrant and refugee populations: A public health and policy perspective on a continuing global crisis. https://core.ac.uk/download/161508312.pdf (accessed on 14th July 2025).

33. Kakkar, M., Shah, N. K., Sekar, N., & Abbas, S. S. (2011). Research options for controlling zoonotic disease in India, 2010–2015. https://core.ac.uk/download/19765602.pdf (accessed on 14th July 2025).

34. Kamat, N. M., & Velho-Pereira, S. (2010). Exploring hidden dimensions of soil fungal biodiversity: A simple technique to detect soil fungi resistant to antifungal compounds. https://core.ac.uk/download/pdf/289013.pdf (accessed on 14th July 2025).

35. Lewnard, J. A., & Reingold, A. L. (2019). Emerging challenges and opportunities in infectious disease epidemiology. https://core.ac.uk/download/323082106.pdf (accessed on 14th July 2025).

36. Matee, M., Mshana, S. E., & Rweyemamu, M. (2013). Antimicrobial resistance in human and animal pathogens in Zambia, Democratic Republic of Congo, Mozambique and Tanzania: An urgent need of a sustainable surveillance system. https://core.ac.uk/download/pdf/18174800.pdf (accessed on 14th July 2025).

37. Putra, A. A. G., Putra, A. A. G., Putra, A. A. G., Putra, A. A. G., Dewi, A. P. M., Chomel, B., Fraser, C., et al. (2013). Designing programs for eliminating canine rabies from islands: Bali, Indonesia as a case study. https://core.ac.uk/download/16463495.pdf (accessed on 14th July 2025).

38. Remais, J. (2010). Modelling environmentally-mediated infectious diseases of humans: Transmission dynamics of schistosomiasis in China. https://core.ac.uk/download/323082019.pdf (accessed on 14th July 2025).

39. Stilianakis, N., & Weber, T. (2008). Risk mapping and mathematical modelling: Assessment tools for the impact of climate change on infectious diseases. https://core.ac.uk/download/38619506.pdf (accessed on 14th July 2025).

40. Todd, K. (2014). The promising viral threat to bacterial resistance: The uncertain patentability of phage therapeutics and the necessity of alternative incentives. https://core.ac.uk/download/213020895.pdf (accessed on 14th July 2025).

OCCUPATIONAL AND ENVIRONMENTAL MEDICINE

11

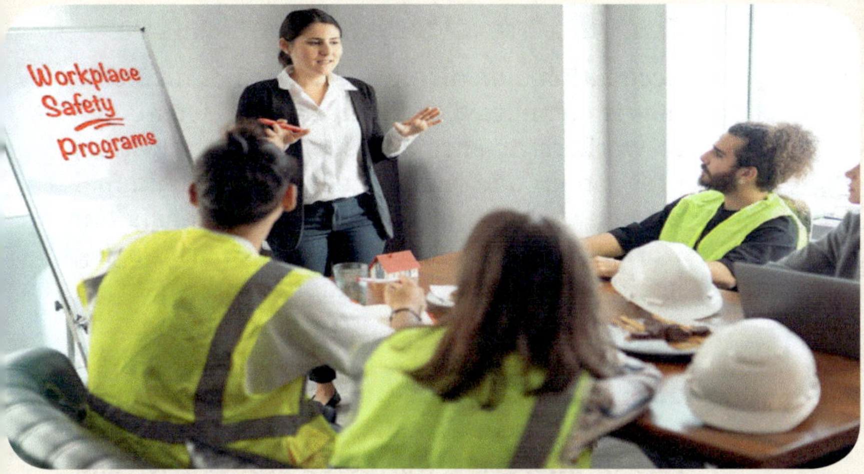

LEARNING OBJECTIVES

After studying this chapter, you will be able to:

1. Describe the common occupational hazards
2. Understand the environmental health risks
3. Describe the regulatory framework governing occupational and environmental medicine
4. Know the prevention and intervention strategies of occupational hazards
5. Understand the current trends and research in occupational and environmental medicine

Introduction

Occupational and Environmental Medicine (OEM) is a significant borderland between public health and healthcare, focusing on the interrelationship between work and environmental conditions and their impact on human health. The field becomes increasingly pertinent as industries evolve and technological advancements alter work environments. OEM addresses short- and long-term conditions of illness by workplace hazards ranging from physical injury to psychological stressors and toxic exposure to chemicals. This interdisciplinary science aims to improve safety and health standards, thereby enhancing the overall well-being of workers across various work sectors. By integrating occupational, social, and biological health factors, OEM enables clinicians and policymakers to develop whole-person approaches to improving workforce health, thereby significantly advancing public welfare. An intrinsic element of Occupational and Environmental Medicine is its use of frameworks such as the International Classification of Functioning, Disability and Health (ICF). The ICF system enables practitioners to understand the intricate relationships among health conditions and more general social and health determinants. It has a vision of health as an active dynamic interaction of biological, psychological, and environmental elements, with a totalistic perspective of patient wellness.

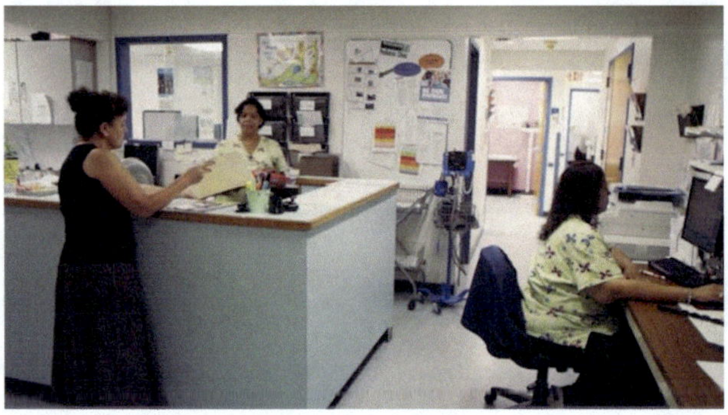

Figure 11.1. Occupational and environmental medicine.

Source: https://www.chartercare.org/globalassets/chartercare/rwmc-occupational.png?width=760&height=425&mode=crop&format=webp&quality=80.

While the ICF has been well accepted by occupational therapists and disability rights activists, its complexity poses a challenge for clinicians in applying it on a broader scale. Notably, the World Health Organization has developed the ICF Core Sets to facilitate ease of use and to enable clinicians to work effectively with the classification without neglecting the broader picture of health (McIntyre et al., 2007). Furthermore, OEMs extend their impact to health surveillance system design and application for monitoring employee health and minimizing the complexities of job-exposure-related risks. Efficacious health maintenance programs play a crucial role in early detection of abnormalities associated with work and in formulating preventive strategies for the industry. For example, a NASA's medical procedure review illustrated the importance of rigorous medical history and toxicological screening for employees in high-exposure environments. By prioritizing the collection and analysis of health data, organizations can establish a safety and health culture that not only protects workers but also improves productivity and overall organizational health. In total, Occupational and Environmental Medicine is key to transcending the challenges of modern work and environmental forces, ultimately leading to healthier workplaces and communities (Figure 11.1).

Definition of Occupational Medicine

Occupational medicine is a branch of medicine that is committed to the health and well-being of workers. It encompasses the investigation, prevention, and management of occupational disease and injury with an emphasis on workplace/health effects dynamics. Encouraging healthy and safe work habits and ensuring that job hazards are controlled are among the primary goals of this branch. By focusing on disease prevention caused by occupational exposure, occupational medicine plays a key role in improving workforce productivity and public health overall. As workplaces shift and the nature of work continues to shift, occupational medicine becomes increasingly vital to deal with through further investigation and adaptation to new health risks associated with various types of work environments. Epidemiology is central to occupational medicine through the application of a wide range of assessment devices and methods to detect and quantify workplace hazards. Job exposure matrices (JEMs) have become a major instrument for this purpose, enabling analysis of exposure to physical demands such as repetitive motion and static strength in tasks. These matrices help identify the relationships between exposures and conditions, such as carpal tunnel syndrome (CTS), thereby bridging the gap between occupational health risk factors and outcomes. While job-title-based exposures introduce a level of misclassification bias, they are helpful in large epidemiological studies where precise data may not be available. Thus, the use of JEMs maximizes occupational medicine's ability to reveal the dangers associated with specific jobs, enabling effective interventions and policy decisions (Dale et al., 2014). In addition, the contemporary approach in occupational medicine emphasizes a comprehensive view that goes beyond mere treatment of disease. This change emphasizes the importance of addressing the causes of conditions within the workplace. Factors such as job design, workload, and organizational climate are key to creating effective health interventions. By applying principles from public health, occupational medicine can broaden its interventions from treatment to proactive prevention of work-related health issues. Such organizations may be able to establish healthier workplaces, with resultant trickle-down advantages for employers and employees. With such a complicated relationship between occupational hazards and health conditions, occupational medicine itself must evolve, coming up with innovative solutions towards maintaining workforce wellness (Karanika-Murray et al., 2013) (Figure 11.2).

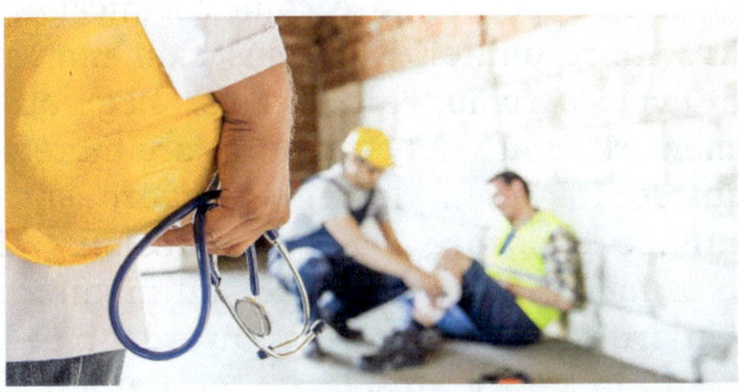

Figure 11.12. Occupational medicine.

Source: https://www.internationalstallions.org/wp-content/uploads/2022/12/Occupational-medicine-doctor.jpg.

Definition of Environmental Medicine

Environmental medicine entails an interdisciplinary investigation of the impact of environmental exposures on human health and well-being. Environmental medicine integrates principles of toxicology, epidemiology, and public health to investigate the relationships between environmental exposures—such as air and water contamination, toxic wastes, and chemical exposure—and associated health consequences. By studying such interactions, environmental medicine seeks to identify high-risk groups and suggest effective interventions, thereby addressing public health issues related to environmental causation. As the prevalence of environmentally induced diseases is on the increase, the role of the field is further emphasized in guiding policy and prevention efforts, highlighting its overarching function in safeguarding community health. The field of environmental medicine is not just broader than simply defining hazards but also encompasses the study of how to minimize exposure and enhance health. These professionals often work with government organizations, health care providers, and neighborhood organizations to develop evidence-based interventions that reduce the risks posed by environmental factors. For example, controlling airborne contaminants can significantly reduce the incidence of respiratory infections and chronic diseases among affected populations. Such comprehensive efforts demonstrate how environmental medicine serves as a bridge between scientific knowledge and public health policy, confirming the need for an integrated concept of health that integrates environmental and occupational determinants. In addition, environmental medicine significantly influences the agenda for future research by emphasizing key knowledge gaps in environmental exposures and their health effects. Using data collected through research on conditions such as traffic-related trauma, researchers can establish links between environmental exposures and public health outcomes. This connection is significant for planning targeted interventions and determines what is most important to prioritize in terms of areas for funding applicable research, as evidenced by the increased volume of studies on traffic medicine-related subjects, where the United States remains at the forefront in published literature (Groneberg-Kloft et al., 2013). The use of instruments such as the International Classification of Functioning, Disability, and Health (ICF) provides assurance that the focus is comprehensive, recognizing the complex interdependence between environmental circumstances and personal health experience (McIntyre et al., 2007). Overall, environmental medicine not only dictates the scope of research but also spearheads progress towards healthier populations and environments.

11.1. Common Occupational Hazards

Learning Outcome

1. Describe the physical hazards in the workplace
2. Know the chemical exposures and their effects
3. Describe the biological hazards and occupational diseases

The occupational hazards scene is multi-dimensional and heterogeneous, and reflects the heterogeneity of work conditions in which workers are engaged. Physical hazards such as noise, vibration, and temperature are some of the most prevalent hazards. They are very hazardous to workers' health, as they can lead to hearing impairment and heat-related diseases. In addition, ergonomic risks present in poorly designed workplaces or repetitive movement contribute to a significant extent of musculoskeletal disease. The physical risks highlight the necessity of workplace assessment to establish mechanisms to prevent injury and disease. Mitigation of these common risks is a critical aspect of occupational and environmental medicine, which seeks to minimize risks and promote workers' health by active intervention and policy-making. Exposure to chemicals is another important occupational risk that cuts across industries, from manufacturing to healthcare. Workers can be exposed to toxic substances, including solvents, heavy metals, and biological agents, that can cause acute or chronic health impacts.

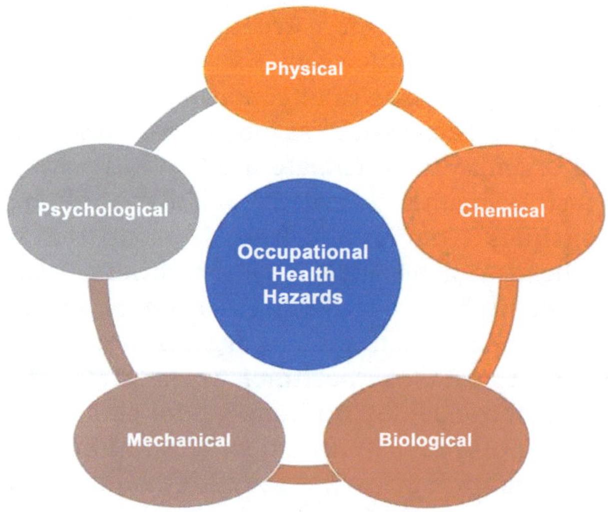

Figure 11.3. Occupational health hazards.

Source: https://www.occucare.co.in/blog/wp-content/uploads/2022/04/3t4w5tg.jpg.

Long-term exposure to certain chemicals has links with respiratory problems, skin ailments, and even carcinogenic effects. Regulatory frameworks and safety measures are therefore required to be implemented rigorously to minimize exposure risks. Emphasizing the role of increased surveillance and monitoring of environmental hazards towards disease prevention policy strategies, the Centers for Disease Control and Prevention (Balmes et al., 2006) points out. On this basis, occupational health professionals play a crucial role in educating workers on handling practices and personal protective equipment, thereby fostering a culture eager to uphold worker health and safety. Also underemphasized but present in the workplace are psychosocial hazards that have severe psychological and social effects, resulting in negative outcomes on mental well-being and even overall productivity. Job stress, harassment, and job insecurity contribute to such states as depression and anxiety. Identification and prevention of such risks entail an integrated approach that encompasses individual and organizational interventions. Occupational physicians are increasingly being called upon to evaluate the psychosocial workplace climate, identify areas of potential concern, and make recommendations for interventions (Demou et al., 2018). Counterbalancing the physical and mental health risks presented to employees enables organizations to create a healthier work climate. Such a focus on psychosocial issues is instrumental in developing a culture of health in organizations that allows employees to flourish both personally and professionally (Figure 11.3).

11.1.1. Physical Hazards in the Workplace

The importance of addressing physical workplace hazards cannot be overstated, as they pose a significant risk to employees' health and safety. Physical hazards include a host of factors such as noise, radiation, heat, and poor ergonomics that can give rise to both acute and long-term health problems. Exposure to high noise levels over a long period of time, for instance, can cause hearing loss or heightened stress levels among employees. Further, poor ergonomic workspace arrangements can lead to musculoskeletal disorders, underscoring the need for preventive measures. Employers must embrace comprehensive methods that prioritize safety training and risk monitoring to manage these hazards efficiently. The programs not only contribute to a healthier working environment but can also boost employee morale and productivity, underlining the interconnection between workplace performance and occupational health at its best. The intersection of physical hazard and work psychosocial climate makes the occupational safety and health scenario even more complex. Physical hazards, sometimes compounded by unsafe working conditions, may lower the overall welfare and job satisfaction of the workers. Thus, there is a need for an integrated strategy that incorporates physical and psychosocial factors to ensure effective risk management.

The literature demonstrates that workplace interventions that address both dimensions produce more substantial improvements in employees' health outcomes than single interventions that focus only on physical risks. Organisations can develop a healthier and safer working environment by addressing such interrelated factors, such as offering stress-reducing programs alongside ergonomic assessments. Psychosocial considerations must be integrated with safety precautions to minimize general workplace well-being and injury rates as part of an effective occupational health system (Pouliakas et al., 2010). Future policy and research would require physical hazard identification to be more closely aligned with general occupational health policies to sustainably improve worker protection. There is existing literature suggesting significant gaps in knowledge about how various physical agents interact in the workplace and about the combined effects of these agents on health outcomes. To resolve these problems, there is a requirement for interdisciplinary research that draws on psychology, economics, and environmental science. An enhanced understanding of the determinants and consequences of physical hazards will inform evidence-based interventions required in specific industries and work environments. Policy-makers can use such evidence to improve policies and develop conditions that not only minimize the occurrence of physical dangers but also promote general occupational safety and health systems. In the long term, improving such infrastructure can yield significant economic and social returns by enhancing the overall standard of living for workers across sectors (Pouliakas et al., 2010) (Figure 11.4).

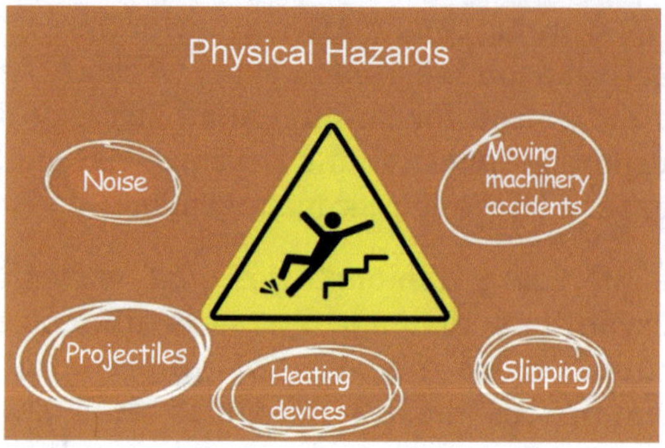

Figure 11.4. Physical hazards.

Source: https://media.licdn.com/dms/image/v2/D5612AQHSvLT_GjqTmg/article-cover_image-shrink_600_2000/article-cover_image-shrink_600_2000/0/1676970626485?e=2147483647&v=beta&t=oSEyWy7FFcwGiywjNT23fp451RUosUih-AbIa4IN4M4.

11.1.2. Chemical Exposures and Their Effects

The complex association between chemical exposures and their resulting health effects in humans is a significant area of investigation in occupational and environmental medicine. Various industries expose people to hazardous chemicals, including solvents, heavy metals, pesticides, and industrial chemicals. Research has proven that repeated exposure to such toxic chemicals may lead to a wide range of diseases, including respiratory diseases, neurological conditions, and even cancer. Surprisingly, studies conducted by organizations such as the Nelson Institute and the Department of Environmental Medicine at New York University emphasize understanding how chemical toxicology affects population health outcomes. With robust epidemiological research and effective training mechanisms, the institute has contributed importantly to identifying the precipitating causes of chemical exposure-related health risks, and to the importance of continuous observation in occupational security and environmental health assurance (Bosland et al., 2024). In explaining the health effects of chemical exposure, it is necessary to explore the physiological mechanisms that result in the adverse effect on health suffered by exposed populations. Occupational and environmental medicine integrates many scientific disciplines to understand how chemical agents disrupt biological systems, leading to diseases such as allostatic load—a chronic stress response. This state is researched in the literature with regard to chronic disease and premature death in working populations.

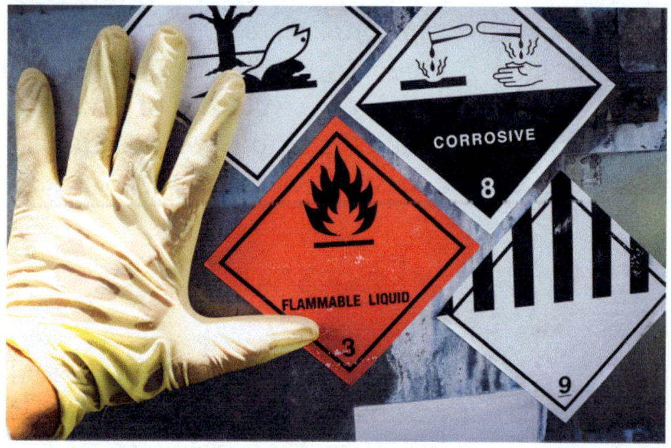

Figure 11.5. Hazardous chemical exposure in the workplace.

Source: https://www.hasnerlaw.com/wp-content/uploads/2024/01/Warning-symbol-for-chemical-hazard.jpg.

As noted by recent research, there are established biomarkers that indicate neuroendocrine and immune system dysregulation, which are indicators of health risks from chemical exposures. Understanding these pathways not only assists in diagnosing existing conditions but also informs preventive interventions to reduce exposure and mitigate long-term health impacts (Bezrukova et al., 2024). Additionally, methodological developments emphasize the role of preventive medicine in managing the health risks posed by chemical exposure. The development of personological diagnostics is an outstanding step toward early intervention for reversible physiological dysregulation. By highlighting the cumulative effects of single exposures to chemicals and interactions with lifestyle factors, clinicians are better placed to assess and manage vulnerabilities in vulnerable groups. While standardizing procedures to define and measure allostatic load remains challenging, the growing evidence of clinical utility points to a promising direction for maximizing workplace health surveillance. Thus, one needs to promote collaboration among policymakers, clinicians, and researchers to enable the development of effective intervention strategies, thereby improving the overall health status of exposed individuals (Bezrukova et al., 2024) (Figure 11.5).

11.1.3. Biological Hazards and Occupational Diseases

Biological hazards are severe in workplaces and lead to numerous diseases with severe health effects on workers. The hazards include pathogens such as bacteria, viruses, fungi, and parasites that can occur in various work environments, especially in industries such as healthcare, agriculture, and waste management. Workers who come into contact with biological material can contract diseases like tuberculosis, hepatitis, and even zoonoses from animals. Research has evidenced that cases of such diseases are frequent when there are lapses in safety procedures and inadequate training, putting the workforce at risk. A study of factory workers and artisans in Nigeria documented excessive cases of respiratory, skin, and musculoskeletal diseases linked to exposure to biological hazards and hazardous working conditions (Dahunsi et al., 2013). The consequences of biological hazards are not just short-term; they can also lead to long-term health issues that may manifest years after the initial exposure. For instance, workers exposed to respiratory pathogens may develop chronic bronchitis or lung infections, which are long-term healthcare costs and quality-of-life losses. Moreover, the psychological impact of such a disease of occupation, such as post-traumatic stress syndrome from severe work-related illness or injury, may introduce another dimension of complexity in managing worker health. Effective intervention methods should include meticulous health surveillance and the implementation of occupational health measures explicitly designed to address these biological hazards. This will facilitate early detection and control of occupational diseases, thereby mitigating their long-term effects on labor and on the general healthcare system (Lethbridge et al., 2008). Conquering biological risk challenges requires not only knowledge but also an effective regulatory system that will enable the application of health and safety measures in the workplace.

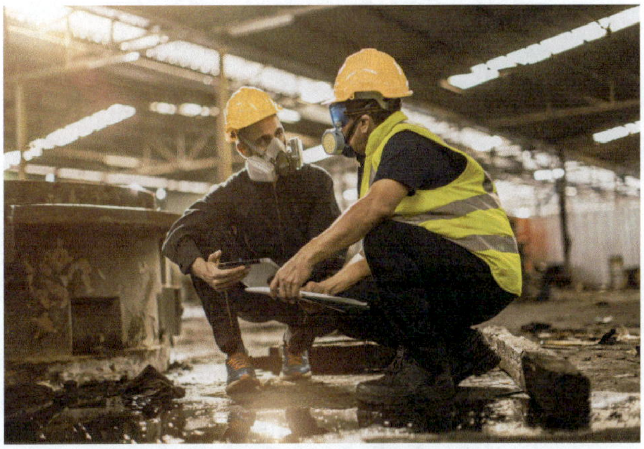

Figure 11.6. Biological hazards.

Source: https://www.certaintysoftware.com/wp-content/uploads/2023/11/Biohazards.webp.

Currently, ratified trade agreements may include occupational health and safety laws, but limitations on applying these serve to undermine their impacts. Weak enforcement measures and minimal political will deter organizations from making efforts towards protecting workers. To effectively combat the prevalence of biological hazards in the workplace, actors such as the government, employers, and workers' unions need to implement robust legislative measures and accountability mechanisms. Research evidence further emphasizes the need for regular training and education programs on personal protective means, thereby able the combat of the risks involved with biological hazards and reducing the incidence of occupational disease (Dahunsi et al., 2013; Lethbridge et al., 2008) (Figure 11.6).

Test Your Knowledge

1. What are the physical hazards in the workplace?
2. What are the effects of chemical exposure?

11.2. Environmental Health Risks

Learning Outcome

1. Describe the air pollution and respiratory diseases
2. Describe the water contamination and public health
3. Know the soil pollution and its impact on agriculture

Environmental health risks are closely related to occupational exposures that transcend industries, with high relevance in the mining sector. Heavy machine operators, especially those operating load-haul-dump machinery, face unique challenges that increase their susceptibility to whole-body vibrations (WBV) and allied musculoskeletal diseases. Emerging evidence highlights the value in assessing such hazards employing standard methods, such as ISO 2631-1:1997 and ISO 2631-5:2018. The latter identifies that, while helpful, conventional approaches to numerically quantifying health hazards could not fully capture the intricacies of prolonged exposure to vibration and shock. Because comparative assessment recognizes the varying risk factors for injury, there is a need to re-evaluate existing guidelines to preserve the health of mining laborers participating in routine work, with the ultimate aim of mitigating the health outcomes of cumulative exposure to such hazardous working conditions (Sharma et al., 2024). Apart from occupational hazards, environmental health risks are also caused by the poor handling of waste, such as fecal sludge. The growing population in urban areas has placed heavy pressure on sanitation facilities, thereby creating a public health issue driven by inefficient disposal. Existing research in Tanzania studies the manufacture of carbonized briquettes as a crucial resource recovery process, with a focus on reducing emissions from the incineration of fecal sludge. The study illuminates varying levels of emissions based on binder materials, pointing out that innovations in waste management not only advance public health but also enhance the quality of the environment. Through the integration of ecological components into waste treatment processes, populations are able to minimize exposure to harmful pollutants significantly, therefore advancing improved public health and reduced environmental degradation (Puig et al., 2024). Finally, occupational and environmental convergence forces consideration of integrative risk assessments that account for exposures at both the workplace and the community levels. From evidence comparing the risks of vibration among mining operators and emissions from sludge handling, an interdisciplinary effort becomes evident. Policy-making success requires balancing occupational and environmental safety to develop a uniform strategy that targets individual as well as aggregate health.

Efforts to promote safe practices, such as the proper use of binders in waste treatment, are excellent examples of how innovations can be incorporated into public health targets. Lastly, designing situations that prioritize workers' health while also addressing environmental problems will result in sustainable development and enhance community well-being (Puig et al., 2024; Sharma et al., 2024) (Figure 11.7).

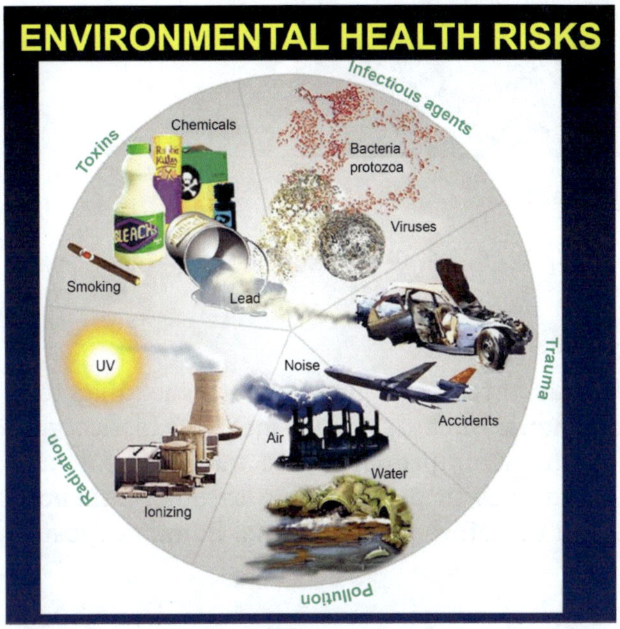

Figure 11.7. Environmental health risks.

Source: https://slideplayer.com/slide/12483076/74/images/4/ENVIRONMENTAL+HEALTH+RISKS.jpg.

11.2.1. Air Pollution and Respiratory Diseases

The relationship between air pollution and respiratory disease is a question of paramount importance in Occupational and Environmental Medicine. Exposure to dangerous pollutants, such as particulate matter and ozone, has been linked with various respiratory diseases, such as asthma, COPD, and lung cancer. The World Health Organization has classified air quality as a critical public health problem, noting that over 7 million premature deaths globally are attributable to air pollution-related diseases. The pathways of occupational exposure, which include highly emitting industries, increase the risk level among employees, particularly those in construction and manufacturing, underscoring the need for rigorous regulatory measures. Naturally, awareness of the impact of air pollution on respiratory health is relevant, since not only does it compromise quality of life, but it is also a significant health care and economic burden on health care systems and economies worldwide. The prevalence of respiratory diseases caused by air pollution underscores the need for public health interventions and policy action. Evidence indicates that deteriorated air quality exacerbates chronic illnesses and contributes to the morbidity and mortality of respiratory diseases. Also, vulnerable groups such as those suffering from chronic health ailments, children, and the elderly are more prone to air pollutants. As more research identifies how air pollution affects respiratory health, more preventive measures at the community level and public education programs become essential. Policymakers must make firm policy choices to implement changes that reduce emissions, including cleaner technologies and stricter air quality standards, to eradicate the adverse effects of poor air quality on vulnerable groups. In recent years, there has been a rising concern regarding the confluence of socioeconomic determinants and health inequities exacerbated by air pollution. Poor communities tend to bear disproportionate burdens of exposure to harmful air pollutants due to their proximity to industrial zones and high-travel roads. This environmental disparity is compounded by inadequate access to healthcare services, leading to delays in diagnosing and treating respiratory conditions. Also, variable utilization of pulmonary function tests, particularly utilizing race and ethnicity, has been called into question for perpetuating health disparities (Bhakta et al., 2021). The use of a more equitable framework for environmental policy and clinical practice may prove highly influential in improving health outcomes. Approaching air pollution mitigation through a social equity lens is necessary to make real strides in reducing respiratory disease rates among diverse groups (Figure 11.8).

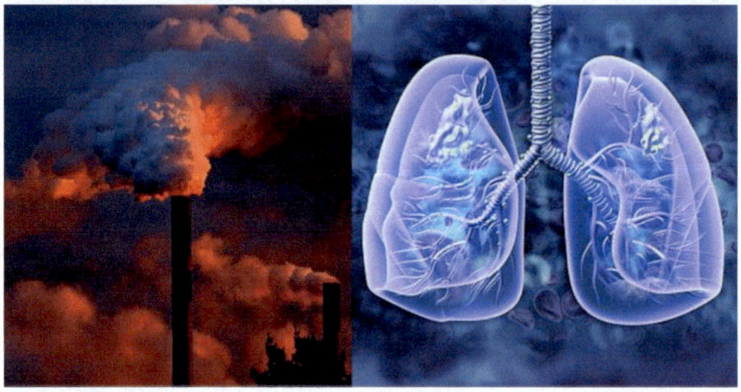

Figure 11.8. Air pollution main cause of respiratory problem.

Source: https://thekabultimes.com/wp-content/uploads/2024/03/lung.jpg.

11.2.2. Water Contamination and Public Health

The broad issue of water contamination poses serious threats to public health, leading to a multitude of diseases and health conditions. Contaminants such as heavy metals, plastics, and pathogens enter water sources through industrial effluent, improper waste management, and agricultural practices. Of particular concern are the additives in plastics that, through enhanced product functionality, become part of water systems and therefore pose potential human exposure via ingestion of contaminated water and food.

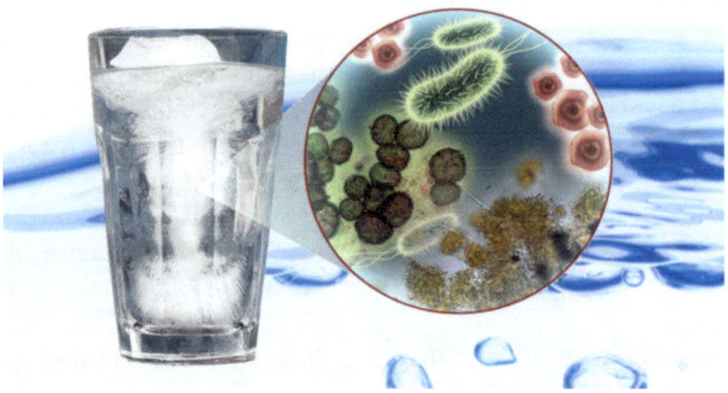

Figure 11.9. Water contamination.

Source: https://apexwaterfilters.com/blogs/wp-content/uploads/2018/09/contaminants-in-water.jpg.

This necessitates significant pollution control and strict regulations to protect water resources. As proposed in the current literature, the proper handling of plastic waste is essential to mitigate its impact not only on the environment but also on human health, exacerbating the issue posed by many contaminants in water resources (Hahladakis et al., 2017). Public health implications of water contamination have become increasingly important as natural systems continue to degrade. Greater urbanization and industrial processes accelerate the discharge of pollutants, creating a cycle that poisons the health of vulnerable populations. In particular, poor communities usually bear the brunt of environmental injustice, with higher levels of exposure to contaminated water. The World Health Organization has reported that a substantial portion of the global disease burden is attributable to modifiable environmental factors, such as unsafe drinking water (Whitmee et al., 2015).

This inequality demands focused public health intervention not only to treat patients exposed to polluted water but also to prevent exposure through safe, sustainable water management. Additionally, the interaction between health and water contamination is dynamic and depends on socioeconomic factors, public policy, and environmental regulation. As natural resources are further used unsustainably by humans, the hazard of health effects from environmental degradation becomes extremely high. Environmental degradation further erodes public health as ecosystems that supply clean water further degrade, indicating a direct link between poor environmental stewardship and increased healthcare expenses (Whitmee et al., 2015). Efforts to improve water quality—ranging from the development of infrastructure to people's movements—are imperative. By fostering intersectoral collaboration and putting health at the heart of environmental policy-making, people's societies can work towards solutions to mitigate the long-term impact of polluted water on public health and reinstate natural water systems for their integrity in the interest of future generations (Figure 11.9).

11.2.3. Soil Pollution and Its Impact on Agriculture

Soil pollution poses a significant hazard to agricultural production, directly affecting crop quality and food safety. Heavy metals, pesticides, and industrial pollutants all pollute the soil, with adverse effects on plant growth and soil diversity. For instance, heavy metals will inhibit root growth and nutrient acquisition, which influences yields and crop quality. Because the agricultural sector relies heavily on soil health for sustainable agriculture, declines in soil health can have wide-ranging effects on farm livelihoods and food safety. To derive strategies to mitigate soil contamination, such an understanding is important. Beyond agricultural productivity, soil pollution has profound long-term implications for environmental health.

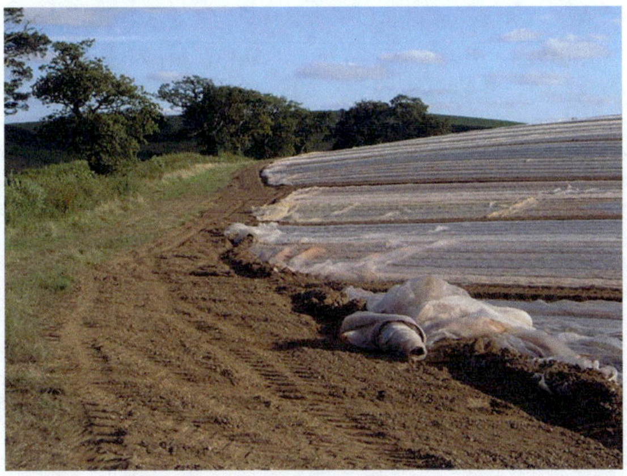

Figure 11.10. Sources of soil pollution and major contaminants in agricultural areas.

Source: https://openknowledge.fao.org/server/api/core/bitstreams/fe5df8d6-6b19-4def-bdc6-62886d824574/content/src/img/CB4894EN_GASP_Fig_3.6.jpg.

Contaminated soils can impact the general ecosystem's well-being by leaching harmful chemicals into nearby water bodies, thus having an impact on aquatic life and contaminating drinking water sources. The synergistic interaction between soil well-being and ecological health is also strained by research efforts to develop a framework to quantify and evaluate these synergistic influences. For example, a new assessment in Malawi highlighted the importance of extensive research to identify priority gaps in environmental health information, such as soil contamination (Lungu et al., 2010). By addressing such gaps, policymakers and scientists are in a better position to comprehend the overall effect of soil contamination consequences in agricultural and environmental contexts. Education and awareness are principal factors to use in managing the effects of soil pollution in agriculture. Use of curricula spanning a range of subjects—from environmental science to food safety—can help future generations acquire the information they need to address these multidimensional challenges. One Health aims to promote the integration of human health, animal health, and environmental health, thereby calling for holistic soil management and agriculture. The Western Institute for Food Safety and Security's subject matter profile is a policy guide for educators and policymakers, assuming that a solution derived from an interdisciplinary approach can foster knowledge and develop efficient strategies for soil health management (Angelos et al., 2017). Interdisciplinary learning helps stakeholders better conserve soil resources while keeping food production sustainable and sound amid pollution problems (Figure 11.10).

Test Your Knowledge

1. What are the respiratory diseases caused by air pollution?
2. What is the impact of soil pollution on agriculture?

11.3. Regulatory Framework

Learning Outcome

1. Understand the Occupational Safety and Health Administration (OSHA) standards
2. Understand the Environmental Protection Agency (EPA) regulations
3. Describe the framework of international guidelines and agreements

The legislative system that governs occupational and environmental medicine is critical to preserving the well-being of workers and the general public from various risks. It forms a mosaic of legislation, guidelines, and standards created by government agencies and professional organizations. At the core of this system are institutions such as the Occupational Safety and Health Administration (OSHA) and the Environmental Protection Agency (EPA), which issue regulations to minimize risks from exposure to toxins in workplaces and the environment. These regulations tend to be based on scientific evidence of the effects of various agents, including chemicals and biological agents, on human health. A robust regulatory system not only ensures that individuals are protected but also places a premium on research in risk analysis, ultimately guiding policy and establishing a culture of safety in occupational and environmental health. In addition, the changing terrain of environmental risks demands a changing regulatory system that responds to emerging scientific knowledge. Particularly, the risk assessment of engineered nanomaterials (ENMs) under regulation is a good example of the need for new risk assessment approaches that can address limited hazard or exposure data. As Bilal et al. (2017) state, existing frameworks cannot effectively serve the interests of policymakers and stakeholders who require timely decision-making capabilities. The call for new risk assessment methodologies emphasizes the importance of an integrated strategy incorporating environmental impact studies alongside occupational health factors. Regulatory agencies, scientists, and industry stakeholders must thus be involved in a cooperative manner to refine existing frameworks and identify priority areas for improvement, thereby enhancing overall intervention effectiveness for occupational and environmental health. In addition to regulating emergent issues, the regulatory system should also take into consideration the additive nature of chemical exposures and their effects on health, particularly regarding cancer hazards. Available evidence indicates that a significant percentage of cases of cancer are attributable to toxic exposures to the environment, and this is a key area for regulation (Hamid et al., 2015). The combination of low-dose chemical exposures and carcinogenic mechanisms necessitates re-examination of existing evaluation processes within the regulatory framework. From existing research evidence, it is clear that most chemicals exhibit low-dose effects without an apparent dose-response threshold, complicating risk assessments and regulatory actions. It is thus imperative to revisit traditional guidelines and to include comprehensive studies on chemical interactions and their biological consequences to enhance public health protections in the workplace. This type of approach would lead to better policy choices, more effectively calibrated to address the multidimensionality of environmental carcinogenesis.

11.3.1. Occupational Safety and Health Administration (OSHA) Standards

In the field of Occupational and Environmental Medicine, policies from the Occupational Safety and Health Administration (OSHA) are critical to establishing safe working conditions. Regulations devised by OSHA are intended to reduce risks and hazards encountered by workers on a day-to-day basis, from chemical exposures to ergonomic concerns. Compliance with these standards is not just for the health and safety of workers but also for the optimal operation of organizations. By imposing policies that mandate safe practices, OSHA prevents work-related injury and illness, in the longterm saving the economic cost of lost productivity and medical treatment. In accordance with OSHA guidelines, employers are responsible for implementing proactive measures to protect their workers, thereby promoting a healthy culture of health and safety in multiracial work environments. The effectiveness of OSHA standards depends on various determinants, including employers' compliance and the training provided to employees. For instance, research highlights that a very high percentage of occupational physicians (OPs) in some regions demonstrate low rates of compliance with OSHA medical surveillance standards, rather turning to local regulations over universal standards. This disparity underscores the necessity of continuous OP education and training in accordance with OSHA standards. Occupational health experts must be conversant with these standards to effectively carry out competency-based assessments, as they directly affect their ability to manage workplace health risks. Failure to meet OSHA standards can mean more incident rates, compromising the workers and the organizations for higher financial and legal consequences, as observed in work-injury economic costs research. Furthermore, integrating OSHA standards into the educational system for occupational health professionals is essential to developing an appropriately trained workforce. Higher learning institutions and training institutions must revise their course curricula and include not just the theoretical aspects but also practical applications of OSHA standards. By creating multidisciplinary approaches that integrate perspectives from different disciplines such as medicine, engineering, and public health, educators can enhance the competencies of future OPs. This integral education will enable professionals to better confront newly arising occupational health issues. Secondly, as the organizations become more integrated with the health professionals, the focus on innovation and following OSHA guidelines can result in the formulation of better safety measures and monitoring mechanisms, in accordance with wider national and global health policies (Azeddoug, 2024). In the end, a commitment to adhering to OSHA standards not only helps the individual employee but also creates a safer and healthier work environment throughout all industries (Figure 11.11).

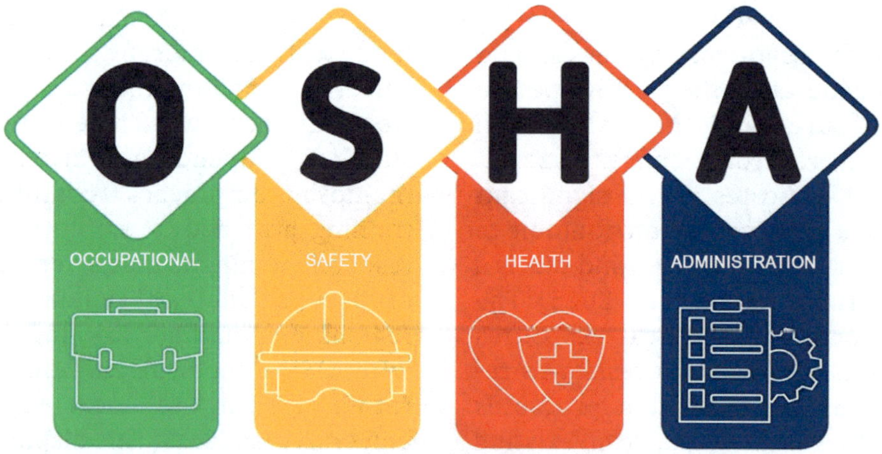

Figure 11.11. OSHA standards for the safety of workers and workplace.

Source: https://keninstitute.com/wp-content/uploads/2023/01/image1.jpg.

11.3.2. Environmental Protection Agency (EPA) Regulations

The Environmental Protection Agency (EPA) plays a basic role at the intersection of environmental and occupational medicine by establishing environmental regulations that provide public as well as environmental protection. The regulations are vital for overseeing how industries conduct business, particularly in sectors such as healthcare, whose environmental impact can be far-reaching. The EPA's regulations encompass many pollutants generated by health facilities, including infectious waste and dangerous substances. For instance, the medical industry's specialized waste disposal problems, such as medical incineration of waste and disposal of hazardous drugs, need to be dealt with using strict regulations in order to prevent environmental degradation and promote community health. By providing enabling infrastructure for the safe disposal of harmful substances and encouraging pollution-prevention techniques, the EPA fosters a cleaner work environment for healthcare workers while safeguarding the surrounding population from potential environmental risks (Davies et al., 2025). Secondly, the EPA's regulations are designed to address the imbalances in environmental risks suffered by minority groups. According to the discourse of risk assessment and allocation, poor communities bear a heightened burden of environmental pollution due to structural imbalances in social and economic status. Regulatory agencies' acknowledgment of heightened risks among minority groups is an indicator of the need for special mechanisms to reverse these impacts. Notably, the EPA's policy measures to move forward in safeguarding vulnerable populations, such as children, the elderly, and pregnant women, emphasize the importance of environmental justice in shaping its policies. These initiatives are essential in the discipline of occupational and environmental medicine, as they make intervention based on EPA regulations effective and fair in reducing health disparities among populations at highest risk (Swanston et al., 1994). In its efforts to promote public health through regulation, the EPA often engages with various stakeholders, including healthcare practitioners, government officials, and community organizations.

Figure 11.12. Environmental protection agency (EPA).

Source: https://encrypted-tbn0.gstatic.com/images?q=tbn:ANd9GcROP8crKrSsentakj_Pe7ZtQY5CiyS1aH8GsA&s.

This comprehensive strategy contributes to increasing environmental policy compliance and public awareness of the health consequences of environmental hazards. Through partnerships, the EPA can communicate crucial information on best practices in waste management and pollution prevention to medical facilities, promoting cleaner operations. Also, ongoing research and data collection is critical in simplifying the EPAs regulatory scheme. With evolving environmental challenges, the agency must remain sensitive to new risks, always maintaining a focus on safeguarding both occupational health and population health through widespread environmental protection measures. The integration of scientific findings into policy making also enhances the effectiveness of the EPA's regulations, ultimately resulting in the general objectives of public health in occupational and environmental medicine (Davies et al., 2025).

11.3.3. International Guidelines and Agreements

The design of international guidelines and agreements plays a significant role in establishing standards for occupational and environmental medicine. The guidelines are vital instruments in establishing standards for safety and health practices, particularly regarding exposure to toxic substances and environmental poisons. By promoting the implementation of evidence-based practices, organizations such as the World Health Organization (WHO) and other international labor institutions lay the groundwork for countries to develop their own regulatory policies. In Italy, for instance, the enactment of new laws following European Union revisions indicates the need for rigorous health surveillance of those exposed to electromagnetic fields, thereby demonstrating how global guidelines naturally influence national legislation (Gobba et al., 2025). An understanding of the specific use of these global guidelines is intricate and involves examining how they align with local settings and adapt to global health issues. The proposals advanced by institutions such as the Italian Association of Medical Radioprotection (AIRM) reflect an integrative approach to workers' health surveillance, taking into account advances in technology and scientific knowledge. The interdisciplinary approach ensures that health practitioners are equipped with the latest information and techniques needed for effective monitoring and evaluation. Moreover, as the guidelines are reviewed systematically in line with global standards such as PRISMA criteria, they are updated to incorporate current studies and emerging health concerns, thereby reflecting the dynamic nature of occupational and environmental medicine (Gobba et al.,

2025). Even in nations like Morocco, where international standards are integrated into domestic schools, this underscores the need to develop innovative occupational health practices. University managers are also at the forefront of this movement, responsible for fostering a culture of safety and health on their respective campuses. By using interdisciplinary task forces and stakeholder participation, these institutions can develop site-specific policies that align with international standards while addressing the specific health issues of their populations. These initiatives not only strive for the welfare of university staff and students but also lay the groundwork for sustainable practices that can be applied in the event of mega-projects, showing commitment towards the incorporation of international standards into local needs.

Test Your Knowledge

1. What are the OSHA standards?
2. What are the EPA regulations?

11.4. Prevention and Intervention Strategies

Learning Outcome

1. Describe the workplace safety programs
2. Understand the community health initiatives
3. Understand the role of education and training

Successful prevention and intervention are critical to reducing occupational risks and improving workers' health status. These are usually extensive efforts incorporating individual behavior as well as systemic processes at the work level. Lifestyle-change-oriented health promotion activities are particularly important in occupational and environmental medicine, emphasizing not only addressing immediate health issues but also promoting long-term productivity and economic viability. Evidence shows that interventions to encourage healthy practice, the offering of individualized health profiles, and having healthy food available on site for staff to have access to reduce issues such as obesity, a concern within the industry, such as transport. Not only do these interventions benefit staff health, but the potential to generate high returns for businesses also underscores the need to integrate work health promotion into work practice (Naweed et al., 2015). Besides, the need for concerted research in environmental health cannot be overemphasized. The identification of lacunae in existing literature is required to provide meaningful intervention actions that are sensitive to targeted groups, e.g., workers in risky occupations. In contexts such as Malawi, where environmental health problems are compounded by socioeconomic status, research must focus primarily on identifying workable strategies that can bridge the gaps. Developing a customized action plan to reduce environmental health issues not only enables better consideration of the local setting but also enhances models for implementing viable interventions. This develops a health and safety culture that transcends sectoral boundaries, particularly where workplace exposure to environmental hazards is a vital issue (Lungu et al., 2010). Implementing these prevention and intervention efforts requires collaboration among stakeholders, including employers, healthcare providers, and policymakers. Through these value-based collaborations of worker well-being, organizations can optimize compliance with health standards and encourage a culture of prevention in workplaces. For instance, regular training and education on health hazards and healthier work practices can empower workers to make informed decisions about their health, thereby ensuring a healthy work environment. Moreover, involving employees in health promotion program design and implementation can maximize participation and outcomes. Thus, integrating evidence-based comprehensive prevention strategies not only addresses current health issues but also develops resilience and a sustainable long-term health model in the workforce that is harmonious with the greater aims of occupational and environmental medicine (Figure 11.13).

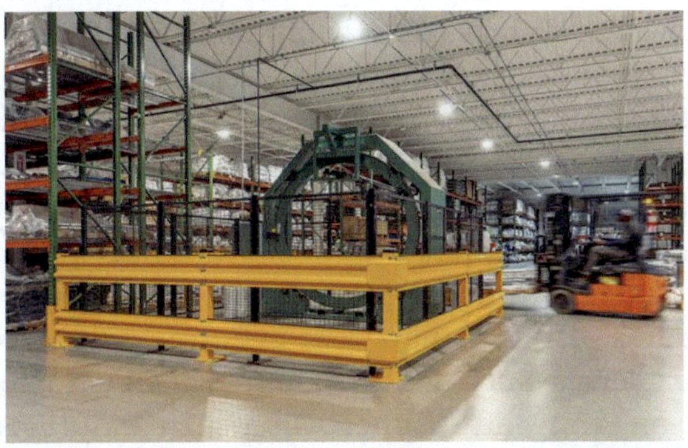

Figure 11.13. Mitigating workplace hazards: Essential strategies for facility safety.

Source: https://www.safetyandhealthmagazine.com/ext/resources/images/WS-bonus/Kee-Safety-Bonus-WS-picture.jpg?t=1716489689&width=696.

11.4.1. Workplace Safety Programs

In Occupational and Environmental Medicine, occupational safety programs are the foundation for safeguarding employees and promoting a healthy work environment. These encompass a wide scope of methods, systems, and practices for preventing workplace illness and injury. By using comprehensive safety measures, organizations not only comply with regulations but also build a health and safety culture. These programs can include regular safety training, ergonomic analysis, and safety committees to involve employees in decision-making, thereby enhancing their participation in safety. Also, the integration of safety programs into the organizational framework has demonstrated positive correlations with employee morale, productivity, and job satisfaction, supporting the contention that safety is an investment worth making rather than an expense. A critical review of workplace safety programs points out that there is always a need to adapt and evolve in response to new challenges and advancements. As Occupational and Environmental Medicine evolves, so must measures be embraced to counteract threats. A case in point is the increasing trend towards remote work, which implies that safety programs also need to be more adaptable and address ergonomic risks in home office setups. Besides, due to the growing application of automation and artificial intelligence at the workplace, safety programs must incorporate training on new technology to prevent potential occupational health hazards. Policymakers and managers within organizations must leverage these opportunities to innovate and update existing programs to make them applicable and effective in a shifting workplace environment. These initiatives not only protect employees but also ensure organizational resilience amid fluctuating market conditions. The success of occupational safety measures largely depends on stakeholder involvement and the implementation of firm policies. Modern occupational health standards recommend collaboration to effectively implement safety measures. Involvement of employees, management, and external professionals in policy formulation and implementation fosters a sense of ownership and accountability among all stakeholders. Also, comprehensive appraisals, such as SWOT analyses, can reveal inherent strengths and weaknesses within existing safety procedures and lay the ground for targeted improvement. In order to maximize the effectiveness of these programs, organizations must establish mechanisms for continued surveillance and evaluation that enable rapid response and adjustment based on feedback and emerging data. By placing greater emphasis on teamwork and ongoing monitoring, occupational health and the final objective of a healthier workforce can be significantly promoted through workplace safety programs, thereby aligning with established human rights norms in respect of workplace health and safety (Arias et al., 2024; Azeddoug, 2024) (Figure 11.14).

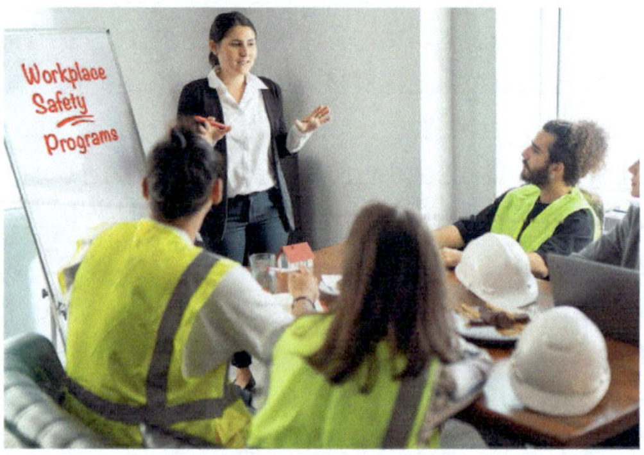

Figure 11.14. Workplace safety programs.

Source: https://www.realtimenetworks.com/hubfs/WPS-PP-top-hero-banner-1200x832-3.jpeg.

11.4.2. Community Health Initiatives

Occupational community health interventions play a significant role in improving occupational health and well-being. Occupational interventions have the potential to address numerous factors influencing workers' overall health, not only physical but also mental health. By designing programs that address employees' particular concerns, organizations can create a healthier occupational environment. This is important because it shifts the focus from mere disease cure to a more holistic understanding that prioritizes prevention and health promotion. Following recent controversies, the incorporation of evidence from public health practice into workplace interventions can be optimized to enhance their efficacy, thereby enabling organizations to prevent and tackle health issues at the root before they reach symptomatic stages (Karanika-Murray et al., 2013). Also, community health programs will prioritize educational elements, significantly shaping employees' understanding of health concerns. For instance, employee programs for educating staff on mental disorders can de-stigmatize conditions based on mental illnesses, thereby fostering an open culture of conversation. As highlighted in the literature, workplaces are optimal settings for promoting awareness of mental health, equipping workers with skills to identify early warning signs, and ensuring access to essential mental health care (Brodniak et al., 2000). Such outreach health education programs can deliver significant dividends in greater productivity and lower healthcare costs, compelling an argument for including health education as part of occupational health mechanisms. Furthermore, the successful implementation of community health programs involves the ability of various stakeholders to collaborate in a multidisciplinary effort, including organizational management, medical professionals, and even the employees themselves. Such multi-stakeholder input fosters an enabling atmosphere in which employees become stakeholders in their own health. The likelihood of workplace culture transforming into a pro-health culture increases significantly through this collaboration, encouraging staff to become more committed and adherent to health programs. Second, the creation of awareness of public health principles within organizations also attests to the recognition of the broad determinants that affect workplace health. Such a conformity of strategy not only enhances the likelihood of effective health interventions but also contributes towards an overall movement towards healthier workplaces (Karanika-Murray et al., 2013). Consequently, community health programs are a core component of occupational and environmental medicine, highlighting interrelations among workplace conditions and public health status (Figure 11.15).

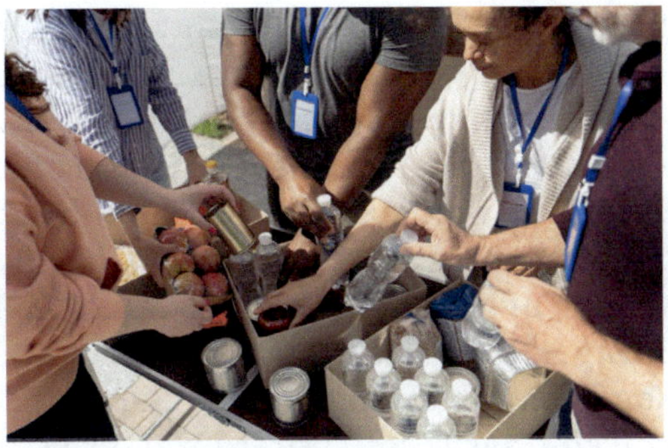

Figure 1.15. Community health initiatives.

Source: https://santhwanamvs.com/wp-content/uploads/2025/02/Blog-3.webp.

11.4.3. Role of Education and Training

In Occupational and Environmental Medicine (OEM), education and training are those pillars on which the expertise of medical specialists, i.e., occupational physicians (OPs), rests. Occupational health problems also evolve in response to the changing nature of work and require a workforce capable and skilled in addressing advanced health issues. The Delphi study found that OPs must possess a broad set of competencies in clinical, academic, and administrative domains. These competencies would be crucial to ensuring effective interventions and promoting best practice in workplace health and safety. Therefore, effectively organized training programs are the sine qua non for equipping OPs to manage the complexity of their role across various practice environments, underlining the authoritative role of organized education within the specialized profession (Demou et al., 2018). Research that determines core competencies serves not just the development of the curriculum but also ongoing professional education for OPs. Identification of the specific skills most relevant across fields of practice enables a more personalized education program, as expressed through the intergroup contrasts of the study. Clinical competencies, for instance, were considered applicable across all fields, but there was diversity in the emphasis placed on environmental issues and communication skills among different OP subgroups. This highlights the necessity of optimizing training programs to address these variances and keep up with evolving demands within the profession, while also accounting for the unique contexts in which OPs are employed. Such targeted educational interventions can, in the long term, contribute to improved occupational health outcomes (Demou et al., 2018). In addition to filling the gaps in practice competencies, OEM education is also critical to bridging the gap between research and practice. Processes such as assessing research priorities in environmental health fields, as in the consultancy for Malawi, underscore the necessity of OPs being aware of both the application of existing knowledge and the identification of areas that require additional research. Equipping practitioners to learn research methods, critically appraise existing literature, and translate findings into practice ensures they can advocate for evidence-based interventions in workplaces. This blended education format establishes a culture of continuous improvement, enables OPs to become change agents who spearhead initiatives for worker health and safety, and, in the long run, reinforces the value of education and training in preventing existing challenges in Occupational and Environmental Medicine.

Test Your Knowledge

1. What are the workplace safety programs?
2. What is community-based initiatives?

11.5. Current Trends and Research

Learning Outcome

1. Understand the emerging occupational health issues
2. Describe the advances in environmental health research
3. Know the impact of climate change on occupational and environmental health

The landscape of occupational and environmental medicine is currently undergoing significant transformation due to heightened awareness of the health risks associated with workplace and environmental exposures. A marked increase in research publications highlights this trend, particularly for diseases such as mesothelioma, which has seen a surge in scholarly interest over the past two decades. Notably, the United States remains the leader in this area of study, with a large share of publications and citations, underscoring the nation's dedication to occupational health issues related to substances such as asbestos. This research interest underscores the necessity of perpetual vigilance and prevention, especially in sectors of work that involve greater risk of exposure. Initiatives to improve regulation and policy implementation are required to mitigate these health hazards at a broader scale (Lai et al., 2023). Alongside the increasing number of publications, current small-scale studies suggest a renewed emphasis on evidence-based approaches within occupational health disciplines. The use of big data analysis in occupational safety protocols represents a new age in which data evidence becomes the focal point for determining health guidelines and interventions. From studies, employing inclusive datasets has been discovered to assist in identifying prevalent health hazards and promoting strategic prevention programs. Furthermore, new methodologies developed in this field have enabled higher precision in health assessments, subsequently optimizing the protection of workers across various industries. Intersectoral collaboration between industry stakeholders and public health officials is needed to harness this data for deriving actionable insights and frameworks in the protection of worker health (Sutanti, 2022). With ongoing developments in occupational and environmental medicine, the need for interdisciplinary collaboration necessitates integrated health measures. For instance, the present research integrates occupational health and safety (OHS) with public health, shifting perceptions of occupational health and how it is addressed within the broader context of community health. The new evidence indicates that factors such as environmental considerations and mental health are increasingly recognized as integral components of workplace safety and worker well-being. This integrated perspective is at the forefront as experts seek to enhance health and disease prevention more effectively, especially amid the challenges posed by public health crises such as the COVID-19 pandemic. Transdisciplinary health promotion programs can enhance occupational wellness and address broader environmental health implications, thereby facilitating an overall public health strategy (Lai et al., 2023) (Figure 11.16).

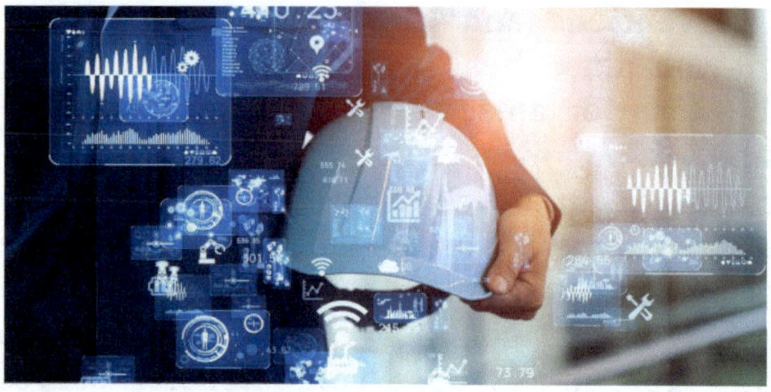

Figure 11.16. Current trends in occupational safety and health.

Source: https://www.columbiasouthern.edu/media/i3fbjzhc/current-trends-in-occupational-health-and-safety.jpg.

11.5.1. Emerging Occupational Health Issues

New technologies and shifting labor patterns are propelling fundamental transformations in occupational health issues. In particular, as work practices become more flexible and digital, traditional employment models become outdated. This development is typified by the proliferation of nonstandard work arrangements, such as gig and contract work, that can lead to job insecurity and limited access to critical health programs. Contemporary occupational health frameworks are not adept at addressing emerging trends in work, leaving most workers exposed and vulnerable. This necessitates the creation of a more integrated and adaptive occupational health system that considers these emerging trends and provides equal access to training in safety, medical checks, and integrated workplace health management, as per existing literature (Ko, 2025). To address the new world of work, occupational health must be approached through a multidisciplinary approach that incorporates diverse disciplines and novel approaches. Legal and institutional reforms are also necessary to ensure that regulations encompass the unique issues of new forms of labor. These would involve revising safety and health standards to address the requirements of new, emerging categories of workers. Additionally, the use of cutting-edge technologies can enable forecasted disease management and individualized healthcare solutions specific to each worker's needs. It is imperative to create a preventive system that harmonizes chronic disease management with mental health care to respond to the psychosocial elements that directly impact worker well-being. Such steps are critical for the institutional transformation of occupational and environmental medicine towards the comprehensive tackling of evolving health issues (Azeddoug, 2024). Moreover, fostering interdisciplinary collaboration across disciplines, including medicine, public health, engineering, and psychology, can encourage research and action to apply innovative solutions to the management of health in the occupational setting. This action can enable the efficient assessment of current practices and emergent issues in occupational health, ultimately leading to more effective intervention strategies. Major stakeholder involvement, including workers and employers, will be critical to identifying and controlling priority health concerns and improving the overall workplace climate. Establishing monitoring and evaluation systems to assess the effectiveness of such interventions will help ensure they succeed in addressing the rapidly changing world of work. By putting occupational health at the center of school and work policies, an integrated policy can be achieved that supports healthier workplaces for all workers in today's dynamic labor market (Ko, 2025).

11.5.2. Advances in Environmental Health Research

In the last two decades, advancements in environmental health research have significantly enhanced the capacity to understand the complexity of environmental effects on human health. The integration of innovative technologies, such as geographic information systems (GIS) and remote sensing, has enabled the detection and probing of environmental threats. These materials enable scientists to map environmental exposures and correlate them with health outcomes in specific populations, resulting in a more informed assessment of how various environmental factors, including air and water quality, affect public health. Moreover, programs initiated by government agencies, such as the CDC's environmental public health tracking program, have developed systems of surveillance and response for environmental health threats, ultimately impacting healthier outcomes at community levels and enabling evidence-based policy making (Balmes et al., 2006). Moreover, cross-disciplinary collaboration has emerged as a key driver of innovation in environmental health research. Through partnerships among environmental scientists, health professionals, and policy-makers, the research community can draw on multidisciplinary expertise to address multidimensional issues. This collaborative system not only elevates the complexity and magnitude of research but also facilitates the better translation of public health implications into practice.

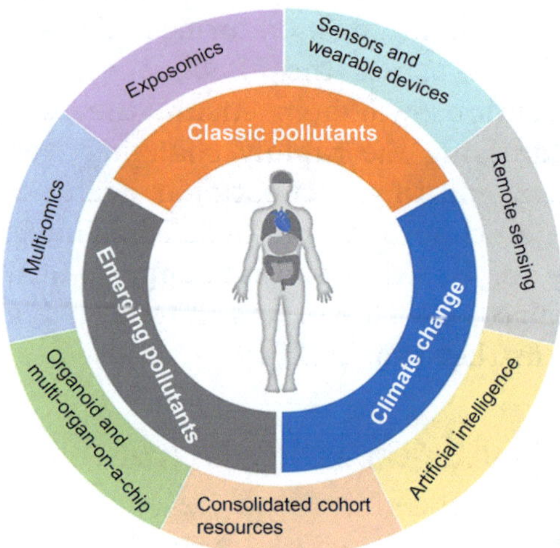

Figure 11.17. Advances and perspectives in environmental health research.

Source: https://media.springernature.com/lw685/springer-static/image/art%3A10.1007%2Fs11783-024-1836-z/MediaObjects/11783_2024_1836_Fig1_HTML.jpg?as=webp.

As has been seen in recent controversies, understanding the implications of genetic-environmental interactions has come to be at the center of crafting environmental health policies. The differentiation between screening and genetic monitoring is what demarcates the potential benefits and risks of forecasting test technologies, necessitating careful notice in policy-making to find equilibrium among innovation and ethical considerations (Jablonski et al., 1999). Finally, as environmental health science advances, there is a greater need to focus on population-level determinants of health. Programs that ensure systematic identification and intervention strategies are essential for reducing the adverse health impacts of environmental hazards. The persistent pursuit of an integrated body of knowledge on environmental factor monitoring prioritizes transparency and stakeholder engagement. Ensuring that the information needs of various stakeholders engaged in environmental health, researchers, and policymakers can be better met to promote public health. Lastly, advances in this field are a key step toward preventive occupational and environmental medicine strategies focusing on the prevention of disease and the maintenance of population health (Balmes et al., 2006) (Figure 11.17).

11.5.3. The Impact of Climate Change on Occupational and Environmental Health

The effects of climate change on occupational and environmental well-being are extensive and multifaceted, cutting across various industries and the workforce within them. When the world temperature goes up, workers working outdoors, like farmers, construction workers, and emergency responders, face higher risks of heat illnesses. The prevalence of heat strain, as observed in research, underscores the need for organizations to implement rigorous cooling measures to safeguard workers' health. Research has established that 99% of first responder organizations cite heat strain as a high hazard, indicating the problem's general concern and the necessity for system-based solutions to correct such issues (International et al., 2018). Employers must realize that preventive measures, such as recognizing frequent multilevel assessments of psychosocial work settings, can significantly reduce occupational health risks associated with climate change, thereby improving employee welfare. Besides, climate change exacerbates environmental pollution, leading to increased respiratory diseases among staff exposed to polluted air.

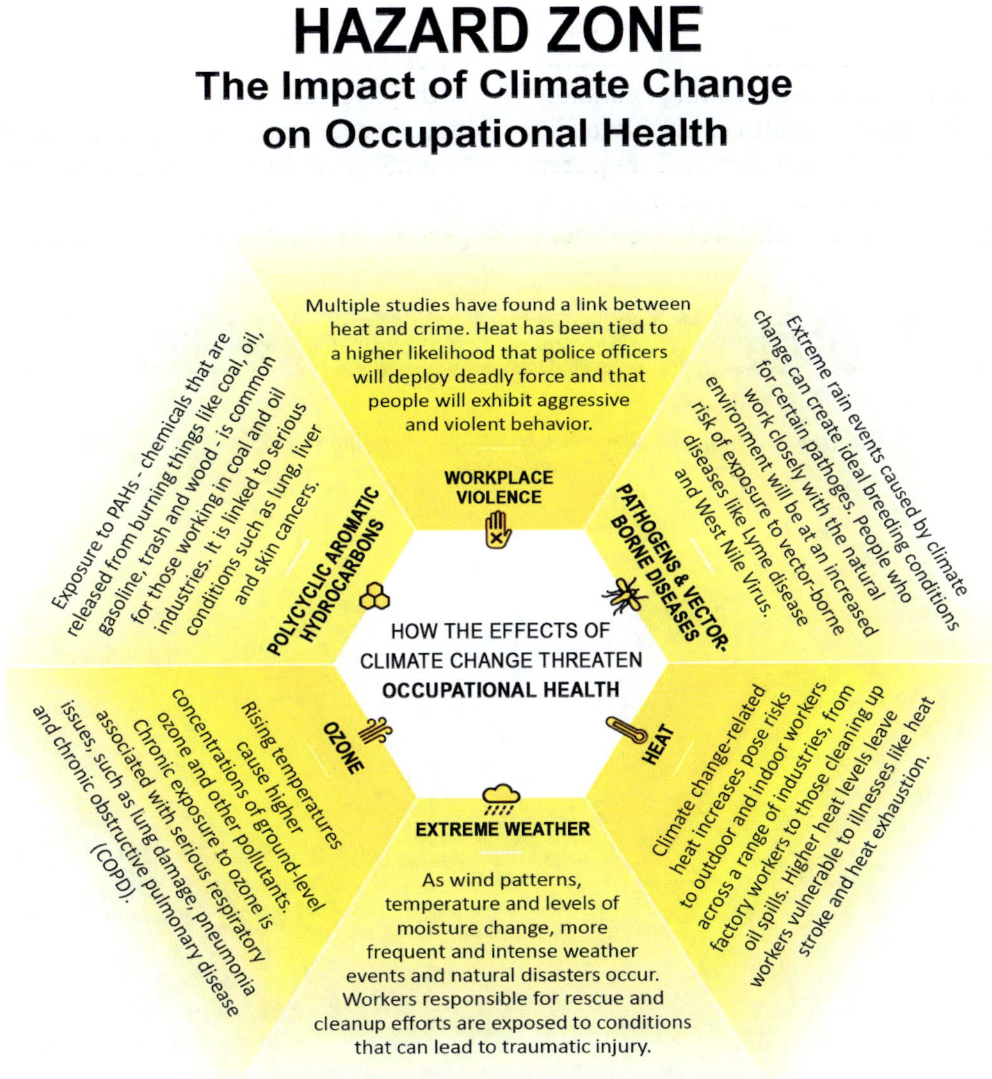

Figure 11.18. The impact of climate change on occupational health.

Source: https://onlinepublichealth.gwu.edu/wp-content/uploads/sites/47/2021/03/infographic_climage-change-and-health-hazards.jpeg.

Studies show that industries such as construction and agriculture have been hit by increased levels of particulate matter, which may lead to long-term health consequences among the workers. The interrelated nature of various factors, from organizational decisions to workgroup dynamics and individual health concerns, calls for a multi-level approach to address these new risks. By incorporating detailed analysis of such complexities, organizational interventions can be more responsive and inclusive, leading to customized strategies to improve immediate and long-term employee health outcomes (International et al., 2018). Such proactive action is critical to addressing the evolving frontier of occupational health amid climate challenges. Also, the long-term effects of climate change extend beyond physical health to encompass employees' mental well-being. Additional stressors such as extreme weather and environmental degradation can significantly affect employee mental health, leading to anxiety and burnout. The mental health crisis, fueled by these external drivers, warrants an integrated approach from organizations to address their health efforts. The use of multilevel assessment approaches enables organizations to identify psychosocial stressors and design effective support systems that foster resilience among employees. Mental health needs to be on par with physical health, given that the effects of climate change on employment sectors continue to emerge and necessitate innovative solutions that address employees' overall well-being (Arnetz et al., 2014) (Figure 11.18).

Test Your Knowledge

1. What are emerging occupational health issues?
2. What is the impact of climate change on occupational and environmental health?

SUMMARY

In short, the practice of Occupational and Environmental Medicine plays a crucial role in public health safety and in enhancing quality of life. From the dominance of the United States in research output in this specialty, as illustrated in Falagas et al. (2010), the boundless pursuit of knowledge has far-reaching policy implications alongside the uptake of health interventions. The leadership of American researchers indicates a concerted effort in the prevention and mitigation of occupational and environmental health hazards. This rigorous scientific scrutiny, beyond merely improving workplace safety measures, also influences the overall framework of public health institutions and thus largely benefits the overall welfare of the population. Moreover, the move towards increasing authorship per article in Occupational Medicine journals, as noted by Aw et al. (2009), represents a mass approach that enriches research quality. The move towards more collaboration demonstrates increased awareness of the multidimensional complexity of occupational health issues, necessitating interdisciplinary perspectives towards successful solutions. This trend also reflects that the complexities of occupational and environmental health require a multiplicity of skills, thereby intensifying debate and enhancing the scientific validity of published literature. The increase in collaborative studies heralds a promising trend towards joint problem-solving, which is critical to addressing priority health concerns. Lastly, the importance of the findings lies in their highlighting the need for international support and cooperation in the practice of Occupational and Environmental Medicine. As developing nations lag in research publications, efforts should be made to build local capacity and increase scientific output, as underscored by Falagas et al. (2010). These initiatives would not only guarantee fairness in health research but also enable nations to respond effectively to their unique occupational and environmental health challenges. With the climate in this region continuing to shift, global cooperation and exchange of information would appear crucial to guarantee sustainable health outcomes and ensure that the progress achieved is for the good of all populations in the world.

Implementation of environmental health education in training healthcare professionals is important, particularly in children's care. The gap is acknowledged in both medical and nursing curricula regarding the impact of environmental exposure on children's health. The rising awareness within health facilities underscores the compelling need for changes in this regard, driven by parents' inquiries about the impact of environmental toxins on their children. Studies have shown that children are biologically, psychologically, and socially distinct from adults, necessitating a specialized area of interest within environmental health education. Working group recommendations have suggested expanding educational material on children's environmental health throughout medical school, residency, and continuing education, with an emphasis on a strategic agenda to effectively prepare future healthcare professionals (Dearry et al., 2004). Moreover, literature reveals the importance of evaluating occupational tasks faced by law enforcers in terms of performance with respect to body armor impacts. A systematic review of existing studies shows that there is insufficient knowledge about how body armor affects both physiological responses and task performance during stressful events. The findings indicate that, while information on marksmanship remains scarce, physical performance indicators related to body armor have been investigated more thoroughly. Results indicate that body armor increases ratings of perceived exertion, task duration times, and decreases fatigue-free functional capacities. This insight inspires a prudent selection of body armor based on its ergonomic design to satisfy the physical demands of law enforcement personnel (Orr et al., 2017). Overall, environmental health education for health professionals and occupational performance evaluation of high-stress jobs, such as law enforcement, indicate the need for a sharply targeted approach in occupational and environmental medicine. By placing educational effort behind pediatric environmental health and considering the physiological impact of occupational equipment like body armor, the field is better able to attack the unique problems of the interplay of occupation and environment. This two-fold method allows for the development of specific strategies to enhance the readiness of healthcare workers and elevate the performance and safety of high-risk employees, thereby contributing to better health outcomes across different populations (Dearry et al., 2004; Orr et al., 2017).

KEY TERMS FROM THIS CHAPTER

- Biological hazards
- Chemical exposure
- Hazardous waste
- Neuroendocrine
- Occupational medicine
- Psychosocial hazards
- Skin diseases
- Carpal tunnel syndrome
- Environmental medicine
- Hepatitis
- Occupational exposure
- Physical hazards
- Public health
- Toxicology

CRITICAL THINKING QUESTIONS

1. **What is the primary focus of occupational medicine?**
   a. Managing chronic diseases
   b. Promoting workplace health and preventing occupational injuries
   c. Providing general healthcare services
   d. Treating environmental allergies
2. **Which of the following is an example of a biological hazard in the workplace?**
   a. Asbestos
   b. Noise pollution
   c. Hepatitis B virus
   d. Silica dust
3. **What is the term for a disease caused by inhalation of asbestos fibers?**
   a. Silicosis
   b. Asbestosis
   c. Coal worker's pneumoconiosis
   d. Farmer's lung
4. **Which of the following is used to measure noise levels in an industrial setting?**
   a. Sphygmomanometer
   b. Dosimeter
   c. Audiometer
   d. Sound level meter
5. **Which occupational disease is associated with prolonged exposure to silica dust?**
   a. Mesothelioma
   b. Pneumoconiosis
   c. Silicosis
   d. Byssinosis

Short Answer Questions

1. Define the occupational medicine.
2. Define the environmental medicine.
3. What are the 3 occupational hazards?
4. What is a biological hazard?
5. What are 3 environmental health risks?

Answer to Critical Thinking Questions

1. (b); 2. (c); 3. (b); 4. (d); 5. (c).

REFERENCES

1. Goodson, W. H., Lowe, L., Carpenter, D. O., Gilbertson, M., Ali, A. M., De Cerain Salsamendi, A. L., Lasfar, A., Carnero, A., Azqueta, A., Amedei, A., Charles, A. K., Collins, A. R., Ward, A., Salzberg, A. C., Colacci, A. M., Olsen, A., Berg, A., Barclay, B. J., Zhou, B. P., . . . Wade, M. (2015). Assessing the carcinogenic potential of low-dose exposures to chemical mixtures in the environment: the challenge ahead. *Carcinogenesis, 36*(Suppl 1), S254–S296. https://doi.org/10.1093/carcin/bgv039Angelos, J. A., Arens, A. L., Cadriel, J. L., Johnson, R., et al. (2017). One Health in food safety and security education: Subject matter outline for a curricular framework. https://core.ac.uk/download/323068605.pdf (accessed on 14th July 2025).
2. Arnetz, B., Bacharach, S., Bamberger, P., Biron, M., Biron, C., Biron, D., Biron, H., et al. (2014). The psychosocial work environment, employee mental health and organizational interventions: Improving research and practice by taking a multilevel approach. https://core.ac.uk/download/30650323.pdf (accessed on 14th July 2025).
3. ASTM International, Bonauto, D., Cadarette, B. S., Carter, R., House, J. R., International Organization for Standardization (ISO), McLellan, T. M., et al. (2018). Occupational cooling practices of emergency first responders in the United States: A survey. https://core.ac.uk/download/288395287.pdf (accessed on 14th July 2025).
4. Aw, T. C., & Shaban, S. (2009). Trend towards multiple authorship in occupational medicine journals. https://core.ac.uk/download/pdf/8261435.pdf (accessed on 14th July 2025).
5. Azeddoug, H. (2024). SPL09 leading innovation for excellence in occupational health in Moroccan universities on the eve of major world-class projects. *Occupational Medicine*. https://www.semanticscholar.org/paper/7487799e6f65c7d1d005246c79e00d5c521b36ea (accessed on 14th July 2025).
6. Balmes, J. R., Buffler, P. A., Kyle, A. D., Lee, C., et al. (2006). Integrating research, surveillance, and practice in environmental public health tracking. https://core.ac.uk/download/323082246.pdf (accessed on 14th July 2025).
7. Bezrukova, G. A., Mikerov, A. N., & Novikov, T. A. (2024). Methodological aspects of using allostatic load analysis in assessing health of working population exposed to adverse occupational factors (Analytical review). *Health Risk Analysis*. https://www.semanticscholar.org/paper/062785a55354679bb48a670f764919b7cb4ac200 (accessed on 14th July 2025).
8. Bhakta, N. R., Kaminsky, D. A., Bime, C., Thakur, N., Hall, G. L., McCormack, M. C., & Stanojevic, S. (2021). Addressing race in pulmonary function testing by aligning intent and evidence with practice and perception. *CHEST Journal, 161*, 288–297. https://doi.org/10.1016/j.chest.2021.08.053 (accessed on 14th July 2025).
9. Bilal, M., Cohen, Y., Godwin, H. A., Romero-Franco, M., et al. (2017). Needs and challenges for assessing the environmental impacts of engineered nanomaterials (ENMs). https://core.ac.uk/download/323076183.pdf (accessed on 14th July 2025).
10. Bosland, M. C., Gordon, T., Solomon, J. J., Shore, R. E., & Lippmann, M. (2024). Seventy-five years of impactful environmental and occupational health research at the Nelson Institute of Environmental Medicine at New York University. *Annals of the New York Academy of Sciences, 1540*, 147–165. https://www.semanticscholar.org/paper/cc4cba37394a2c64a4c64c26350f79bff8910eba (accessed on 14th July 2025).

11. Brodniak, W., Czabala, J. C., Dudek, B., International Labor Office, et al. (2000). *Mental Health in the Workplace: Situation Analyses, Poland*. https://core.ac.uk/download/5129369.pdf (accessed on 14th July 2025).

12. Caraballo Arias, Y., & Saito, K. (2024). O-099 Future of global OEM: Challenges and opportunities. *Occupational Medicine*. https://www.semanticscholar.org/paper/35b1018ed771c09b429330c7c07d855f7395a54c (accessed on 14th July 2025).

13. Dahunsi, S. O., Idowu, S. A., & Oranusi, S. U. (2013). Assessment of occupational diseases among artisans and factory workers in Ifo, Nigeria. https://core.ac.uk/download/18295285.pdf (accessed on 14th July 2025).

14. Dale, A. M., Evanoff, B. A., Franzblau, A., Zeringue, A., et al. (2014). Using job-title-based physical exposures from O*NET in an epidemiological study of carpal tunnel syndrome. https://core.ac.uk/download/80494858.pdf (accessed on 14th July 2025).

15. Davies, J. C., & Lowe, A. (2025). Environmental implications of the health care service sector. https://core.ac.uk/download/pdf/9307987.pdf (accessed on 14th July 2025).

16. Dearry, A., Rogers, B., Roberts, J., Paulson, J., McCurdy, L. E., Lindberg, M. A., Witherspoon, N. O., et al. (2004). Incorporating environmental health into pediatric medical and nursing education. https://core.ac.uk/download/pdf/3775759.pdf (accessed on 14th July 2025).

17. Demou, E., Lalloo, D., & MacDonald, E. B. (2018). Differences in opinions of occupational physicians on the required competencies by field of practice: Results of an international Delphi study. https://core.ac.uk/download/151395562.pdf (accessed on 14th July 2025).

18. Falagas, M. E., & Soteriades, E. S. (2010). A bibliometric analysis in the fields of preventive medicine, occupational and environmental medicine, epidemiology, and public health. https://core.ac.uk/download/28934732.pdf (accessed on 14th July 2025).

19. Gobba, F., & Modenese, A. (2025). [New approaches and criteria for the development of the new guidelines of the Italian Association of Medical Radioprotection (AIRM) for the protection of the workers exposed to EMF related risks:]. *Giornale Italiano di Medicina del Lavoro ed Ergonomia*. https://www.semanticscholar.org/paper/dec3b28b9b2c0aeb9c3a5bd46bea0ddfef4277f4 (accessed on 14th July 2025).

20. Groneberg-Kloft, B., Klingelhöfer, D., Scutaru, C., Zitnik, M., et al. (2013). Traffic medicine–related research: A scientometric analysis. https://core.ac.uk/download/16213823.pdf (accessed on 14th July 2025).

21. Hahladakis, J. N., Velis, C. A., Weber, R., Iacovidou, E., & Purnell, P. (2017). An overview of chemical additives presents in plastics: Migration, release, fate and environmental impact during their use, disposal and recycling. *Journal of Hazardous Materials, 344*, 179–199. https://doi.org/10.1016/j.jhazmat.2017.10.014 (accessed on 14th July 2025).

22. Jablonski, R., Musham, C., & Trettin, L. (1999). Genetic monitoring in the workplace: A tool not a solution. https://core.ac.uk/download/72056451.pdf (accessed on 14th July 2025).

23. Karanika-Murray, M., & Weyman, A. K. (2013). Optimizing workplace interventions for health and wellbeing: A commentary on the limitations of the public health perspective within the workplace health arena [forthcoming]. https://core.ac.uk/download/30633930.pdf (accessed on 14th July 2025).

24. Ko, S. (2025). Perspectives from the new president of the Korean Society of Occupational and Environmental Medicine: Future strategies for occupational and environmental medicine. *Annals of Occupational and Environmental Medicine, 37*. https://www.semanticscholar.org/paper/61cc9c30305fde9edf40134bc9371cf82746602d (accessed on 14th July 2025).

25. Lai, H., Hu, C., Qu, M., Liu, X., Xue, Y., Xu, P., & Hao, D. (2023). Mesothelioma due to workplace exposure: A comprehensive bibliometric analysis of current situation and future trends. *International Journal of Environmental Research and Public Health, 20*. https://www.semanticscholar.org/paper/81ecc37decad93c0d58a2e29d7f12f6ab17b9588 (accessed on 14th July 2025).

26. Lethbridge, J. (2008). Occupational health regulations and health workers: Protection or vulnerability? https://core.ac.uk/download/67329.pdf (accessed on 14th July 2025).

27. Lungu, K., Morse, T., & Taulo, S. (2010). Gap analysis of environmental health research in Malawi: Report to the National Commission of Science and Technology. https://core.ac.uk/download/19610167.pdf (accessed on 14th July 2025).

28. McIntyre, A., & Tempest, S. (2007). Two steps forward, one step back? A commentary on the disease-specific core sets of the International Classification of Functioning, Disability and Health (ICF). https://core.ac.uk/download/335602.pdf (accessed on 14th July 2025).

29. Naweed, A., & Chapman, J. (2015). Health initiatives to target obesity in surface transport industries: Review and implications for action. https://core.ac.uk/download/pdf/30671333.pdf (accessed on 14th July 2025).

30. Orr, R. M., Pope, R., & Tomes, C. (2017). The impact of body armor on physical performance of law enforcement personnel: A systematic review. https://core.ac.uk/download/196605080.pdf (accessed on 14th July 2025).

31. Pouliakas, K., & Theodossiou, I. (2010). An inquiry into the theory, causes and consequences of monitoring indicators of health and safety at work. https://core.ac.uk/download/177141.pdf (accessed on 14th July 2025).

32. Rovira Puig, M., Mbonaga, S. S., Seco, J., & Chacha, N. (2024). P-453 Assessing gas emissions from fecal sludge fuel briquettes; good practices for tackling occupational safety and health concerns in Tanzania. *Occupational Medicine*. https://www.semanticscholar.org/paper/21bdc594b29c1e2a94a9ee8e66b85ff5b2664c35 (accessed on 14th July 2025).

33. Sharma, A., & Mandal, B. B. (2024). A critical assessment of boundary limits of health risks associated with WBV exposure based on field studies on LHD vehicles in Indian underground coal mines. *Indian Journal of Occupational and Environmental Medicine, 28*, 198–206. https://www.semanticscholar.org/paper/657517549f9e945622ffa4ecaa926b283860dfea (accessed on 14th July 2025).

34. Sutanti, Y. S. (2022). Message. *Acta Medica Philippina*. https://www.semanticscholar.org/paper/a1a54dbdf7784834dbd8709fe00dbe66cda221f9 (accessed on 14th July 2025).

REHABILITATION MEDICINE

12

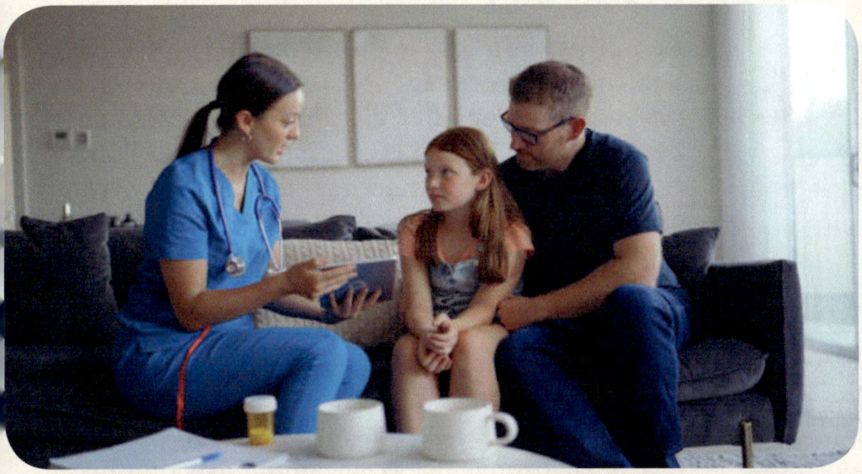

LEARNING OBJECTIVES

After studying this chapter, you will be able to:

1. Describe the types of rehabilitation
2. Understand the goals of rehabilitation medicine
3. Know the multidisciplinary approach in rehabilitation medicine
4. Describe the treatment modalities in rehabilitation medicine

Introduction

Rehabilitation medicine is a multi-disciplinary approach that attempts to improve the patient's quality of life with multiple disabilities or chronic illnesses. Rehabilitation medicine integrates the efforts of healthcare professionals such as physiatrists, occupational therapists, and rehabilitation nurses who pool their expertise to create patient-tailored interventions. Rehabilitation medicine is not merely a matter of restoring physical function but also maximizing emotional and social rehabilitation. By taking a comprehensive approach, rehabilitation practitioners collaborate with patients to create realistic, achievable goals that target independence and participation in activities of daily living. This patient-centered approach is critical to building resilience and enhancing outlook, which can significantly influence rehabilitation outcomes. Rehabilitation therapy not only requires clinical expertise but also empathetic understanding of the unique issues of rehabilitation patients, a departure from standard medicine that has a tendency to focus on curing diseases. A major component of rehabilitation medicine is the acceptance of standardized systems, such as the International Classification of Functioning, Disability and Health (ICF). The ICF provides a comprehensive model that enables health professionals to communicate effectively and ensure that all areas of a patient's health—physical, mental, and environmental—are addressed. According to the recent literature, the use of the ICF is in its infancy stage, especially in North America, where the uniform application of its concepts is minimal (Bruyere et al., 2005).

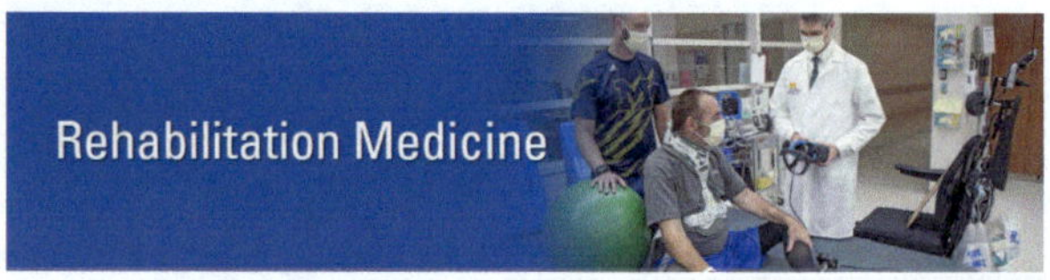

Figure 12.1. Rehabilitation medicine.

Source: https://www.uofmhealth.org/sites/default/files/rehabilitation_main.jpg.

This inconsistency emphasizes the importance of promoting awareness and provider education in optimal use of the ICF model. By shared language regarding function and disability, the ICF can foster collaboration among caregivers and enhance rehabilitation practice. With the rehab community increasingly adopting the ICF, ongoing research will be required to determine optimal practice for applying the model in practice settings. Culturally responsive rehabilitation practice is critical in addressing the diverse needs of patients with diverse backgrounds, particularly in the context of rising immigrant populations in the United States. Cultural perceptions of disability and health may influence patients' responses to rehabilitation interventions. For instance, providers must recognize that individuals with disabilities in other cultures may hold different assumptions and priorities that affect their engagement with health systems (Hasnain et al., 2008). Intercultural understanding between service providers and patients requires involvement to ensure better treatment outcomes. This awareness calls professionals to customize their practices to serve the specific needs of groups, for instance, Muslims with disabilities. By incorporating cultural competence into rehabilitation medicine, providers will be more likely to provide access to the relevant services, and thus quality of care and patient satisfaction will follow (Figure 12.1).

Importance of Rehabilitation in Healthcare

Rehabilitation is a fundamental part of healthcare because it supports not only physical recovery but also psychological well-being. Rehabilitation is a complex process and is extremely important for the patient with chronic disease, e.g., multiple sclerosis. Pain is a frequent and sometimes disabling symptom in this patient population that can have an intrusive impact on functioning and satisfaction with life and result in high levels of depression and anxiety. The use of cognitive-behavioral therapy (CBT) as part of rehabilitation models has been promising as an adjunctive therapy. Evidence indicates that such interventions might assist participants in reducing pain intensity and its impact on activities of daily living, along with addressing psychological distress simultaneously. By incorporating rehabilitation interventions that integrate physical and psychosocial therapy, healthcare providers can create an improved support system, thereby facilitating overall patient improvement and highlighting the importance of rehabilitation in delivering holistic care (Beauvais et al., 2019). Rehabilitation is also important in facilitating patient safety during transitions between different levels of care. Accurate medication reconciliation, particularly between skilled nursing facilities and acute care hospitals, is one of the cornerstones of good communication practices in rehabilitation. Inappropriate medication management upon transfer has been associated with increased risks for medical errors that yield adverse drug events, placing vulnerable groups at heightened risk. A quality improvement project determined the need to establish robust protocols that ensure precision in the medication administration record. By embracing systematic medication reconciliation processes, healthcare workers can reduce medication errors and, in the process, enhance patient safety, as evidenced by improved clinical outcomes. The practice is part of the recovery process, which not only entails healing but also patient wellness throughout medical treatment (Blake et al., 2017).

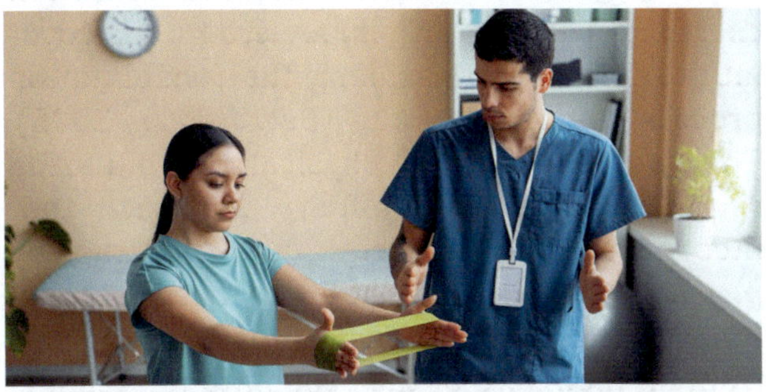

Figure 12.2. Importance of rehabilitation in healthcare.

Source: https://nursesgroup.co.uk/assets/images/blog/rehabilitation-types-uk.jpg.

The function of rehabilitation in medicine extends beyond patient treatment plans to encompass social comprehension of the collective problems of patient recovery. Effective rehabilitation programs restore not just function but also facilitate patients' return to society, thereby promoting social reintegration and overall quality of life. Rehabilitation programs incorporating physical therapy along with psychosocial intervention are central in addressing the physical as well as the emotional challenges of the patients. Furthermore, through interdisciplinary partnerships, rehabilitation professionals can tailor interventions to unique patient needs, which, in turn, results in independence and self-efficacy. Not only does this combined approach advantage patients, but it also pressures healthcare systems as it enhances patient satisfaction and reduces readmission into the hospital. Hence, rehabilitation is a necessary component of contemporary health care as a unifying journey between disease and wellness that facilitates health equity and community integration (Figure 12.2).

12.1. Types of Rehabilitation

Learning Outcome

1. Understand the physical rehabilitation
2. Understand the occupational rehabilitation
3. Describe the speech and language rehabilitation

Rehabilitation medicine encompasses various modalities tailored to patients' needs across physical, cognitive, and emotional dimensions. The most common mode is physical rehabilitation, which is employed primarily to rehabilitate musculoskeletal trauma, neurological conditions, and surgery. Therapeutic exercises, manual therapy, and modalities such as ultrasound and electrical stimulation are the techniques of first choice. Ideal physical rehabilitation aims to restore mobility and function, treat pain, and prevent further harm. Recent advances in knowledge of neuroplasticity—our brains' ability to reorganize itself—have had a profound impact on the practice of physical rehabilitation. Given the implications set forth in recent discussions, the implementation of evidence-based treatments rather than traditional models has been critical to achieving optimal patient outcomes in the discipline (Scheets et al., 2020). Cognitive rehabilitation is also an essential aspect of rehabilitation medicine, but more precisely focused on assisting patients with brain injuries, strokes, or degenerative diseases that impair cognitive abilities such as memory, attention, and problem-solving. Treatment can include cognitive training, compensation methods, and environmental modifications to improve activities of daily living. The evidence attesting to the efficacy of cognitive rehabilitation underscores the necessity for treatment programs tailored to the individual's specific cognitive impairments and daily difficulties. With growing research emphasizing the promise of cognitive rehabilitation, clinicians in the field are increasingly adopting evidence-based methods that are designed to maximize patient quality of life through the integration of rehabilitation into routine care (Hill et al., 2020). Emotional rehabilitation is also necessary, addressing the psychological impacts of illness and trauma. Patients who have suffered physical trauma usually develop emotional setbacks such as depression, anxiety, and low self-esteem, which can interfere with their rehabilitation. Therapeutic interventions such as counseling, support groups, and behavioral therapy help patients recover from these emotional challenges and provide a holistic rehabilitation process. The recognition of mental health as inseparable from physical recovery has spawned an increasingly comprehensive model of rehabilitation based on the significance of interdisciplinary collaboration between medicine, psychology, and social services. As rehabilitation medicine has evolved, the combination of emotional and mental health care with rehabilitation programs is paramount in helping to foster overall recovery in patients with complex, multifaceted problems (Scheets et al., 2020) (Figure 12.3).

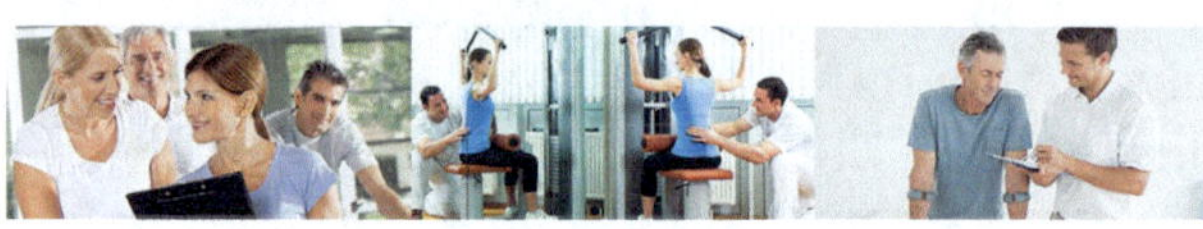

Figure 12.3. Types of rehabilitation.

Source: https://blog.rehabselect.net/hs-fs/hub/281126/file-591641784-jpg/Website/BlogBannerRS.jpg?width=1440&name=BlogBannerRS.jpg.

12.1.1. Physical Rehabilitation

Physical rehabilitation is a key component of rehabilitation medicine, serving as a transitional step from injury or disease to restored function. It is a wide-ranging set of interventions aimed at augmenting a patient's physical function, thereby promoting independence and improving quality of life. In recent years, technological advancements have enabled the implementation of new rehabilitative techniques, including the development of tailored equipment tailored to individual therapeutic needs. The development of programs like Music Maker illustrates how technology can assist individuals with physical disabilities in regaining motor functions through encouraging and innovative ways. With the integration of music into rehabilitation exercises, patients are empowered to discover motivation and joy, making the rehabilitation process effective and fun (Betke et al., 2005). The sophistication of physical rehabilitation requires a multidisciplinary approach that incorporates interdisciplinary working by physical therapists, occupational therapists, and other medical professionals. Different expertise from all members of the rehabilitation team is brought to assess and treat patients' various needs. Physical rehabilitation is particularly essential for patients who are recovering from surgery, stroke, or trauma, where regaining function may be a lengthy process. Individually tailored interventions that are based on specific rehabilitation goals have been shown to reduce recovery time and enhance outpatient outcomes. Furthermore, hospital services such as physical medicine and rehabilitation indicate that economies of scale can contribute to the effectiveness and efficiency of care delivery (Barros et al., 2025). Through the ongoing advancement of these services, health systems can deliver improved patient outcomes and experiences. The integration of new approaches into physical rehabilitation can be highly effective in therapy. As new therapeutic modalities evolve, therapists must stay current with developments to optimize patient care. The use of technology, for example, camera-based systems that translate body movements into music, is the further development of rehabilitation aides. Not only do these interdisciplinary aides provide sensory feedback directly to patients, but they can also be systematically measured for their impact on recovery processes. This is associated with the necessity of continuous evaluation of the rehabilitation process; studying outcomes allows healthcare providers to adjust interventions appropriately. A patient-centered paradigm ultimately facilitates maximal recovery of physical function but is also associated with global well-being and sustainable health (Betke et al., 2005) (Figure 12.4).

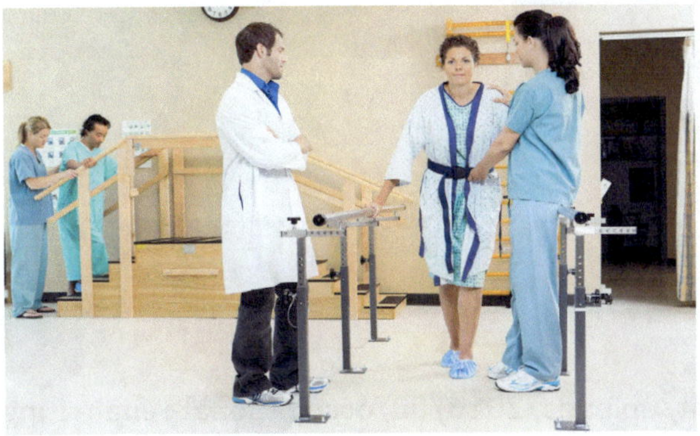

Figure 12.4. Physical rehabilitation.

Source: https://sukinohealthcare.com/wp-content/uploads/2023/06/Physical-Rehabilitation.webp.

12.1.2. Occupational Rehabilitation

Occupational rehabilitation is a necessary component of rehabilitation medicine with the goal of facilitating individuals' return to work and activities of daily living following recovery from injury or illness. It encompasses a variety of interventions, including assessments, adaptation strategies, and skill learning, designed to facilitate individuals' return to their functional potential. One of the distinguishing characteristics of occupational rehabilitation is the use of standardized tests, which provide objective measures of patients' progress and direct tailoring of rehabilitation protocols. In particular, movement-based tests such as the Berg and Fugl-Meyer Assessment have been found to be valuable tools for establishing baseline levels and tracking improvement. However, research has indicated that occupational therapists, unlike their physical therapy counterparts, make less use of these assessments, and that the problem with their proper use and impact on patient outcomes stems from this (Bosch et al., 2019). Occupational therapists' role in meeting both patient and caregiver needs is naturally intertwined with successful occupational rehabilitation. Family caregivers of stroke survivors often struggle after discharge, describing themselves as not being adequately prepared to deal with the changed caregiving rhythms. Occupational therapists are uniquely qualified to assess and respond to these unmet caregiver needs, which has been shown to enhance patient outcomes overall. While therapists understand the importance of formal caregiver assessment, they employ informal methods due to systemic barriers such as pressure on productivity and compensation rates that are too low. All these problems must be handled because the utilization of robust caregiver assessment tools introduced can make assistance more inclusive in the rehabilitation process (Clymer et al., 2020). Lastly, closer integration between occupational rehabilitation and caregiver readiness enhances the overall impact of rehabilitation medicine. Moreover, technological advances and the internet are revolutionizing the landscape of occupational rehabilitation. Therapists are increasingly using electronic media to reference a series of standardized measurements and interventions that may enhance the value of their clinical work. The acclamation of internet-based resources has been keenly felt in the field of stroke rehabilitation, with therapists employing these resources frequently to acquire more information and improve patient care. The Rehabilitation Measures Database is a goldmine for monitoring and understanding standardized measures, for instance. However, while such resources have been helpful, their use is uneven across physical and occupational therapists.

This shortage can potentially restrict the optimization of occupational rehabilitation practice and underscores the need for a systemic overhaul toward a more standardized process for harnessing assessments by profession (Bosch et al., 2019). In light of continued advances in rehabilitation medicine, greater cooperation and cross-professional information sharing will be crucial to ensuring optimal patient outcomes in occupational rehabilitation (Figure 12.5).

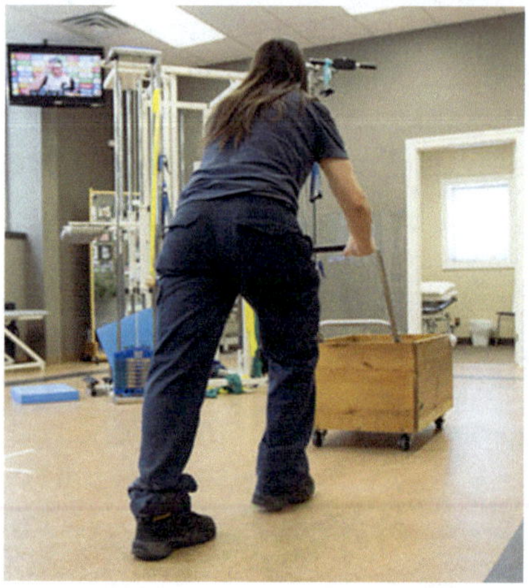

Figure 12.5. Occupational rehabilitation.

Source: https://www.totalphysiotherapy.ca/wp-content/uploads/2016/08/occupational-rehab-1.jpg.

12.1.3. Speech and Language Rehabilitation

Speech and language rehabilitation is one of the most important clinical fields in rehabilitation medicine, particularly for patients recovering from neurological diseases. The latter tend to impair motor skills, language, and cognition, which can drastically interfere with communication abilities. Due to improvements in rehabilitation, the use of noninvasive brain stimulation techniques, such as transcranial direct current stimulation and transcranial magnetic stimulation, is increasingly popular. Recent studies indicate that such neuromodulation devices can potentially augment traditional treatments and therefore improve speech-language pathology outcomes. Second, the complexity of applying the techniques in the clinical setting highlights the need for standardization across methodologies, patient groups, and treatment parameters to effectively translate the benefits of higher technology into actual gains in rehabilitation (Sebastian et al., 2023). Music therapy has also emerged as an advanced approach to speech and language rehabilitation, with particularly high promise for cochlear implant patients. Research conducted between 2016 and 2021 identifies the utility of music therapy in optimizing auditory rehabilitation for these patients. By the inclusion of sound-musical activities in speech therapy interventions, therapists have observed considerable progress not only in music-related aspects of auditory perception but also in oral language comprehension following implantation. This indicates that systematic, incremental auditory rehabilitation can yield large gains in frequency and phonological discrimination, resulting in improved quality-of-life measures among patients. The addition of holistic methods, such as music therapy, demonstrates the multidimensional range of practices employed in rehabilitation for speech and language disorders (Fuentes et al., 2022). The addition of traditional and emerging practices demonstrates a multifaceted conceptualization of speech and language rehabilitation in practice today. While traditional approaches focus on one-on-one formal speech therapy sessions based on the patient's needs, newer advancements like noninvasive brain stimulation and music therapy offer extra benefits. As rehabilitation medicine continues to advance, evidence-based practice must be emphasized, and therapists must be provided with a robust armamentarium in managing speech and language impairments. Lastly, an integrative treatment program that combines diverse methods can maximize patient rehabilitation, facilitating greater overall improvement in communication and quality of life. Integrated, such as this, underscores the dynamic nature of rehabilitation medicine, where interprofessional collaboration can offer unique solutions to problems arising from speech and language interruption (Figure 12.6).

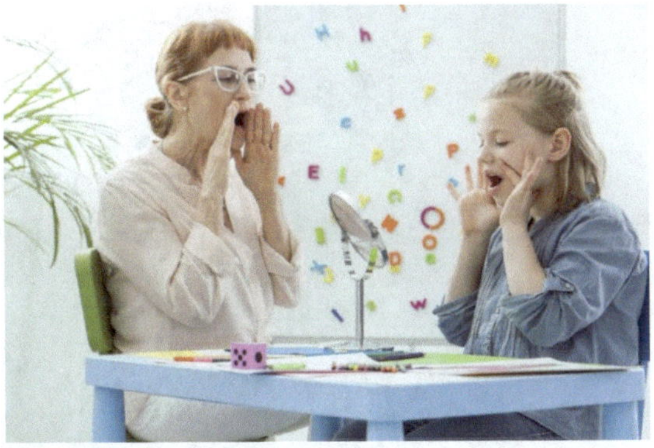

Figure 12.6. Speech and language rehabilitation.

Source: https://wellknox.com/wp-content/uploads/2022/12/Speech-therapy-rehabilitation-center-for-childrens.webp.

Test Your Knowledge

1. What is physical rehabilitation?
2. What is occupational rehabilitation?

12.2. Goals of Rehabilitation Medicine

Learning Outcome

1. Understand the restoration of function in rehabilitation medicine
2. Describe the role of rehabilitation in the improvement of quality of life and the prevention of further disability

The overall goals of rehabilitation medicine are to restore function, support independence, and enhance quality of life in patients recovering from injury, illness, or disability. Most prominent among these goals is the emphasis on individualized care, with treatment strategies tailored to each patient's unique needs. Rehabilitation begins with a complete evaluation that not only establishes the patient's medical background and physical abilities but also considers psychosocial determinants that affect rehabilitation. Functional goals are then individualized and made realistic and achievable, which enhances motivation and active involvement throughout the course of rehabilitation. By knowing the personal needs and aspirations of the patients, rehabilitation professionals can create an environment where they can continue striving for recovery (Computational and Methods in Medicine, 2023). Another significant goal of rehabilitation medicine is to enable patients to be readmitted to their community and daily life. That is not physical recovery alone; it also addresses the emotional and social facets of health. Enhancing patients' level of functioning is fundamental to enabling them to participate in activities that are meaningful to them, whether at home, at work, or in social life.

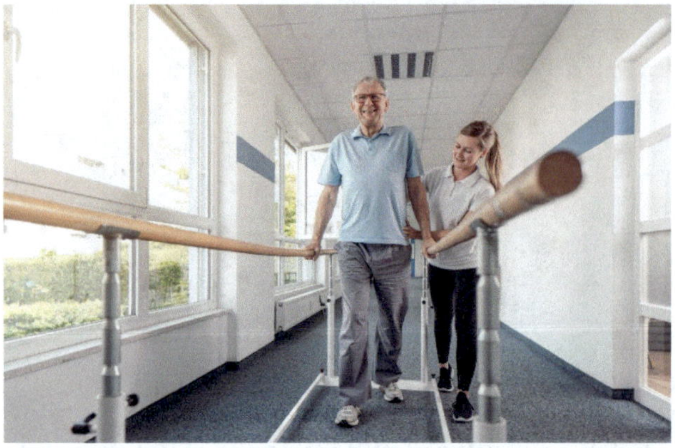

Figure 12.7. Goals of rehabilitation.

Source: https://kingstonresidenceofperrysburg.com/wp-content/uploads/sites/3/2024/08/What-Is-The-Goal-Of-Rehabilitation-Hero.jpg.

For instance, certain therapy interventions aimed at facilitation of mobility or communication can be a significant factor towards changing a patient's level of independence and satisfaction. Further, the development of relationships, stimulation of community activity, and the provision of adequate resources are critical in the pursuit of long-term health outcomes. The importance of a positive social network cannot be overstated, as it is key to the long-term effectiveness of rehabilitation programs and helps prevent feelings of depression or loneliness among patients (O'Brien et al., 2022). The application of advanced technology in rehabilitation medicine also plays a central role in its success. The use of wearable technology and movement sensors enhances the accuracy and effectiveness of rehabilitation therapy by providing real-time feedback on a patient's improvement. For example, studies have indicated that adding wearable motion-sensor feedback can improve predictions of post-stroke ambulatory capacity. By using machine learning algorithms to analyze biomechanical data, clinicians can plan more targeted treatments tailored to customized recovery patterns. This new approach not only supplements traditional rehabilitation models but also enables clinicians to set more realistic and well-informed objectives for their patients. Lastly, technological advancement and patient-centered care in rehabilitation medicine join forces to transform recovery outcomes and individualize the rehabilitation process (O'Brien et al., 2022) (Figure 12.7).

12.2.1. Restoration of Function

Rehabilitation of function in rehabilitation medicine is a multifaceted process that involves physical and neurological intervention aimed at recovery after injury, such as stroke, spinal cord injury, or head injury. Traditionally defined as a static phase after injury, recent research suggests that recovery is not only possible but can produce miraculous improvements in motor function. Neurobiological research has highlighted the exploitation of the nervous system's regenerative capacity through diverse strategies to enhance functional recovery. For instance, novel neuro-engineering techniques, such as brain-machine interfaces, are being developed to address gaps caused by lesions and restore motor function.

This interdisciplinary approach emphasizes that restoration of function is not just a matter of physical therapy but also requires a well-rounded understanding of the neurological mechanisms of recovery and how multiple rehabilitation approaches can be applied synergistically to optimize patient outcomes (Edgerton et al., 2016). Interest has emerged over the past several years regarding the role of low-frequency oscillatory (LFO) activity in the primary motor cortex in skilled motor ability. Experiments have identified that restoration of these oscillatory dynamics after stroke is necessary to achieve maximal recovery. Observational data indicate that diminished LFOs are associated with impaired motor capacity in animal models as well as stroke-afflicted human patients. Notably, with spontaneous recovery, LFO activity in the perilesional cortex has also normalized in parallel. These findings suggest that neuromodulation of cortical oscillatory patterning is an interesting candidate for neuromodulation treatments to regain upper-limb function.

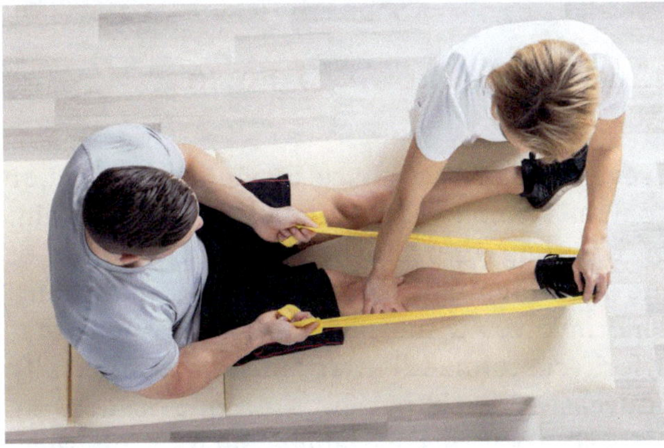

Figure 12.8. Functional restoration program for recovery.

Source: https://www.advantagehcs.com/wp-content/uploads/2022/11/func-res-big-img.jpg.

Thus, integrating this information into rehabilitation protocols can significantly enhance the effectiveness of interventions and provide patients with additional opportunities for functional recovery (Berényi et al., 2018). Effective rehabilitation requires a multi-modal treatment plan that includes physical, cognitive, and neuromodulatory treatments. Task-oriented rehabilitation combined with neurofeedback appears to promote neural connectivity and enhance motor function recovery. Particularly, interventions that are consistent with the body's own neural intentions and aligned with cortical function can enhance the brain's capacity to change and reorganize. The dynamic interplay between conscious action and neural repair is one area of investigation, but it too underscores the necessity of patient involvement in the rehabilitation process. By integrating an array of methodologies, ranging from cellular neuronal repair strategies to sophisticated neurorehabilitative practices, clinicians can develop tailored plans that suit the individual needs of the patient. As science advances, the challenge remains how these new approaches can be woven together into concerted rehabilitation programs that achieve maximal restoration of function across a wide variety of patient populations (Edgerton et al., 2016) (Figure 12.8).

12.2.2. Improvement of Quality of Life

The process of rehabilitation medicine significantly enhances the life span of patients with physical disability due to a wide range of diseases. Rehabilitation medicine emphasizes an integrative approach that combines physical therapy, occupational therapy, and psychosocial guidance. Rehabilitation tailored to the patient's individual needs maximizes the effectiveness and applicability of interventions. It has been shown that successful rehabilitation restores physical function but also improves mental health and social interaction. The multi-dimensionality of rehabilitation, for example, the significance of nutrition and medication management, also contributes significantly to patients' quality of life. Reducing drug-induced functional impairments by proper pharmacotherapy in older patients further optimizes outcomes of recovery. With an eye on both psychological and physical etiology, rehabilitation medicine aims to optimize patients' independence, enhancing their ability to perform daily activities and quality of life (Yoshimura et al., 2022). Cardiovascular disease (CVD) is one of the biggest threats to quality of life, and successful rehabilitation methods aimed at recovery and prevention are a necessity. As the leading global cause of death, ischemic heart disease and stroke impose a vast burden on patients' daily activity, causing extra disability-adjusted life years and reduced well-being. CVD rehabilitation typically consists of exercise training, nutritional counseling, and ongoing medical care. Not only do these treatments result in recovery of physical capacity, but they also assist in educating patients about lifestyle change, reducing the likelihood of recurrent negative events.

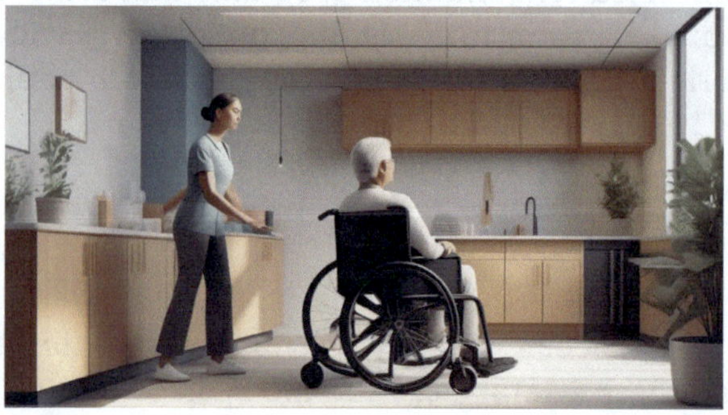

Figure 12.9. Rehabilitation techniques for improved quality of life.

Source: https://cdn.prod.website-files.com/6300a3e1148cfc395accfea9/660b7da735de51fcfd5df05d_post-15.webp.

With the growing burden of CVD, rehabilitation must evolve to cater to this population of patients. Spending on intensive rehabilitation interventions can reverse the disease-related destruction, support recovery, and significantly improve quality of life by enhancing physical function and psychological resilience (Roth et al., 2020). Also, implementation of a multidisciplinary model in rehabilitation medicine is needed to facilitate continuous enhancement of quality of life. Interdisciplinary collaboration among healthcare professionals—physicians, pharmacists, physical therapists, and nutritionists—is needed to ensure that all aspects of a patient's recovery are taken into account. It is particularly important in the treatment of complex cases with comorbidities and medication-related complications. Evidence shows that rehabilitation is enhanced by a pharmacist-led model, maximizing therapeutic interventions and improving medication safety, leading to improved health outcomes. By focusing on medication management alongside physical rehabilitation, health teams can greatly improve patients' activities of daily living and overall well-being. The goal remains the same: to empower patients through customized rehabilitation regimes, thereby facilitating long-term improvements in their quality of life and, ultimately, better health and autonomy (Yoshimura et al., 2022) (Figure 12.9).

12.2.3. Prevention of Further Disability

Prevention of secondary disability is a major goal in rehabilitation medicine with the aim of bringing improvement in the quality of life in individuals with existing impairment. This involves a multidisciplinary system that offers customized interventions specifically addressing each patient's unique issues. By assessing various variables, such as physical, psychological, and social environments, health practitioners can design individualized rehabilitation interventions that support recovery of function and independence.

It is believed that early intervention following an event of disability, such as stroke or trauma, significantly reduces the occurrence of secondary complications and further deterioration of health status. These preventive measures not only enhance chances of recovery but also confer resilience upon the patients and caregivers, creating an atmosphere of healing and readjustment. Additionally, emerging evidence indicates that metabolic and inflammatory factors are primary mediators of disability avoidance.

Specifically, comorbid conditions like obesity have the impact of expediting the onset of disabling diseases in a vicious cycle, which is difficult to break. For instance, a recent paper outlined distinct profiles in at-risk obese individuals that were characterized by increased comorbidities and widespread functional deficits. By clustering patients, clinicians can target effective interventions specifically tailored to reverse these risks, both against obesity and its complementary barriers such as sarcopenia, depression, and chronic inflammation. Addressing these co-occurring causes holistically can lead to improved outcomes and ensure a holistic approach to preventing further disability in at-risk groups (Carretero-Gómez et al., 2022). In addition, the integration of novel therapeutic modalities, such as rehabilitation technologies, holds the promise of complementing traditional rehabilitation techniques.

Technologies such as tele-rehabilitation, wearable technology, and gamified interventions enable real-time monitoring and adaptation of rehabilitation programs, providing patients with greater autonomy and control over their recovery. These technologies can potentially implement self-management strategies that encourage patients to take an active role in their own health, thereby improving adherence to rehabilitation protocols. Further, the development of therapies targeting molecular mechanisms of disability avoidance has the potential to revolutionize paradigms for treatment in rehabilitation medicine. The potential of such technologies to strike at fundamental cellular processes engaged in recovery makes it increasingly important that continuous research and realignment of clinical practice take place to prevent further disability as well as to enable optimal function in recuperating individuals from incapacitating disease (Chen et al., 2024) (Figure 12.10).

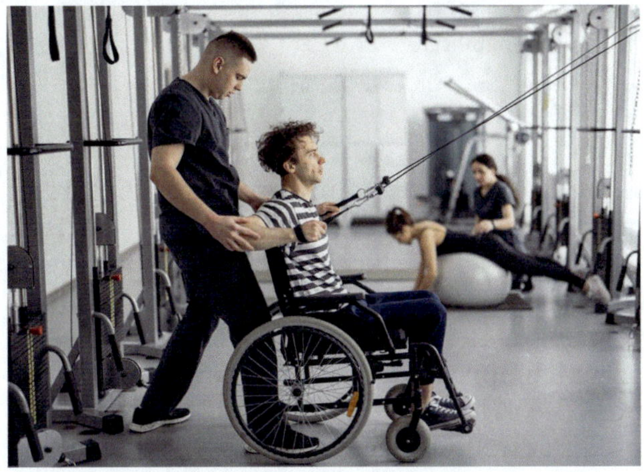

Figure 12.10. Physical disability.

Source: https://leafcare.co.uk/alovoocm/uploads/2022/12/Physical-Disability-1024x683.jpg.

Test Your Knowledge

1. What is the restoring function?
2. What is the role of rehabilitation in disability?

12.3. Multidisciplinary Approach

Learning Outcome

1. Describe the role of physicians in rehabilitation
2. Understand the involvement of therapists in the rehabilitation process
3. Understand the importance of support staff in rehabilitation medicine

A multidisciplinary approach in rehabilitation medicine is central to better patient outcomes, particularly with stroke recovery. In a healthcare system where specialists collaborate to share their domains of knowledge, more comprehensive, tailored care becomes possible. The literature identifies that HCPs prefer accredited, classroom-based educational interventions but also recognize the necessity for hybrid approaches to both uni- and multidisciplinary requirements. Specifically, stroke unit professionals express a high level of interest in assuming leadership roles within the multidisciplinary team, with a focus on teamwork as the linchpin of rehabilitation (Craig et al., 2008). Through a forum that provides opportunities for HCPs to share expertise and gain advanced skills, a multidisciplinary strategy will ultimately translate into more effective stroke treatment and a better understanding of patients' holistic needs. In addition, integrating models such as the International Classification of Functioning, Disability and Health (ICF) into neurorehabilitation is a step in the right direction toward implementing multidisciplinary practice. This international model, though widely accepted, requires careful local adaptation to meet local service needs before becoming an effective key to enhancing practice. Stroke and neurorehabilitation literature recognizes at least 35 diverse applications of the ICF in clinical practice, unveiling its potential to advance HCPs' communication and establish team roles. In action research, participants have noted that employing the ICF encourages holistic thinking and enables clinicians to discuss a patient's recovery process in its entirety (Jefferson et al., 2015). The intermingling of several professionals through a structured platform like the ICF is the quintessence of the success of multidisciplinary approaches in rehabilitation medicine. Ultimately, proper execution of a multidisciplinary approach in rehabilitation medicine relies on continuous education and collaboration among medical teams. Because research demonstrates that training interests differ across professions and demand the development of educational models that produce shared information and professional knowledge, HCPs may focus on multidisciplinary education to take up a broader set of competencies and become more familiar with how social, emotional, and physical factors influence rehabilitation outcomes. Having accepted that multidisciplinary team working is conducive to good stroke care, health systems must strive to establish an education and training system conducive to this approach. As has been observed in more recent studies, bridging such education gaps and facilitating interprofessional working across various categories of health professionals can make a big impact towards enhancing the quality of care provided to patients in rehabilitation settings (Craig et al., 2008).

12.3.1. Role of Physicians in Rehabilitation

The role of physicians in rehabilitation medicine is multifaceted, comprising clinical evaluation, planning, and multidisciplinary coordination. Physicians are central figures who assess patients' physical and psychological conditions to develop a comprehensive understanding of their rehabilitation needs. The initial evaluation is pivotal in designing individualized treatment plans that are proportional to each patient's individual circumstances. Furthermore, doctors have a duty to coordinate interventions with various healthcare professionals, such as occupational therapists, physical therapists, and psychologists. This is a team model that ensures all aspects of a patient's recovery are catered for, making it a healing- and functional improvement-conducive environment. The doctors are also the team leaders who monitor progress and adjust treatment plans as needed to ensure optimal results and prevent relapses. Apart from performing their clinical functions, physicians are also supposed to recognize and address psychological obstacles that may hinder a patient's rehabilitation. Research has noted the significance of factors such as fear of re-injury, particularly following procedures such as ACLR, where psychological health would play an important part in the recovery rate. The identification of these psychological factors is important because quite a few athletes, having physically recovered, will struggle with returning to previous activity levels owing to persisting fears. By including psychological assessment in rehabilitation plans, doctors can better match interventions to address patients' emotional and mental health alongside their physical recovery. This integrated approach not only improves the outcomes of rehabilitation but also develops a stronger patient-physician bond, optimizing trust and cooperation in the rehabilitative process (Mcveigh et al., 2015). Furthermore, the evolving nature of rehabilitation medicine demands that physicians remain up to date on the latest evidence and best practices. Ongoing professional development through literature review and adherence to updated guidelines ensures that clinicians practice with the most effective rehabilitation methods. For instance, recent updates to evidence-based guidelines have highlighted trends and inequalities in critical illness rehabilitation, necessitating an examination of care protocols. The application of such evidence in practice has the potential to significantly enhance the quality of rehabilitation care provided to patients convalescing from a variety of ailments, including those requiring intensive critical care (Gibson et al., 2010). By staying current with the latest research discoveries and through dedication to ongoing education, physicians can maximize rehabilitation outcomes, ensuring patients receive care based on today's best standards (Figure 12.11).

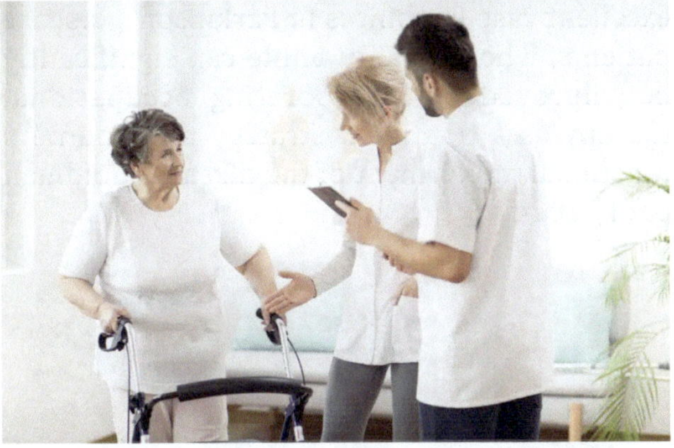

Figure 12.11. Role of physicians in rehabilitation.

Source: https://wp05.cdn.ihealthspot.com/wp-content/uploads/sites/30/2019/11/iStock-1147159539-1024x683.jpeg.webp.

12.3.2. Involvement of Therapists (Physical, Occupational, Speech)

The work of physical, occupational, and speech therapists plays a pivotal role in the rehab process, significantly enhancing patient outcomes across various settings due to injury, illness, or disability. Each discipline of therapy has various approaches unique to the requirements of patients. Physical therapists, for instance, focus on maintaining mobility and function. They use concentrated workouts and modalities to improve strength and stamina, as required for patients whose physical abilities have been threatened, as evidenced by return-to-work rehabilitation protocols among cancer survivors, where experts effectively collaborate to enable a patient to return to work (Teramatsu et al., 2024). This inter-disciplinary process not only assists in the return of physical functioning but also fosters patient confidence, enabling more effective integration into activities of daily living and work places. Occupational therapy is also significant, as it aims to help individuals perform daily activities important to them. Therapists assess patients' individual needs and develop tailored interventions to improve functioning in daily tasks at work or at home. An excellent case in point is in Parkinson's disease patients, whose quality of life can significantly be improved by incorporating occupational therapy as a treatment strategy that counters functional impairment of the disease (Goldman et al., 2024).

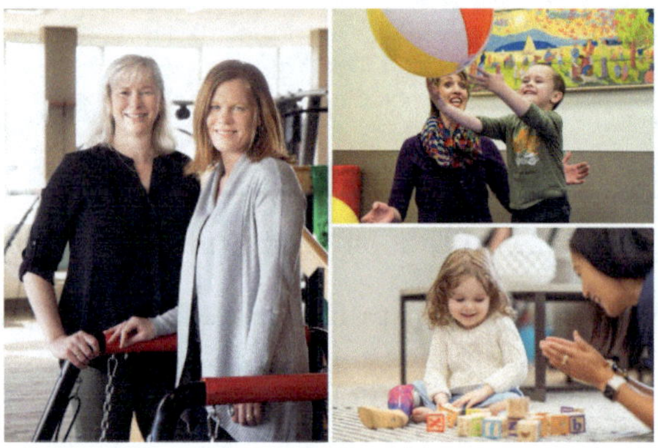

Figure 12.12. Exploring the three disciplines of rehabilitation therapy: physical, occupational and speech therapy.

Source: https://islandhealth.org/wp-content/uploads/2024/05/blog-size-graphics17.jpg.

By further fostering independence-building skills, occupational therapy allows the person to redevelop their ability to work and play and offers a comprehensive recovery process that advances beyond physical rehabilitation. Speech therapy assists these efforts by addressing communicative and swallowing abilities that are often impaired by neurological or physical trauma. It is focused on issues that can arise as a direct consequence of certain conditions, such as stroke or disabling diseases like multiple sclerosis. Speech therapists apply various techniques to develop articulation, fluency, and cognitive skills for communication, thereby facilitating effective work and social relationships. The communication among physical, occupational, and speech therapists creates a comprehensive rehabilitation process that empowers patients in a multidimensional manner. This integrated approach, in addition to enhancing recovery, fosters an enabling environment that empowers people with the resources needed to complete their rehab and regain independence. Their independence in the workplace and daily living is also regained (Goldman et al., 2024) (Figure 12.12).

12.3.3. Importance of Support Staff (Nurses, Social Workers)

The role of support staff, including nurses and social workers, cannot be overstated in rehabilitation medicine. These are the backbone of the health care system, delivering care that is not only compassionate but also clinically expert. Nurses, for instance, play a pivotal role in the day-to-day management of patients, reviewing vital signs, writing prescriptions, and coordinating general patient care. Their consistent presence ensures that the rehabilitation process is not only effective but also tailored to the specific needs of individual patients, thereby enhancing recovery outcomes. Additionally, training courses that organizations undertake ensure that the incorporation of best practices in infection prevention and antimicrobial stewardship is integral to all their work, with immediate impact on the safety and effectiveness of rehabilitation interventions (Fleming et al., 2025). By doing so, nurses can adapt their practice to evolving healthcare demands and patient expectations, making their services valuable in rehabilitation settings. Social workers play a vital role in addressing the psychological and social barriers patients face during rehabilitation. Their background in making IDT member communication effective ensures that families and patients are active stakeholders in the care process within a recovery-supportive work environment. This importance is further supported by evidence showing that pre-meeting engagement and participation in family meetings are critical to successful rehabilitation outcomes (Donnelly et al., 2024). Social workers not only advocate for patient-centered interventions but also relate medical treatment to emotional care, settling issues such as mental illness, economic struggles, and family dynamics.

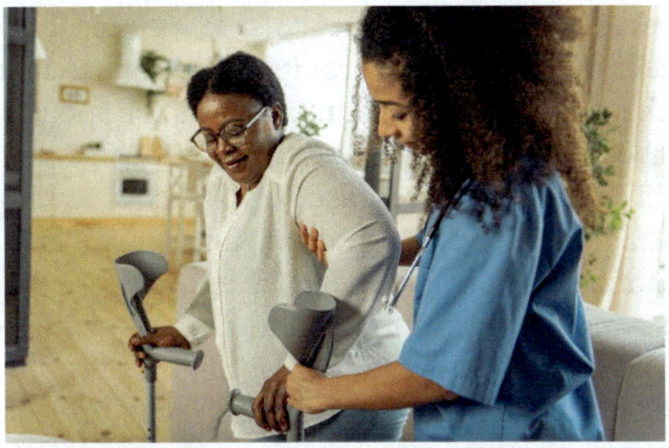

Figure 12.13. Role of the rehabilitation nurse.

Source: https://www.myamericannurse.com/wp-content/uploads/2024/02/shutterstock_1705398322-Rehabilitation-Nursing-scaled.jpg.

Their complete understanding of these interconnected aspects triggers more effective rehabilitation strategies, ultimately contributing to an improved holistic model of patient care that actually enhances the rehabilitation process. The integration of support staff, such as nurses and social workers, into rehabilitation medicine further expands the scope of individualized care plans. In their participation alongside physicians and therapists, they provide helpful input on patient progress and support the team-based recovery process. For example, the application of mandated family meetings by social workers can improve communication and collaborative decision-making, thereby further involving patients in their own rehabilitation. This not only empowers the family but also creates a sense of community support that can enhance motivation and adherence to rehabilitation guidelines (Donnelly et al., 2024). Furthermore, ongoing training and education for such roles, as promoted in recent initiatives, create a culture of continuous enhancement in rehabilitation settings. These collaborative efforts are central to creating a more integrated patient care experience in rehabilitation medicine, with a focus on the value of support staff in achieving total healthcare outcomes (Figure 12.13).

Test Your Knowledge

1. What is the role of physicians in rehabilitation?
2. What is the importance of support staff in rehabilitation medicine?

12.4. Treatment Modalities

Learning Outcome

1. Describe the therapeutic exercises and physical therapy
2. Know the assistive devices and technology
3. Discuss the psychological support and counseling in rehabilitation medicine

Treatment modalities in rehabilitation medicine encompass a broad array of techniques used to restore function and mitigate pain following disease or injury. Physical therapy, one of the oldest of these modalities, uses techniques such as manual therapy, exercise, and modalities like ultrasound and electrical stimulation to enable recovery. These modalities offer practitioners the versatility to tailor intervention to the specific needs of the patient, thus optimizing therapeutic results. Furthermore, the application of technology, such as telehealth and virtual reality, has altered the delivery of these therapies, leading to greater access and patient engagement. With advances in biomechanical understanding and patient-specific conditions, rehabilitation professionals can now create more effective and precise programs that maximize healing and prevent future harm, as outlined in new models of sports medicine. Rehabilitative innovative approaches extend beyond bodily treatments and encompass modalities such as pharmacologic intervention and psychological support. Pharmacologic interventions include anti-inflammatory medications, painkillers, and supplemental treatments that help reduce pain and facilitate physical rehabilitation. Psychological support, aside from these interventions, has been an important component of treatment regimens, particularly for individuals who are undergoing chronic pain or extended recovery processes. The psychological aspect of rehabilitation cannot be overestimated, as psychological resilience directly impacts physical outcomes. The interactive nature of physical and psychological treatment methodologies underscores the multidimensional nature of rehabilitation medicine, where interdisciplinary care leads to integrated healing and improved quality of life for the patient. Emphasis on this harmonized conception accords with the upcoming trends in rehabilitation, pointing to the expansion of comprehension concerning the patient's overall state of affairs. The role of evidence-based protocols to rehabilitation medicine cannot be overemphasized, particularly in the case of treatment modalities for sport and active clients. Sports medicine protocols outline disciplined, evidence-based approaches to injury management, rehabilitation, and performance optimization. Strict adherence to these protocols ensures that treatment methods are grounded in the most up-to-date research and tailored to each athlete's individual needs. These protocols generally combine treatment modalities, including physical therapy, strength training, and preventive measures. What is important is that the application of sports medicine protocols has led to advancements in recovery times and return-to-play decisions, further underscoring their significance in rehabilitation and performance enhancement. Through a focus on personalized care and evidence-based practice, practitioners can promote athletes' well-being and recovery efficiently, as highlighted by recent developments in the field (Chauhan, 2024; Leong et al., 2024).

12.4.1. Therapeutic Exercises and Physical Therapy

Rehabilitation medicine encompasses a wide array of methods designed to regain function and enhance quality of life for patients with disabilities, injuries, or chronic diseases. Among these methods, therapeutic exercises are an integral part of physical therapy and foster recovery by improving strength, flexibility, and physical performance. Systematic use of therapeutic exercises aims to target specific areas affected by illness or injury, promoting both physical recovery and mental well-being.

Evidence shows that a customized exercise program can result in dramatic improvements in mobility and pain relief, maximizing the ability of the patients to manage everyday activities. In addition, engagement in formal physical activity has been shown to enable mental health benefits, reducing symptoms of anxiety and depression that now mark recovery processes. Therapeutic exercises are therefore a cornerstone in the varied regime of rehabilitation medicine. Physical therapy extends beyond classic therapeutic exercise to include a variety of modalities designed to maximize outcomes. Methods such as trigger point dry needling illustrate some of the new strategies used to overcome muscle tightness and pain, two of the most prevalent obstacles to effective rehabilitation. Dry needling involves the insertion of non-medicated needles into precise areas of muscle called trigger points, which can result in muscle relaxation and increased range of motion. Evidence holds that integrating dry needling into typical therapeutic exercises could be the key to improved gains, significantly reducing distress, and improving mobility for the individuals undergoing rehabilitation. The volume of research on the practice underscores its potential impact when integrated with current physical therapy practices. Therefore, physical therapists are increasingly using such modalities in treatment, creating comprehensive treatment plans that are sensitive to the patient's individual needs and reactions, maximizing a more individualized response in rehabilitation medicine. In addition, interdisciplinary teamwork is emphasized in rehabilitation medicine. Adding therapeutic exercises and newer methods, such as dry needling, is best done through the combined efforts of various healthcare providers, such as physical therapists, occupational therapists, and fitness trainers. This cross-disciplinary collaboration yields integrated treatment and assessment plans that address the multidimensional nature of patient rehabilitation. For instance, physical therapy can initiate treatment protocols that incorporate exercise therapy while integrating supplementary modalities, such as dry needling, to address specific muscle groups optimally. Multidisciplinary management enhances not only the therapeutic outcomes of physical therapy but also presents patients with comprehensive interventions tailored to their respective clinical presentations. As research continues to demonstrate the efficacy of these combined methodologies, the future of rehabilitation medicine appears to lie increasingly in the synergy among numerous health professionals, ultimately resulting in improved patient outcomes and quality of life (Figure 12.14).

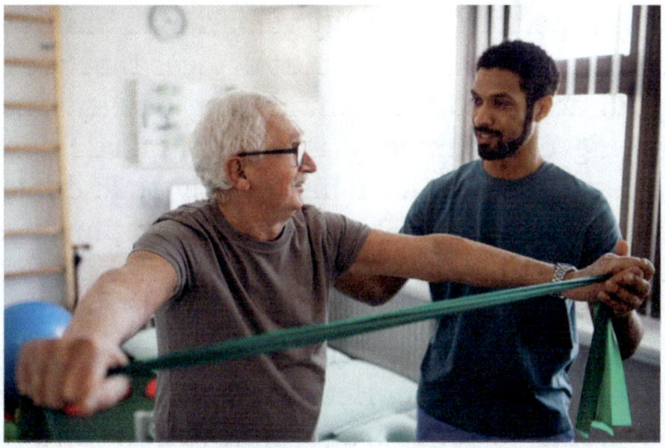

Figure 12.14. Therapeutic exercise in physical therapy.

Source: https://www.caryortho.com/wp-content/uploads/2022/10/physical-therapist-leading-patient-through-therapeutic-exercise.jpg.

12.4.2. Assistive Devices and Technology

The landscape of rehabilitation medicine has been significantly changed by the advent of assistive devices and technology, which enhance patients' functional capacity and facilitate recovery. These technologies range from straightforward mobility aids, such as wheelchairs and walkers, to sophisticated wearable devices that monitor health parameters or aid in rehabilitation training. Wearable technology, in particular, has revolutionized neurorehabilitation, facilitating real-time data collection and personalized feedback. This philosophy promotes which ultimately leads to improved outcomes. Increasing utilization of advanced devices in rehabilitation is an indication of a shift toward an individualized and data-driven approach to treatment, with scientists and clinicians already starting to investigate how these devices can be optimally employed to meet the unique needs of patients (Reinkensmeyer et al., 2019). In assistive technology, there is a common push towards making advances accessible to larger segments, evidence of a concern for inclusivity in practice rehabilitation. Among the advances of the last period, especially remarkable has been the introduction of low-cost devices that are as useful at the cost of diminishing quality. Such leveling of technology is critical, particularly for segments that have historically been denied access to rehabilitation services. By emphasizing usability and cost, health professionals can enable patients to regain control of their lives. Furthermore, state interventions, as illustrated in the Department of Health's report, emphasize the need to encourage innovation and to have assistive devices address diverse user needs (Burton et al., 2011). By emphasizing research and development with this goal, the final potential of assistive technology for rehabilitation is optimally achieved. Future rehabilitation medicine will be characterized by further advances in assistive devices and technology, driven by expanding research and the application of data analytics to treatment strategies. As neurorehabilitation progresses, big data will play an integral part in tailoring intervention to dramatically enhance patient outcomes. Intelligent, networked devices integrated seamlessly into patients' day-to-day lives can transform rehabilitation. Technologies such as virtual reality and augmented reality environments also come into view as essential devices for skill learning and recovery. Ultimately, the continued push for assistive technology fosters a paradigm shift towards more individualized, user-focused approaches in rehabilitation medicine, reflecting a greater understanding of patients' specific experiences and the complexity of their rehabilitation needs (Reinkensmeyer et al., 2019) (Figure 12.15).

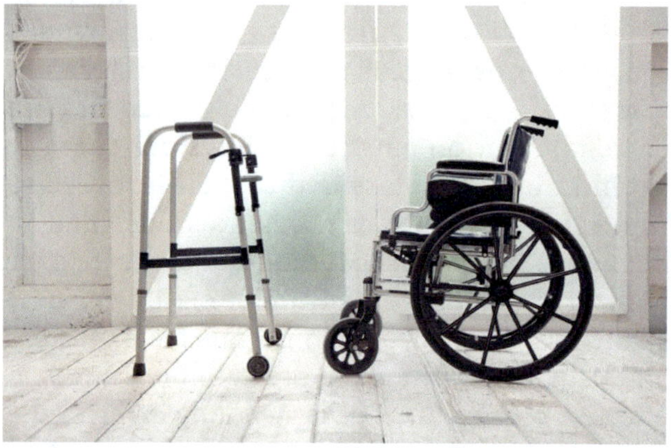

Figure 12.15. Assistive devices for spinal cord injury (SCI) rehabilitation.

Source: https://propelphysiotherapy.com/wp-content/uploads/2019/08/assistive-devices-sci-rehabilitation-propel-physiotherapy.jpg.

12.4.3. Psychological Support and Counseling

Psychiatric counseling and care are also a significant aspect of rehabilitation medicine in patients with serious physical and mental issues following diseases or surgery. The psychological impact of disease usually contributes to the physical condition, generating anxiety, depression, and stress. For example, patients after lung cancer surgery are usually subject to psychological trauma while adapting to health and social role changes, which negatively impacts their recovery. Psychological demands should be addressed in these situations since the quality of life for patients can be significantly improved, along with overall rehabilitation outcomes, through proper mental health treatment. Mental function rehabilitation procedures, therefore, have to encompass not just bodily recovery but also a comprehensive treatment of emotional health, developing resilience and coping mechanisms in patients for significant life changes, especially following intrusive medical procedures (Cao et al., 2025). When discussing the psychological support system offered in rehab centers, there is no doubt that integrating counseling services is central to effective patient management. For instance, support systems for empowerment, such as peer counseling or institutional mental health care, may be critical in the provision of resources for stress and anxiety management. The Nairobi church ministers' case study emphasizes the intricacies of emotional labor and organizational demands as reasons for constructing accessible support networks. The outcomes show that ministers, like other professionals under pressure, highly value formal counseling and peer support groups. The diversity in the availability and efficacy of such services necessitates a rethinking of the delivery of mental health care within rehabilitation facilities so that all patients can access the psychological support they need for better outcomes (Kibuh, 2025). Second, the potential of holistic approaches to contribute to psychiatric care in rehabilitation medicine cannot be overemphasized. The synergy among spiritual practice, counseling, and peer support can promote resilience and improve coping behaviors among patients. Furthermore, strategies that integrate traditional psychiatric interventions with alternative healing techniques such as meditation and prayer have shown promise to enhance global well-being. The combination of these diverse methods is particularly pertinent to populations that are experiencing unique stressors, such as religious officials or patients recuperating from very dangerous medical conditions. To properly implement these new approaches, medical professionals need first to conduct thorough assessments of their patients' emotional and psychological needs. By addressing these factors within the umbrella of rehabilitation medicine, clinicians can greatly improve cure rates and provide a healing-conducive environment (Cao et al., 2025; Kibuh, 2025) (Figure 12.16).

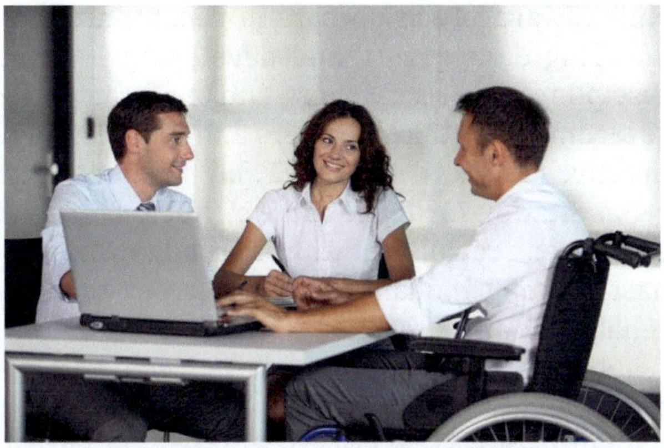

Figure 12.16. Rehabilitation counseling.

Source: https://res.cloudinary.com/dqtmwki9i/image/fetch/https://project-alpine.com/assets/ca85b6eb-3d24-4608-84df-9b28d05f014e?width=780&height=520.

Test Your Knowledge

1. What is a therapeutic exercise?
2. Which are assistive devices?

SUMMARY

The chapter summary is a crucial condensation of the main arguments developed during the discussion, particularly in rehabilitation medicine. As the field develops with the growth of technology and methods, it becomes increasingly necessary to assess the implications of such developments critically. The incorporation of evidence-based approaches, as noted in the latest guidelines for idiopathic pulmonary fibrosis, reflects the necessity for rehabilitation professionals to remain current on new protocols. Perhaps more significantly, conditional recommendations regarding the use of nintedanib emphasize the priority of individualized patient care, which is an essential element of effective rehabilitation in this arena. Hence, the future of rehabilitation medicine lies in its capacity to grow and adapt with the new evidence and clinical research, offering patients the best possible care based on the most up-to-date evidence (Raghu et al., 2022). In addition, new developments in artificial intelligence (AI) technologies present both opportunities and challenges for rehabilitation medicine. As outlined in recent literature, AI is increasingly applied in predictive medicine to aid decision-making and enhance patient outcomes. The potential of AI to assist physicians in personalizing treatment regimens and enhancing diagnostic capabilities speaks to an elemental shift toward precision care in rehabilitation settings. With this, however, comes the challenge of ensuring data quality and developing interdisciplinary approaches that integrate studies across disciplines. As researchers and medical professionals collaborate, they should exercise vigilance regarding the ethical matters and knowledge required for effective implementation of AI in clinical practice (Secinaro et al., 2021). The effective integration of these technologies will eventually make rehabilitation medicine more efficacious. The evolving situation of rehabilitation medicine demands permanent reconsideration and adaptation to provide effective patient care. The intersection of past therapy modalities with current technologies, such as AI, holds vast potential to improve rehabilitation outcomes. But it is critical that decision-makers, researchers, and clinicians come together to issue evidence-based guidelines while navigating the intricacies introduced by new technological advancements. With the growing specialty, education, interdisciplinary practice, and patient care will be critical to breaking barriers and achieving the greatest good of rehabilitation medicine. Future research should be directed under these principles so practice can advance both scientifically based and patient needs-focused (Raghu et al., 2022; Secinaro et al., 2021).

In rehabilitation medicine, it is imperative to understand the varied patterns of recovery among patients to optimize treatment protocols and enhance health outcomes. A major study across 10 European countries on geriatric rehabilitation after COVID-19 emphasized the pivotal role of variable recovery rates among patients. These ratios were influenced by varying referral and patient-specific selection criteria, underscoring the value of harmonized measurements in the rehabilitation of the elderly. Harmonization would enable more robust comparative research, beneficial for optimizing rehabilitation processes and, ultimately, rehabilitation and patient care across diverse populations (van Tol et al., 2024). Another critical area of rehabilitation medicine is the management of dysphagia, particularly in older patients with CVD. Research conducted in Japan revealed that dysphagia in this population is prevalent and has a significant impact on their recovery and quality of life. The outcome revealed that the application of integrated dysphagia rehabilitation would dramatically improve oral intake and body mass index and enhance independence in activities of daily living. This suggests that rehabilitation programs should specifically incorporate dysphagia management as an integral part of more comprehensive cardiovascular rehabilitation and better overall recovery for older patients (Obata et al., 2024). The significance of these findings in rehabilitation medicine extends beyond clinical recovery to more general health outcomes. Both analyses validate the applicability of individualized and comprehensive approaches within rehabilitation frameworks, advocating the necessity of addressing isolated patient needs and recovery barriers. Differences in patient responses and performance across rehabilitation maneuvers justify scrutiny of existing protocols. With the grasp and synthesis of the main outcomes among various studies, rehabilitation professionals are able to tailor interventions that not only hasten recovery but also improve patients' overall welfare and functional independence, setting the foundation for subsequent development in the field (Obata et al., 2024; van Tol et al., 2024).

KEY TERMS FROM THIS CHAPTER

- Brain injuries
- Degenerative diseases
- Memory
- Musculoskeletal injuries
- Physical rehabilitation
- Psychological distress
- Rehabilitation services
- Cognitive-behavioral therapy
- Manual therapy
- Multiple sclerosis
- Occupational rehabilitation
- Problem-solving
- Rehabilitation medicine
- Strokes

CRITICAL THINKING QUESTIONS

1. **What is the primary goal of rehabilitation medicine?**
   a. Cure chronic illnesses
   b. Prevent all future disabilities
   c. Optimize function and improve quality of life
   d. Provide acute medical treatment
2. **Which of the following is a key component of a rehabilitation program?**
   a. Surgery
   b. Pharmacotherapy alone
   c. Physical therapy and occupational therapy
   d. Exclusive use of assistive devices
3. **What is the term for the ability to perform tasks necessary for independent living?**
   a. Functional mobility
   b. Activities of Daily Living (ADLs)
   c. Instrumental Activities of Daily Living (IADLs)
   d. Rehabilitation goals
4. **Which of the following conditions is most likely to require rehabilitation after acute treatment?**
   a. Common cold
   b. Stroke
   c. Migraine headache
   d. Mild dehydration
5. **A patient with hemiparesis after a stroke is being trained in ADLs. This is an example of:**
   a. Cognitive therapy
   b. Physical therapy
   c. Occupational therapy
   d. Speech therapy

Short Answer Questions

1. What is the meaning of rehabilitation medicine?
2. Why is rehabilitation important in healthcare?
3. List the types of rehabilitation.
4. What are the goals of rehabilitation medicine?
5. What is the multidisciplinary approach in rehabilitation?

Answer to Critical Thinking Questions

1. (c); 2. (c); 3. (b); 4. (b); 5. (c).

REFERENCES

1. McLean, S. M., Burton, M., Bradley, L., & Littlewood, C. (2010). Interventions for enhancing adherence with physiotherapy: A systematic review. *Manual Therapy, 15*(6), 514–521. https://doi.org/10.1016/j.math.2010.05.012Barros, P. P., & Gonçalves, R. (2025). Economies of scale and scope in the provision of diagnostic techniques and therapeutic services in Portuguese hospitals. https://core.ac.uk/download/pdf/6262270.pdf (accessed on 14th July 2025).
2. Beauvais, J., Beenken, B., Czlapinski, R., Gromisch, E. S., et al. (2019). Cognitive behavioral therapy for the management of multiple sclerosis–related pain: A randomized clinical trial. https://open.bu.edu/bitstream/2144/34298/1/CBT%20for%20MS%20Pain%20Merged%20PDF.pdf (accessed on 14th July 2025).
3. Berényi, A., Delorme, A., Bansal, A. K., Taplin, A. M., Hishinuma, A. K., Fritsch, B., Lafon, B., et al. (2018). Low-frequency cortical activity is a neuromodulator target that tracks recovery after stroke. https://core.ac.uk/download/323062172.pdf (accessed on 14th July 2025).
4. Betke, M., Gorman, M., Lahav, A., Saltzman, E., et al. (2005). Music Maker–A camera-based music making tool for physical rehabilitation. https://open.bu.edu/bitstream/2144/1858/1/2005-032-music-maker.pdf (accessed on 14th July 2025).
5. Black, A. E., Halvari, A. E. M., Murray, A., Hall, A. M., Walker, B. F., Craig, C., Leonhardt, C., et al. (2012). Communication style and exercise compliance in physiotherapy (CONNECT). A cluster randomized controlled trial to test a theory-based intervention to increase chronic low back pain patients' adherence to physiotherapists' recommendations: Study rationale, design, and methods. https://core.ac.uk/download/pdf/9837538.pdf (accessed on 14th July 2025).
6. Blake, R. W. (2017). Reducing medication errors through workflow redesign. https://core.ac.uk/download/84064373.pdf (accessed on 14th July 2025).
7. Bosch, P. R., Fasoli, S. E., Langan, J., Lin, C., et al. (2019). Use of standardized assessments and online resources in stroke rehabilitation. https://core.ac.uk/download/232209260.pdf (accessed on 14th July 2025).
8. Bruyere, S. M., Peterson, D., & VanLooy, S. (2005). The International Classification of Functioning, Disability and Health: Contemporary literature overview. https://core.ac.uk/download/5124461.pdf (accessed on 14th July 2025).
9. Burton, A. K., Christian, J., & Wickizer, T. (2015). A community-focused Health & Work Service (HWS). https://core.ac.uk/download/30734111.pdf (accessed on 14th July 2025).
10. Burton, M., Chamberlain, P., Mountain, G., Reed, H., et al. (2011). Future bathroom: A study of user-centred design principles affecting usability, safety and satisfaction in bathrooms for people living with disabilities. https://core.ac.uk/download/9426427.pdf (accessed on 14th July 2025).
11. Cao, L., Wang, Z., Wang, X., Zhu, G., Zhang, Y., & Li, J. (2025). Effectiveness of traditional Chinese medicine in psychological rehabilitation after lung cancer surgery: Systematic review and meta-analysis protocol. *Integrative Cancer Therapies, 24*. https://www.semanticscholar.org/paper/caa9bf143a7bd8825e5e57ed47be8e6a3127b6f7 (accessed on 14th July 2025).
12. Carretero-Gómez, J., Pérez-Martínez, P., Seguí-Ripoll, J. M., Carrasco-Sánchez, F., Martínez, N. L., Fernández Pérez, E., Pérez Hernández, O., et al. (2022). High-risk obesity phenotypes: Target for multimorbidity prevention at the ROFEMI study. *Journal of Clinical Medicine, 11*.

https://www.semanticscholar.org/paper/8c4dab3ca44eb636b1b3992e75a3d646a4aaa8f9 (accessed on 14th July 2025).

13. Chauhan, A. (2024). Sports medicine: Advances in injury prevention, treatment, and rehabilitation. *Innovations in Sports Science*. https://www.semanticscholar.org/paper/99a507be38ce6a681e1df51cac201d8d9771e565 (accessed on 14th July 2025).
14. Chen, Y., Shan, Y., Cao, W., Cao, Y., & Pu, J. (2024). The role of PDZ in cerebral ischemia. *Modern Chemistry*. https://www.semanticscholar.org/paper/27d288db75696a5f74c0bc6a44f90d008b0c6624 (accessed on 14th July 2025).
15. Chopra, V., Flanders, S. A., O'Malley, M., Malani, A. N., & Prescott, H. C. (2020). Sixty-day outcomes among patients hospitalized with COVID-19. *Annals of Internal Medicine, 174*, 576–578. https://doi.org/10.7326/m20-5661 (accessed on 14th July 2025).
16. Clymer, D. R., Fields, H. A., & Kniepmann, K. (2020). Assessing unmet needs of caregivers after stroke: Occupational therapist practices and perspectives. https://core.ac.uk/download/304636394.pdf (accessed on 14th July 2025).
17. Computational and Mathematical Methods in Medicine. (2023). Retracted: Effect of acupuncture and rehabilitation therapy on the recovery of neurological function and prognosis of stroke patients. *Computational and Mathematical Methods in Medicine, 2023*. https://www.semanticscholar.org/paper/5821e3764b1437bc645c77687c654f1e95825a75 (accessed on 14th July 2025).
18. Craig, L. E., McAlpine, C. H., Smith, L. N., Weir, C. J., et al. (2008). Stroke education for healthcare professionals: Making it fit for purpose. https://core.ac.uk/download/90007.pdf (accessed on 14th July 2025).
19. Donnelly, S., Butler, P., O'Loughlin, A., Russell, E., & Carroll, P. (2024). Interdisciplinary team members' experiences of family meetings in an Irish rehabilitation hospital: A social work action-research project. *European Social Work Research*. https://www.semanticscholar.org/paper/216753a9a68e226d82b3ea0fd2515bf6825b0cf7 (accessed on 14th July 2025).
20. Edgerton, V. R., Krucoff, M. O., Rahimpour, S., Slutzky, M. W., et al. (2016). Enhancing nervous system recovery through neurobiologist, neural interface training, and neurorehabilitation. https://core.ac.uk/download/323078214.pdf (accessed on 14th July 2025).
21. Fleming, N., Bowler, S., Ahearn, L., Matereke, S., & Marshall, F. (2025). P03 Antimicrobial stewardship nurses—the story so far. *JAC-Antimicrobial Resistance, 7*. https://www.semanticscholar.org/paper/bd53e6493d4cebfa9328913d4e104660447a54af (accessed on 14th July 2025).
22. Gibson, V., Griffiths, J., Kishen, R., Morris, C., et al. (2010). 2010 Annual evidence update on critical illness rehabilitation. https://core.ac.uk/download/4146014.pdf (accessed on 14th July 2025).
23. Goldman, J. G., Volpe, D., Ellis, T. D., Hirsch, M. A., Johnson, J., Wood, J., Aragon, A., et al. (2024). Delivering multidisciplinary rehabilitation care in Parkinson's disease: An international consensus statement. *Journal of Parkinson's Disease, 14*, 135–166. https://www.semanticscholar.org/paper/3c9f30b506e7af7c1981056f948d1e82f0ea9739 (accessed on 14th July 2025).
24. Hasnain, R., Shaikh, L. C., & Shanawani, H. (2008). Disability and the Muslim perspective: An introduction for rehabilitation and health care providers. https://core.ac.uk/download/5127570.pdf (accessed on 14th July 2025).

25. Hernández Fuentes, A., & Fernández Company, J. F. (2022). Study on the efficacy of harmonic frequencies applied through music therapy intervention techniques in cochlear implant patients. *International Physical Medicine & Rehabilitation Journal*. https://www.semanticscholar.org/paper/e3680a45a7d7e692f2a0487afdf223a6f87fa356 (accessed on 14th July 2025).
26. Herrera, J. E., Niehaus, W., Whiteson, J., Azola, A., Baratta, J. M., Fleming, T. K., Kim, S. Y., et al. (2021). Multidisciplinary collaborative consensus guidance statement on the assessment and treatment of fatigue in post-acute sequelae of SARS-CoV-2 infection (PASC) patients. *PM&R, 13*, 1027–1043. https://doi.org/10.1002/pmrj.12684 (accessed on 14th July 2025).
27. Hill, M. A., Mantzoros, C. S., & Sowers, J. R. (2020). Commentary: COVID-19 in patients with diabetes. *Metabolism, 107*, 154217. https://doi.org/10.1016/j.metabol.2020.154217 (accessed on 14th July 2025).
28. Jefferson, R., & Tempest, S. E. (2015). Engaging with clinicians to implement and evaluate the ICF in neurorehabilitation practice. https://core.ac.uk/download/30339922.pdf (accessed on 14th July 2025).
29. Kibuh, S. (2025). Availability and effectiveness of support systems for church ministers in Nairobi County. *The American Journal of Management and Economics Innovations*. https://www.semanticscholar.org/paper/66949b3ef029f78fae81d00e4c5b48f2fa56652a (accessed on 14th July 2025).
30. Kotze, K. (2019). The pairing of trigger points dry needling with rehabilitation techniques. https://core.ac.uk/download/213463742.pdf (accessed on 14th July 2025).
31. Leitão, J. R., Rosado, I. R., Menezes, T. T. P., Lopes, M. G., & Alves, E. G. L. (2025). Plate rod in humerus fracture in *Caracara plancus*: Challenges and outcomes of a case. *Arquivo Brasileiro de Medicina Veterinária e Zootecnia*. https://www.semanticscholar.org/paper/6313bd884d23608dbb7d36213035a57a6c3ce6ec (accessed on 14th July 2025).
32. Leong, W. Y., Leong, Y. Z., & Leong, W. (2024). Sports medicine protocols: A comprehensive guide to injury management and rehabilitation. *2024 IEEE 6th Eurasia Conference on Biomedical Engineering, Healthcare and Sustainability (ECBIOS)*. https://www.semanticscholar.org/paper/a2042fad714d53443d21bb362bbcc5786321b6df (accessed on 14th July 2025).
33. McVeigh, F., & Pack, S. (2015). An exploration of sports rehabilitators and athletic rehabilitation therapists' views on fear of re-injury following anterior cruciate ligament reconstruction. https://core.ac.uk/download/29852312.pdf (accessed on 14th July 2025).
34. Morton, S., & Dunn, W. (2015). Addressing the health needs of an aging America: New opportunities for evidence-based policy solutions. https://core.ac.uk/download/75783019.pdf (accessed on 14th July 2025).
35. O'Brien, M. K., Shin, S. Y., Khazanchi, R., Fanton, M., Lieber, R., Ghaffari, R., Rogers, J. A., et al. (2022). Wearable sensors improve prediction of post-stroke walking function following inpatient rehabilitation. *IEEE Journal of Translational Engineering in Health and Medicine, 10*, 1–11. https://www.semanticscholar.org/paper/11f632de516a119af81fee23cca7f4e71368b3a6 (accessed on 14th July 2025).
36. Obata, H., Izumi, T., Ishizuka, M., Yamaguchi, K., Hao, N., Yagihara, N., Abe, S., et al. (2024). Impact and management of integrated dysphagia rehabilitation within cardiac care programs for older patients with cardiovascular disease. *European Geriatric Medicine, 15*, 1657–1668. https://www.semanticscholar.org/paper/073eb6b16f670a5af4da9eeb275215335b3e701c (accessed on 14th July 2025).

37. Raghu, G., Rémy-Jardin, M., Richeldi, L., Thomson, C. C., Inoue, Y., Johkoh, T., Kreuter, M., et al. (2022). Idiopathic pulmonary fibrosis (an update) and progressive pulmonary fibrosis in adults: An official ATS/ERS/JRS/ALAT clinical practice guideline. *American Journal of Respiratory and Critical Care Medicine, 205*, e18–e47. https://doi.org/10.1164/rccm.202202-0399st (accessed on 14th July 2025).

38. Reinkensmeyer, D. J. (2019). JNER at 15 years: Analysis of the state of neuroengineering and rehabilitation. https://core.ac.uk/download/286362777.pdf (accessed on 14th July 2025).

39. Roth, G. A., Mensah, G. A., Johnson, C. O., Addolorato, G., Ammirati, E., Baddour, L. M., Barengo, N. C., et al. (2020). Global burden of cardiovascular diseases and risk factors, 1990–2019. *Journal of the American College of Cardiology, 76*, 2982–3021. https://doi.org/10.1016/j.jacc.2020.11.010 (accessed on 14th July 2025).

40. Samoy, Y., Saunders, J., & Van Ryssen, B. (2016). Physiotherapy in small animal medicine. https://core.ac.uk/download/154408470.pdf (accessed on 14th July 2025).

41. Scheets, P. L., Hornby, T. G., Perry, S. B., Sparto, P. J., Riley, N., Romney, W., Fell, D. W., et al. (2020). Moving forward. *Journal of Neurologic Physical Therapy, 45*, 46–49. https://doi.org/10.1097/npt.0000000000000337 (accessed on 14th July 2025).

42. Sebastian, R., Cherry-Allen, K. M., Pruski, A. D., Sinkowitz, J., Stilling, J., Anaya, M., Cantarero, G., et al. (2023). Clinical implementation of noninvasive brain stimulation in an outpatient neurorehabilitation program. *American Journal of Physical Medicine & Rehabilitation, 102*(2S Suppl 1), S79–S84. https://www.semanticscholar.org/paper/6ed5e3870cc8932b2c0d7522e919864ec04ec701 (accessed on 14th July 2025).

43. Secinaro, S., Calandra, D., Secinaro, A., Muthurangu, V., & Biancone, P. (2021). The role of artificial intelligence in healthcare: A structured literature review. *BMC Medical Informatics and Decision Making, 21*. https://doi.org/10.1186/s12911-021-01488-9 (accessed on 14th July 2025).

44. Teramatsu, H., Hachisuka, A., Nagata, M., Kohi, S., Hamada, M., Kuhara, S., Takemoto, A., et al. (2024). Perioperative rehabilitation in collaboration with the Department of Occupational Medicine for patients with cholangiocarcinoma: A case report. *Physical Therapy Research, 27*, 108–114. https://www.semanticscholar.org/paper/744c07242af7bf55d34b654092b813500f7cca9b (accessed on 14th July 2025).

45. van Tol, L. S., Lin, T., Caljouw, M., Cesari, M., Dockery, F., Everink, I., Francis, B. N., et al. (2024). Post-COVID-19 recovery and geriatric rehabilitation care: A European inter-country comparative study. *European Geriatric Medicine, 15*, 1489–1501. https://www.semanticscholar.org/paper/c25653aa79ba0ef88fe2db3606aa2786e0d78053 (accessed on 14th July 2025).

46. Yoshimura, Y., Matsumoto, A., & Momosaki, R. (2022). Pharmacotherapy and the role of pharmacists in rehabilitation medicine. *Progress in Rehabilitation Medicine, 7*. https://doi.org/10.2490/prm.20220025 (accessed on 14th July 2025).

FUTURE TRENDS IN FAMILY MEDICINE

13

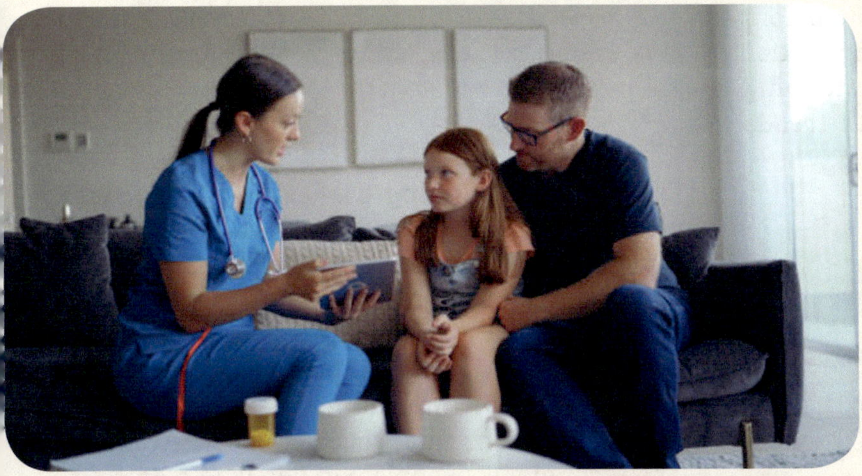

LEARNING OBJECTIVES

After studying this chapter, you will be able to:

1. Understand the technological advancements in family medicine
2. Describe the patient-centered care in family medicine
3. Understand the preventive care and wellness in family medicine
4. Know the interprofessional collaboration in family medicine
5. Understand the health equity and access in family medicine
6. Understand the policy and regulation changes in family medicine

Introduction

The face of family medicine is undergoing a revolutionary transformation marked by the integration of new technology and the latest treatment approaches. The force behind this transformation is the growing interest in patient-centric medicine, with a focus increasingly on individualized treatment processes. As health systems cope with the challenges of chronic disease and a multitudinous patient population, medical genetics offers promising avenues for increasingly accurate diagnostic and therapeutic methods. With knowledge of the role of genetic information in structuring interventions, family medicine clinicians are better equipped to manage and prevent conditions that have a disproportionate impact on their patient populations. The use of genetic information in everyday practice is an emerging trend that underscores the need for healthcare workers to continually adapt and improve, staying skilled in their work as the profession evolves (Orlova et al., 2024). In addition to the promise of medical genetics, another underlying trend shaping family medicine is the increasing recognition of cardio-renal-metabolic diseases as high-priority targets. As prevalence to fight these conditions effectively. Present educational interventions in family medicine residency programs have identified the importance of personalized curricula for enhancing knowledge and skills related to these interlinked diseases. There is evidence that residencies with integrated educational modules on cardio-renal-metabolic disorders achieve significant improvements in residents' knowledge and patient care practices. This strategy not only prepares new doctors for the intricacies of managing comorbidities but also reaffirms the importance of continuing education to keep up with new health trends (Pesqueira et al., 2024).

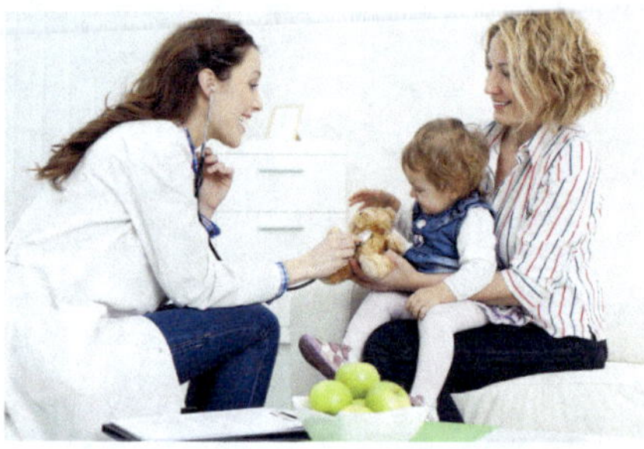

Figure 13.1. Future of family medicine.

Source: https://cdn.hswstatic.com/gif/familymedicine-1200x800.jpg.

Family medicine's future relies on an abiding commitment to innovation and flexibility, with practitioners equipped to deliver changing healthcare needs to their communities. As the discipline progresses, the focus will shift to personalized medicine, fueled by advances in genetics and strengthened educational platforms. Family medicine is more than treating individual conditions; it involves a more conceptual approach to understanding the biological, social, and environmental determinants that affect health. The interaction of these factors will inform practitioners in creating successful strategies for disease prevention and control, ultimately improving patient outcomes. Thus, as the profession falls behind in aligning technology and know-how, it paves the way for more extensive and effective patient care in the coming years (Figure 13.1).

13.1. Technological Advancements

Learning Outcome

1. Describe the telemedicine and remote patient monitoring
2. Know the artificial intelligence in diagnostics
3. Understand the electronic health records and data management

Emerging technological innovations are increasingly shaping the field of family medicine, primarily by connecting artificial intelligence (AI) and telemedicine. AI technologies, such as advanced diagnostic algorithms and machine learning algorithms, enable physicians to process patient information in an improved manner, leading to improved clinical outcomes. The technologies enable personalized medicine by creating treatment plans based on specific patient properties and predictive analytics. Moreover, the application of electronic health records (EHRs) enhances continuity of care by making full patient histories available to family doctors, which facilitates more effective clinical decisions. The rapid evolution of these technologies not only facilitates the effective management of chronic conditions but also enhances preventive efforts in care. By adopting AI-powered software that streamlines routine procedures, family medicine clinics can spend more time on in-person interactions with patients, thereby enhancing the doctor-patient relationship. The age of telemedicine has transformed the delivery of health into a more convenient and accessible process for both patients and healthcare practitioners. Remote consultations have been particularly helpful in enhancing access to care, especially among the marginalized or remote communities. With video conferencing, family medical practitioners can consult with patients without the need to travel, which is also time-consuming and costly. Telehealth services not only eliminate barriers to care, such as transportation issues, but also enable constant patient contact and follow-up. With advancements in telemedicine, the capability to incorporate health-monitoring devices into these consultations would enhance the sophistication of care delivery.

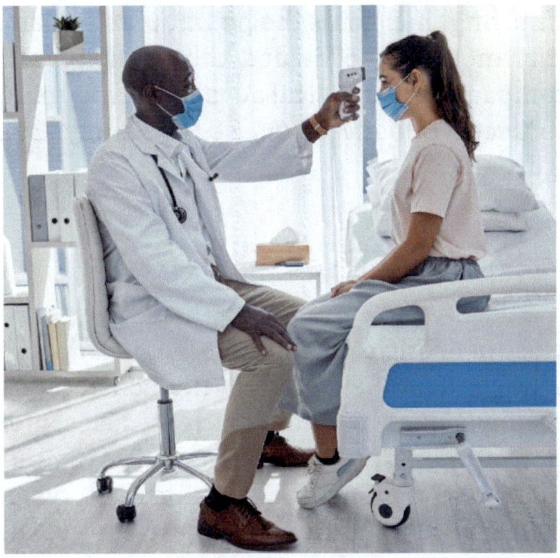

Figure 13.2. Technologies shaping the future of family medicine.

Source: https://drstevensukhokim.com/wp-content/uploads/2025/04/dr-steven-sukho-kim-also-oversees-all-clinical-operations-at-his-clinic.jpg.

Remote patient monitoring technology allows physicians to monitor patients' vital signs in real-time, enabling timely intervention, adherence to treatment plans, and reduced hospital visits, ultimately leading to improved patient outcomes. Other than AI and telemedicine, the application of wearable health technology offers promising avenues for the evolution of family medicine. Wearable devices that monitor healthcare parameters such as heart rate, blood pressure, and blood glucose levels foster active patient participation in their healthcare. Wearables not only facilitate real-time data capture but also enhance patient-physician communication. The flow of continuous data from wearables can facilitate treatment planning, enabling healthcare providers to make evidence-based decisions on a timely basis. However, the adoption of such technologies does come with issues, among them reservations about data protection and privacy. It is crucial that the medical community is aware of these and advocates for the benefits of wearable technology in enhancing patient monitoring and overall health. By acknowledging and addressing such complexities, family medicine can utilize technological advancements to create a more proactive patient-centered healthcare climate (Figure 13.2).

13.1.1. Telemedicine and Remote Patient Monitoring

Telemedicine and remote patient monitoring have emerged as essential parts of family medicine, driven largely by the growing demand for convenient healthcare. The revolution introduces punctual medical consultations and check-ups via electronic media channels, thereby doing away with geographical limitations and enhancing patient involvement. With the development of technology, patients can now visit their doctors from the comfort of their homes, which is especially crucial for individuals who reside in underserved or rural areas. The COVID-19 pandemic provided an impetus to the use of such telehealth services, demonstrating their ability to reduce the burden on healthcare systems and provide good avenues for managing chronic diseases. As telemedicine advances, it will not only facilitate more streamlined clinical processes but also enable patients to be engaged participants in their own health, positioning it as a key component of the future of family medicine. Remote patient monitoring (RPM) complements telemedicine by enabling healthcare professionals to collect important health information via wearable sensors and mobile health apps on consumers' existing mobile devices. This innovation enhances the chronic disease care paradigm by providing real-time information on patients' status, enabling timely interventions and tailored care. Through real-time data capture, health professionals will be better positioned to address fluctuations in patients' health, a method that is particularly relevant for diabetes, hypertension, and cardiovascular disease.

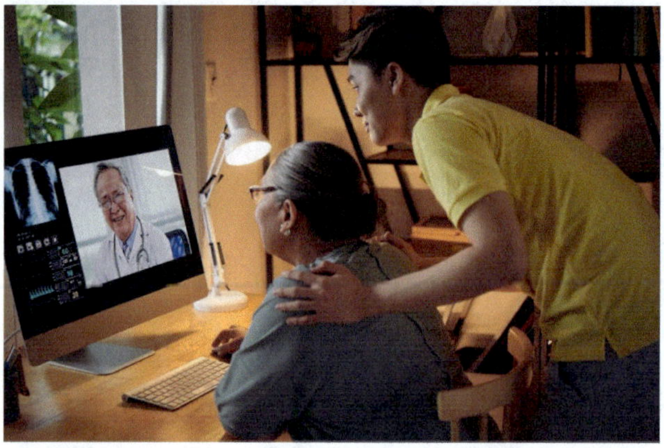

Figure 13.3. Remote patient monitoring and telehealth.

Source: https://www.ominext.com/storage/files/1/Blog/IMG%2004-01-2024/how-remote-patient-monitoring-and-telehealth-work-together.jpg.

Moreover, remote patient monitoring enhances patient independence as patients are more informed concerning their treatment and health condition. The integration of RPM into day-to-day practice is a fundamental shift towards active management of healthcare, aligning with patient-centered care, which is central to existing family medicine strategies. Gazing towards the future, the convergence of telemedicine and remote patient monitoring brings a new model to family medicine, focused on efficiency, accessibility, and individualized care. The integration of artificial intelligence (AI) within these technologies promises to further increase their effectiveness, enhancing diagnostic accuracy and treatment planning as amply supported by recent reviews of AI in medicine. By drawing on vast volumes of patient data, AI can help clinicians predict and identify trends in patient needs, with a view to improving outcomes. With the potential of these innovations so great, however, challenges related to data privacy, algorithmic bias, and regulatory environments must be addressed to ensure their safe use in clinical settings. The future of telehealth and remote patient monitoring thus holds the potential to transform family medicine, provided the challenges that accompany technological advancements are fully embraced (Bobade et al., 2024; Fahmy, 2024) (Figure 13.3).

13.1.2. Artificial Intelligence in Diagnostics

The use of Artificial Intelligence (AI) in diagnostics is a key milestone in family medicine, altering how physicians conduct patient assessments and treatment. By leveraging large amounts of data and advanced algorithms, AI systems can interpret medical images, lab results, and patient histories with high precision and speed. This ability not only improves diagnostic accuracy but also reduces the time patients wait for diagnoses, resulting in more timely interventions. Studies have shown that AI systems can help identify diseases such as diabetes and certain cancers at their earliest stages, which is crucial for patient outcomes. As captured by the changing higher education landscape, the versatility and effectiveness of AI reflect its transformative potential for healthcare treatment and diagnostics, opening doors to a more proactive model of patient care in family medicine (Rudolph et al., 2023). In addition, the diagnostic potential of AI extends to personalized medicine, where treatments can be tailored to individual genetic profiles. Family practice often calls for a delicate understanding of family trends and patient history; AI solutions can assist professionals with identifying trends that may not be immediately apparent to the naked eye. For instance, machine learning enables computer programs to assess the risk that a patient will develop particular diseases based on family history, lifestyle, and other medical information. This predictive capacity aids practitioners in creating preventive treatment plans and facilitates patient engagement in health. With growing evidence of the application of AI in healthcare, it is increasingly important that healthcare professionals embrace these new technologies to improve the standard of care provided to families (Burton et al., 2021).

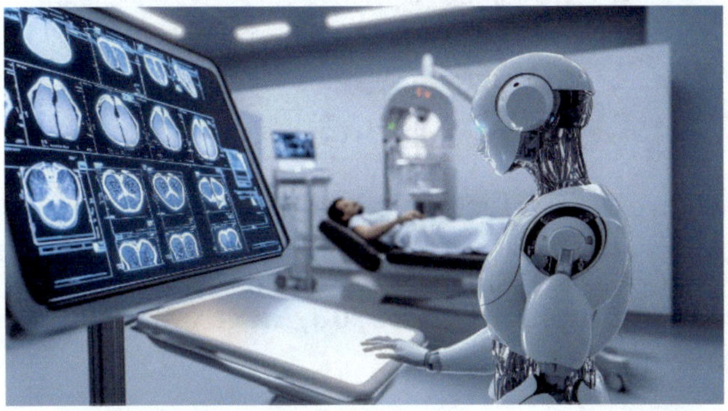

Figure 13.4. AI in medical diagnostics.

Source: https://media.licdn.com/dms/image/v2/D4E12AQHTFHXEe3ffjA/article-cover_image-shrink_720_1280/article-cover_image-shrink_720_1280/0/1725296210279?e=2147483647&v=beta&t=vJuoE7zYATsz0yPgcK5h2DIr8IVBw6BaR7Z8UrMhsiw.

However, AI applications in diagnosing are not without difficulty and ethical consequences. Prioritizing the accuracy and trustworthiness of AI instruments is the most important aspect, especially given varying data quality and algorithmic bias. Issues of patient confidentiality, consent, and the implications of AI errors all need to be monitored closely as family medicine further adopts these technologies. Secondly, physicians must be trained and equipped to interpret AI outputs meaningfully, thereby creating synergy between human knowledge and machine processing. The debate is continuously ongoing in the field of the potentiality of AI, and the need for human intervention in medicine underscores the need for balanced practice that considers patient welfare while seeking technological answers (Rudolph et al., 2023). Solving these problems will ultimately pave the way for the adoption of a future in which AI is a central collaborator in diagnostics for family medicine (Figure 13.4).

13.1.3. Electronic Health Records and Data Management

The landscape of family medicine is evolving at a rapid rate, particularly by the building of Electronic Health Records (EHRs) and data handling technology. Since the healthcare system recognizes the importance of efficient patient data handling, Electronic Health Records form the basis for streamlining clinical processes and improving patient care. Smart Health Records (SHRs) bring about a paradigm shift in integrating Artificial Intelligence (AI) into traditional EHRs, enabling real-time data sharing, predictive analytics, and improved clinical decision-making. Medical professionals can now access comprehensive patient profiles and medical history data in a timely manner, enabling targeted treatment plans tailored to individual needs. This interactive model increases the effectiveness of proactive care management and puts EHRs in the spotlight of the constant quest for optimized delivery of healthcare in family medicine (Arnold, 2025). Moreover, the integration of AI into EHR systems has enabled significant advancements in data management, which can transform family medicine. With techniques such as machine learning and natural language processing, physicians can more effectively analyze complex datasets, identifying trends and anomalies that would otherwise go unreported. This capability enhances diagnosis not only by being more precise but also preventive care through early intervention and ongoing monitoring of one's well-being. But unifying these technologies is not without problems; for instance, the challenges of data privacy, algorithmic bias, and the interpretability of AI models. To exploit the full potential of AI-based EHR systems, stakeholders must address these challenges in advance so that patient data remains secure while fostering trust and transparency throughout the health care ecosystem (Wang, 2025). In the future, family medicine will become more dependent on the smooth integration of EHRs and innovative data management approaches. As emerging technologies become available, attention must be directed to developing inclusive systems that foster collaborative care and elevated patient participation. Advances in federated learning and generative AI will open new avenues for developing more sophisticated EHR systems that can offer findings relevant to specific populations and individual patient needs. That such advances accompany the complete training of medical professionals is significant, as their knowledge will remain valuable in interpreting results and making highly informed clinical judgments. Lastly, the harmonious integration of electronic health records and advanced data processing techniques will transform family medicine, paving the way for improved, patient-centered care (Arnold, 2025) (Figure 13.5).

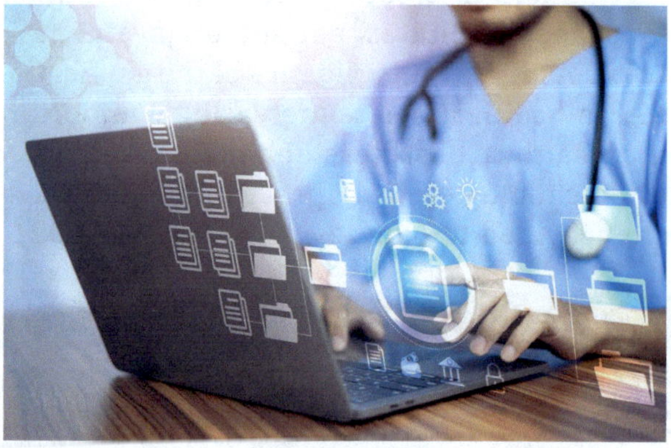

Figure 13.5. Electronic health records.

Source: https://hospitalsmagazine.com/wp-content/uploads/2023/08/Electronic-Health-Records.jpg.

Test Your Knowledge

1. What do you mean by telemedicine?
2. How is AI used in diagnostics?

13.2. Patient-Centered Care

Learning Outcome

1. Emphasize on personalized treatment plans
2. Understand the role of patient engagement and education
3. Integrate the behavioral health services

During the last few years, the inherent shift towards patient-centered care has been a crucial trend in family medicine, a sign of broader changes in the provision of health care. It is concerned with the function of recognizing the unique needs, preferences, and values of individual patients to establish a participatory partnership between physicians and patients. By involving patients in decisions about their own care, family practitioners can improve compliance, patient satisfaction, and ultimately healthier outcomes.

The integration of technology, such as telehealth platforms, also facilitates patient involvement, allowing them to be part of their care while remaining at home. With patient-centered care growing ever more prominent, family medicine must adapt training and practice standards that fully meet this paradigm shift, and healthcare providers are well-placed to meet their patients' shifting expectations (Thibault, 2020). During the age of personalized medicine, patient-centered care has become even more important in family medicine. By considering genetic, environmental, and lifestyle determinants, clinicians can more precisely tailor treatments to individual patients. By expanding their vision this way, they not only improve the effectiveness of clinical treatments but also foster a greater appreciation of the patient's context, which is central to the treatment of complex medical conditions.

Focusing on disease prevention and health promotion, patient-centered care helps family medicine practitioners promote healthier behavior and assist patients in goal setting and achieving individual health goals. This shift from reactive to proactive practice is one future model of family medicine that places patient-centered care at the basis of high-quality provision of healthcare, addressing patient empowerment and health equity (Tillu et al., 2020).

In the years to come, patient-centered care in family medicine will be sustained due to the success of interprofessional collaboration. The blending of multiple healthcare perspectives enables a complete understanding of patient needs, allowing decisions to be made together and care to be coordinated more efficiently.

As family medicine increasingly collaborates with specialists, mental health professionals, and community agencies, the horizon for patient-centered care will widen, enabling more comprehensive management of health. Furthermore, embracing novel educational paradigms, such as interprofessional education and simulation-based education, can prepare future physicians to prioritize and apply these values effectively.

In doing so, family medicine can set the pace for a healthcare system that not only looks but also acts on the priority of patient-centered care as an intrinsic aspect of future practice (Thibault, 2020) (Figure 13.6).

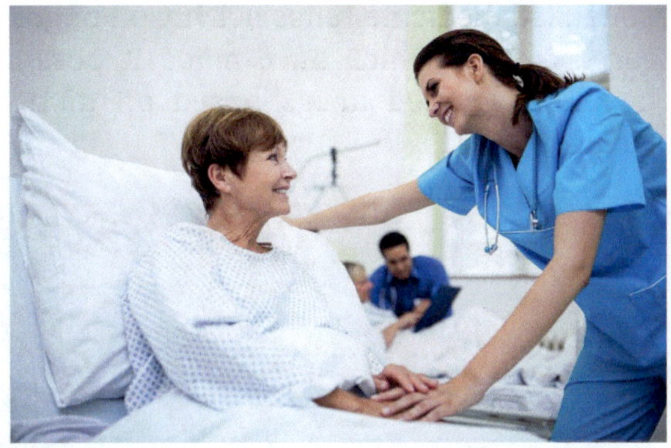

Figure 13.6. Patient-centered care.

Source: https://www.austco.com/wp-content/uploads/2019/04/post-patientCentered.jpg.

13.2.1. Emphasis on Personalized Treatment Plans

With the evolving nature of family medicine, tailored treatment plans are the state-of-the-art approach that is centered on the unique needs of each patient. A tailored treatment plan takes into account an infinite number of details, ranging from genetic inclinations to external influences, lifestyle, and personal preferences. It is an enhanced, integrated wellness experience, rather than the traditional one-size-fits-all model. By virtue of the integration of technological and analytical advances, healthcare providers may design individualized interventions that not only treat illness but the patient's overall well-being, fostering a collaborative dynamic between provider and patient when it comes to regulating health outcomes. A shift towards individualized treatment reflects a broader movement in medicine, where patient-centered care can enhance patient satisfaction and compliance rates. The incorporation of genetic testing and other diagnostic tests into customized treatment protocols further increases the precision of care delivered in family medicine. The ability to research genetic markers and variants' expressions allows physicians to identify the most advantageous treatment plans for diseases such as cancer and chronic diseases.

Personalized medicine relies heavily on ongoing research efforts, which have made it possible to develop targeted drugs based on distinct molecular profiles.

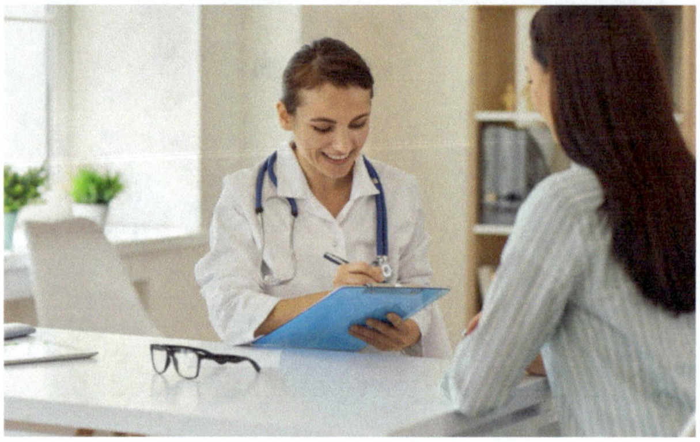

Figure 13.7. Personalized treatment plans.

Source: https://kineticrehabspine.com/wp-content/uploads/2023/07/personalized-treatment-1080x675.png.

For instance, targeted medication therapy, immunotherapy, and other interventions point out developments in the approach, suggesting the method is normalizing for treatment protocols. Through implementation of these strategies, practitioners not only optimize patient outcomes but also optimize systemic knowledge of disease dynamics, further shaping future treatment interventions in family medicine (Anand et al., 2022). The integration of machine learning and artificial intelligence in the formulation of personalized treatment plans also highlights the revolutionary path that family medicine is taking. Advanced algorithms can process vast amounts of information, identifying patterns and predicting patients' responses to treatments. These advances in technology present significant opportunities to achieve maximum treatment efficacy and minimize side effects, thereby transforming how family medicine practitioners treat patients. Among the general ethical issues, the relationship between human doctors and AI systems poses major problems for patient trust and information confidentiality. These problems will need to be resolved as AI applications in family medicine evolve. Thus, not only does the convergence of AI and personalized medicine portend a trend toward more individualized care, but also the era of healthcare in the immediate future will be much more responsive and agile to patient needs heterogeneity (Dwivedi et al., 2023) (Figure 13.7).

13.2.2. Role of Patient Engagement and Education

The role of patient education and activation continues to become an increasingly important factor in shaping the future of family medicine. With health care systems shifting toward shared decision-making models, it is essential to provide patients with critical information about their conditions and treatment options. Engaged patients will increasingly demonstrate greater compliance with recommended therapies and preventive practices, ultimately leading to improved health outcomes. Such a transition not only maximizes the effectiveness of care but also promotes a culture of collaboration between patients and providers, which is crucial since diseases such as Alzheimer's require prolonged strategies to manage them. The educational drive towards chronic disease management, particularly in complex cases, enhances the critical necessity of patient involvement in care plans, aligning with the trends anticipated to define family medicine in the future, like personalized and patient-centered. With the impact of the COVID-19 pandemic, patient education also underwent a remarkable transformation, with an emphasis on technology to enhance engagement. Telehealth services became widely accepted, providing real-time interaction between the patients and the providers, as necessary for ongoing education and care. With virtual platforms, patients can access educational materials, attend webinars, and join online support groups, thereby enhancing their knowledge of health conditions and self-management skills. This digital innovation not only enables continuity of care but also democratizes access to information across diverse populations, reducing health literacy disparities. Future family medicine clinics will have such technological equipment and make sure that patients are not only consumers of treatment but also agents who take an active role, creating a culture of empowerment and accountability in their own health care management (Thibault, 2020).

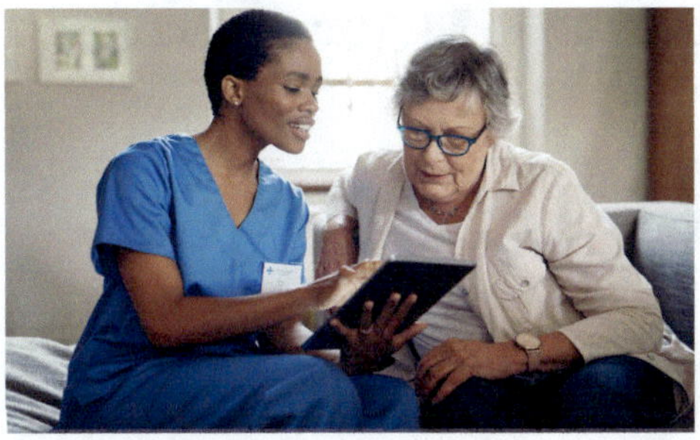

Figure 13.8. Enhancing patient education through video-based solutions.

Source: https://www.enghousevideo.com/wp-content/uploads/2024/08/Study-Patients-need-better-tools-for-education-and-engagement-scaled-1.jpg.

Moreover, studies continue to show that integrating social determinants of health into patient education programs is likely to significantly improve family medicine outcomes. By equipping patients with information that is sensitive to their socio-economic and environmental contexts, healthcare providers can most effectively tailor interventions to meet individual needs. For instance, culturally sensitive educational interventions that leverage community resources can lead to more sustainable health habits among diverse patient populations. As holistic models of care continue to evolve, talking with patients regarding lifestyle, environment, and personal values will become standard practice. This combined approach represents a departure from traditional models, aligning with the overall mission of family medicine to deliver quality, fair care that considers the whole person, thereby improving not only satisfaction but also health outcomes for patients (Figure 13.8).

13.2.3. Integration of Behavioral Health Services

The combination of primary care with behavioral health care is a historic advance in family medicine that is the growing recognition of the interconnectedness of mind and body. Traditionally, the two have operated in a kind of silo, isolating them and leading to fragmented care that often fails to address the full set of patients' needs. By integrating behavioral health care, primary care clinicians can address the mental health aspects of chronic illness and thereby enhance the overall patient experience. The model aims to increase access to prevention care and enhance comorbid condition management that commonly torments mentally ill patients, thereby encouraging better health outcomes and patient satisfaction. Thus, creating synergies among healthcare specialties is not a matter of modifying logistics; it is a call for more coordinated patient care in the 21st century. In addition, the proposed model of integrated care emphasizes collaboration between mental health professionals and primary care physicians as the solution to successful implementation. Education is at the heart of this model: education of providers in both fields to grasp and manage mental health issues is critical to the expansion of the integrative model. The model necessitates broad-based education programs directed at current practitioners and future practitioners in medical school and residency training programs. Through developing a strong knowledge of behavioral health in the primary care environment, physicians will be better equipped to make appropriate referrals or offer services in integrated clinic settings. The model's multi-faceted approach is designed not only to address fundamental health problems but also to decrease healthcare expenditure by developing preventive services and mitigating overuse of emergency care, with a specific focus on high-risk populations (Read et al., 2016). Psychologists are increasingly becoming an integral part of pediatric primary care, and their role is critical to the overall management of the child's and family's health. Some of their roles include individual and family therapy, screening for mental illness, and offering consultation to healthcare staff. Having them integrated not only provides an instant response but also enhances the overall quality of care by facilitating interdisciplinary communication. Of particular interest, psychologists often provide education and supervision to health professionals to augment overall competence in successfully meeting behavioral health needs. Nevertheless, as chronicled in recent studies, a number of clinical activities performed by psychologists within primary care sites are repeatedly unbilled, reflecting a structural deficit that can erode the economic viability of behavioral health integration. Further investigation and study in this field are necessary to maximize the integration of models of care and make family medicine sustainable (Cammarata et al., 2017).

Test Your Knowledge

1. What is a personalized treatment plan?
2. What is the role of patient engagement and education?

13.3. Preventive Care and Wellness

Learning Outcome

1. Know the shift from reactive to proactive healthcare
2. Understand the importance of lifestyle medicine
3. Describe the community health initiatives

The evolution of family medicine is facing numerous challenges, but prevention and wellness are poised to become central pillars in enhancing patient outcomes. With the shift in the healthcare landscape towards value-based care, an increasing focus on prevention is needed to offset chronic disease and reduce healthcare expenditures. Wellness programs place significant importance on lifestyle modification—healthy nutrition, regular physical activity, and stress reduction—as central to disease prevention. Interventions such as community-based health education activities and preventive care at affordable prices can bridge the healthcare disparity gap among vulnerable groups. For instance, addressing the epidemic of obesity by offering policy recommendations at the public level and targeted health interventions can lead to improvements in population health and reductions in healthcare costs (Juliano et al., 2006). Hence, integrating preventive care in family practice not only adds value to personal health but also to the efficiency of the healthcare system as a whole. One significant trend in preventive care is the supremacy of technology in promoting health. Telehealth and mobile health applications are transforming how patients access and engage with preventive care. These technologies enable more personalized care, with the patients remaining connected to healthcare professionals irrespective of geographical distances. Wearable health technology integration enables real-time monitoring of key health indicators and facilitates proactive health maintenance. Family medicine doctors are increasingly able to utilize data analytics to determine high-risk populations and tailor preventive interventions as a consequence. With an aging population and a growing proportion living with chronic health conditions, the role of technology in preventing care will be paramount in optimizing health outcomes (Bruyere et al., 2013). In this context, technology combined with evidence-based practice will be essential in shaping the future of family medicine. Additionally, the focus of preventive care will need to adapt to an aging population, which presents unique challenges for family medicine. As the workforce ages and people live longer, healthcare providers will need to prioritize strategies targeted specifically at the elderly. Preventive care measures, such as routine health screenings, cognitive function, and fall assessment, become key to maintaining seniors' health and independence. By adopting policies that support flexible work arrangements and healthy aging for older employees, family medicine has a role to play in serving the needs of the group (Bruyere et al., 2013). Speaking of management of chronic disease in this age group through holistic nature preventive care interventions not only highlights the applicability of wellness in older populations, but also ensures the importance of family medicine taking an integrated approach in its practice in order to provide better outcomes both for individuals and the health care system (Figure 13.9).

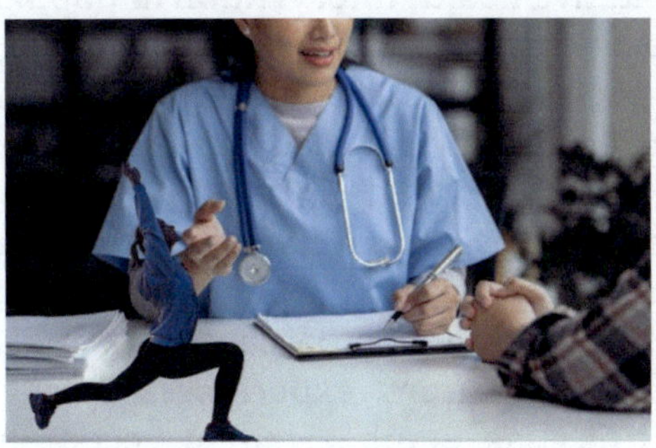

Figure 13.9. Preventive care and wellness.

Source: https://jainnursinghome.in/wp-content/uploads/sites/50/2025/05/Preventive-Care-Wellness-13.jpg

13.3.1. Shift From Reactive to Proactive Healthcare

The transition from reactive to proactive care represents a significant transformation in the provision of family medicine. Traditionally, healthcare systems operated on a reactive model, in which care was largely provided after the disease had set in. This not only raised the cost of healthcare but also resulted in poorer outcomes for patients, especially in chronic disease care. With lifestyle diseases escalating and the aging population going up, newer models that emphasize early detection and prevention have become imperative. Proactive healthcare would aim to shift the focus towards ongoing health maintenance and patient activation, leading to a much lower disease burden and improved quality of life for families and individuals. The integration of technology innovations and prevention strategies is necessary to make this vision a reality, creating a model for the future of family medicine focused not only on disease management but also on patient health. As the healthcare landscape continues to evolve, proactive strategies are increasingly evidence-based. Technologies such as telemedicine, wearable medical devices, and electronic health records (EHR) help gather and monitor patient data, allowing health professionals to anticipate potential health issues before they become severe. Clinicians can identify risk groups and implement targeted interventions to promote wellness using predictive analytics. For example, regular screening and health examinations can lead to earlier diagnosis, enhancing treatment efficacy and reducing reliance on costly acute care. Incorporating personalized medicine, particularly through genetic insights, is another proactive area of healthcare. With insight into individual health profiles, practitioners are able to generate tailored personal health plans specific to patients' individual genetic tendencies, thus optimizing health results and a strategy for prevention in family practice (Mittler-Matica et al., 2024). In child practice, change towards an active model of healthcare is aptly demonstrated through initiatives like Precision Child Health (PCH). It puts genomic sequencing at its core, enabling practitioners to tailor preventive interventions based on unique genetic information. With the identification of genetic markers for common and rare health disorders, clinicians are in a position to facilitate informed conversations with families about risk and prevention. It optimizes the quality of care and enhances patient safety, as early detection enables timely interventions tailored to individual needs. Besides, the broader implications of PCH also address the value of adopting evidence-based approaches in other healthcare settings, with learnings from genomic approaches being applicable to other active interventions. On the whole, the transition towards proactive healthcare not only improves the efficacy of family medicines but also facilitates a higher-order, knowledge-driven collaboration between patients and clinicians (Costain et al., 2020).

13.3.2. Importance of Lifestyle Medicine

The integration of lifestyle medicine into family practice is emerging as a trend-making phenomenon in the fast-paced world of medicine. With chronic illnesses on the rise, the emphasis on treating root causes of lifestyle problems—diet, physical fitness, and mental health—has come a long way among physicians. This mode of operation not only shifts attention from the cure of symptoms alone to prevention but also promotes a healthier lifestyle. By engaging patients in their own health journeys, lifestyle medicine gives individuals the power to make decisions that can lower the risk of chronic disease. The need for prevention is something that very much resonates with family medicine, where physicians understand the imperative of treating patients with an entire context in mind that involves both physical and emotional. As families deal with complex health issues, lifestyle medicine offers a promising path to achieving better health outcomes and greater long-term wellness. Current research underscores the importance of lifestyle medicine in addressing those conditions prevalent in family health, such as obesity, diabetes, and cardiovascular disease. For instance, the implementation of lifestyle interventions in primary care settings has proven effective in enhancing patients' engagement in healthier lifestyles, which in turn leads to improved clinical outcomes. The interventions usually entail patient-specific counseling, dietetic advice, and exercise recommendations according to their needs. By applying evidence-based methods, family physicians can establish effective treatment relationships with their patients by involving them in serious conversations about lifestyle choices. Also, the increasing use of technology in lifestyle medicine, such as mobile health applications and telemedicine, provides more avenues for monitoring and support. These activities are well aligned with patients, allowing the incorporation of direction, healthy lifestyle changes into daily routines, and enhancing overall quality of life. With the ongoing demographic transitions and increasing prevalence of lifestyle diseases, lifestyle medicine will lead the way in the future of family medicine. Not only does this new way of thinking potentially provide higher quality care for patients, but it puts preventative health intervention in populations at the center stage. When family physicians adopt such interventions, preventive healthcare measures are prioritized, and coordination with caregivers and public health agencies becomes even more critical. For example, campaigns promoting awareness of disease conditions like dementia can really maximize patients' and carers' experiences during care transitions, as emphasized in recent health guidelines (Livingston et al., 2020). In addition, addressing physical health in a holistic manner allows healthcare providers to fulfill their ethical obligations, as identified in the family practice guidance documents (Mach et al., 2019). Lastly, embracing lifestyle medicine as family medicine underscores the position of lifestyle choices in disease prevention but also charts the course towards holistic, patient-centered care in the 21st century (Figure 13.10).

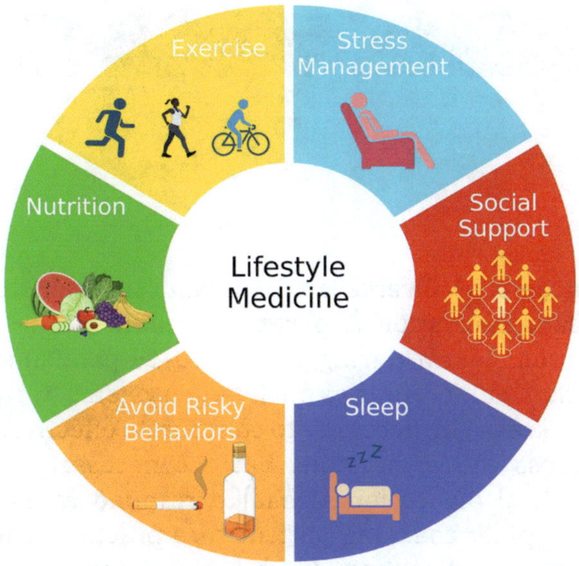

Figure 13.10. The components of lifestyle medicine.

Source: https://www.researchgate.net/publication/372410795/figure/fig1/AS:11431281239280526@1714299815734/The-components-of-lifestyle-medicine-Lifestyle-medicine-focuses-on-six-pillars-of-a.tif.

13.3.3. Community Health Initiatives

With the evolving terrain of family medicine, community health programs are offered as critical components that help enhance the quality and accessibility of health care. Community health programs focus on addressing the social determinants of health, such as income, education, and the environment, which strongly influence health outcomes. By creating connections between healthcare providers, local governments, and community organizations, these programs aim to make the healthcare system equitable. In this manner, community health programs assist in population health management by recognizing and addressing particular health issues in populations. The incorporation of such programs could help alleviate health access and outcome disparities, an issue of urgency in contemporary medicine. This paradigm shift towards community care is matched by the broader trend of investing in preventive care and in more general strategies of health management, which are key to improving public health as a whole in an increasingly complex healthcare environment. The future of family medicine is inextricably entwined with the evolution of integrated models of care, a subset of the broader class of community health programs. These models enable primary care providers to work in tandem with specialty providers, particularly in the care of medical comorbidities in vulnerable populations. Notably, integrating mental health services into primary care can yield large health outcome benefits among severely mentally ill patients, whose health deteriorates due to the fact that they do not have coordinated care. Interventions promoting efficient referral systems and collaboration can significantly enhance preventative care measures, enabling such patients to receive timely intervention and attention. Education of current and future healthcare professionals can be an area of focus through which such interventions could transform the delivery of care in family medicine, creating a more integrated healthcare system with priorities toward comprehensive, patient-oriented care (Read et al., 2016). Besides, community health programs also act to neutralize market forces that challenge conventional models of healthcare provision. As healthcare systems converge into consumer-centric models, an increased need for family practices to innovate towards new governance forms and economic imperatives arises. The interdependence of healthcare providers is being put to the test as efforts aim to reconcile efficiency with quality of care. Focus on community health also strengthens the relationship between family medicine and hospitals, ensuring they collaborate to improve patient outcomes. As outlined in the current health policy discourse, the potential to integrate care while remaining responsive to patients' needs will determine whether this shift is successful. These trends emphasize innovation and flexibility in family practice, putting community health efforts at the forefront of its future effectiveness and sustainability in meeting the challenges that lie ahead.

Test Your Knowledge

1. What is the importance of lifestyle medicine?
2. What is community health initiatives?

13.4. Interprofessional Collaboration

Learning Outcome

1. Describe the team-based care models in family medicine
2. Understand the role of family physicians in multidisciplinary teams
3. Describe the benefits of collaborative practice

As the practice of family medicine continues to evolve, interprofessional collaboration stands out as a critical element for enhanced patient outcomes. The nature of the modern practice of medicine, grounded in an interdisciplinary practice, shifts from fragmented health services towards the incorporation of various healthcare professionals into a single unit. This concern is especially pertinent in family medicine, where providers are likely to encounter multifaceted health problems that span multiple specialties. Effective interprofessional care not only improves communication among health professionals but also facilitates a shared approach to patients' complex needs. Specifically, studies indicate that care delivered in teams leads to better patient participation and satisfaction, thereby shaping the future of family medicine. With healthcare becoming more holistic, teamwork will be essential in developing comprehensive treatment plans that encompass diverse opinions and experiences. Team innovation is particularly influenced by lessons learnt during the COVID-19 pandemic, when vulnerabilities in health systems were revealed. The necessity to collaborate effectively across the professions became necessary as medical professionals had to respond rapidly to rapidly changing patient care practices and resource allocation. In this, the emphasis on collaborative practice has grown stronger, as the pandemic underscored the importance of collaboration in confronting challenges in the healthcare sector. The need for education institutions and agencies is now established to integrate collaborative competency training within their curricula so that future healthcare professionals are prepared. Furthermore, the development of new ways of working together, such as through technology and virtual conferences, has opened up new opportunities for cross-disciplinary collaboration, witnessed in the expansion of web-based training modules focused on teamwork and non-technical skills. This attitudinal shift is a positive trend towards stronger interprofessional collaborations in the future, anchored in flexibility and resilience. The recurring development of evidence-based interventions to improve interprofessional collaboration is imperative to the best delivery of family medicine outcomes. Evidence has shown that evidence-based team interventions, such as those evaluated using the Grading of

Recommendations, Assessment, Development, and Evaluation Scale, are indispensable for shaping effective collaborative care practices. Training interventions such as TeamSTEPPS and simulation-based training have been highly effective in improving team performance and communication in healthcare settings. Increased training aimed at developing non-technical skills allows various health professionals to work more coordinated care strategies, filling any potential gaps in the provision of services and ultimately leading to improved patient safety and satisfaction. The future of family medicine will largely depend on developing such coordinated systems to ensure healthcare teams can adequately address the evolving health landscape. Highlighting interprofessional collaboration as a necessary pillar will help ensure the overall care patients expect and deserve more and more (Figure 13.11).

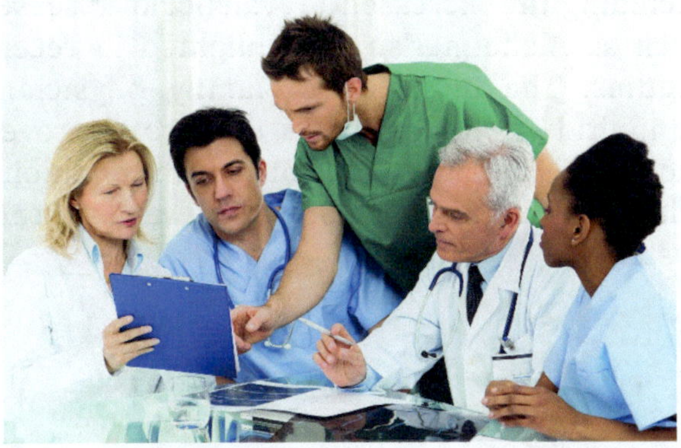

Figure 13.11. Interprofessional collaboration.

Source: https://www.myamericannurse.com/wp-content/uploads/2021/12/shutterstock_138847457-scaled.jpg.

13.4.1. Team-Based Care Models

The evolution of family medicine team-based model care is a milestone innovation in health care provision, particularly given the growing complexity of patients' needs. Team-based models aim to deliver multilateral care that leverages the expertise of various healthcare practitioners, such as physicians, nurses, social workers, and behavioral health clinicians, to provide comprehensive coverage. The overlap of different disciplines allows for a more holistic perspective, enabling both physical and psychosocial issues to be addressed. A case in point is the application of family-centered care guidelines in settings like neonatal intensive care units, which has confirmed the benefits of involving relatives in decision-making about their care, potentially leading to improved health outcomes. As healthcare institutions increasingly recognize the significance of interprofessional teamwork, there is a strong prospect for enhancing the patient experience, improving continuity of care, and mitigating barriers to service utilization, ultimately reconfiguring the family medicine landscape into an integrative model (Cho et al., 2025). When healthcare emergencies intensify, particularly with the rising prevalence of chronic diseases, team-based models of care offer an appropriate alternative for management and prevention. As opposed to relying exclusively on specialty care, these models foster a coordinated effort that integrates the professional skills of diverse health workers in a single procedure. Chronic disease management in team-based care focuses not only on filling clinical requirements but also on recognizing the impact of social determinants of health. For example, involving behavioral health experts in primary care centers enhances the ability to treat diabetes and hypertension more effectively by allowing patients to incorporate treatment routines into their day-to-day lives (Olowomeye, 2025). Additionally, the models facilitate integration and joint decision-making, empowering patients to become integral components of their own treatment. This is a transition towards an interdisciplinary practice that, in addition to enhancing patient outcomes, reduces the overall burden on health systems by promoting prevention and best disease management. In the future, the implementation of team-based care models of family medicine necessitates structural and systemic changes to provide a setting where there is teamwork. The key to success lies in developing coordinated electronic health record systems that facilitate seamless interaction among team members and in extensive training programs to enhance teamwork capabilities. Through the application of such measures, shared obstacles such as professional role boundaries and communication deficits will be minimized to discourage seamless collaboration. Furthermore, value-based reimbursement systems can promote team-based models with incentives aligned to improved patient outcomes and satisfaction. With family medicine moving towards more integrated and team-based practice, opportunities for such models to offer effective and equitable solutions to healthcare problems become increasingly clear, paving the way for an era where integrated and humane care becomes the priority (Olowomeye, 2025) (Figure 13.12).

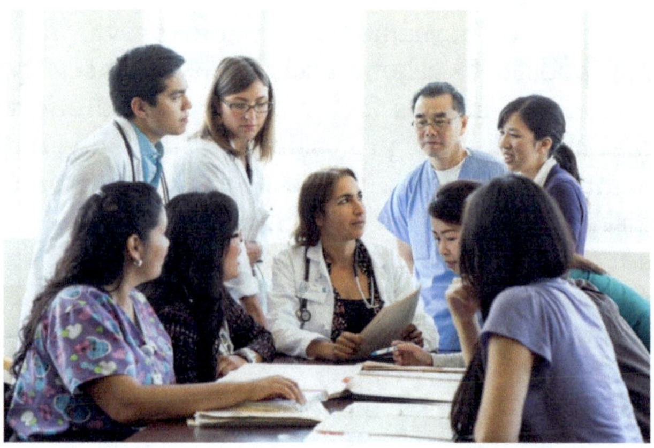

Figure 13.12. Team-based care models.

Source: https://www.ucsf.edu/sites/default/files/styles/2014_wysiwyg_full/public/fields/field_insert_file/news/vener-huddle.jpg?itok=PcJyC_6d.

13.4.2. Role of Family Physicians in Multidisciplinary Teams

The role of family physicians in multidisciplinary teams becomes more critical as healthcare systems evolve to meet the complex and heterogeneous needs of patients. Family physicians naturally play a role not only as first-line providers of care but also as coordinators of care across various specialties. Their thorough understanding of the social determinants of health and patient history enables them to collaborate with other healthcare professionals, including allied health workers, specialists, and nurses. This integrated approach ensures that all aspects of a patient's care are addressed, provoking holistic treatment plans and better health outcomes. With more chronic diseases and an aging population, the need for family physicians to work in multidisciplinary teams will increase, in line with future trends in family medicine that emphasize coordinated, patient-centered care.

Moreover, family physicians play a critical function in public health management, including the increased prevalence of diseases such as Alzheimer's, as highlighted in recent studies. The inclusion of family physicians in multidisciplinary teams enables improved monitoring and management of such conditions, with implications for a more proactive healthcare system.

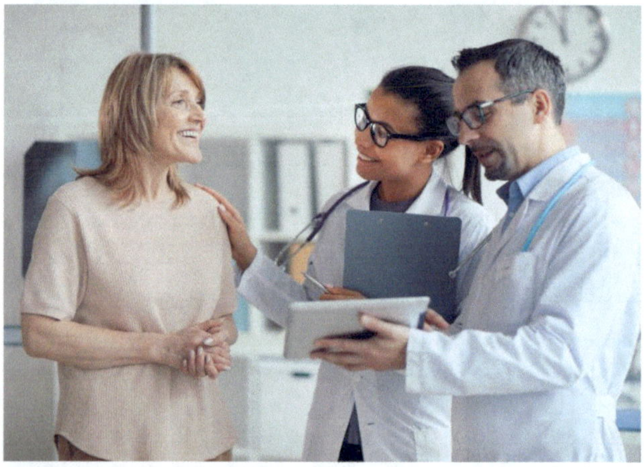

Figure 13.13. Family physicians

Source: https://api.myfamilymd.org/uploads/blogs/photo_1734681494539.JPG.

Chronic illness burdens extend beyond the individual to reach the family and community, as is evidenced in the increasing strains on family caregivers, who provided an estimated 18 billion hours of care in 2022 to those with Alzheimer's. By incorporating family medicine into the multidisciplinary team, health systems can facilitate more holistic, community-oriented approaches that address not only the patient's medical condition but also the emotional and logistical strain on caregivers. On addressing evolving healthcare demands, the integration of family physicians into multidisciplinary teams is similarly essential in solving clinician burnout and enhancing workforce resilience, especially as seen during the COVID-19 pandemic. The compounded stressors faced by health professionals require a supportive, integrated workspace that can be provided by family physicians (Dewey et al., 2020). By fostering clinician well-being and bringing best practices in mental health care to their practice settings, family physicians can help create more resilient healthcare teams. As trends in family medicine continue to move toward greater levels of interdisciplinary teamwork, family physicians will be responsible for applying their specialized skills to promote team building, thereby improving both clinician retention and patient care in ever-more complex healthcare settings (Figure 13.12).

13.4.3. Benefits of Collaborative Practice

As family medicine evolves, the benefits of collaborative practice are a basis for healthcare delivery and improved patient outcomes. By promoting a multidisciplinary approach, collaborative practice unites professionals from disciplines such as medicine, nursing, pharmacy, and social work to form an extensive care team. This team environment not only addresses diverse patient needs but also facilitates the sharing of experiences and knowledge, ultimately leading to more informed decision-making. Enhanced team communication helps buffer mistakes and the replication of effort and is thus particularly useful in the instance of complex conditions. such as chronic disease management. Since family medicine is increasingly collaborative in practice, health professionals can harness the strengths of others, thereby promoting a patient-centered model attuned to community needs. Collaborative practice also comes along with the growing emphasis on patient-centered care, which is at the heart of the study of family medicine. Including patients as active participants in their care encourages closer relationships between healthcare professionals and those they serve, ultimately improving treatment plan compliance and health outcomes. Through cooperation, healthcare professionals can better appreciate each patient's unique circumstance, adapting interventions to meet individual tastes and cultural heritage. This not only heightens patient satisfaction but also enables patients to take ownership of their health, thereby facilitating preventive care. As health systems move towards models centered on the patient experience, embracing collaborative practice can significantly help build a culture of shared decision-making, which translates to mutual understanding and commitment between providers and patients. Finally, integration of collaborative practice in family medicine has serious benefits as far as resource management and efficiency are concerned. When various professionals work together, there is potential to streamline processes, eliminate waste, and boost overall efficiency in the provision of health care. For instance, when every job is clearly defined within a collaborative team, healthcare providers can optimize their time by performing what they excel at, thus preventing unnecessary delays in patient treatment. Additionally, solving shared health care issues, such as the opioid crisis, through collective action offers a unique benefit that is inherent to collaborative practice in family medicine. As outlined in recent literature, the integration of multiple healthcare perspectives not only meets current clinical demand but also advances the sustainability of healthcare systems through resource synergism, and hence forms integrated solutions that meet the needs of populations at large (Becker et al., 2020; Kruk et al., 2018) (Figure 13.14).

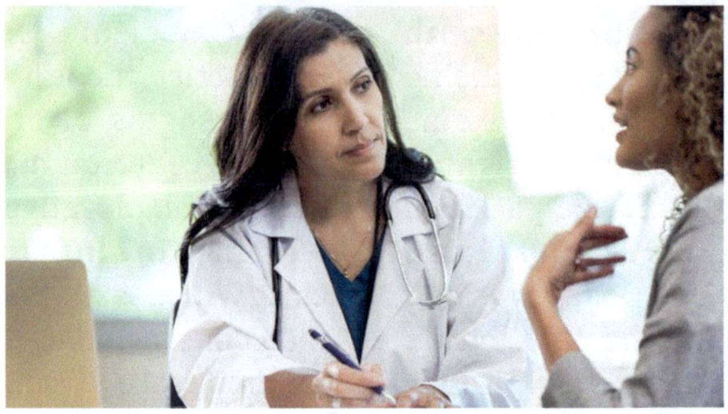

Figure 13.14. Benefits of collaborative practice.

Source: https://animosanopsychiatry.com/wp-content/uploads/2023/05/feature-image.jpg.

Test Your Knowledge

1. What is the team-based care model?
2. What are the benefits of collaborative practice?

13.5. Health Equity and Access

Learning Outcome

1. Address disparities in healthcare
2. Know the strategies for improving access to care
3. Understand the role of family medicine in underserved communities

Historically, in the United States, health equity has been nothing but a far-off dream, with gross disparities in access to care across segments. To a large extent, such disparities are well-entrenched in cases of populations affected with chronic diseases, such as Alzheimer's disease, where an aggregate of 6.7 million Americans aged 65 and older live with this disease. The projected rise to 13.8 million by 2060 underscores the imperative for health solutions that are fair and equal in response to this mounting need. Furthermore, family caregivers, disproportionately women and minorities, experience higher emotional burden and health harm from the overwhelming caregiving demands for loved ones with dementia. The imperative of innovative healthcare policies with provisions for fair access to care, and especially in the handling of chronic diseases, becomes increasingly paramount as trends in healthcare shift towards combating such ingrained disparities. Telehealth, which gained popularity during the COVID-19 pandemic, presents a key pathway to advancing health access and equity in family medicine. The convenience of virtual care promises to activate patients and manage disease, particularly for vulnerable populations. But this shift comes with new challenges as well; broadband availability disparities and techno-savviness could exacerbate existing inequities.

Studies have demonstrated that marginalized patients often distrust telehealth services due to historical abuses and a lack of prior relationship with healthcare providers. To overcome these challenges, it is critical to design telehealth systems that prioritize patient-clinician relationships, establishing proximity and trust through deliberate deployment. Enhancing these interactions may eventually lead to improved health outcomes and greater acceptance of telehealth services across diverse populations, potentially reshaping family medicine's future landscape (Yee et al., 2022). As family medicine responds to these changing healthcare dynamics, closing health equity and access gaps must be at the core of its strategic efforts.

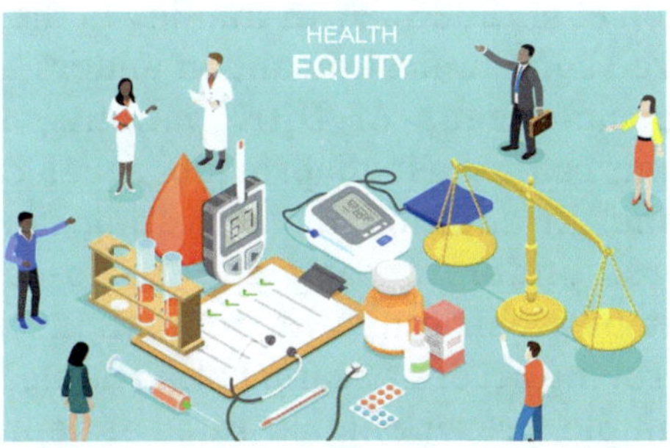

Figure 13.15. Health systems creating a benchmark for health equity.

Source: https://demo.smart-hospital.in/uploads/gallery/media/health-equity.jpg.

This is to be done with a multi-pronged approach, including community outreach to ensure that healthcare policy deliberations are informed by the needs of different populations. Education and training of healthcare workers should also change to place greater emphasis on cultural competence and on establishing trust across diverse patient populations. Integrating equitable practices into medical education, including implicit bias training, will be essential to empower the future generation of physicians to address the needs of patient care in today's increasingly digital landscape. By facilitating equitable access and enhancing health literacy among vulnerable groups, family medicine can play a vital role in promoting health equity—a key factor for making the healthcare system more just and efficient (Yee et al., 2022) (Figure 13.15).

13.5.1. Addressing Disparities in Healthcare

In contemporary discourse on healthcare, the eradication of disparities has emerged as a key component of family medicine, specifically as a response to shifting practice trends. Disparities can present in various ways, including socioeconomic status, geographic location, and access to information. As healthcare professionals strive to offer inclusive care, the reliance on credible sources of information takes precedence.

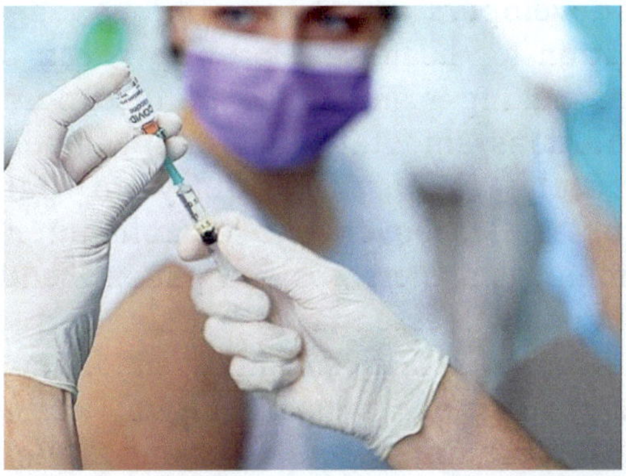

Figure 13.16. Addressing healthcare disparities: Strategies for ensuring equal access to health.

Source: https://thecsrjournal.in/wp-content/uploads/2021/11/CSR-Healthcare.jpeg.

A study on differences in CAM information sources among oncology patients and health professionals corroborates this. Patients most commonly access CAM information from friends and relatives (82.6%), whereas healthcare practitioners most frequently access it from internet sources (61.4%) (Aleksandar et al., 2025). This disparity underscores the need for standardized educational approaches that effectively bridge the gap, enabling informed decision-making and ultimately improving patient care among multicultural populations. To move towards equitable health care delivery, the technology component, such as artificial intelligence (AI), plays a role. AI technology brings disruptive possibilities, such as improved diagnostic accuracy, personalized treatment pathways, and greater ease of access to healthcare.

For instance, AI-powered applications can identify at-risk populations and create targeted interventions for specific health issues, thereby mitigating disparities. AI also demands attention to ethical issues such as algorithmic bias and transparency, as these may inadvertently reproduce existing healthcare disparities (Basubrin, 2025). Hence, emphasis on inter-disciplinary collaboration among physicians and developers of AI, as well as ongoing education for healthcare providers, can be of epoch-making significance in incorporating AI solutions smoothly into family medicine, ultimately supporting equity in patient outcomes. Moreover, the establishment of community partnerships and patient-centered care models is essential in working to reduce healthcare disparities. Family medicine can make good strides toward equity by extending to local communities and assessing the unique health problems and cultural contexts of such communities. Outreaching in this manner builds trust and enhances care compliance among underserved communities. Interventions that focus on culturally sensitive care and community education have the potential to empower patients to make informed health decisions. Further, integrating feedback mechanisms into health care organizations can enable tailored services to address community-specific needs. All these combined can fortify the healthcare system so that there is quality, equitable care available to everybody, eradicating disparities and opening doors to a more inclusive future for family medicine (Figure 13.16).

13.5.2. Strategies for Improving Access to Care

Efficacious strategies to improve access to care through family medicine are essential for addressing rising disparities across patient groups. Expanding communication with marginalized groups, such as Deaf and Hard of Hearing (DHH) patients, is a huge opportunity for family medicine providers. Aiming to improve healthcare providers' cultural competence through educational interventions can reduce barriers to effective communication and, in turn, improve patient-provider interactions. There is evidence that DHH patients receive unequal care with longer waiting times and limited access to appropriate diagnostic services (Johnson et al., 2025). With training in the use of preferred communication and in understanding the special needs of DHH patients, family medicine can adjust to provide equal care to everyone. In addition to alleviating language barriers, understanding the socio-cultural context between different populations is key to improving access to care. Latina adolescents, for example, present higher rates of depressive symptoms but experience significant obstacles in pursuing treatment, like stigma and financial limitations (Werder et al., 2022). Family doctors are able to apply this knowledge by developing specially targeted outreach programs that educate families about mental health care and the necessity to seek treatment. Working with community groups and advocating culturally responsive systems of service delivery can make the general mental health climate more robust for these groups. Modifying interventions to address specific barriers faced by various groups ensures the ongoing applicability and responsiveness of family medicine to the needs of the community. Moreover, the adoption of technological solutions can be a vital part of expanding access to care, particularly for underserved populations. Telemedicine has been recognized as an emerging tool in family medicine, offering remote consultations that reduce transportation barriers and make scheduling appointments more flexible. This digital model has been advantageous during the COVID-19 pandemic by providing ongoing access to care for patients who may otherwise have encountered barriers to in-person services. In addition, incorporating digital health resources into everyday practice can empower patients by providing information and tools to help them proactively manage their health. With changing family medicine, it is advisable to invest in new access strategies first to transform healthcare delivery and enhance health outcomes among various populations.

13.5.3. Role of Family Medicine in Underserved Communities

Family medicine is the leading provider of care for vulnerable populations, specifically by delivering holistic, accessible, and culturally competent care. These groups are likely to encounter numerous systemic barriers, including economic constraints, limited health insurance coverage, and limited access to specialty care. Family medicine physicians possess the ability to deliver comprehensive care, not merely physical, but also mental and social care related to the determinants of health. Through the formation of solid doctor-patient relationships, such doctors are able to instill trust and encourage patients from disadvantaged groups to access care on a regular basis, reducing preventable conditions and admissions to the hospital. It is an active step, as it can reduce long-term healthcare costs by managing chronic diseases, ultimately leading to healthier populations and reduced overall healthcare costs. In addition, the family medicine role is more urgently needed in the context of addressing public health emergencies such as the COVID-19 pandemic. Public health emergencies such as the pandemic have disproportionately impacted underserved populations, with increased rates of severe illness that result from underlying health disparities, which are compounded by the socio-economic circumstances they face. Family doctors have emerged as frontline warriors, offering basic services such as vaccination campaigns, health education, and care for chronic conditions amid these unforgiving times.

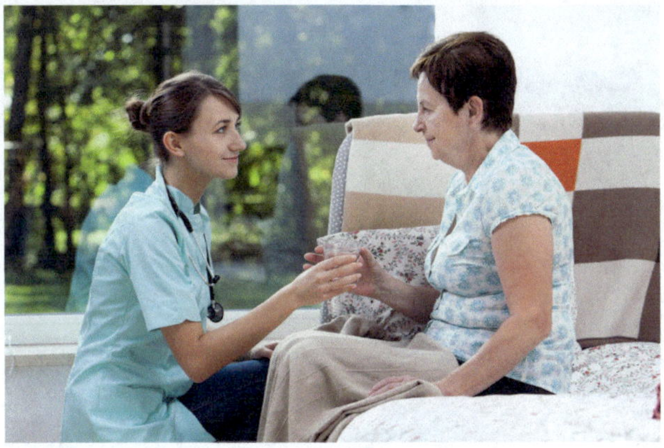

Figure 13.17. The role of the family nurse practitioner in underserved communities.

Source: https://onlinenursing.cn.edu/sites/default/files/2024-03/serving-underserved-community-health-nurse-1.jpg.

In the process, they are serving a crucial purpose in combating not only the immediate effects of the pandemic but also in erasing the longstanding gap in access to and outcomes in health. Family medicine practices that prioritize responsiveness to locally relevant matters are more likely to shape future trends, underscoring the significance of responsive, sustainable health systems for vulnerable populations (Browne et al., 2020). Integration of technology into family medicine makes it even more efficient for implementation in vulnerable communities. Telemedicine has also emerged as a revolutionary tool, opening care to those who may be geographically or physically unable to receive in-office visits. By employing telehealth functions, family medicine doctors can address patient needs in a convenient and timely manner, increasing their scope and ensuring continuity of care, especially for chronic disease patients. Furthermore, technology can be employed to augment health education and awareness campaigns specifically targeted to the requirements of these heterogeneous populations. As family medicine continues to evolve and incorporates technological advancements such as telehealth, it is imperative that professionals are cognizant of the specificity of issues and the cultural sensitivities involved among underserved populations, so that they provide equal and effective healthcare interventions for everyone (Figure 13.17).

Test Your Knowledge

1. Describe the strategies for improving access to care.
2. What is the role of family medicine in underserved communities?

13.6. Policy and Regulation Changes

Learning Outcome

1. Know the impact of healthcare legislation on family medicine
2. Understand the future of insurance models and reimbursement
3. Describe the advocacy for family medicine at the policy level

The destiny of family medicine hangs in the balance on the scales of grand policy and regulatory reforms seeking to address the evolving healthcare needs of a multiracial, multigenerational society. To respond to increasing demand for primary care, the reforms are required to create a more equitable and effective healthcare system. Directions in the future will be toward increased care coordination and prevention services that place patient results at the forefront. This diversion would be guided by policies that promote value-oriented models of care and integrated health services. Furthermore, technology uptake in the healthcare sector will also be supported by policy reforms that facilitate telemedicine and electronic health interventions. This provision will be imperative in bridging geographical constraints and improving access to care, essential building stones in the continuum of family medicine. In light of such previous precedent, the trajectory of health workforce research calls for policy intervention. Decades-long waves of research have repeatedly pointed out the need for proper health workforce planning, particularly in the context of imminent health crises. Current research identifies the means through which technological innovation and changes in the scope of practice legislation influence provider capacity and performance in their delivery of services. Specifically, the licensure law reforms have enabled greater flexibility in the workforce, allowing professionals to practice to the full extent of their training. This change in policy results from greater awareness of how pressures on family physicians and other practitioners in the system necessitate innovative solutions to address community needs and enhance the overall health delivery system (Dower et al., 2011). As the regulatory context evolves, future migration and workforce development will play a key role in determining family medicine. Historical examination reveals stages in health workforce policy, with a transition from mid-20th-century planning models to current frameworks focusing on resource optimization and efficiency. The ongoing scarcity of health workers in both the industrialized and developing world has led countries to pay more attention to the international movement of health workers. Such policies to cause this migration can alleviate local shortages and hence cater to underserved populations. Further, integrating global health perspectives into local policies could offer learning opportunities for effective recruitment and retention strategies, ultimately leading to an effective family medicine system that can respond satisfactorily to future healthcare demands (Bloom et al., 2025).

13.6.1. Impact of Healthcare Legislation on Family Medicine

Healthcare legislation plays a pivotal role in reshaping family medicine, significantly impacting the accessibility of care and the level of service delivered. The enactment of legislation such as the Affordable Care Act (ACA) in the USA is a stark example of how legislative intervention can expand insurance coverage among the previously uninsured and, as a result, increase demand for family medicine practitioners. By mandating essential health benefits and preventive services, the ACA did not just increase access to healthcare but also placed a high priority on primary care. The shift establishes the importance of family medicine in improving public health outcomes and meeting the complex demands of diverse patient populations. Because family physicians have become the first point of entry into healthcare systems, legislative policies that prioritize investment in primary care reflect broader trends toward integrated health services and patient care overall (Kruk et al., 2018). Nevertheless, healthcare legislation is a problem that cannot be disregarded. While policies like the ACA opened access, they also introduced complexities, such as value-based reimbursement models rather than volume-based. This change means that family medicine physicians need to adapt to new fiscal incentives that are based on quality outcomes rather than volume. The pressure to meet performance targets can lead to higher patient numbers for family physicians, in opposition to the patient-centered care required for effective primary care. Secondly, reimbursement policies can be perverse for rural family practice, where resource limitations already constrain capacity for greater service delivery. Thus, policymakers need to collaborate with medical professionals to simplify legislation sustainability, in addition to sustaining the fundamental values of family medicine (Manyi-Loh et al., 2018). In the future, the influence of healthcare legislation on family medicine will continue to evolve as new public health issues emerge.

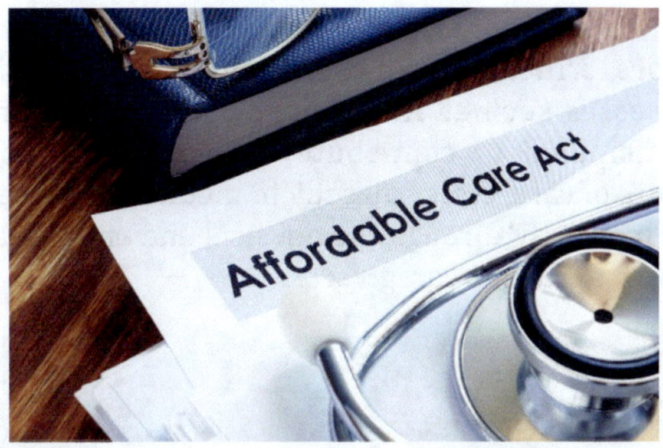

Figure 13.18. Affordable Care Act (ACA).

Source: https://www.sanabenefits.com/wp-content/uploads/2022/03/iStock-1141247654.jpg.

Legislative proposals focused on meeting global health priorities, such as the COVID-19 pandemic, are an indication of the necessity for an adaptive and responsive family medicine paradigm to shift between states of crisis. The move towards telemedicine and digital health technologies, preceded by policy changes that boosted emergency legislation, is a sign of an upward trajectory in technology adoption in primary care. But ensuring universal coverage of such innovation is the key to not making current health disparities worse. As family medicine adapts to meet legislative reforms, ongoing advocacy for policies that support complete, high-quality care will be needed to serve the population's diverse healthcare needs while affirming the specialty's role as a foundation of the health system (Kruk et al., 2018) (Figure 13.18).

13.6.2. Future of Insurance Models and Reimbursement

As family medicine shifts and evolves, so must the insurance models and payment structures that support it. Fee-for-service payment systems are giving way to value-based care systems that reward patients for outcomes instead of services. These novel forms of care are focused on comprehensive patient management, are more critical in the management of chronic illnesses such as Alzheimer's disease, and are anticipated to contribute enormously to the costs of care, either directly in medical expenses or indirectly through the physical and emotional costs to family caregivers.

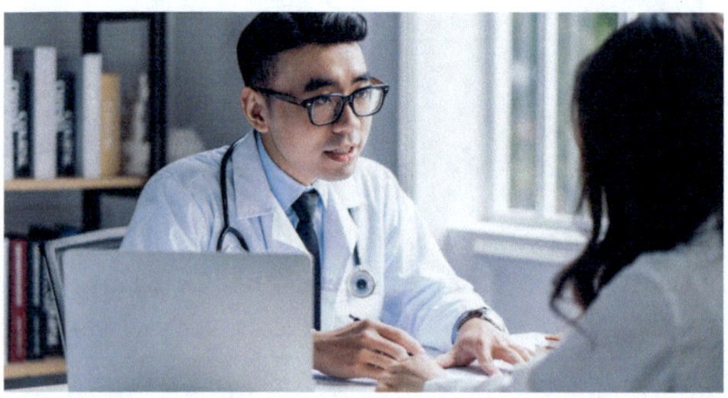

Figure 13.19. Guide to healthcare reimbursement.

Source: https://www.sermo.com/wp-content/uploads/2023/05/insurance-reimbursement-img1-min-1050x555.jpg.

In the future, healthcare policy will increasingly reward those providers who successfully integrate care coordination, prevention, and continuous patient engagement into their business models. These measures not only benefit patients but also help reduce the cost pressure on the overall health system. With the projected rise in demand for healthcare services because of an increased population of the elderly and a proliferation of chronic illnesses, insurance payment models need to be revised. New steps, such as the bundled payment model, in which one payment is made for a series of services for a particular condition or episode of care, can maximize the delivery of healthcare while creating efficiency and responsibility in providers. This is particularly relevant, as Medicare payment for demented patients, for instance, can be nearly three times that for non-disadvantaged patients. In addition, expanding access to data through such comprehensive health databases, as in Denmark, may more suitably examine insurance models and reimbursement strategies, facilitating well-informed policy-making and decision-making that accurately reflects the complexities of family medicine patient care. The future of insurance designs will also involve paying attention to the integration of technology into patient care, thereby creating an integrated process that boosts reimbursement programs. Telemedicine, for example, has gained momentum in the post-COVID-19 era by providing an affordable way to manage patient consultations and extend access to care. Reimbursement designs that encourage and support telehealth interventions can boost the efficiency of healthcare delivery, especially among low-income segments. Moreover, as family medicine doctors increasingly adopt electronic health records and other health information technologies, there is a need to restructure reimbursement policies that acknowledge the value of technology in enhancing care quality. In short, insurance model innovation and dynamic reimbursement strategies are crucial in building the future of family medicine with value, access, and improved patient outcomes for diverse populations (Figure 13.19).

13.6.3. Advocacy for Family Medicine at Policy Level

Family medicine advocacy on the policy level plays a vital role in shaping future healthcare systems amidst shifting demographics and health concerns. As the pillars of primary care, family medicine doctors play a pivotal role in advocating for preventive care and chronic disease management while ensuring health services are accessible and fair. Engaging policymakers in discussions of the need for a strong family medicine system can give the push needed to implement flexible policies that support patient-focused care. The discussion will also assist in addressing systemic issues, such as disparities in healthcare access and the increasing burden of chronic diseases, that need a strong family medicine workforce in a bid to effectively control. This campaigning is not only vital to public health but to the functioning of health systems in general, particularly in a system increasingly dominated by health crises like the COVID-19 pandemic. Due to the massive demographic changes, among which are higher incidence rates of chronic diseases and an aging population, the role of family medicine has never been as significant. It allows providers to establish policies that effectively meet these changing needs. Policymakers, aware that healthcare systems are becoming progressively overloaded, can benefit from integrating the principles of family medicine into overall health policy. For instance, broadening the scope of family physician practice can lead to reduced costs in healthcare and improved patient outcomes, as they are the first point of entry within the health system. As has been demonstrated by the increasing significance of preventive care in diseases like Alzheimer's, family medicine should be appropriately represented in health policymaking so that it can innovate and adapt to emerging health concerns, as a testament to its commitment to delivering high-quality care to diverse populations . Furthermore, advocacy for family medicine must increasingly form alliances that cross several sectors beyond the traditional boundaries of healthcare. By working with schools, civil society organizations, and even as far-reaching sectors as housing and transport, family medicine can ensure that support is provided to integrated health approaches that tackle the social determinants of health. Such integrated systems are pivotal for healthier outcomes, particularly among disadvantaged groups where inequalities are more prevalent. Policies that underpin these partnerships not only enhance community health but also encourage health system resilience, making family medicine a leader in innovative, whole-person care models. Lastly, a strong policy advocacy framework for family medicine ensures that professionals are prepared to respond to the exigencies of future healthcare demands while advocating for the equitable distribution of healthcare resources essential to achieving successful healthcare outcomes for populations (Kruk et al., 2018).

Test Your Knowledge

1. What is the impact of healthcare legislation on family medicine?
2. What is the future of insurance models and reimbursement?

SUMMARY

As family medicine progresses, it is important to recognize the complex determinants that shape future directions. One such revolutionary shift in the direction towards care models of integration has been recognized, with an emphasis on streamlined access to the health system. The integration of general practice cooperatives and NHS Direct, as reflected in the current literature, indicates the benefits that can be gained from such integrations. While the studies are successful to some extent in lowering aggregate demand for care, they also show that many patients still face access barriers, requiring multiple calls just to get assistance. This indicates that integration can reduce redundancies, but has still not delivered on its promise of integrated care. Therefore, emphasizing the need for coordinated approaches towards expanding access and efficiency in patient care remains of paramount significance as the future of family medicine is mapped out (Burgess et al., 2005). Technology's contribution to revolutionizing family medicine cannot be overemphasized, with developments on course to redefine the provider-patient relationship and service delivery. Telemedicine, among other emerging technologies, is quickly becoming a pivotal instrument for overcoming geographical and logistical challenges to access. This kind of shift aligns with evidence on the supply and distribution of the primary care core workforce, which indicates growing demand for accessible health services that can meet the health needs of populations (Dower et al., 2011). In this way, integrating technology into family medicine clinics will most likely empower patients by giving them greater control over their health care choices. As practitioners embrace these innovations, provision must also be made for how technology enhances and complements modalities of customary care and not replaces them. In summary, family medicine's future will be the precarious balance between innovation and access. The success of the integrated models of care, as well as new technology, will shape healthcare policy and practice in the future. Continued examination of the effects of these trends will be crucial to developing more effective strategies to maximize patient outcomes. Stakeholders will need to take an active role in anticipating and filling service gaps in order to enable a healthcare system as equitable as it is advanced. Thus, setting patient-centered care policies at the top of the agenda will not only enhance satisfaction but will ultimately fortify the system of family medicine against threats presented by an evolving health care environment (Burgess et al., 2005; Dower et al., 2011).

Understanding significant trends in family medicine indicates a changing environment influenced by various socioeconomic, technological, and healthcare delivery determinants. One significant trend is the increased emphasis on patient-centered care, in which patients' needs and desires are prioritized in treatment options. This trend has resulted from health systems' efforts to enhance patient participation and satisfaction, leading to better health outcomes. Besides, the synergy between telemedicine and data analytics has transformed family physicians' engagement with patients, making it more accessible and efficient. Data-driven practice being the new norm, family medicine should embrace more technologies that facilitate the provision of care from afar, particularly vital in rural or disadvantaged areas. Another crucial trend is the added focus on prevention using health measures in family medicine. Practices are being redirected toward chronic disease management and early intervention, as evidenced by the adoption of comprehensive health screenings and lifestyle modification programs. It's a forward-looking policy that aims to control risk factors before they progress to severe diseases, thus reducing long-term healthcare costs and improving population health. The integration of behavioral health into family practice is also growing, with physicians more aware of the connection between body and mind. Such trends reflect a general increase in respect for comprehensive healthcare that focuses on healing the whole patient rather than isolated symptoms. Lastly, the role of family medicine in public health initiatives is more prominent than ever before. With pandemics, environmental stressors, and health inequities as universal challenges, family physicians are particularly well-positioned to lead community-based health initiatives. Being the initial contact most patients have with the medical system, they possess a great opportunity to learn valuable hints regarding community health needs and crises. The World Health Organization's Essential Medicines List is a best-practices model for family medicine, with a focus on access to essential pharmaceuticals as a public health force for advancement (Cavicchi et al., 2011). In addition, the development of measurable indicators of child safety, permanency, and well-being has the potential to enhance the efficacy of family-focused public health intervention (Gibbons et al., 2003). This new position places a greater responsibility on family medicine to shape public health policy and outcomes.

KEY TERMS FROM THIS CHAPTER

Artificial intelligence
Blood pressure
Electronic health records
Machine learning models
Natural language processing
Personalized medicine
Smart health records
Blood glucose levels
Data management
Heart rate
Medical genetics
Patient-centered care
Remote patient monitoring
Telemedicine

CRITICAL THINKING QUESTIONS

1. **What is one of the most significant advancements shaping the future of family medicine?**
   a. Reduced use of electronic medical records
   b. Integration of artificial intelligence in diagnostics
   c. Elimination of telemedicine
   d. Sole reliance on traditional treatment methods
2. **How is telemedicine expected to transform family medicine?**
   a. By reducing patient access to healthcare
   b. By enabling remote consultations and follow-ups
   c. By replacing in-person visits entirely
   d. By focusing solely on urban healthcare
3. **Which of the following is a benefit of personalized medicine in family practice?**
   a. One-size-fits-all treatment protocols
   b. Treatment based on individual genetic profiles
   c. Ignoring lifestyle factors in treatment plans
   d. Uniform prescription practices
4. **What role will wearable technology play in future family medicine?**
   a. Making healthcare less accessible
   b. Reducing patient engagement in their health
   c. Tracking patient health metrics in real time
   d. Eliminating the need for regular check-ups
5. **Artificial intelligence in family medicine can assist with:**
   a. Reducing patient interactions
   b. Automated diagnosis and clinical decision-making support
   c. Replacing physicians entirely
   d. Eliminating the need for patient histories

Short Answer Questions

1. What is technological advancement in family medicine?
2. What is the electronic health record?
3. What is patient-centered care?
4. What is preventive care and wellness?
5. Describe the role of family physicians in multidisciplinary teams.

Answer to Critical Thinking Questions

1. (b); 2. (b); 3. (b); 4. (c); 5. (b).

REFERENCES

1. Abela, J. C., & Bugeja, M. (2014). Continuity of information and care: A pilot study in a health center. https://core.ac.uk/download/46602484.pdf (accessed on 14th July 2025).
2. Anand, U., Dey, A., Chandel, A. K. S., Sanyal, R., Mishra, A., Pandey, D. K., De Falco, V., Upadhyay, A., Kandimalla, R., Chaudhary, A., Dhanjal, J. K., Dewanjee, S., Vallamkondu, J., & De La Lastra, J. M. P. (2022). Cancer chemotherapy and beyond: Current status, drug candidates, associated risks and progress in targeted therapeutics. *Genes & Diseases*, *10*(4), 1367–1401. https://doi.org/10.1016/j.gendis.2022.02.007Arnold, N. (2025). Smart health records: Integrating AI for efficient data management. *Newport International Journal of Research in Medical Sciences*. https://www.semanticscholar.org/paper/98feac9c92610dd866e5345edeca410bbec11935 (accessed on 14th July 2025).
3. Basubrin, O. (2025). Current status and future of artificial intelligence in medicine. *Cureus, 17*. https://www.semanticscholar.org/paper/e68f6724c968166658ebecc499861e5c521524df (accessed on 14th July 2025).
4. Becker, W. C., & Fiellin, D. A. (2020). When epidemics collide: Coronavirus disease 2019 (COVID-19) and the opioid crisis. *Annals of Internal Medicine, 173*, 59–60. https://doi.org/10.7326/m20-1210 (accessed on 14th July 2025).
5. Bloom, D., & Bärnighausen, T. (2025). Changing research perspectives on the global health workforce. https://core.ac.uk/download/pdf/6617062.pdf (accessed on 14th July 2025).
6. Bobade, S., & Asutkar, S. (2024). Current trends and future directions in surgery: A brief scoping review. *Multidisciplinary Reviews*. https://www.semanticscholar.org/paper/dce2c942973a655c14274c2b83fe57f226e4ca91 (accessed on 14th July 2025).
7. Browne, N. T., Snethen, J., Greenberg, C. S., Frenn, M., Kilanowski, J. F., Gance-Cleveland, B., Burke, P. J., et al. (2020). When pandemics collide: The impact of COVID-19 on childhood obesity. *Journal of Pediatric Nursing, 56*, 90–98. https://doi.org/10.1016/j.pedn.2020.11.004 (accessed on 14th July 2025).
8. Bruyere, S. M., Erickson, W., Malzer, V. B., et al. (2013). Absence and disability management practices for an aging workforce. https://core.ac.uk/download/19958865.pdf (accessed on 14th July 2025).
9. Buljac-Samardžić, M., Doekhie, K. D., & van Wijngaarden, J. D. H. (2020). Interventions to improve team effectiveness within health care: A systematic review of the past decade. *Human Resources for Health, 18*. https://doi.org/10.1186/s12960-019-0411-3 (accessed on 14th July 2025).
10. Burgess, A., George, S., Gerard, K., Lathlean, J., et al. (2005). Integrated out-of-hours care arrangements in England: Observational study of progress towards single call access via NHS Direct and impact on the wider health system. https://core.ac.uk/download/2709866.pdf (accessed on 14th July 2025).
11. Burns, N., de Brun, T., Dowrick, C., Lionis, C., et al. (2013). Communication in cross-cultural consultations in primary care in Europe: The case for improvement. The rationale for the RESTORE FP 7 project. https://core.ac.uk/download/16458188.pdf (accessed on 14th July 2025).

12. Burton, M. J., Ramke, J., Marques, A. P., Bourne, R., Congdon, N., Jones, I., Ah Tong, B. A. M., et al. (2021). The Lancet Global Health Commission on global eye health: Vision beyond 2020. *The Lancet Global Health, 9*, e489–e551. https://doi.org/10.1016/s2214-109x(20)30488-5 (accessed on 14th July 2025).

13. Cammarata, C., Grennan, A. O., Hoffses, K. W., Menousek, K., et al. (2017). Professional practices, training, and funding mechanisms: A survey of pediatric primary care psychologists. https://core.ac.uk/download/83050024.pdf (accessed on 14th July 2025).

14. Cavicchi, J. R., & Kowalski, S. P. (2011). Preliminary report on patent literature, search methodology and patent status of medicines on the WHO EML 2009. https://core.ac.uk/download/72052453.pdf (accessed on 14th July 2025).

15. Cho, I. Y., & Kim, C. H. (2025). Topics and trends in neonatal family-centered care: A text network analysis and topic modeling approach. *Computers, Informatics, Nursing: CIN*. https://www.semanticscholar.org/paper/88adc62bdbee6a51a665e4b53c376373583cc4f6 (accessed on 14th July 2025).

16. Costain, G., Cohn, R., & Malkin, D. (2020). Precision child health: An emerging paradigm for pediatric quality and safety. *Current Treatment Options in Pediatrics, 6*, 317–324. https://www.semanticscholar.org/paper/bc3b698db045a18a6f4bf3b5d3045680408ad881 (accessed on 14th July 2025).

17. Dewey, C. M., Hingle, S., Goelz, E., & Linzer, M. (2020). Supporting clinicians during the COVID-19 pandemic. *Annals of Internal Medicine, 172*, 752, 753. https://doi.org/10.7326/m20-1033 (accessed on 14th July 2025).

18. Dower, C., & O, E. (2011). Primary care health workforce in the United States. https://core.ac.uk/download/71358775.pdf (accessed on 14th July 2025).

19. Dwivedi, Y. K., Kshetri, N., Hughes, L., Slade, E., Jeyaraj, A., Kar, A. K., Baabdullah, A. M., et al. (2023). Opinion paper: "So what if ChatGPT wrote it?" Multidisciplinary perspectives on opportunities, challenges and implications of generative conversational AI for research, practice and policy. *International Journal of Information Management, 71*, 102642–102642. https://doi.org/10.1016/j.ijinfomgt.2023.102642 (accessed on 14th July 2025).

20. Fahmy, A. (2024). Opportunities and challenges of applying artificial intelligence in healthcare. *Premier Journal of Artificial Intelligence*. https://www.semanticscholar.org/paper/059803ce4a08a9fafdc24ace9e4a95644f394a39 (accessed on 14th July 2025).

21. Ferrel, M., & Ryan, J. (2020). The impact of COVID-19 on medical education. *Cureus*. https://doi.org/10.7759/cureus.7492 (accessed on 14th July 2025).

22. Gibbons, A., Moore, K. A., & Chalk, R. (2003). The development and use of child well-being indicators in the prevention of child abuse and neglect. https://core.ac.uk/download/71347454.pdf (accessed on 14th July 2025).

23. Johnson, L., Smetana, S., Hall, W., Weaver, A. D., & Rotoli, J. (2025). Dos and don'ts of taking care of deaf patients. *Journal of Education & Teaching in Emergency Medicine, 10*, L1–L8. https://www.semanticscholar.org/paper/949a01476656fc016fc18f1b6e5877ed418416d9 (accessed on 14th July 2025).

24. Juliano, C., Levi, J., & Segal, L. M. (2006). *F as in Fat: How Obesity Policies are Failing in America, 2006*. https://core.ac.uk/download/71351406.pdf (accessed on 14th July 2025).

25. Kruk, M. E., Gage, A., Arsenault, C., Jordan, K., Leslie, H. H., Roder-DeWan, S., Adeyi, O., et al. (2018). High-quality health systems in the Sustainable Development Goals era: Time for a revolution. *The Lancet Global Health, 6*, e1196–e1252. https://doi.org/10.1016/s2214-109x(18)30386-3 (accessed on 14th July 2025).

26. Livingston, G., Huntley, J., Sommerlad, A., Ames, D., Ballard, C., Banerjee, S., Brayne, C., et al. (2020). Dementia prevention, intervention, and care: 2020 report of the Lancet Commission. *The Lancet, 396*, 413–446. https://doi.org/10.1016/s0140-6736(20)30367-6 (accessed on 14th July 2025).

27. Mach, F., Baigent, C., Catapano, A. L., Koskinas, K. C., Casula, M., Badimón, L., Chapman, M. J., et al. (2019). 2019 ESC/EAS guidelines for the management of dyslipidemias: Lipid modification to reduce cardiovascular risk. *European Heart Journal, 41*, 111–188. https://doi.org/10.1093/eurheartj/ehz455 (accessed on 14th July 2025).

28. Manyi-Loh, C. E., Mamphweli, S., Meyer, E. L., & Okoh, A. I. (2018). Antibiotic use in agriculture and its consequential resistance in environmental sources: Potential public health implications. *Molecules, 23*, 795–795. https://doi.org/10.3390/molecules23040795 (accessed on 14th July 2025).

29. Mittler-Matica, R., & Friebe, M. (2024). Healthspan horizon–Pioneering preventive care as the new standard of healthcare. *Qeios*. https://www.semanticscholar.org/paper/949a1d5f52f5ffd4d5709bb319f56eb54499670e (accessed on 14th July 2025).

30. Olowomeye, E. (2025). Exploring interdisciplinary family medicine approaches to improve chronic disease management and patient centered outcomes. *International Journal of Research Publication and Reviews*. https://www.semanticscholar.org/paper/1aba97ef4fa650cde7a2b57a3245a9763fe5e6d4 (accessed on 14th July 2025).

31. Orlova, I., Abramchuk, O., Babik, I., Borysiuk, I., & Dats-Opoka, M. (2024). Future trends in genetic research and their implications for public health: A literature review. *Futurity Medicine*. https://www.semanticscholar.org/paper/cbf38d491bb297c5d994d65bc9a0b9895fabff44 (accessed on 14th July 2025).

32. Pesqueira, J. P., Singh, P., & VELEZ-DALLA TOR, M. (2024). 1829-LB: Cardiorenal-metabolic educational program for family medicine residents (CARE ME). *Diabetes*. https://www.semanticscholar.org/paper/a78e72d80c766de489744c1c6bf331fd528b2b5f (accessed on 14th July 2025).

33. Racz, A., Vanja, V., Rukavina, T., Hošnjak, A. M., & Armano, L. (2025). Sources of information about complementary and alternative medicine commonly used by oncology patients and healthcare professionals. *Edelweiss Applied Science and Technology*. https://www.semanticscholar.org/paper/9737d32a14490e60b5538137565ca7a3451478e3 (accessed on 14th July 2025).

34. Read, T. L. (2016). Emerging needs in behavioral health and the integrated care model. https://open.bu.edu/bitstream/2144/17694/1/Read_bu_0017N_11995.pdf (accessed on 14th July 2025).

35. Rudolph, J., Tan, S., & Tan, S. (2023). ChatGPT: Bullshit spewer or the end of traditional assessments in higher education? *Journal of Applied Learning & Teaching, 6*. https://doi.org/10.37074/jalt.2023.6.1.9 (accessed on 14th July 2025).

36. Schmidt, M., Schmidt, S. A. J., Adelborg, K., Sundbøll, J., Laugesen, K., Ehrenstein, V., & Sørensen, H. T. (2019). The Danish health care system and epidemiological research: From health care

contacts to database records. *Clinical Epidemiology, 11*, 563–591. https://doi.org/10.2147/clep.s179083 (accessed on 14th July 2025).

37. Thibault, G. E. (2020). The future of health professions education: Emerging trends in the United States. *FASEB Bio Advances, 2*, 685–694. https://doi.org/10.1096/fba.2020-00061 (accessed on 14th July 2025).

38. Tillu, G., Chaturvedi, S., Chopra, A., & Patwardhan, B. (2020). Public health approach of Ayurveda and Yoga for COVID-19 prophylaxis. *The Journal of Alternative and Complementary Medicine, 26*, 360–364. https://doi.org/10.1089/acm.2020.0129 (accessed on 14th July 2025).

39. Wang, W. (2025). AI for medical application: Current trends, challenges, and future directions. *International Journal of Artificial Intelligence for Science (IJAI4S)*. https://www.semanticscholar.org/paper/7d161d0896ebfbd3d508ac81568cecf34fbdf142 (accessed on 14th July 2025).

40. Werder, K., Curtis, A., & Abufarsakh, B. (2022). APNA 35th annual conference, October 13–16, 2021: Mini concurrent session abstracts. *Journal of the American Psychiatric Nurses Association, 28*, NP28–NP44. https://www.semanticscholar.org/paper/6315ff02d6d0548e5b6637c194008cf5fd31ce47 (accessed on 14th July 2025).

41. Yee, V., Bajaj, S. S., & Stanford, F. C. (2022). Paradox of telemedicine: Building or neglecting trust and equity. *The Lancet Digital Health, 4*, e480–e481. https://doi.org/10.1016/s2589-7500(22)00100-5 (accessed on 14th July 2025).

INDEX

D

E

N

O

P